Index to emergency topics

Oxford Handbook of
Respiratory Medicine

Third Edition

Stephen Chapman
Consultant and Senior Lecturer in Respiratory Medicine,
Oxford University Hospitals, Oxford

Grace Robinson
Consultant in Respiratory Medicine,
Royal Berkshire Hospital, Reading

John Stradling
Professor of Respiratory Medicine,
University of Oxford, Oxford

Sophie West
Consultant in Respiratory Medicine,
Freeman Hospital, Newcastle

John Wrightson
Specialist Registrar, Respiratory Medicine,
Oxford Rotation, Oxford

OXFORD
UNIVERSITY PRESS

OXFORD
UNIVERSITY PRESS

Great Clarendon Street, Oxford, OX2 6DP,
United Kingdom

Oxford University Press is a department of the University of Oxford.
It furthers the University's objective of excellence in research, scholarship,
and education by publishing worldwide. Oxford is a registered trade mark of
Oxford University Press in the UK and in certain other countries

© Oxford University Press 2014

The moral rights of the authors have been asserted
First Edition published in 2005
Second Edition published in 2009
Third Edition published in 2014

Impression: 1

Published in the United States of America by Oxford University Press
198 Madison Avenue, New York, NY 10016, United States of America

British Library Cataloguing in Publication Data
Data available

Library of Congress Control Number: 2014931103

ISBN 978–0–19–870386–0

Printed in China by
C&C Offset Printing Co. Ltd

Forewords

I'm always full of awe for the Herculean efforts of the authors when asked to write a foreword to a book. The long hours that the authors of the *Oxford Handbook of Respiratory Medicine* put into the first edition, published in 2005, have been compensated by the book's clear value and popularity. Since 2005, research has increased our understanding of respiratory disease, particularly in the areas of airway disease, lung cancer and interstitial lung disease. Large robust clinical trials have also informed our clinical practice, and there have been subsequent modifications in national and international guidelines to reflect these. Our practice on the respiratory ward and clinic has been influenced as a result.

Nationally the burden of respiratory disease is being increasingly recognised. The government responses to the harmful effects of cigarette smoke, currently focused on banning smoking in cars carrying children, and considering plain packaging for cigarettes, highlight the ongoing prominence of smoking in respiratory health.

This third edition reflects many of these updates and changes, and is therefore a reliable and useful information source. The same authors across the three editions bring consistency (and reflects admirable stamina); and the need to keep it 'user friendly' for the respiratory trainee has been recognised and a new author has been added to provide a trainee's perspective.

Ian Pavord MA DM FRCP
Professor of Respiratory Medicine
NDM Research Building
University of Oxford

This respiratory medicine handbook provides reliable and up-to-date information for the respiratory trainee. Its format is designed so that information is easily accessible and practical, with useful tips for investigation and management in the outpatient clinic and the ward. It summarizes the most recent guidelines from the British Thoracic Society when applicable in each chapter, along with a detailed discussion of each condition, pertinent research and common practice. As such, it could be used as a learning resource when preparing for the MRCP Speciality Certificate Examination in Respiratory Medicine, or other respiratory assessments. The practical procedures section is particularly useful, with step-by-step 'how to' guides for all procedures encountered by the trainee, such as pleural aspiration, chest drains, thoracoscopy, and bronchoscopy.

Dr Adam Hill
Consultant Respiratory Physician and Honorary Reader
Royal Infirmary of Edinburgh Specialist Advisory Committee Chair
Respiratory Associate PG Dean SE Scotland (Quality Management)

Prefaces

This *Handbook of Respiratory Medicine* has been written largely by specialist registrars, for specialist registrars. Three of the four authors, Stephen Chapman, Grace Robinson, and Sophie West, are specialist registrars on the Oxford rotation and John Stradling is Professor of Respiratory Medicine in Oxford. It is in a format that the authors would like to have had when they started their specialist registrar training. However, we hope that any health worker or student with an interest in respiratory medicine will find this text a rapid and useful reference source.

The layout of the book tries to fulfil the requirement to be able to look up a topic quickly when the clinical need arises, but also to provide a bit more insight into the more difficult areas. Therefore, the chapters are of necessity different in style and reflect the authors' own views on how to best approach and understand an area.

The handbook is divided into five sections: clinical presentations and approaches to symptoms and problems; the clinical conditions themselves; supportive information; procedures; and useful appendices (also on the inside covers), containing more technical and reference information.

We hope you find it helpful. Feedback on errors and omissions would be much appreciated. Please post your comments via the OUP website: ℘ http://www.oup.com/uk/medicine/handbooks.

June 2005

The second edition of this book has allowed us to make several improvements in response to readers' suggestions. We have changed the order of chapters within each section to alphabetical and improved the index, to make the contents more rapidly accessible. We have added new content such as more detailed radiology, pandemic influenza, and pulmonary complications of sickle cell disease. In addition, we have updated and enhanced topics where there have been new guidelines and relevant publications. The overall aim of the book, to provide a rapid and comprehensive resource for all those involved in respiratory medicine, has remained paramount.

October 2008

The third edition has allowed us to review and update all the existing chapters and include new clinical guidelines and significant research. New sections on thoracic ultrasound and indwelling pleural catheters reflect changes in routine clinical practice since the previous editions. There are also new chapters on safe sedation and cardiopulmonary exercise testing. We welcome the contribution of our new co-author, John Wrightson, who has helped maintain the specialist registrar perspective.

September 2013

Acknowledgements

We would like to offer our grateful thanks to the following friends and colleagues for their reviewing and advice on various sections of this book.

First edition
Dr Nicholas Bates, Dr Lesley Bennett, Dr Rachel Bennett, Dr Malcolm Benson, Dr Penny Bradbury, Mrs Debbie Buttar, Dr James Calvert, Dr Jane Collier, Dr Graham Collins, Dr Chris Conlon, Dr Chris Davies, Dr Helen Davies, Dr Rob Davies, Dr Thearina de Beer, Mrs Joan Douglass, Dr Rachael Evans, Dr Fergus Gleeson, Dr Maxine Hardinge, Dr Ling Pei Ho, Dr Andrew Jeffreys, Dr Nick Maskell, Dr Phil Mason, Dr Kim McAnaulty, Dr Fiona McCann, Dr Sarah Menzies, Dr Annabel Nickol, Dr Jayne Norcliffe, Dr Jeremy Parr, Mrs Lisa Priestley, Dr Naj Rahman, Dr Catherine Richardson, Mrs Jo Riley, Dr Peter Sebire, Mrs Gerry Slade, Dr Mark Slade, Dr S Rolf Smith, Dr Catherine Swales, Dr Denis Talbot, Dr David Taylor, Dr Catherine Thomas, Dr Estée Török, Dr David Waine, Dr Chris Wathen, Dr John Wiggins, and Dr Eleanor Wood.

Second edition: additional acknowledgements
Dr Luke Howard, Dr Clare Jeffries, Dr Stuart Mucklow, Dr Andrew Stanton, and Mrs Jan Turner-Wilson. Dr Fergus Gleeson and Dr Rachel Benamore provided considerable help with the radiology section.

Third edition: acknowledgements
Dr Henry Bettinson, Mr Peter Close, Dr Helen Davies, Mrs Julia De Soyza, Dr Prosenjit Dutta, Dr Rachael Evans, Dr Julia Fuller, Dr Helmy Haja-Mydin, Dr Bernard Higgins, Dr Ling-Pei Ho, Dr Rachel Hoyles, Ms Elaina Jamieson, Dr Alastair Moore, Dr Ben Prudon, Dr Naj Rahman, Mrs Jo Riley, Professor John Simpson, Dr Catherine Thomas, Mrs Jan Turner-Wilson, Dr Ann Ward.

Contents

Symbols and abbreviations

►►	don't dawdle
↓	decreased
↑	increased
→	leading to
♀	female
♂	male
1°	primary
2°	secondary
~	approximately
≈	approximately equal to
±	plus/minus
>	greater than
<	less than
≥	equal to or more than
°	degree
°C	degree celsius
α	alpha
β	beta
γ	gamma
+ve	positive
£	pound sterling
®	registered trademark
α1-AT	α1-antitrypsin
A–a	alveolar to arterial gradient
Ab	antibody
ABG	arterial blood gas
ABPA	allergic bronchopulmonary aspergillosis
ACCP	American College of Chest Physicians
ACE	angiotensin-converting enzyme
AChR	acetylcholine receptor
ACTH	adenocorticotropic hormone
ADH	antidiuretic hormone
A&E	accident and emergency
AF	atrial fibrillation
AFB	acid-fast bacillus; autofluorescent bronchoscopy
AFP	alpha-fetoprotein
AIA	aspirin-induced asthma
AIDS	acquired immune deficiency syndrome
AIP	acute interstitial pneumonia
AJCC	American Joint Committee on Cancer

ALP	alkaline phosphatase
ALT	alanine aminotransaminase
AMTS	abbreviated mental test score
ANA	antinuclear antibody
ANCA	antinuclear cytoplasmic antibody
ANP	atrial natriuretic peptide
APC	argon–plasma coagulation
APTT	activated partial thromboplastin time
ARDS	acute respiratory distress syndrome
ART	antiretroviral therapy
AST	aspartate aminotransferase
ASV	adaptive servo-ventilation
ATRA	all-trans retinoic acid
ATS	American Thoracic Society
AV	arteriovenous
AVM	arteriovenous malformation
BHCG	beta human chorionic gonadotrophin
BAL	bronchoalveolar lavage
BCG	bacille Calmette–Guérin
bd	twice a day
BDP	beclomethasone
BHR	bronchial hyperreactivity or hyperresponsiveness
BiPAP	bi-level positive airways pressure
bLVR	bronchoscopic lung volume reduction
BMI	body mass index (kg/m^2)
BNP	B-type natriuretic peptide
BOOP	bronchiolitis obliterans organizing pneumonia
BOS	bronchiolitis obliterans syndrome
BP	blood pressure
BPD	bronchopulmonary dysplasia
bpm	beats per minute
BSAC	British Sub-Aqua Club
BTS	British Thoracic Society
CABG	coronary artery bypass graft
CAP	community-acquired pneumonia
CCB	calcium channel blocker
CCF	congestive cardiac failure
CCPA	chronic cavitary pulmonary aspergillosis
CF	cystic fibrosis
CFA	cryptogenic fibrosing alveolitis
CFT	complement fixation test
CFTR	cystic fibrosis transmembrane conductance regulator
cfu	colony-forming unit
CHART	continuous hyperfractionated accelerated radiotherapy

Chr	chromosome
CI	contraindication
CK	creatine kinase
Cl⁻	chloride ion
CLD	chronic lung disease
CLL	chronic lymphocytic leukaemia
cm	centimetre
cmH_2O	centimetre of water
CMV	cytomegalovirus
CNS	central nervous system
CO	carbon monoxide
CO_2	carbon dioxide
COHb	carboxyhaemoglobin
COP	cryptogenic organizing pneumonia
COPD	chronic obstructive pulmonary disease
CPAP	continuous positive airway pressure
CPD	continuous professional development
CPET	cardiopulmonary exercise testing
CPK	creatine phosphokinase
CPPE	complicated parapneumonic effusion
CRP	C-reactive protein
CSA	central sleep apnoea
CSF	cerebrospinal fluid
CT	computed tomography
CTPA	computed tomographic pulmonary angiogram
CTEPH	chronic thromboembolic pulmonary hypertension
CVA	cerebrovascular accident
CVD	cardiovascular disease
CVP	central venous pressure
CXR	chest radiograph
2D	two-dimensional
3D	three-dimensional
DEXA	dual-energy X-ray absorptiometry
DFA	direct fluorescent antibody
DIC	disseminated intravascular coagulation
DIF	direct immunofluorescence test
DIOS	distal intestinal obstructive syndrome
DIP	desquamative interstitial pneumonitis
dL	decilitre
DM	dermatomyositis
DNA	deoxyribonucleic acid
DOT	directly observed therapy (usually tuberculosis)
DPI	dry powder inhaler
dsDNA	double-stranded DNA
DVLA	Driver and Vehicle Licensing Agency

DVT	deep vein thrombosis
dyn	dyne
EBUS	endoscopic bronchial ultrasound
EBV	Epstein–Barr virus
ECG	electrocardiogram
echo	echocardiogram
ECOG	Eastern Cooperative Oncology Group
EEG	electroencephalogram
eGFR	estimated glomerular filtration rate
EGFR	epidermal growth factor receptor
EGPA	eosinophilic granulomatosis with polyangiitis (Churg–Strauss syndrome)
EIA	enzyme immunoassay
ELCAP	Early Lung Cancer Action Project
ELISA	enzyme-linked immunosorbent assay
EMG	electromyogram
EMU	early morning urine
ENA	extractable nuclear antigen
ENT	ear, nose, and throat
EOG	electro-oculogram
EPAP	expiratory positive airways pressure
ERA	endothelin receptor antagonist
ERS	European Respiratory Society
ESR	erythrocyte sedimentation rate
ESS	Epworth sleepiness scale/score
EUS-FNA	endoscopic ultrasound fine-needle aspiration
EVLP	ex vivo lung perfusion
FBC	full blood count
FDA	Food and Drug Administration
FDG-PET	18-fluorodeoxyglucose positron emission tomography
feNO	fraction of nitric oxide
FEV_1	forced expiratory volume in 1s
$FiCO_2$	fractional inspired carbon dioxide
FiO_2	fractional inspired oxygen
FNA	fine-needle aspirate
FOB	fibre optic bronchoscopy
FPAH	familial pulmonary arterial hypertension
FRC	functional residual capacity
ft	foot
FVC	forced vital capacity
g	gram
GABA	G-aminobutyric acid
GBM	glomerular basement membrane
GCS	Glasgow coma scale
GI	gastrointestinal

GMC	General Medical Council
GM-CSF	granulocyte-macrophage colony-stimulating factor
GORD	gastro-oesophageal reflux disease
GP	general practitioner
GPA	granulomatosis with polyangiitis (Wegener's)
GVHD	graft-versus-host disease
Gy	gray
h	hour
H^+	hydrogen ion
H2	histamine receptors, type 2
HAART	highly active antiretroviral therapy
HACE	high altitude cerebral oedema
HADS	Hospital Anxiety and Depression score
HAPE	high altitude pulmonary oedema
Hb	haemoglobin
HCG	human chorionic gonadotrophin
HCO_3^-	bicarbonate ion
HDU	high dependency unit
HFOV	high-frequency oscillatory ventilation
HHT	hereditary haemorrhagic telangiectasia
HIV	human immunodeficiency virus
HLA	human leucocyte antigen
HOCF	Home Oxygen Consent Form
HOOF	home oxygen order form
HP	hypersensitivity pneumonitis
HPLC	high-performance liquid chromatography
HPOA	hypertrophic pulmonary osteoarthropathy
HPS	hepatopulmonary syndrome
HPV	human papillomavirus
HR	heart rate
HRCT	high resolution computed tomography
HRT	hormone replacement therapy
HSCT	haematopoietic stem cell transplant
HSV	herpes simplex virus
Hz	hertz
IBD	inflammatory bowel disease
ICSI	intracytoplasmic sperm injection
ICU	intensive care unit
IFN-G	interferon gamma
IgE	immunoglobulin E
IgG	immunoglobulin G
IgM	immunoglobulin M
IGRA	interferon G release assay
IIP	idiopathic interstitial pneumonia

IL	interleukin
ILD	interstitial lung disease
IM	intramuscular
in	inch
INR	international normalized ratio
IPAH	idiopathic pulmonary arterial hypertension
IPAP	inspiratory positive airways pressure
IPC	indwelling pleural catheter
IPF	idiopathic pulmonary fibrosis
IRIS	immune reconstitution inflammatory syndrome
ITU	intensive therapy unit
IU	international units
IV	intravenous
IVAD	implantable venous access device
IVC	inferior vena cava
IVDU	intravenous drug user
JVP	jugular venous pressure
K^+	potassium ion
kCO	carbon monoxide transfer factor coefficient
kg	kilogram
kHz	kilohertz
km	kilometre
kPa	kilopascal
L	litre
LABA	long-acting B$_2$ agonist
LAM	lymphangioleiomyomatosis
LCH	Langerhans cell histiocytosis
LDH	lactate dehydrogenase
LEMS	Lambert–Eaton myasthenic syndrome
LFT	liver function test
LIP	lymphoid interstitial pneumonia
LMWH	low molecular weight heparin
LOS	lower oesophageal sphincter
LPA	lasting power of attorney
LTOT	long-term oxygen therapy
LV	left ventricle/ventricular
LVF	left ventricular failure
LVRS	lung volume reduction surgery
m	metre
MAC	*Mycobacterium avium* complex
MAI	*Mycobacterium avium intracellulare*
M,	C, & S microscopy, culture, and sensitivity
MCV	mean corpuscular volume
MDI	metered dose inhaler

MDR-TB	multidrug-resistant TB
MDT	multidisciplinary team
MEN	multiple endocrine neoplasia
meq	milliequivalent
MERS	Middle East respiratory syndrome
MERS-CoV	Middle East respiratory syndrome coronavirus
mg	milligram
MGUS	monoclonal gammopathy of uncertain significance
MHRA	Medicines and Healthcare products Regulatory Agency
MHz	megahertz
MI	myocardial infarction
min	minute
mL	millilitre
MMF	mycophenolate mofetil
mmHg	millimetre of mercury
mmol	millimole
MND	motor neurone disease
mosmol	milliosmole
MPA	microscopic polyangiitis
MPO	myeloperoxidase
MRC	Medical Research Council
MRI	magnetic resonance imaging
mRNA	messenger ribonucleic acid
MRSA	meticillin (or multiply) resistant *Staphylococcus aureus*
ms	millisecond
mSv	millisievert
MTB	*Mycobacterium tuberculosis*
mTOR	mammalian target of rapamycin
MU	megaunit
MVV	maximum voluntary ventilation
6MWT	6 minute walking test
N	newton
Na^+	sodium ion
NaCl	sodium chloride
NEWS	National Early Warning Score
ng	nanogram
NG	nasogastric
NHS	National Health Service
NICE	National Institute for Health and Care Excellence
NCEPOD	National Confidential Enquiry into Patient Outcome and Death
NIMV	non-invasive mechanical ventilation
NIPPV	non-invasive positive pressure ventilation
NIV	non-invasive ventilation
nmol	nanomole
NNRTI	non-nucleoside reverse transcription inhibitor

NO	nitric oxide
NO_2	nitrogen dioxide
non-REM	non-rapid eye movement sleep
NPSA	National Patient Safety Agency
NRT	nicotine replacement therapy
NSAID	non-steroidal anti-inflammatory drug
NSCLC	non-small cell lung cancer
NSIP	non-specific interstitial pneumonia
NTM	non-tuberculous mycobacteria
NT-proBNP	N-terminal pro-B type natriuretic peptide
NYHA	New York Heart Association
O_2	oxygen
OCP	oral contraceptive pill
od	once a day
OGD	oesophagogastroduodenoscopy
OP	organizing pneumonia
OSA	obstructive sleep apnoea
OSAH	obstructive sleep apnoea/hypopnoea
OSAS	obstructive sleep apnoea syndrome
p	probability
PA	posteroanterior
$PaCO_2$	arterial carbon dioxide tension
PAF	platelet-activating factor
PAH	pulmonary arterial hypertension
PAN	polyarteritis nodosa
PaO_2	arterial oxygen tension
PAP	pulmonary artery pressure
PAS	para-aminosalicylic acid
PAVM	pulmonary arteriovenous malformation
PC_{20}	provocative concentration (of histamine or methacholine) causing a 20% fall in FEV_1
PCD	primary ciliary dyskinesia
PCO_2	carbon dioxide tension
PCP	*Pneumocystis carinii* (now *jirovecii*) pneumonia
PCR	polymerase chain reaction
PDE	phosphodiesterase
PDE-5	phosphodiesterase type-5 inhibitor
PDT	photodynamic therapy
PE	pulmonary embolus
PEEP	positive end expiratory pressure
PEF	peak expiratory flow
PEFR	peak expiratory flow rate
PEG	percutaneous endoscopic gastrostomy
PESI	pulmonary embolism severity index
PET	positron emission tomography

PFT	pulmonary function test
PHT	pulmonary hypertension
Pi	protease inhibitor
PM	polymyositis
PMF	progressive massive fibrosis
PO	orally/by mouth
PO_2	oxygen tension
PO_4^-	phosphate ion
POPH	porto-pulmonary hypertension
ppb	part per billion
PPH	primary pulmonary hypertension
PPI	proton pump inhibitor
PPO	predicted post-operative
PR	pulmonary rehabilitation
PR3	proteinase 3
PRF	pulse repetition frequency
prn	as required
PSA	prostate-specific antigen
PSB	protected specimen brush
PSG	polysomnography
PSI	Pneumonia Severity Index
PT	prothrombin time; percutaneous tracheostomy
PTH	parathyroid hormone
PVL-SA	Panton-Valentine leukocidin-producing *Staphylococcus aureus*
QALY	quality-adjusted life year
qds	four times a day
QoL	quality of life
RA	rheumatoid arthritis
RAD	right axis deviation
RAST	radioallergosorbent test
RBBB	right bundle branch block
RB-ILD	respiratory bronchiolitis-associated interstitial lung disease
RCP	Royal College of Physicians
RCT	randomized controlled trial
REM	rapid eye movement
RER	respiratory exchange ratio
RFA	radiofrequency ablation
RHC	right heart catheterization
RhF	rheumatoid factor
RNA	ribonucleic acid
RQ	respiratory quotient
RNP	ribonuclear protein
RR	respiratory rate
RSV	respiratory syncytial virus

Part 1

Clinical presentations— approaches to problems

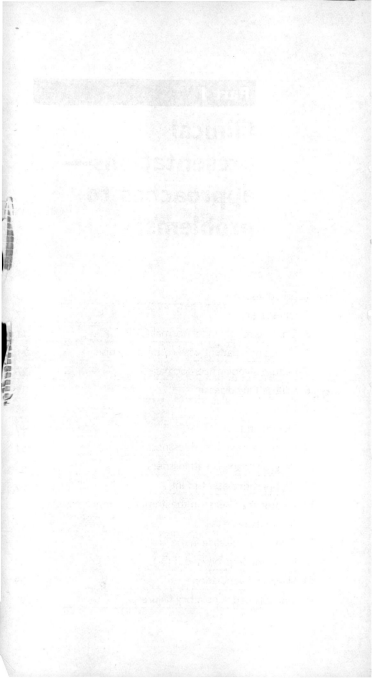

Chapter 1

Breathlessness

Clinical assessment and causes

Physiological mechanisms of breathlessness

Dyspnoea refers to the abnormal and uncomfortable awareness of breathing. Its physiological mechanisms are poorly understood; possible afferent sources for the sensation include receptors in respiratory muscles, juxta-capillary (J) receptors (sense interstitial fluid), and chemoreceptors (sensing $\uparrow CO_2$ and $\downarrow O_2$).

Clinical assessment

All patients need a full history and examination. Key points in the assessment are:

- *Duration and onset* of breathlessness. Box 1.1 groups the causes of breathlessness by speed of onset, although, in practice, some variability and overlap exist. Patients often underestimate the duration of symptoms—enquiring about exercise tolerance over a period of time is a useful way of assessing duration and progression
- *Severity* of breathlessness. Assess the level of handicap and disability by asking about effects on lifestyle, work, and daily activities
- *Exacerbating factors.* Ask about rest and exertion, nocturnal symptoms, and body position. The timing of nocturnal breathlessness may provide clues to the likely cause: left ventricular failure (LVF) causes breathlessness after a few hours of sleep and resolves after about 45min; asthma tends to occur later in the night; laryngeal inspiratory stridor causes noisy breathlessness of very short duration (<1min); and Cheyne–Stokes apnoeas result in breathlessness that is recurrent and clears each time in <30s. Orthopnoea is suggestive of LVF or diaphragm paralysis, although it is also common in many chronic lung diseases. Breathlessness during swimming is characteristic of bilateral diaphragm paralysis. Trepopnoea refers to breathlessness when lying on one side as a result of ipsilateral pulmonary disease
- *Associated symptoms*, such as cough, haemoptysis, chest pain, wheeze, stridor, fever, loss of appetite and weight, ankle swelling, and voice change. Wheeze may occur with pulmonary oedema, pulmonary embolism (PE), bronchiolitis, and anaphylaxis, in addition to asthma and chronic obstructive pulmonary disease (COPD)
- *Personal and family history* of chest disease
- Lifetime employment, hobbies, pets, travel, smoking, illicit drug use, medications
- *Examination* of the cardiovascular and respiratory systems. Observe the pattern and rate of breathing. Assess for signs of respiratory distress. Look for paradoxical abdominal movement if the history suggests diaphragmatic paralysis. A useful bedside test is to exercise the patient (e.g. by stepping on and off a 15–20cm block) until their breathlessness occurs, and then measure oximetry immediately on stopping when the finger is still; a fall in O_2 saturation is expected with organic causes of dyspnoea.

RT-PCR	reverse transcriptase polymerase chain reaction
RV	residual volume; right ventricle/ventricular
RVH	right ventricular hypertrophy
s	second
SABR	stereotactic ablative radiotherapy
SaO$_2$	arterial oxygen saturation (usually a percentage)
SAP	serum amyloid P
SARS	severe acquired respiratory syndrome
SARS-CoV	SARS-coronavirus
SBE	subacute bacterial endocarditis
SBOT	short-burst oxygen therapy
SBRT	stereotactic body radiation therapy
SC	subcutaneous
SCIT	subcutaneous allergen immunotherapy
SCL-70	scleroderma antibody (to topoisomerase 1)
SCLC	small cell lung cancer
SCUBA	self-contained underwater breathing apparatus
SE	side effect
SEMAS	self-expanding metal airway stent
SF-36	Short Form-36
SIADH	syndrome of inappropriate secretion of ADH
SLE	systemic lupus erythematosus
SO$_2$	sulphur dioxide
SO$_4^-$	sulphate ion
SOB	shortness of breath
spp.	Species
SPPE	simple parapneumonic effusion
SUV	standardized uptake value
SVC	superior vena cava
SVCO	superior vena caval obstruction
SWT	shuttle walk test
TB	tuberculosis
TBB	transbronchial biopsy
TBNA	transbronchial needle aspiration
tds	three times a day
TENS	transcutaneous electrical nerve stimulation
TFT	thyroid function test
TGC	time gain compensation
TGF	transforming growth factor
Th2	T helper 2 cell
TIA	transient ischaemic attack
TIPS	transjugular intrahepatic portosystemic shunt
TLC	total lung capacity
TLCO	total lung carbon monoxide transfer factor

TNF	tumour necrosis factor
tPA	tissue plasminogen activator
TPMT	thiopurine methyltransferase
TR	tricuspid regurgitation
TRALI	transfusion-related acute lung injury
TSH	thyroid-stimulating hormone
TTR	transthyretin
TU	tuberculin unit
TUS	thoracic ultrasound
U	unit
UACS	upper airway cough syndrome
U&E	urea and electrolytes
UICC	Union for International Cancer Control
UIP	usual interstitial pneumonia
UK	United Kingdom
URTI	upper respiratory tract infection
US	ultrasound
USA	United States of America
USS	ultrasound scan
UTI	urinary tract infection
VAP	ventilator-associated pneumonia
VAPSP	volume-assured pressure support ventilation
VATS	video-assisted thoracoscopic surgery
VC	vital capacity
VCD	vocal cord dysfunction
VKA	vitamin K antagonist
V/Q	ventilation-perfusion ratio
vs	versus
VTE	venous thromboembolism
WCC	white cell count
WHO	World Health Organization
XDR-TB	extensively drug-resistant tuberculosis
y	year
YAG	yttrium–aluminium–garnet
ZN	Ziehl–Neelsen

Investigations

Initial investigations typically include resting oximetry, peak flow and spirometry, CXR, and ECG. Further tests depend on clinical suspicion; options include full pulmonary function tests (PFTs) with measurement of lung volumes lying and standing, gas transfer and flow–volume loop, bronchial hyperresponsiveness or reversibility testing, maximal mouth or inspiratory sniff pressures, arterial blood gases (ABGs) (with measurement of alveolar to arterial (A–a) gradient (see ➲ p. 826), exercise oximetry, ventilation-perfusion (V/Q) scanning and computed tomographic pulmonary angiography (CTPA), high-resolution CT (HRCT), blood tests (FBC and TSH), echocardiogram (echo), exercise ECG, and cardiac catheterization.

Box 1.1 Causes of breathlessness grouped by speed of onset

Instantaneous
- Pneumothorax
- PE.

Acute (minutes to hours)
- Airways disease (asthma, exacerbation of COPD, upper airways obstruction)
- Parenchymal disease (pneumonia, pulmonary oedema, pulmonary haemorrhage, acute hypersensitivity pneumonitis (HP))
- Pulmonary vascular disease (PE)
- Cardiac disease (e.g. acute myocardial infarction (MI), arrhythmia, valvular disease, tamponade, aortic dissection)
- Metabolic acidosis
- Hyperventilation syndrome.

Subacute (days)
- Many of the above, plus:
  - Pleural effusion
  - Lobar collapse
  - Acute interstitial pneumonia
  - Superior vena caval obstruction (SVCO)
  - Pulmonary vasculitis.

Chronic (months to years)
- Some of the above, plus:
  - Obstructive airways disease (COPD, asthma)
  - Diffuse parenchymal disease (including idiopathic pulmonary fibrosis (IPF), sarcoidosis, lymphangitis carcinomatosis)
  - Pulmonary vascular disease (chronic thromboembolic disease, idiopathic pulmonary hypertension (PHT), veno-occlusive disease)
  - Hypoventilation (chest wall deformity, neuromuscular weakness, obesity)
  - Anaemia
  - Thyrotoxicosis.

Specific situations

Causes of breathlessness with a normal CXR

- Airways disease (asthma, upper airways obstruction, bronchiolitis)
- Pulmonary vascular disease (PE, idiopathic PHT, intrapulmonary shunt)
- Early parenchymal disease (e.g. sarcoid, interstitial pneumonias, infection—viral, *Pneumocystis jirovecii* pneumonia (PCP))
- Cardiac disease (e.g. angina, arrhythmia, valvular disease, intracardiac shunt)
- Neuromuscular weakness
- Metabolic acidosis
- Anaemia
- Thyrotoxicosis
- Hyperventilation syndrome.

Causes of episodic/intermittent breathlessness

- Asthma
- Pulmonary oedema
- Angina
- PE
- HP
- Vasculitis
- Hyperventilation syndrome.

Distinguishing cardiac and respiratory causes of breathlessness

This can be difficult. Many of the clinical features of left heart failure are non-specific and easily confused with respiratory disease (e.g. orthopnoea, wheeze). In chronic cardiac failure, crackles on auscultation and radiological features of pulmonary oedema may be absent, even when the pulmonary capillary wedge pressure is significantly raised (due to adaptive changes from vascular remodelling). The presence of emphysema may also render crackles inaudible and lead to atypical CXR appearances of pulmonary oedema. Chronic left heart failure commonly leads to a restrictive ventilatory defect and reduced gas transfer on PFTs and may also result in PHT. HRCT features of left heart failure include septal and peribronchovascular interstitial thickening, ground-glass shadowing, pleural effusions, and cardiomegaly. Resting ECG is useful—in practice, a cardiac cause of breathlessness is unlikely in the setting of a completely normal ECG. Exercise ECG, echo, and cardiac catheterization may be required. Elevated natriuretic peptide levels predict the likelihood of heart failure as well as the prognosis from this condition. Cardiac and respiratory diseases can, of course, coexist.

Chapter 2

Chest pain

Introduction to chest pain

The majority of patients with chest pain referred for a respiratory opinion have either acute pleuritic pain or persistent, well-localized pain. Cardiac pain rarely presents in this manner, although it should be considered in exertional pain or in the presence of risk factors for ischaemic heart disease. Within the respiratory system, pain may arise from the parietal pleura, major airways, chest wall, diaphragm, and mediastinum; the lung parenchyma and visceral pleura are insensitive to pain. Processes involving the upper parietal pleura cause a pain localized to that part of the chest. The lower parietal pleura and outer region of the diaphragmatic pleura are innervated by the lower six intercostal nerves, and pain here may be referred to the abdomen. The central region of the diaphragm is supplied by the phrenic nerve (C3, 4, and 5), and pain may be referred to the ipsilateral shoulder tip. Tracheobronchitis tends to be associated with retrosternal pain.

Acute pleuritic chest pain

- Pleuritic pain is sharp, well localized, worse on coughing and inspiration, and the subsequent limitation of inspiration often leads to a degree of breathlessness
- Causes of acute pleuritic chest pain include:
  - Pulmonary infarction (following embolism)
  - Pneumonia
  - Pneumothorax
  - Pericarditis
  - Pleural infection (empyema, tuberculous)
  - Autoimmune disease (e.g. systemic lupus erythematosus (SLE), rheumatoid arthritis (RA))
  - Musculoskeletal
  - Fractured rib
- In addition, consider atypical presentations of serious conditions such as MI, aortic dissection, oesophageal rupture, and pancreatitis. Consider angioinvasive fungi, such as *Aspergillus*, as a cause of pleuritic chest pain in the immunocompromised
- Diagnosis is typically based on 'pattern recognition' of clinical features, followed by selected investigations. Initial investigations typically include CXR, ECG, ABGs, serum inflammatory markers, and D-dimers. Further investigations may include V/Q scanning or CTPA, pleural aspiration, and measurement of serum autoantibodies
- PE (see ➲ pp. 398–9) commonly presents with pleuritic pain, and exclusion of this diagnosis is the usual reason for referral. Assess risk factors for thromboembolic disease. Normal O_2 saturations and PaO_2 in the 'normal' range do not exclude the diagnosis; calculate the A–a gradient (see ➲ p. 826). The presence of a pleural rub is a non-specific sign that occurs with pleural inflammation of any cause
- In young adults, pneumococcal pneumonia may present with acute-onset pleuritic chest pain, although systemic symptoms, such as fever, usually predate the pain by hours
- The pain from pericarditis is pleuritic, but central, and relieved on leaning forward; there may also be a pericardial rub, characteristic ECG features, and a small pericardial effusion on echo
- Musculoskeletal pain may occur as a result of cervical disc disease, arthritis of the shoulder or spine, a fractured rib, or costochondritis (Tietze's syndrome), which often follows a viral infection
- The presence of chest wall tenderness does not invariably indicate a benign musculoskeletal cause; tenderness may be seen in malignant chest wall infiltration and sometimes following pulmonary infarction
- Other features besides pleurisy that may suggest a diagnosis of SLE include rash, photosensitivity, oral ulcers, arthritis, pericarditis, renal or neurological disease, cytopenia, positive ANA, and dsDNA.

Chronic chest pain

- Persistent chest pain that is well localized is typically caused by chest wall or pleural disease. Causes include:
  - Malignant pleural disease or chest wall infiltration
  - Benign musculoskeletal pain
  - Pleural infection (empyema, tuberculous)
  - Benign asbestos-related pleural disease
  - Autoimmune disease (e.g. SLE, RA)
  - Recurrent pulmonary infarction (emboli, vasculitis)
- Pain from malignant chest wall infiltration is often 'boring' in character and may disturb sleep; it is frequently not related to respiration. Causes include 1° lung cancer, 2° pleural malignancy, mesothelioma, and rib or sternal involvement from malignancy (including myeloma and leukaemia)
- Chronic thromboembolic disease tends to present with breathlessness; when chest pain occurs, it is usually episodic, rather than persistent
- As with acute pleuritic pain, investigations are directed by initial clinical suspicion. Consider CT chest, bone scan, serum autoantibodies, FBC and film, serum electrophoresis. CXR may appear normal in malignant chest wall disease.

Chapter 3

Chronic cough and a normal CXR

Aetiology and clinical assessment

Cough is a frequent symptom of many respiratory diseases and is often associated with underlying lung pathology and an abnormal CXR. Cough can occur in otherwise healthy people and is often a self-limiting symptom. Persistent coughing can be a socially disabling and distressing symptom, for which help is often sought. *Cough syncope* is loss of consciousness following violent coughing, a Valsalva-type manoeuvre, which impairs venous return to the heart and provokes bradycardia and vasodilatation (similar to an ordinary faint). Important as car drivers must cease driving until liability to cough syncope has ceased, confirmed by medical opinion; commercial drivers must cease driving and have no cough syncope or pre-syncope for 5y if they have a chronic respiratory condition, including smoking. If they have asystole due to cough, driving can be considered after pacemaker insertion.

- *Acute cough* = cough lasting <3 weeks, usually due to viral upper respiratory tract infection (URTI). May linger for 3–8 weeks as a 'post-viral cough' or subacute cough
- *Chronic cough = cough lasting >8 weeks*
- Patients with a normal CXR and persistent cough are often grouped under the heading *'chronic cough'*
- It can sometimes be difficult to determine the underlying cause
- Susceptible individuals have a heightened cough reflex (therefore coining the term 'cough hypersensitivity syndrome')
- Investigation is warranted, but successful response to therapeutic trials may aid determination of the underlying cause. Centres vary in their approach to this
- Specialist cough clinics suggest they achieve diagnosis and effective treatment in over 80% of patients referred with chronic cough.

Aetiology In practice, over 90% of cases of chronic cough with a normal CXR are caused by one or more of:
- Cough variant asthma or eosinophilic bronchitis
- Gastro-oesophageal reflux disease (GORD)
- Post-nasal drip (or upper airway cough syndrome), due to perennial or allergic rhinitis, vasomotor rhinitis, or chronic sinusitis.

In clinic Full history can be unhelpful. Although cough is most commonly due to asthma, reflux, or post-nasal drip, there may be no specific symptoms to suggest these diagnoses.
- Duration of cough
- When it tends to occur—night or early morning, after exertion, on exposure to dust, pollen, aerosols, cold air (asthma), after meals or on sitting or bending over (GORD), nocturnal (post-nasal drip and asthma)
- Non-productive or productive and, if so, how much sputum and colour. Significant amounts of sputum usually indicate a 1° lung pathology
- Haemoptysis
- Fever
- Associated symptoms:
  - Shortness of breath (SOB) or wheeze
  - Throat clearing or sensation of post-nasal drip
  - Chest pain

- Ankle swelling/orthopnoea/paroxysmal nocturnal dyspnoea
- Dyspepsia
- Previous respiratory disease such as childhood asthma, eczema, or hay fever
- History of sinus disease or perennial rhinitis
- History of previous severe respiratory infections, such as whooping cough, that may have caused bronchiectasis
- Known cardiac disease or valvular heart disease
- Drug history ?ACE inhibitor
- Occupation ?Workplace irritants
- Pets/birds
- Smoker (common cause of persistent cough, dose-related, improves on stopping)
- Use of recreational drugs.

Examination can also be unhelpful, as it is usually normal. Look for signs of underlying lung disease or other medical conditions such as heart failure, neurological disease (particularly bulbar involvement). Significant tonsillar enlargement should be excluded, as this is a recognized cause of cough which can respond to tonsillectomy.

Investigations

Initially

- *Ensure CXR is normal*
- *Spirometry* may indicate restrictive or obstructive defect. Performance of spirometry may provoke cough and bronchospasm
- *Methacholine challenge test* (see ⮞ p. 776) provides the best positive predictive value for cough due to asthma. Lack of response means cough variant asthma is extremely unlikely. PC_{20} is normal in eosinophilic bronchitis
- *Serial peak flow recordings* twice daily for 2 weeks. >20% diurnal variation suggests asthma. Can be normal in cough variant asthma
- *Induced sputum examination*, if available, for eosinophil count, to suggest either asthma or eosinophilic bronchitis.

Later

- *Consider chest HRCT* if any features suggestive of lung cancer or interstitial lung disease (ILD), as a small proportion may present with a normal CXR (central tumour)
- *Consider ENT examination* if predominantly upper respiratory tract disease, resistant to treatment. Consider sinus CT
- *Consider bronchoscopy* if foreign body possible, or history suggestive of malignancy, small carcinoid, endobronchial disease. Perform after CT to help guide bronchoscopist
- *Consider 24h ambulatory oesophageal pH monitoring*
- *Consider oesophageal manometry* for oesophageal dysmotility.

Treatment

The initial treatment of patients with a chronic cough is determined by what the most likely underlying cause is, based on the history and investigations. The key is to give any drug treatment at a high enough dose, and for a long enough time (such as 2–3 months), to be effective.

Symptomatic treatment for cough

Over-the-counter medicines may provide relief, although there is little evidence of a specific pharmacological effect. Below is a list of possible treatments:

- *Honey and lemon*—home remedies
- *Dextromethorphan*—a non-sedating non-opiate. Component of many over-the-counter cough remedies. Dose response, with maximum cough reflex suppression at 60 mg (Benylin® preparations, Actifed® preparations, Vicks Vaposyrup® preparations, Sudafed Linctus®, Night Nurse®)
- *Menthol*—short-lived cough suppressant (Benylin® preparations, Vicks Vaposyrup® preparations)
- *Sedative antihistamines*—suppress cough but cause drowsiness. Good for nocturnal cough
- *Codeine or pholcodine*—opiate antitussives—codeine requires prescription. No greater efficacy than dextromethorphan and greater side effect profile
- *Opiates*—prescription. Low-dose morphine sulfate 5–10mg showed significant improvement in patients with intractable cough in randomized controlled trial (RCT) (Morice AH *et al. Am J Crit Care Med* 2007). Side effect profile of opiates, so should be used with caution
- *Gabapentin*—prescription. Neuromodulator used for chronic pain. Not yet licensed for cough, but RCT treatment success in Leicester Cough Questionnaire, with side effects mostly of nausea and fatigue in 31% on gabapentin, managed with dose reduction (Ryan NM *et al. Lancet* 2012). Starting dose 300mg/day, with gradual increases until cough suppressed, side effects, or maximum 600mg tds. Other side effects include diarrhoea, emotional lability, sleepiness, nystagmus, tremor, weakness, peripheral oedema
- *Thalidomide*—used in cough due to IPF, with RCT showing significant improvements in cough quality of life (QoL) questionnaires (Horton MR *et al. Ann Intern Med* 2012). Side effects in 74% on thalidomide vs 22% placebo, with constipation, dizziness, and fatigue (for IPF, see ➔ pp. 270–1).

Assessing treatment response

Several measures have been developed and validated such as:

- Cough visual analogue scale
- Leicester Cough Questionnaire—cough-specific QoL
- Cough reflex sensitivity measurements—primarily a research tool; subjects inhale increasing doses of either capsaicin or citric acid, with the sensitivity recorded as the dose to cause two or five coughs.

Causes of cough (with or without CXR abnormality)

Respiratory
- Infection: viral upper and lower respiratory tract infection, bacterial pneumonia, tuberculosis (TB), pertussis
- Chronic bronchitis
- Obstructive airways disease: COPD, asthma
- Cough variant asthma
- Eosinophilic bronchitis
- Obstructive sleep apnoea (OSA) (nocturnal only)
- Lung cancer
- Bronchiectasis, cystic fibrosis (CF)
- ILD
- Airway irritants: smoking, dusts and fumes, acute smoke inhalation
- Airway foreign body.

Mediastinal
- External compression of trachea by enlarged lymph nodes (e.g. lymphoma, TB)
- Mediastinal tumours/cysts/masses.

Cardiac
- LVF
- Left atrial enlargement (e.g. severe mitral stenosis).

ENT
- Upper airway cough syndrome, including:
  - Acute or chronic sinusitis
  - Post-nasal drip due to perennial, allergic, or vasomotor rhinitis.

GI
- GORD
- Oesophageal dysmotility, stricture, or pharyngeal pouch causing repeated aspiration
- Oesophago-bronchial fistula.

CNS
Neurological disease affecting swallowing, causing repeated aspiration, such as stroke, multiple sclerosis, motor neurone disease (MND), or Parkinson's disease.

Drugs
- ACE inhibitors
- Some inhaled preparations can cause cough—particularly ipratropium.

Other
- Idiopathic
- Ear wax (vagal nerve stimulation)
- Psychogenic/habitual.

Causes of chronic cough: asthma, GORD

Asthma or 'cough variant asthma', 'cough-predominant asthma'. This represents one end of the asthma spectrum, with airway inflammation, but may have minimal bronchoconstriction. There is not always a typical asthma history, but ask about wheeze, atopy, hay fever, or childhood asthma or eczema. Cough may be the only symptom. Cough is typically worse after exercise, in cold air, after exposure to fumes or fragrances, or in the mornings.

- *Spirometry* may be normal, without evidence of airflow obstruction. There may be typical asthmatic diurnal peak flow variability of >20%, or peak flows may be stable
- *Methacholine challenge* should be positive for asthma but does not rule out a steroid-responsive cough. If negative, other causes of cough should be sought
- *Treatment* should be for at least 2 months, with high-dose inhaled steroids. Response may take days or weeks. Bronchodilators may make little difference. If inhaled steroid therapy has been tried unsuccessfully, ensure inhaler technique is optimal and a high dose has been used. Alternatively, prescribe a 2-week course of oral prednisolone 30mg/day, and assess response. If the cough improves, high-dose inhaled steroids should be continued and slowly reduced after about 2 months. There is a small trial showing leukotriene receptor antagonists decreased cough in people with cough variant asthma; consider using in patients who want to avoid inhaled steroids or in whom they are ineffective
- *Eosinophilic bronchitis* Airway eosinophilia, rarely with peripheral blood eosinophilia, causing heightened cough reflex, but no bronchial hyperresponsiveness/wheeze or peak flow variation. Diagnosis based on negative asthma investigations and induced sputum eosinophilia. Improves with inhaled corticosteroids, usually after 2–3 weeks, or trial of oral prednisolone. Sputum eosinophil count also reduces with treatment. If there is no response, the cough is unlikely to be due to eosinophilic airway inflammation.

GORD

Cough may be related to distal reflux at the lower oesophageal sphincter (LOS) or due to micro-aspiration of acid into the trachea. There may be associated oesophageal dysmotility. LOS reflux is often long-standing and is associated with a productive or non-productive daytime cough, and minimal nocturnal symptoms. It is worse after meals and when sitting down, due to increased intra-abdominal pressure being transmitted to the LOS. Micro-aspiration is associated with more prominent symptoms of reflux or dyspepsia, although these are not always present. Patients may have an intermittent hoarse voice, dysphonia, and sore throat. Cough may be the only symptom of reflux.

Laryngoscopy may reveal posterior vocal cord inflammation, but this is not a reliable sign.

A trial of treatment for both is recommended. This is with a high-dose proton pump inhibitor (PPI) for at least 2, usually 3, months, although longer treatment may be required to control cough. H2 receptor blockers are also effective, and prokinetics like metoclopramide may help as an addition if cough improves but has not gone completely. Other reflux avoidance measures should be carried out: avoiding caffeine, fatty foods, chocolate, excess alcohol, acidic drinks like orange juice, red wine, stop smoking, loose-fitting clothes, sleeping with an empty stomach (avoid eating <4h before bed), sleeping propped up, weight loss if overweight. Surgical fundoplication for reflux-associated cough resistant to drug therapy is not widely used but may be effective in carefully selected cases.

Investigation, if required, due to either treatment failure or because of diagnostic uncertainty, is with 24h ambulatory pH monitoring, which determines the presence of reflux events, and event markers allow correlation with cough. These may not necessarily be responsible for the cough, so it is not a very specific or sensitive test. Oesophageal manometry can be used to measure the LOS pressure and oesophageal contractions after swallowing to determine the presence of oesophageal dysmotility.

Causes of chronic cough: rhinitis, post-infectious, ACE inhibitors, idiopathic

Rhinitis and post-nasal drip

The term *upper airway cough syndrome (UACS)* is now being used to include all upper airway abnormalities causing cough and is replacing post-nasal drip. *Rhinitis* is defined as sneezing, nasal discharge, or blockage for >1h on most days for either a limited part of the year (seasonal) or all year (perennial). Rhinitis may be allergic (e.g. hay fever), non-allergic, or infective. The associated nasal inflammation may irritate cough receptors directly or produce a post-nasal drip. These secretions may pool at the back of the throat, giving a sensation of liquid dripping into the back of the throat, which requires frequent throat clearing, or drip directly into the trachea, initiating cough. There may be frequent nasal discharge. A history of facial pain and purulent nasal discharge suggests sinusitis, which can also predispose to post-nasal drip. Symptoms of cough can occur on lying but can be constant, regardless of position. Rhinosinusitis describes inflammation and infection within the nasal passages and paranasal sinuses, with chronic rhinosinusitis defined as symptoms persisting for more than 12 weeks.

ENT examination may reveal swollen turbinates, 'cobblestone' nasopharyngeal mucosa, nasal discharge, or nasal polyps.

Treatment Nasal preparations should be taken by kneeling with the top of the head on the floor ('Mecca' position) or lying supine with the head tipped over the end of the bed. Improvements in cough should be found within 2 weeks. Duration of treatment is unclear.

- *Non-allergic rhinitis* Trials suggest the best results are with an initial 3 weeks of nasal decongestants with first-generation antihistamines (which have helpful anticholinergic properties) and pseudoephedrine. Alternatives are nasal ipratropium bromide or xylometazoline. This is then followed by 3 months of high-dose nasal steroids, which are ineffective when used as first-line treatment. Second-generation antihistamines (i.e. non-sedating) are of no use in non-allergic rhinitis
- *Allergic rhinitis* Second-generation oral antihistamine (e.g. cetirizine, loratadine, fexofenadine) and high-dose nasal steroids for 3 months at least
- *Vasomotor rhinitis* Nasal ipratropium bromide for 3 months; nasal steroids may also have a role
- *Chronic rhinosinusitis* Nasal steroids and saline lavage, which should have an effect by 4 weeks, and, if so, treatment should continue, although optimal duration unclear.

Sinusitis is an infection of the paranasal sinuses, which may complicate an URTI and is frequently caused by *Haemophilus (H.) influenzae* or

Streptococcus (S.) pneumoniae. It causes frontal headache and facial pain. Chronic sinusitis may require further investigation with CXR or CT, which shows mucosal thickening and air-fluid levels. Surgery may be indicated.

- *Chronic sinusitis* Treat as for non-allergic rhinitis, but include 2 weeks of antibiotics active against *H. influenzae* such as doxycycline or co-amoxiclav.

Post-infectious Respiratory tract infections, especially if viral in nature, can cause cough. This may take weeks or months to resolve spontaneously, although most settle within 8 weeks. There may be a post-nasal drip contribution. The cough is related to a heightened cough reflex. Associated laryngospasm can occur, which is a sudden hoarseness, with associated stridulous inspiratory efforts and a sensation of being unable to breathe.

Treatment with antitussives, such as codeine linctus, may ease the symptoms. Inhaled steroids have been tried for the transient bronchial hyperactivity, but there is no trial evidence that these work. Inhaled ipratropium has also been tried, with one report of effectiveness.

ACE inhibitor cough occurs with any ACE inhibitor and is related to bradykinin not being broken down by angiotensin-converting enzyme and accumulating in the lung. Occurs in 10–15% of people on ACE inhibitors; more frequent in women. Can occur within weeks of starting the drug, but up to 6 months; the cough may be initiated by a respiratory tract infection but persists thereafter. Cough usually settles within a week of stopping the drug but may take months. Avoid all ACE inhibitors thereafter and may need to change to an angiotensin receptor antagonist. Stop ACE inhibitor in any patient with a troublesome cough.

Idiopathic chronic cough accounts for 20% of referrals to a specialist cough clinic. It is diagnosed after a thorough assessment. Typically, there is lymphocytic airway inflammation, but there may also be a history of reflux cough. Typically, the patients are middle-aged women with a long-standing dry cough, often starting around the time of the menopause and triggered by an URTI. Organ-specific autoimmune disease is present in up to 30%, particularly hypothyroidism. Treatment is often ineffective.

Further information

BTS guidelines. Recommendations for the management of cough in adults. *Thorax* 2006;**61**(suppl 1). Ⓜ http://www.thoraxjnl.com.

Review series on cough. Morice A, Kastelik J. *Thorax* 2003;**58**:901–5; Fontana GA, Pistolesi M. *Thorax* 2003;**58**:1092–5; Dicpinigaitis PV. *Thorax* 2004;**59**:71–2; McGarvey LP. *Thorax* 2004;**59**:342–6.

Birring SS *et al.* Development of a symptom specific health status measure for patients with chronic cough: Leicester Cough Questionnaire. *Thorax* 2003;**58**:339–43.

Birring SS *et al.* Eosinophilic bronchitis: clinical features, management and pathogenesis. *Am J Resp Med* 2003;**2**:169–73.

Irwin RS, Madison JM. The diagnosis and treatment of cough. *N Engl J Med* 2000;**343**:1715–21.

Chapter 4

Critically ill patient with respiratory disease

Introduction

Patients often present critically ill to the emergency or the acute medical department with respiratory disease. This may be due to a deterioration or exacerbation of an existing condition, a first presentation of a previously undiagnosed disease, or respiratory involvement of an acute systemic disease. As with any critically ill patient, standard management is required initially to stabilize, with the focus moving to diagnosis and treatment. Often these need to take place in parallel. Depending on the presence of any pre-existing respiratory disease and the nature and severity of this, it may be important to determine disease-specific treatment and/or treatment limitations, and senior physician input should be sought for this.

Initial assessment

Airway—is the patient maintaining their airway? Is there snoring or gurgling? Tilt head; lift chin; use suction if good views. Is an airway adjunct necessary? Consider inserting Guedel airway or nasopharyngeal airway if GCS reduced <8 (see ➜ p. 742). Consider calling ITU if intubation and ITU care likely to be necessary, or if the patient is rapidly deteriorating/peri-arrest and full assessment has not yet been possible (see ➜ p. 688).

Breathing—cyanosis? What is the SaO_2 and associated FiO_2?
- Exclude tension pneumothorax clinically (see ➜ p. 380)
- What is the respiratory rate (RR)?
- Has a blood gas been taken, and what does it show? (see ➜ p. 826)
- Oxygenation adequate? If not, likely to need increased FiO_2 (see ➜ pp. 704–6), or, if this is already maximal, need ventilatory support—involve ITU
- Is the CO_2 low? If hyperventilation, already working hard breathing to maintain O_2 at current level. May need to increase FiO_2, or, if already maximal, need ventilatory assistance—involve ITU
- Is the CO_2 high (see ➜ p. 826)? Hypoventilating, tiring, or CO_2 narcosis in COPD—consider ventilatory support
- Request an urgent portable CXR.

Circulation—what is pulse rate, BP, rhythm on cardiac monitor/ECG? What is fluid balance status? Aim to optimize. Ensure IV access secured and blood tests sent. Look at BP, JVP, urine output, peripheral perfusion (capillary refill time). If they are hypotensive, are they underfilled? Consider fluids (crystalloid). If they are euvolaemic/overfilled, but hypotensive, with poor urine output, they may need inotropic support. Likely to need central venous access to enable CVP monitoring, and this will aid drug administration.

Disability—Conscious level: GCS or AVPU (alert, responsive to verbal commands, responsive to pain, unresponsive). Are they confused? Check blood glucose, temperature, pupils, signs of acute neurological disease—neck stiffness, plantar reflexes, tone.

Examination—temperature, sputum, asterixis, chest signs (pneumothorax, wheeze, silent chest, effusion, consolidation, pulmonary oedema), cardiac murmurs, palpable abdominal organomegaly, skin/nail signs, rash.

Investigations—immediate tests include FBC, clotting screen, CRP, U&E, blood cultures before antibiotics.

Underlying cause

If known respiratory disease, this will enable more targeted therapy. Try and obtain recent hospital notes. Ask patient or their relatives about disease severity, current treatment, plans of clinicians for long-term care (immuno-suppression, transplant list, home non-invasive ventilation (NIV), advance directive, lasting power of attorney, etc.). What is their usual current health status—exercise tolerance, activities of daily living? What has caused this deterioration—a potentially reversible process (e.g. infection, drugs, pneu-mothorax, PE) or gradual progression of underlying disease? Review CXR, and compare with old films, if possible.

* For more details regarding exacerbations of chronic lung diseases, see → p. 125 (asthma), → p. 169 (COPD), → p. 209 (CF), → p. 153 (bronchiectasis), → p. 265 (IPF), → p. 283 (lung cancer), → p. 565 (sickle cell).

If no known respiratory disease, full history required to obtain diagnosis. The patient's cardiovascular status and illness severity will determine how brief/full this is. Ask about recent symptoms, travel, contact illness, risk factors for immunocompromise, usual health status, drugs.

For presentation-based differential diagnoses and initial investigation plans, see → p. 3 (breathlessness), → p. 7 (chest pain), → p. 43 (haem-optysis), → p. 73 and p. 83 and → p. 95 (immunocompromise), → p. 95 (unexplained respiratory failure), → p. 31 (diffuse lung disease), → p. 27 (diffuse alveolar haemorrhage), → p. 49 (pleural effusion), → p. 65 (preg-nancy), → p. 61 (post-operative), → p. 417 (pneumonia), → p. 397 (PE), → p. 371 (pneumothorax), → p. 597 (toxic agents), → pp. 641 and → pp. 644–5 (upper airway disease and anaphylaxis), and → pp. 302–4 (SVCO).

Treatment aims

In patients with known severe respiratory disease, with poor pre-morbid state (e.g. very limited exercise tolerance, comorbidities, severe dementia), intubation and invasive ventilation may not be appropriate. The patient may have their own views on this or have made a living will/advance directive. Old notes should be reviewed, if possible, and this decision should be discussed with their respiratory consultant or the consultant on call. NIV (see ➔ p. 691) may be appropriate.

In patients with known respiratory disease, with an acute exacerbation (infective or non-infective), respiratory and organ support may be indicated to enable them to survive this episode. This should be discussed with their respiratory consultant or the consultant on call and ITU.

In patients with no known respiratory disease, respiratory and organ support may well be indicated to enable them to survive this episode. This should be discussed with the consultant on call and ITU. If they have significant pre-existing comorbidity from a non-respiratory disease (severe cardiac failure, severe dementia), the details of this should be ascertained and discussed with their usual consultant, if possible.

If there is any doubt about a patient's usual health status, or no previous history or notes available, or they are deteriorating before full assessment can be made, they should be considered for full ventilatory and organ support.

Chapter 5

Diffuse alveolar haemorrhage

Causes

Has multiple causes (see Box 5.1). A triad of:
- Diffuse alveolar infiltrates
- Haemoptysis (although not always present)
- A fall in Hb or haematocrit.

Bleeding into the alveoli is often a feature of a small-vessel vasculitis of the lungs. Most of this blood tends to remain in the lungs and is not expectorated. Patients with diffuse alveolar haemorrhage may have a background history of vasculitis over the preceding weeks to months. They can present with slowly progressive dyspnoea with haemoptysis or be acutely unwell with hypoxia. They may require ventilatory support.

Box 5.1 Causes of alveolar haemorrhage

First three are most common:
- Goodpasture's disease*   see  p. 659
- GPA (Wegener's)*   see pp. 654–5
- SLE*   see pp. 194–5
- RA   see pp. 192–3
- Microscopic polyangiitis (MPA)*   see p. 658
- Progressive systemic sclerosis   see pp. 198–9
- Polyarteritis nodosa (PAN)   see p. 662
- Mixed connective tissue disease
- Antiphospholipid syndrome
- Behçet's disease
- Essential mixed cryoglobulinaemia
- Endocarditis- or tumour-related vasculitis
- Idiopathic rapidly progressive glomerulonephritis
- Idiopathic pulmonary haemosiderosis
- Leptospirosis
- Isolated pauci-immune pulmonary capillaritis
- Coagulopathy such as disseminated intravascular coagulation (DIC)
- Mitral valve disease
- Bone marrow transplantation (usually within 1 month)
- Drugs: abciximab, ATRA, sirolimus, PTU, penicillamine, cocaine
- Chemicals: trimellitic anhydride, pyromellitic dianhydrate.

*Indicates conditions commonly considered in the differential diagnosis of *pulmonary-renal syndrome* (diffuse alveolar haemorrhage with glomerulonephritis). Note: conditions causing diffuse CXR infiltrate and renal failure may mimic these, e.g. severe cardiac failure, severe pneumonia, leptospirosis.

Clinical features and investigations

Presentation Abrupt-onset haemoptysis is the most common symptom, although this is not present in one-third of cases. Also cough, dyspnoea, low-grade fever, weight loss, arthralgia, myalgia. There may be a history of chronic sinusitis and other ENT symptoms (granulomatosis with polyangiitis; GPA ≈ Wegener's).

Examination May be non-specific or may have signs of underlying vasculitis with skin rashes, nail fold infarcts, digital gangrene. Episcleritis, corneal ulceration, epistaxis, nasal crusting, or deafness may be present. Neurological signs, including mononeuritis multiplex, should raise the possibility of vasculitis. Patients may be breathless. Haematuria and proteinuria on urine dip.

Investigations
- May be hypoxic—check SaO_2 ± ABG
- FBC—?falling Hb, clotting profile
- CRP/ESR
- Creatine kinase (CK)
- CXR showing bilateral alveolar infiltrates—difficult to distinguish from pulmonary oedema or infection
- Consider chest HRCT
- Raised kCO, as increased intra-alveolar Hb is available to combine with carbon monoxide (CO). Abnormal if raised by >30%. If breathless at rest, they will not be able to perform this test, as it requires breath-holding of an air, CO, and helium mixture for 10s. This test can be used to monitor disease progress
- BAL shows bloodstained lavage, which becomes sequentially more so with each washing. Cytology shows haemosiderin-laden macrophages
- Renal involvement: blood and/or protein in the urine, red cell casts, raised urea, and creatinine
- Send blood for urgent complement levels, ANA, ANCA (PR3 and MPO), anti-GBM Ab, anti-dsDNA Ab, antiphospholipid Ab, and rheumatoid factor (RhF)
- Consider biopsy of lung, kidney (if acute glomerulonephritis present), or other affected site if well enough to make a tissue diagnosis. Transbronchial biopsy (TBB) specimens are usually insufficient to make a diagnosis of vasculitis, and a surgical lung biopsy may be required. Capillaritis (a neutrophilic vasculitis of capillaries and venules), haemorrhage, or diffuse alveolar damage with haemorrhage seen on lung biopsy.

Key questions
- Is this isolated lung disease?
- Is there accompanying renal disease?
- Are there other features of an underlying disease?—ENT, joints, etc.?

Management

▶▶ **Management of alveolar haemorrhage**

- Admit to hospital
- Supportive treatment, with IV fluids, blood transfusion, and O_2, if necessary
- Monitor, paying particular attention to O_2 saturations and keeping them above 92% with O_2 therapy. May need respiratory support with intubation and ventilation or CPAP. Monitor Hb, and transfuse, if necessary. Monitor urine output and renal function
- Aim to establish the underlying diagnosis, usually with tissue biopsy
- Treatment with plasma exchange, high-dose steroids and cyclophosphamide, and dialysis, if required.

Chapter 6

Diffuse lung disease

Causes

Diffuse lung disease is common, and its diagnosis is frequently challenging. This chapter describes a diagnostic approach, based on clinical features, imaging, and other investigations; more detailed descriptions of the diseases themselves are presented later in the book. The term 'diffuse lung disease' is used here to describe any widespread pulmonary disease process. Patients typically present with breathlessness and bilateral CXR shadowing. The rate of onset and severity of breathlessness are extremely variable, however, and presentations range from an asymptomatic patient with long-standing radiological changes to an acute onset of breathlessness over a period of days, leading rapidly to respiratory failure and death.

Anatomy of diffuse lung disease

An understanding of lung anatomy is helpful when considering the causes of diffuse lung disease and their appearance on HRCT. Many diffuse lung diseases primarily affect the interstitium ('interstitial lung disease', also described as 'diffuse parenchymal lung disease'), a poorly defined term that refers to the connective tissue fibrous framework of the lung. Centrally, connective tissue surrounds bronchovascular bundles (each consisting of a bronchus and its accompanying pulmonary artery) that originate at the hila. Peripherally, these connective tissue sheaths are in continuity with fibrous interlobular septa, which organize the lung into units called '2° pulmonary lobules', polyhedral structures with approximately 2cm sides (see Fig. A4.4, ➔ p. 851). Interlobular septa, which define and separate 2° pulmonary lobules, contain lymphatics and venules. A 2° pulmonary lobule contains around 5–12 acini and is supplied at its centre by a bronchiole and pulmonary arteriole.

The term 'interstitial lung disease' is potentially confusing, because many primarily interstitial processes also involve the airways, vasculature, and alveolar airspaces. Disease processes that primarily affect the airways (e.g. bronchiectasis), vessels (e.g. vasculitis), or airspaces (e.g. pneumonia) may also present with diffuse CXR shadowing.

Causes

There are several hundred causes of diffuse lung disease, and it is useful to divide these into groups, based on their rate of onset and aetiology/disease mechanism (see Table 6.1).

Further information

British Thoracic Society. Interstitial lung disease guideline. *Thorax* 2008;**63**(suppl. V):v1–v58.

Table 6.1 Causes of diffuse lung disease

Disease onset	Cause/ mechanism	Examples (common conditions in bold)
Acute (days–weeks)	Infection	**Bacterial** (pneumococcal, staphylococcal, Gram-negative, anaerobic, TB, atypical), viral (influenza, parainfluenza, adeno, respiratory syncitial virus (RSV), cytomegalovirus (CMV), measles, varicella, hanta), fungal (aspergillosis, histoplasmosis, PCP)
	Miscellaneous	**Adult respiratory distress syndrome (ARDS)**, acute interstitial pneumonia (AIP), acute HP
Acute or chronic	Drugs	Immunosuppressants (methotrexate, azathioprine, cyclophosphamide); treatment of connective tissue disease (gold, penicillamine, sulfasalazine); cytotoxics (chlorambucil, melphalan, busulfan, lomustine, carmustine, bleomycin, mitomycin); antibiotics (nitrofurantoin, cephalosporins); anti-arrhythmics (amiodarone); illicit (cocaine inhalation, heroin, methadone, talc)
	Toxins	Radiotherapy, high-concentration O_2, paraquat
	Vasculitis/alveolar haemorrhage	Wegener's granulomatosis, Churg–Strauss syndrome, Goodpasture's syndrome, SLE, MPA, idiopathic haemosiderosis
	Pulmonary venous hypertension	**Cardiogenic pulmonary oedema**, pulmonary veno-occlusive disease
	Miscellaneous	**Sarcoidosis**, organizing pneumonia (OP), eosinophilic pneumonia, lipoid pneumonia
Chronic (months–years)	Idiopathic interstitial pneumonias (IIPs)	**IPF**, non-specific interstitial pneumonia (NSIP), desquamative interstitial pneumonia (DIP), lymphocytic interstitial pneumonia (LIP), respiratory bronchiolitis-associated interstitial lung disease (RB-ILD)
	Inhalational Inorganic	Asbestosis, coal worker's pneumoconiosis, silicosis, metals, e.g. cobalt, aluminium
	Organic	Hypersensitivity pneumonitis, e.g. bird fancier's lung, farmer's lung
	Connective tissue disease	RA, SLE, scleroderma, poly- and dermatomyositis, ankylosing spondylitis, Sjögren's syndrome, Behçet's disease
	Malignancy	Lymphangitis carcinomatosa, bronchoalveolar cell carcinoma, pulmonary lymphoma
	Miscellaneous	**Bronchiectasis**, Langerhans cell histiocytosis (LCH), amyloidosis, lymphangioleiomyomatosis (LAM), alveolar proteinosis, microlithiasis

Clinical assessment and imaging

History

Clinical features may provide useful clues to the underlying diagnosis. Key points in the history are:

Presenting symptoms

- Breathlessness is the most common symptom, and its rate of onset may be useful diagnostically (see Table 6.1)
- Causes of truly *episodic* breathlessness and CXR shadowing include eosinophilic pneumonia, vasculitis, alveolar haemorrhage, Churg–Strauss syndrome, HP, cryptogenic organizing pneumonia (COP), allergic bronchopulmonary aspergillosis (ABPA), and pulmonary oedema
- Cough may occur, although its diagnostic value is uncertain; it may be a prominent symptom in IPF, lymphangitis carcinomatosis, HP, OP, sarcoid, and eosinophilic pneumonia. Chronic production of purulent sputum suggests bronchiectasis. Bronchorrhoea (production of large volumes of sputum) may occur with bronchoalveolar cell carcinoma. Haemoptysis suggests alveolar haemorrhage, malignancy, or pulmonary venous hypertension
- Wheeze may occur in asthma associated with eosinophilic pneumonia or Churg–Strauss syndrome
- Weight loss and fever are non-specific symptoms associated with many diffuse lung diseases.

Other medical conditions, e.g. malignancy, connective tissue disease, HIV infection, other immunosuppression.

Drugs

- Common drug causes of diffuse lung disease are listed in Table 6.1; refer to ℘ http://www.pneumotox.com for a comprehensive database
- Delays of months, or even years, may occur between starting the drug and developing lung involvement
- Illicit drug abuse (crack cocaine or heroin—pulmonary oedema, eosinophilic pneumonitis, diffuse alveolar haemorrhage, interstitial pneumonia; IV drug use—IV talcosis, septic emboli)
- Oily nose drops (lipoid pneumonia).

Occupation, lifestyle, hobbies, and pets

- May involve inhalation of inorganic or organic dusts. Document lifelong employment history, including probable exposure levels, use of protective equipment, and names of employers
- Inorganic dusts associated with development of diffuse lung disease include asbestos, silica, cobalt, beryllium, aluminium, isocyanates, copper sulfate, iron, tin, barium, and antimony
- HP may result from inhalation of organic dusts, such as *Thermoactinomycetes* in mouldy hay (farmer's lung), avian proteins or feathers (bird fancier's lung), mushroom compost, mouldy cheese, cork or sugar cane, and isocyanates

- Risk factors for immunocompromise (opportunistic infection, LIP, lymphoma)
- Smoking history (LCH, RB-ILD, DIP, and Goodpasture's syndrome are more common in smokers).

Evidence of extrapulmonary disease

Manifestations of connective tissue disease, vasculitis, sarcoidosis, e.g. arthralgia, skin rash or thickening, ocular symptoms, muscular pain and weakness, Raynaud's, nasal/sinus disease, sicca symptoms, haematuria. Infertility in ♂ (immotile cilia syndrome, CF).

Travel

TB, pulmonary eosinophilia from parasites (tropics), histoplasmosis (north and central USA, parts of South America and Africa), hydatid disease (Middle East, Australasia, Mediterranean).

Family history

α1-antitrypsin (α1-AT) deficiency, rare familial forms of usual interstitial pneumonitis (UIP), and sarcoidosis.

Examination

- Cyanosis and signs of cor pulmonale in severe disease
- Clubbing (IPF, asbestosis, bronchiectasis)
- Basal crackles (IPF, asbestosis, connective tissue disease, pulmonary oedema, lymphangitis, drugs); crackles in bronchiectasis are characteristically coarse
- Absence of crackles, despite a significant CXR abnormality, may be suggestive of sarcoidosis, pneumoconiosis, HP, or LCH
- Squeaks suggest the presence of bronchiolitis and may occur in HP
- Skin, joint, and eye disease (connective tissue disease, sarcoidosis, vasculitis).

Imaging

CXR is an essential test although is rarely diagnostic. Up to 10% of patients with biopsy-proven diffuse lung disease have a normal CXR. Previous CXRs are helpful in assessing disease duration and progression.

Chest HRCT is more sensitive and specific than CXR for diagnosing diffuse lung disease (for HRCT diagnosis, see ➋ pp. 36–7 and Appendix 4). HRCT is often, in itself, diagnostic and should always precede biopsy in the investigation of diffuse lung disease. HRCT also enables assessment of disease extent and optimal biopsy site, if required. HRCT appearance correlates to some extent with disease activity in the interstitial pneumonias: a predominantly 'ground-glass' appearance may signify a steroid-responsive inflammatory state, whereas reticulation and honeycombing are often associated with fibrosis, poor response to treatment, and a worse prognosis.

⌐Γ diagnosis

⌐ΙRCT (and, to a limited extent, CXR) appearances can be classified, according to the pattern and distribution of disease and the presence of additional features (see also Appendix 4).

Imaging pattern

Reticular (or linear) pattern
Causes include:
- Interstitial pulmonary oedema
- UIP (reticular shadowing is typically patchy, subpleural, and basal; other features include loss of architecture of 2° pulmonary lobules, honeycombing, traction bronchiectasis)
- Asbestosis (similar features to UIP, often with pleural plaques)
- Connective tissue disease associated fibrosis (similar features to UIP)
- Chronic HP (often associated with regions of ground-glass change, air trapping on expiration, and centrilobular micronodules)
- Drug-induced fibrosis
- Sarcoidosis.

Nodular pattern consists of numerous discrete, round opacities 0.1–1cm in diameter.
- Interstitial processes result in nodularity within interlobular septa, around bronchovascular bundles, and subpleurally (e.g. sarcoidosis, which may demonstrate associated perihilar reticular shadowing and lymphadenopathy)
- Airspace diseases may lead to affected acini becoming visible as nodules (e.g. HP, miliary TB, COP, malignancy).

Ground-glass change is an increase in lung density through which pulmonary vasculature is still visible (compare the lung density with that of air within the bronchi). May occur as a result of airspace or interstitial disease and may be patchy or diffuse. Causes include:
- Pulmonary oedema or haemorrhage, ARDS
- HP
- Drugs
- Certain IIPs (NSIP, RB-ILD, DIP, AIP)
- PCP
- Sarcoidosis
- Bronchoalveolar cell carcinoma
- Alveolar proteinosis.

Ground-glass appearance may be artefactual, the increased density resulting from breath-holding during expiration. It may also be confused with 'mosaic perfusion' where densities vary in different regions of the lung as a result of either variable perfusion (e.g. in chronic thromboembolic disease) or gas trapping (small airways disease).

Consolidation (or airspace shadowing) is an increase in attenuation, characterized by air bronchograms (air-filled bronchi superimposed against opacified alveoli) and the loss of visibility of adjacent vessels. It occurs as disease processes infiltrate and fill alveolar airspaces, e.g. with water, blood, pus, malignant cells, or fibrous tissue. Causes include:

- Pneumonia
- Pulmonary oedema or haemorrhage, ARDS
- Drugs
- OP
- Bronchoalveolar cell carcinoma, lymphoma
- Other rare conditions (e.g. eosinophilic pneumonia, alveolar proteinosis).

Cystic change refers to well-defined airspaces with a thin wall. Causes include:

- LCH (bizarrely shaped cysts and nodules, apical predominance)
- UIP (subpleural honeycombing)
- PCP
- LIP
- Septic emboli
- LAM (thin-walled cysts, otherwise normal lung)
- Centrilobular emphysema may simulate cystic disease, but there is absence of a well-defined wall.

Interlobular septal thickening occurs as a result of processes affecting the lymphatics or venules within interlobular septa such as:

- Pulmonary oedema (smooth thickening)
- Lymphangitis carcinomatosis (irregular, nodular thickening of interlobular septa and bronchovascular bundles, no architectural distortion)
- Sarcoidosis
- UIP.

Imaging distribution

- Upper zone: silicosis, pneumoconiosis, chronic sarcoidosis, HP, ankylosing spondylitis, TB, LCH
- Lower zone: UIP, connective tissue diseases, asbestosis
- Mid-zone: sarcoidosis, pulmonary oedema, PCP
- Peripheral: UIP, eosinophilic pneumonia, drugs (amiodarone), COP
- Sharp borders: radiation pneumonitis.

Additional imaging features

- Lymphadenopathy: sarcoidosis, lymphoma, malignancy, infection, silicosis, berylliosis, LIP
- Pleural effusion/involvement: pulmonary oedema, connective tissue diseases, infection, malignancy, asbestosis, drugs, LAM.

Further investigations

Urine and blood tests

Consider the following investigations:
- Urine dipstick and microscopy for detection of renal disease associated with vasculitis/connective tissue disease
- ESR, CRP, FBC (look specifically at the eosinophil count), renal and liver function, CK (?myositis), calcium (increased in >10% of patients with sarcoidosis)
- Autoantibodies (RhF, ANA, ENAs (Ro, La, RNP, Scl-70, Jo-1, Sm))
- ANCA (vasculitis), anti-GBM (Goodpasture's syndrome)
- Serum precipitins (to antigens in HP; poor specificity)
- Serum ACE levels may be increased in sarcoidosis, but this is a non-specific and relatively insensitive test and is unhelpful diagnostically
- HIV testing.

Sputum

- Cytology may be diagnostic in bronchoalveolar cell carcinoma
- Induced sputum may be useful in the diagnosis of PCP and TB.

PFTs

- Useful in assessing progression and severity of disease and response to treatment, but often unhelpful diagnostically
- Typically show restrictive pattern with reduced vital capacity (VC) and transfer factor. Normal values do not exclude mild, early lung disease
- Obstructive pattern rare but may be seen in sarcoidosis, LCH, and LAM; may see mixed picture if coexisting COPD
- Transfer factor may be increased transiently (days) in alveolar haemorrhage. Reduced transfer factor with preserved lung volumes is suggestive of pulmonary vascular disease (pulmonary arterial hypertension (PAH) or vasculitis) or coexistent emphysema
- Disease progression and response to treatment are best assessed by serial measurements of vital capacity and transfer factor
- Check O_2 saturation, and consider ABGs. A fall in O_2 saturation on simple exercise may be performed in the clinic setting and is a useful clue to underlying lung disease in patients with normal saturation and lung function at rest and an unremarkable CXR.

Cardiac investigations

- *ECG* Conduction abnormality in sarcoidosis; cardiogenic pulmonary oedema is unusual in the presence of a completely normal ECG
- *Echo* Assess LV and valvular function if cardiac pulmonary oedema suspected, and measure pulmonary arterial pressure (PAP) (e.g. in scleroderma or suspected pulmonary veno-occlusive disease). The presence of a tricuspid regurgitation jet is required in order to assess PAP on echo.

BAL

- Most useful in diagnosis of opportunistic infection (bacterial or fungal pneumonia, TB, PCP), eosinophilic pneumonia, malignancy, alveolar proteinosis, and alveolar haemorrhage
- BAL differential cell counts usually unhelpful diagnostically, although BAL lymphocytosis is typical of HP, sarcoidosis, and LIP, and eosinophilic BAL occurs in eosinophilic pneumonia or drug-induced lung disease.

Lung biopsy

Which patients need a lung biopsy?

In cases of uncertain aetiology, despite clinical assessment and HRCT, lung biopsies often provide a definitive diagnosis. Ideally, they should be taken before treatment is started. The decision to biopsy varies amongst clinicians and should take into account the individual patient's clinical condition and wishes, and the likely benefit of a definitive diagnosis in terms of predicting treatment response and prognosis. Some take a pragmatic approach when a diagnosis (or group of diagnoses with the same treatment) is likely, but not biopsy-proven, and treat empirically. In some cases, the patient may be too unwell for biopsy and require empirical treatment. Lung biopsy is not usually recommended in patients with typical clinical and HRCT features of IPF, and biopsy of end-stage fibrosis is in general unhelpful in eliciting an underlying aetiology.

Biopsy techniques

TBB provides small samples but relatively high diagnostic yield in diseases with a 'centrilobular' distribution, e.g. sarcoidosis, HP, malignancy, infection (fungi, TB), and OP. Take 4–6 samples. Additional blind endobronchial biopsies may be diagnostic in sarcoidosis.

Open lung biopsy via thoracotomy or video-assisted thoracoscopic (VATS) biopsy provides larger samples than TBB and have diagnostic yields of at least 90%. Both require general anaesthesia. VATS probably has a lower morbidity and is generally preferred in stable patients; open biopsy is required in ventilator-dependent patients. Open or VATS biopsy is required for histological confirmation of IIPs, vasculitis, lymphoma, LAM, and LCH— the yield of TBB in these conditions is very low.

Percutaneous image-guided biopsy may be useful in the diagnosis of well-localized and dense peripheral infiltrates. A cutting needle biopsy technique is best and, if the lesion(s) abuts the pleural surface, pneumothorax is uncommon.

Diffuse lung disease presenting with acute respiratory failure

The management of patients presenting with diffuse lung disease—particularly ILD—and acute respiratory failure is challenging. These patients are often critically ill with rapidly progressive disease, and a variety of diverse conditions can underlie the typically non-specific presentation with breathlessness, hypoxia, raised inflammatory markers, and diffuse ground-glass infiltrates on HRCT. There is little evidence to guide management, which needs to be on a case-by-case basis. Assessment is largely as outlined earlier in this chapter but with particular emphasis on prompt identification and treatment of reversible causes and early consideration of appropriate ceilings of care/ICU admission.

Causes/differential diagnosis

- Diffuse infection (community-acquired pneumonia (CAP)—including 'atypical', PCP, other fungi, viral, TB)
- LVF
- ARDS
- Drug-induced pneumonitis
- Diffuse alveolar haemorrhage/vasculitis
- Fulminant OP
- AIP
- Acute exacerbation of previously subclinical IPF
- Acute HP
- Acute eosinophilic pneumonia
- Malignancy.

Key points in assessment and treatment

- Have a low threshold for treating *infection*, which, in practice, is difficult to distinguish from many non-infectious causes. Consider PCP. Subacute presentations of infection, such as fungal disease or TB, may rarely mimic ILD
- Look for evidence of *extrapulmonary disease*, particularly involving kidneys (urine dipstick and microscopy), heart, eyes, ENT, skin, muscles, joints. Active disease in these sites may, in some cases, provide a safer biopsy target than the lungs, if histology is required
- Actively consider *drug-induced* lung disease (see ℰ http://www.pneumotox.com): review current and previous medications carefully, and discontinue potentially offending drugs
- *Bloods* FBC (?eosinophilia), renal and liver function, CRP, ESR, CK, urgent immunology (RhF, ANA, ENA profile—including antisynthetase antibodies (anti-Jo-1 (see ➋ p. 203), ANCA (vasculitis), anti-GBM (Goodpasture's), serum precipitins (to antigens in HP)), HIV testing
- The presence of an antisynthetase antibody, in combination with one or more of interstitial pneumonitis, myositis, and arthritis, is characteristic of *antisynthetase* syndrome. Fever, Raynaud's phenomenon, and mechanic's hands (thick, cracked skin on palms and fingers) may also occur, or pneumonitis may be the sole clinical manifestation.

Check anti-Jo-1, which may be positive in myositis-associated acute pneumonitis, even in the setting of a negative ANA. Other antisynthetase antibodies, such as anti-PL-7 and anti-PL-12, and anti-CADM-140 may underlie rapidly progressive pneumonitis, with or without myositis, but are not yet routinely available

- Consider *echo* to assess LV and valvular function if cardiac pulmonary oedema suspected
- Further *imaging* PEs may coexist with ILD, and CTPA with HRCT slices is usually the radiological investigation of choice
- *BAL* is useful in excluding infection but may decompensate seriously ill, hypoxic patients; it is often safer to wait and perform after patients are ventilated. TBBs may increase diagnostic yield, but risk probably outweighs benefit in the majority of patients. *Surgical lung biopsy* may yield a diagnosis that alters management in carefully selected individuals, particularly those with *de novo* lung disease. It can be performed in the ICU on mechanically ventilated patients
- Consider empirical high-dose *steroids* (e.g. IV methylprednisolone 750mg–1g on 3 consecutive days, followed by maintenance therapy with 0.5–1mg/kg/day prednisolone). Fulminant COP is frequently steroid-responsive, and, although robust evidence is lacking, the outcome in AIP may be more favourable following early use of high-dose steroids. Assess the response to steroids over 5–7 days, and then consider further *immunosuppression*, particularly if there is any suggestion of underlying connective tissue disease: IV cyclophosphamide 600–650mg/m^2 is usually favoured because of relatively rapid onset (often <1 week), with mesna protection against bladder toxicity if total dose exceeds 1g; a second dose can be given 7–10 days later (depending upon white blood count) or 2-weekly. Empirical 'upfront' treatment with cyclophosphamide, alongside initial IV methylprednisolone, increases the infection risk but may be indicated in severe disease or in suspected severe vasculitis/Wegener's. Rituximab (a monoclonal antibody that targets peripheral B lymphocytes) or tacrolimus may be of benefit in severely ill patients with connective tissue disease-associated interstitial pneumonitis, particularly antisynthetase syndrome
- Consider *ceiling of care*. High-flow O_2 is almost always needed, and ICU admission and mechanical ventilatory support are usually required. ICU admission is usually appropriate for patients with *de novo* ILD, and it is appropriate to support patients with mechanical ventilation whilst awaiting a possible response to steroids/immunosuppression. Note that mechanical ventilation is usually considered an absolute contraindication to lung transplantation in the UK. The outcome of mechanical ventilation in patients with IPF is typically very poor, and ICU admission is rarely appropriate in the setting of underlying IPF/extensive fibrotic change.

Further information

British Thoracic Society. Interstitial lung disease guideline. *Thorax* 2008;**63**(suppl. V):v1–v58.

Chapter 7

Haemoptysis

Clinical assessment and causes

Haemoptysis is a common and non-specific symptom and can be a sign of significant underlying lung disease. However, in up to one-third of cases, no cause is found. An early assessment of the likely underlying cause needs to be made and investigations planned accordingly.

Diagnostic approach to haemoptysis Small-volume haemoptysis is a commonly encountered problem in the outpatient department. It can be safely and efficiently investigated as an outpatient. Massive haemoptysis is usually encountered in the accident and emergency department or in a patient already on the ward with known underlying lung disease. The approaches to small-volume and massive haemoptysis are different.

History
- Past history of lung disease?
- Document volume of blood and whether old (altered) or fresh
- Time course (intermittent, constant)
- Definitely from the airway, and not from the nose or mouth, or haematemesis? (haemoptysis may be swallowed and then vomited)
- Presence of systemic features—associated infection, symptoms consistent with underlying malignancy or vasculitis?

Examination May be normal or show signs of underlying lung disease, e.g. bronchiectasis, bronchial carcinoma, or symptoms of circulatory collapse.

Causes of haemoptysis

Common
- Bronchial tumour (benign, e.g. carcinoid, or malignant). Haemoptysis is a common presenting feature of bronchogenic malignancy, indicating endobronchial disease, which is usually visible endoscopically
- Bronchiectasis and CF (see ➜ p. 224). Small-volume haemoptysis is a common feature of bronchiectasis, particularly during exacerbations. It can be a cause of massive haemoptysis from dilated and abnormal bronchial artery branches that form around bronchiectatic cavities
- Active TB. Haemoptysis occurs in cavitating and non-cavitating disease, active disease and inactive disease (e.g. from an old bronchiectatic cavity, which might contain a mycetoma)
- Pneumonia (especially pneumococcal disease)
- Pulmonary thromboembolic disease
- Vasculitides/alveolar haemorrhage syndromes, e.g. GPA (formerly Wegener's), SLE, anti-GBM disease (Goodpasture's syndrome)
- Warfarin with any of the above causes.

Rare
- Lung abscess
- Mycetoma
- Fungal/viral/parasitic infections
- Fat embolism
- Foreign body
- Pulmonary endometriosis
- Arteriovenous malformation (AVM), e.g. in hereditary haemorrhagic telangiectasia (HHT) (see ➔ pp. 636–7)
- Severe PHT (see ➔ p. 383)
- Mitral stenosis
- Congenital heart disease
- Aortic aneurysm
- *Aspergillus*—invasive fungal disease (intracavity mycetoma) can be a cause of massive haemoptysis
- Coagulopathy, including DIC
- Endometriosis
- Pulmonary haemosiderosis
- Pseudoaneurysm post-aortic surgery
- Iatrogenic, e.g. post-lung biopsy, bronchoscopy.

Investigations

The investigation of haemoptysis can be carried out as an outpatient, but patients with significant bleeding or a likely serious underlying cause should be admitted if there is clinical concern. Note: beware of the apparently small bleed, which is a sentinel/herald bleed for massive haemoptysis. This is fortunately rare. Massive haemoptysis is more likely to be from a bronchial artery bleed (at systemic pressure) than from a pulmonary artery bleed (low pressure). See Box 7.1.

Outpatient investigations and management

First-line investigations
- *Blood tests* FBC, clotting, group & save. If systemic vasculitis is suspected, renal function and a urine dip, with microscopy for casts, are necessary, as well as autoantibodies—start with ANCA, anti-GBM, and ANA
- *Sputum* M, C, & S and AFB if infection suspected
- *CXR* may show mass lesion, bronchiectasis, consolidation, or an AVM
- *CT chest* should be done prior to bronchoscopy; prior knowledge of site of abnormality leads to increased pick-up at bronchoscopy. Similarly, a definitive diagnosis, e.g. AVM, may be made from the CT, obviating the need for further investigations. This depends on local resources; CT may miss an upper airway lesion, but bronchoscopy should not. Bronchial artery dilatation may be large enough to be visible on CT with contrast
- *Bronchoscopy* to visualize the airways and localize the site of bleeding. May also be therapeutic, e.g. if a bleeding tumour can be injected with a vasoconstricting agent (adrenaline) or a catheter inserted for tamponade (see Box 7.1)
- *TBB*—if vasculitis suspected.

Second-line investigations
Usually done if first-line investigations fail to demonstrate a cause.
- *CTPA* to exclude PE. Bronchial artery dilatation may be large enough to be visible on a CTPA
- *Bronchial angiogram* Diagnostic and therapeutic. Rare for the actual bleeding site to be identified; more often, the bleeding site is assumed from visualizing a mesh of dilated and tortuous vessels, e.g. around a bronchiectatic cavity. Usually done during an episode of bleeding to maximize the chance of identifying the site of bleeding
- *Bronchial artery embolization* Therapeutic approach to embolize the bleeding artery, usually with coils or glue (specialist centre only). There is a small risk of paraplegia (<1%) if the anterior spinal artery originates from the bronchial arterial circulation and is inadvertently embolized
- *ENT review* The source of the bleeding may be the upper airway
- *Echo* Moderate/severe PHT can cause haemoptysis, especially in a patient on anticoagulants.

Cryptogenic haemoptysis In about one-third of cases, despite appropriate investigations as described previously, no cause for the haemoptysis can be found. This has a good prognosis. Often the haemoptysis will settle without treatment and will become less worrying to the patient over time, especially as investigations have failed to determine the cause.

▶▶ Box 7.1 Management of massive haemoptysis

Massive haemoptysis (100–600mL blood in 24h) is a life-threatening emergency, with a mortality of up to 80%. It is extremely distressing for the patient, relatives, and medical staff but is fortunately rare. Investigations will follow treatment, which may be difficult, and is often unsuccessful. In some cases, active treatment may be inappropriate, and palliative treatment with O_2 and diamorphine may be warranted.

- Airway protection and ventilation:
  - Protection of the non-bleeding lung is vital to maintain adequate gas exchange. This may involve either sitting the patient up or lying on the bleeding side (to prevent blood from flowing into the unaffected lung), or intubation with a double-lumen tube. If intubation is not needed or not appropriate, give high-flow O_2
- Cardiovascular support:
  - Large-bore/central IV access
  - Cross-match blood
  - Fluid resuscitation ± transfusion
  - Correct clotting, e.g. vitamin K 10mg od; give platelets
  - Inotropes may be required
- Nebulized adrenaline (1mL of 1:1,000 made up to 5mL with NaCl 0.9%)
- Oral or IV tranexamic acid (1g tds, not if in severe renal failure)
- IV terlipressin, 2mg IV, then 1–2mg every 4–6h if continued bleeding
- CXR ± chest CT (depending on stability of patient)
- Early bronchoscopy—diagnostic and therapeutic
- Rigid bronchoscopy (with general anaesthesia) is preferable. May allow localization of the site of bleeding; balloon tamponade with a Fogarty catheter
- Bronchial artery embolization—therapeutic approach to embolize bleeding artery, usually with coils or glue (specialist centre only)
- Surgery—resection of bleeding lobe (if all other measures have failed).

Chapter 8

Pleural effusion

Clinical assessment

Pleural effusion is a common presentation of a wide range of different diseases. Commonest causes in the UK and USA (in order): cardiac failure, pneumonia, malignancy, PE.

Priority is to make a diagnosis and relieve symptoms, with minimum number of invasive procedures. The majority of patients do not require a chest drain and can be managed as outpatients. Procedures, such as therapeutic thoracentesis, may be performed readily on a day unit. Consider admission and chest drain insertion for:

- Patients with malignant effusions who are candidates for pleurodesis
- Empyema (pus) or complicated parapneumonic effusion (pleural fluid pH <7.2)—the majority of these effusions are unlikely to resolve without drainage and antibiotics
- Patients who are unwell with an acute massive effusion.

Key steps in the management of the patient with a pleural effusion follow and are also detailed in the diagnostic algorithm in Fig. 8.1.

History, examination, CXR, and pleural USS Including a drug history (see ⅍ http://pneumotox.com).

Does the patient have an obvious cause for transudative effusions? (e.g. heart failure, hypoalbuminaemia, dialysis) If so, this should be treated, with no need for thoracentesis unless atypical features (such as very asymmetrical bilateral effusions, unilateral effusion, echogenicity/septations/nodularity on pleural USS, chest pain, or fever) or failure to respond to therapy.

Thoracentesis (= 'pleural tap' or pleural fluid aspiration) may be diagnostic and/or therapeutic, depending on the volume of fluid removed. See ➲ p. 798 for procedure details and ➲ p. 56 for pleural fluid analysis. Following diagnostic tap:

- Note pleural fluid *appearance*
- Send sample to biochemistry for measurement of *glucose*, *protein*, and lactate dehydrogenase (*LDH*)
- Send a fresh 20mL sample in sterile pot to *cytology* for examination for malignant cells (yield ~60% in malignancy) and differential cell count
- Send samples in sterile pot to *microbiology* for Gram stain and microscopy, culture. For suspected pleural infection, also send pleural fluid in blood culture bottles. Low threshold for AFB stain and TB culture
- Process non-purulent, heparinized samples in ABG analyser for *pH*
- Consider measurement of cholesterol, triglycerides, chylomicrons, haematocrit, adenosine deaminase, and amylase, depending on the clinical circumstances.

If the patient is breathless, they may benefit from removal of a larger volume of fluid (therapeutic thoracentesis, see ➲ p. 800).

Is the pleural effusion a transudate or an exudate? Helpful in narrowing the differential diagnosis. In patients with a normal serum protein, pleural fluid protein <30g/L = transudate, and protein >30g/L = exudate. In borderline cases (protein 25–35g/L) or in patients with abnormal serum protein, apply Light's criteria—effusion is exudative if it meets one of following criteria.

- Pleural fluid protein/serum protein ratio >0.5
- Pleural fluid LDH/serum LDH ratio >0.6
- Pleural fluid LDH > two-thirds the upper limit of normal serum LDH.

These criteria are very sensitive in the diagnosis of exudative effusions although may occasionally falsely identify transudates as being exudates, e.g. patients with partially treated heart failure on diuretics may be misidentified as exudates. N-terminal pro-brain natriuretic peptide (NT-proBNP) may be of use in these cases.

Further investigations if the diagnosis remains unclear:
- CT chest with pleural phase contrast (ideally scan prior to complete fluid drainage to improve images of pleural surfaces; useful in distinguishing benign and malignant pleural disease, see ⊃ p. 344)
- Further pleural fluid analysis (see ⊃ pp. 58–9), e.g. cholesterol, triglyceride, chylomicrons, haematocrit, adenosine deaminase, amylase, fungal stains
- Pleural tissue biopsy for histology and TB culture using image-guided or thoracoscopic biopsies. These techniques are superior to Abrams' closed pleural biopsy for malignant disease and TB (thoracoscopy has sensitivity of ~100% for TB and >90% for malignancy and allows therapeutic talc pleurodesis at the same time). Use Abrams' biopsy only when TB is strongly suspected and thoracoscopy not available
- Reconsider PE and TB.

Bronchoscopy has no role in investigating undiagnosed effusions, unless the patient has haemoptysis or a CXR/CT pulmonary abnormality. Pleural fluid may compress the airways and limit bronchoscopic views, and so, if bronchoscopy is indicated, it is best performed following drainage of the effusion.

Further information

Light RW. Pleural effusion. *N Engl J Med* 2002;**346**:1971–7.

Hooper C *et al.* Investigation of a unilateral pleural effusion in adults: British Thoracic Society pleural disease guideline 2010. *Thorax* 2010;**65**(Suppl. 2):ii4–17.

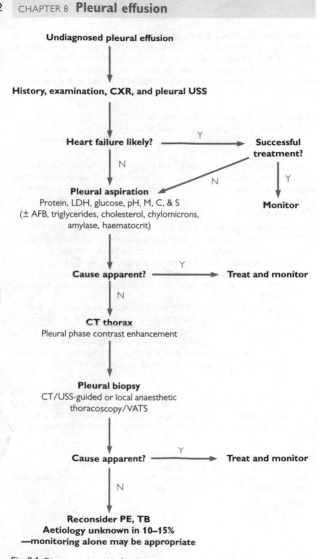

Undiagnosed pleural effusion

History, examination, CXR, and pleural USS

Heart failure likely? ——Y——→ **Successful treatment?**

N

Pleural aspiration
Protein, LDH, glucose, pH, M, C, & S
(± AFB, triglycerides, cholesterol, chylomicrons,
amylase, haematocrit)

N   Y

Monitor

Cause apparent? ——Y——→ **Treat and monitor**

N

CT thorax
Pleural phase contrast enhancement

Pleural biopsy
CT/USS-guided or local anaesthetic
thoracoscopy/VATS

Cause apparent? ——Y——→ **Treat and monitor**

N

Reconsider PE, TB
Aetiology unknown in 10–15%
—monitoring alone may be appropriate

Fig. 8.1 Diagnostic algorithm for the patient with a pleural effusion.

Transudative pleural effusions

Mechanisms involve either increased hydrostatic pressure or reduced osmotic pressure (due to hypoalbuminaemia) in the microvascular circulation.

Differential diagnosis See Table 8.1.

Treatment of transudative effusions is directed at the underlying cause; consider further investigation if fails to respond.

Table 8.1 Causes of transudative pleural effusions

Cause	Notes
Common	
LVF	Investigate further if atypical features (very asymmetrical bilateral effusions, unilateral effusion, chest pain, fever); may be complicated by PE (up to 1/5 of cases at autopsy)
Atelectasis	Common on ITU or post-operatively (also, hypoalbuminaemia); usually small effusion, may be bilateral; rarely needs investigation
Cirrhotic liver disease ('hepatic hydrothorax')	Ascites often, but not invariably, present; majority right-sided; remove ascites and treat hypoalbuminaemia (see ➲ pp. 248–9)
Hypoalbuminaemia	
Peritoneal dialysis	Pleural fluid analysis resembles dialysis fluid, with protein <10g/L and glucose >17mmol/L
PE	10–20% are transudates (see ➲ p. 397)
Nephrotic syndrome	Usually bilateral; consider 2° PE if atypical features
Less common	
Constrictive pericarditis	May be unilateral or bilateral
Hypothyroidism	May be transudate or exudate; pleural effusions occur most commonly in association with ascites, pericardial effusion, and cardiac failure, although may be an isolated finding
Malignancy	Up to 5% are transudates
Meigs' syndrome	Unilateral (often right-sided) or bilateral pleural effusions and ascites; occurs in women with ovarian or other pelvic tumours; resolves following removal of tumour
Mitral stenosis	
Urinothorax	Effusion ipsilateral to obstructed kidney with retroperitoneal urine leak, resolves after treatment of obstruction; pleural fluid smells of urine, pH usually low; pleural fluid creatinine > serum creatinine is diagnostic

Exudative pleural effusions

Mechanisms involve an increase in capillary permeability and impaired pleural fluid resorption.

Differential diagnosis
See Table 8.2.

Table 8.2 Causes of exudative pleural effusions

Cause	Notes
Common	
Simple parapneumonic effusion (SPPE)	Occurs in 40% of bacterial pneumonias; commonest exudative effusion in young patients (see ➔ p. 418)
Malignancy	Commonest exudative effusion in patients >60y (see ➔ p. 283)
TB	Typically lymphocytic effusion; pleural fluid AFB smear positive in <5% of cases, culture positive in 10–20%, thoracoscopic biopsy histology sensitivity ~100% (see ➔ p. 488). Adenosine deaminase may be a useful 'rule out' test.
Less common	
Complicated parapneumonic effusion (CPPE) and empyema	CPPE defined by pleural fluid pH <7.2 and clinical features of infection, e.g. fever, sweats (see ➔ pp. 350–1); empyema defined by pleural pus
Other infections	Rare; include viral, parasitic, rickettsial, and fungal (e.g. *Aspergillus*, histoplasma, coccidioidomycosis)
PE	80–90% are exudates (see ➔ p. 397)
RA	Typically low pleural fluid glucose, often <1.6mmol/L (see ➔ pp. 192–3)
SLE	Lupus erythematosus cells in fluid are diagnostic; may respond quickly to prednisolone
Other autoimmune diseases	Eosinophilic granulomatosis with polyangiitis (Churg–Strauss syndrome; intensely eosinophilic fluid), Sjögren's syndrome, scleroderma, dermatomyositis, GPA (Wegener's)
Sarcoidosis	Effusions uncommon
Hepatic, splenic, or subphrenic abscess	
Oesophageal rupture	Initially sterile exudate, followed by empyema; pH <7.2, ↑ salivary amylase, often history of vomiting
Pancreatitis	Pleural fluid pancreatic amylase may be raised
Post-cardiac injury syndrome (Dressler's syndrome) and post-CABG surgery	Pleural effusions common; may be bloodstained (see ➔ p. 359)

(Continued)

Table 8.2 (Continued)

Cause	Notes
Less common	
Radiotherapy	May cause small, unilateral effusions up to 6 months after treatment
Uraemia	Effusions frequently resolve after starting dialysis
Chylothorax	Presence of chylomicrons or pleural fluid triglyceride level >1.24mmol/L (see ➋ pp. 58–9)
Benign asbestos-related pleural effusion	(See ➋ pp. 114–5)
Drug-induced	Drugs include amiodarone, β-blockers, bromocriptine, methotrexate, nitrofurantoin, and phenytoin; see ℐ http://www.pneumotox.com for full list; effusions usually resolve following discontinuation of drug
Other, rare causes	Include yellow nail syndrome, COP, amyloidosis, familial Mediterranean fever

Treatment of exudates involves treatment of the underlying cause, as well as measures to improve breathlessness and remove pleural fluid, e.g. therapeutic thoracentesis (see ➋ p. 800), intercostal drainage (see ➋ p. 761), and pleurodesis (see ➋ p. 783).

Pleural fluid analysis 1

'Routine' pleural fluid analysis comprises assessment of:
• Pleural fluid appearance and other characteristics (see Table 8.3)
• Biochemistry (glucose, protein, and LDH)
• pH measured using a heparinized syringe in a blood gas analyser
• Cytology (for malignant cells and differential cell count (see Table 8.4); ideally fresh 20mL sample)
• Microbiology (Gram stain and culture). Also send blood culture bottles, each inoculated with 5mL of pleural fluid, if pleural infection likely (increases yield). Low threshold for AFB stain and TB culture

Although considered routine, some of these investigations may be unnecessary, and even misleading, depending on the clinical picture (e.g. microbiological analysis on patients suspected as having transudates).

Additional pleural fluid investigations, such as measurement of cholesterol and triglycerides, haematocrit, glucose, adenosine deaminase, and amylase, may be helpful in certain clinical circumstances.

Table 8.3 Relevance of pleural fluid characteristics

Characteristics	Possible causes
Bloody	Trauma, malignancy, pulmonary infarction, pneumonia, post-cardiac injury syndrome, pneumothorax, benign asbestos-related pleural effusion, aortic dissection/rupture; defined as haemothorax if pleural fluid haematocrit >50% of peripheral blood haematocrit (see ➔ pp. 358–9)
Turbid or milky	Empyema, chylothorax, pseudochylothorax (clear supernatant after centrifuging favours empyema; cloudy after centrifuging suggests chylothorax or pseudochylothorax, see ➔ p. 58)
Viscous	Mesothelioma
Food particles	Oesophageal rupture
Bile-stained	Cholothorax (biliary fistula)
Black	Aspergillus infection
Brown, 'anchovy sauce'	Amoebic liver abscess draining into pleural space
Urine odour	Urinothorax
Putrid odour	Anaerobic empyema

Table 8.4 Relevance of pleural fluid differential cell count

Predominant cell type	Possible causes
Neutrophils	Any acute effusion, e.g. parapneumonic, PE
Mononuclear cells	Any chronic effusion, e.g. malignancy, TB
Lymphocytes	TB, especially if >80%; other causes include cardiac failure, malignancy, sarcoidosis, lymphoma, rheumatoid pleurisy, post-CABG, chylothorax
Eosinophils	Often unhelpful; associations include air or blood in pleural space (haemothorax, pulmonary infarct, pneumothorax, previous tap), malignancy, infection (parapneumonic, tuberculous, fungal, parasitic), drug- and asbestos-induced effusions, Churg–Strauss syndrome, or idiopathic
Mesothelial cells	Predominate in transudates; variable numbers in exudates, typically suppressed in inflammatory conditions, e.g. TB
Lupus erythematosus cells	Diagnostic of SLE

Pleural fluid analysis 2

Pleural fluid pH and glucose Pleural fluid pH may be measured using an arterial blood pH analyser. The sample should be appropriately heparinized, e.g. aspirate a few mL of pleural fluid into a pre-heparinized blood gas syringe. Pleural fluid pH is affected by exposure to air (increases pH) or local anaesthetic (decreases pH). Frankly purulent samples should not be analysed—it is unnecessary and might damage the machine.

Normal pleural fluid pH is about 7.6. An abnormally low pH (<7.3) suggests pleural inflammation and is often associated with a low pleural fluid glucose (<3.3mmol/L or pleural fluid/serum glucose ratio <0.5). The mechanism probably involves increased neutrophil phagocytosis and bacterial or tumour cell breakdown, resulting in the accumulation of lactate and CO_2.

Causes of low pH and low glucose effusions
- CPPE and empyema (pH <7.2 indication for drainage of pleural space, as unlikely to resolve spontaneously; this is not an absolute cut-off—values can vary in each locule of a multiloculated effusion)
- Rheumatoid pleuritis (glucose <1.7mmol/L in 66% and <2.8mmol/L in 80% of cases)
- Malignant pleural effusion (associated with advanced disease and poor survival, higher sensitivity of pleural fluid cytological analysis, and failure of pleurodesis)
- Tuberculous pleural effusion
- Oesophageal rupture
- Lupus pleuritis.

Urinothorax is the only transudative effusion that can cause a pH <7.3. An abnormally high (alkaline) pH may rarely occur in the setting of *Proteus* pleural infection.

Pleural fluid triglyceride and cholesterol Measure in turbid or milky effusions or where chylothorax is suspected.

Chylothorax occurs following disruption of the thoracic duct, and pleural fluid may appear turbid, milky, serous, or bloodstained. The presence of pleural fluid chylomicrons or a pleural fluid triglyceride level >1.24mmol/L confirms the diagnosis. Causes of chylothorax:
- Trauma or following thoracotomy
- Malignancy (particularly lymphoma)
- Pulmonary LAM
- TB.

Pseudochylothorax occurs due to cholesterol crystal deposition in chronic effusions, most commonly due to rheumatoid pleurisy or TB, and may cause a milky effusion; raised pleural fluid cholesterol (>5.17mmol/L) and cholesterol crystals at microscopy distinguish it from chylothorax.

Pleural fluid amylase Abnormal if pleural fluid amylase > upper normal limit for serum amylase, or if amylase pleural fluid/serum ratio >1.0. Causes include:

- Pleural malignancy and oesophageal rupture (both associated with raised *salivary* amylase)
- Pancreatic disease (acute and chronic pancreatitis, pancreatic pseudocyst; associated with raised *pancreatic* amylase).

Note—may be normal early in the course of acute pancreatitis or oesophageal rupture.

Chapter 9

Post-operative breathlessness

Introduction

The respiratory physician is often asked to see patients post-operatively who have become dyspnoeic following an operative procedure. The risk of pulmonary complications is greatest with thoracic or upper abdominal surgery, when a degree of pulmonary dysfunction and consequent breathlessness due to atelectasis is inevitable. Always rule out upper airway obstruction. See Table 9.1 for possible causes and management.

The four most likely common causes are:
- Infection/atelectasis
- PE
- LVF (fluid overload)
- Exacerbation of underlying lung disease such as COPD or UIP.

Initial assessment

- Is the patient acutely unwell, needing immediate resuscitation and ventilatory support?
- Comorbid disease and past medical history, especially pulmonary, cardiac, or thromboembolic disease
- Type of surgery:
  - *Thoracic surgery* Consider lobar gangrene (torsion of the remaining lobe causing vascular occlusion) leading to pulmonary infarction with fever and haemoptysis, bronchopleural fistula, often associated with an infected pleural space, leading to sepsis and failure of the underlying lung to re-expand
- Time since surgery:
  - *Early complications (hours)* related to residual anaesthetic effect not adequately reversed, atelectasis, respiratory failure, hypovolaemic shock, infection, PE, fat embolism, air embolism, LVF and fluid overload, myocardial ischaemia
  - *Later complications (hours to days)* related to PE, ARDS, infection, myocardial ischaemia.

Table 9.1 Management of post-operative dyspnoea

Possible cause of dyspnoea	Management options
Basal atelectasis (commoner in smokers and following abdominal or trans-thoracic procedures. Mucus in bronchial tree causes small airway obstruction, subsequent alveolar air reabsorption, and collapse of lung segments); collapsed lobe—mucus plugging	Adequate analgesia to encourage expectoration, nebulized saline, chest physiotherapy, deep breathing. If lung does not reinflate, consider bronchoscopy to suction out secretions
Pneumonia—follows atelectasis and collapse. Possible aspiration also	If fever and chest signs, give antibiotics for hospital-acquired pneumonia (see ⊃ pp. 434–5), adequate analgesia to encourage expectoration, chest physiotherapy
Thromboembolic disease	O_2 as required. Measure A–a gradient on blood gas. Start treatment dose of unfractionated heparin (if not contraindicated by the operation); arrange V/Q scan or CTPA; check D-dimers (although unhelpful unless negative). If in extremis, consider urgent CT or echo and thrombolysis (see ⊃ pp. 409–10)
Respiratory failure	Opiate overdose or anaesthetic agents causing neuromuscular block not reversed. Undiagnosed respiratory muscle weakness
Metabolic acidosis	Check U&E; look for underlying problem such as renal failure or sepsis
Myocardial ischaemia	O_2, check 12h troponin. Sublingual or IV glyceryl trinitrate, if required for pain. Start prophylactic heparin (if not contraindicated by the operation)
MI or acute coronary syndrome	Thrombolysis likely to be contraindicated by recent surgery, so consider referral for 1° angioplasty. Consider aspirin, clopidogrel, low molecular weight heparin (LMWH)
Cardiac failure/fluid overload	O_2, IV furosemide, central line, and inotropes if required. Echo to assess LV
ARDS	Supportive, likely to need mechanical ventilatory assistance (see ⊃ pp. 108–9)
Phrenic nerve damage causing diaphragmatic paralysis. May occur with thoracic operations such as CABG	Diagnose on lung function tests, CXR, and clinically decreased diaphragm movement. Advise to tilt whole bed (head up) when sleeping. Phrenics may recover but can take 2+ years
Fat embolism following long bone fracture, especially with reaming and manipulation	O_2, IV fluids, supportive care
Laryngeal spasm	Reassurance, O_2 if required
Anaemia	Cross-match and transfuse. Identify if ongoing bleeding source
Myasthenia gravis crisis precipitated by anaesthetic agents	May need intubation and ventilation. Stop all anticholinesterases. Consider plasma exchange and IV immunoglobulin. Urgent neurology input

Initial investigations

- O_2 saturations and ABG breathing room air and on O_2
- ECG
- CXR—compare with preoperative CXR, if available
- FBC and clotting screen
- U&E and bicarbonate
- See if they had preoperative oximetry and spirometry performed. There should be a record of the O_2 saturation in the anaesthetic room.

A D-dimer level is unhelpful, as it will be raised by many different intra- and post-operative mechanisms.

CRP and WCC are also largely unhelpful, as these are frequently raised post-operatively.

Chapter 10

Pregnancy and breathlessness

Causes

Normal physiological changes of pregnancy

- Elevated serum progesterone levels stimulate respiratory drive and lead to an increased tidal volume and raised minute ventilation, with only a modest increase in O_2 consumption. The subsequent fall in maternal pCO_2 facilitates foetal CO_2 transfer across the placenta; any cause of maternal hypercapnia leads quickly to foetal respiratory acidosis. Respiratory rate is unaffected by pregnancy. Elevation of the diaphragm occurs due to the enlarging uterus, leading to a reduced functional residual capacity (FRC), although diaphragm function is normal and VC is unaffected. Peak flow and FEV_1 are unaffected by pregnancy
- Increased cardiac output occurs due to an increase in heart rate (HR) (by about 15 beats/min) and stroke volume; peripheral resistance falls. BP is reduced in the first and second trimesters by 10–20mmHg but is normal at term. Peripheral pulses tend to be increased in volume. Dependent oedema is common. Third heart sound and ejection systolic murmurs are commonly heard. May hear venous hums in the neck
- Raised levels of coagulation factors and impaired fibrinolysis, combined with venous stasis, result in a 5-fold increased risk of venous thromboembolism (VTE)
- Upper airway oedema, particularly in the setting of pre-eclampsia, may predispose to upper airways obstruction during sleep, but rarely frank OSA. OSA tends to occur in obese women and may be associated with impaired foetal growth and pre-eclampsia. Snoring in pregnancy is a poor predictor of OSA.

Causes of breathlessness in pregnancy

Causes are listed in Box 10.1. In general, breathlessness may be due to:
- Normal physiological changes of pregnancy. Up to 70% of pregnant women experience a degree of breathlessness, perhaps as a result of the increase in ventilation. Tachypnoea is a useful sign, as it is abnormal in pregnancy and suggests an underlying disease process
- New disease process. PE is the commonest and is a major cause of maternal death. Other rare, but serious, causes include amniotic fluid embolism and ARDS
- Exacerbation of chronic respiratory or cardiac disease. Asthma is the commonest. Unsuspected underlying disease may present for the first time in pregnancy, e.g. structural heart disease such as mitral stenosis, LAM. PHT is associated with a particularly poor prognosis during pregnancy. Patients with ILD and VC <1L should also consider avoiding pregnancy. In patients with CF, the presence of PHT or FEV_1 <60% predicted are associated with a poor outcome.

Box 10.1 Causes of breathlessness in pregnancy

Pulmonary
- Exacerbation of pre-existing lung disease, e.g. asthma, CF, LAM
- Pneumonia
  - Bacterial, including TB, aspiration
  - Viral, particularly varicella, influenza
  - Fungal, particularly coccidioidomycosis
- Aspiration pneumonitis
- Pulmonary metastases from choriocarcinoma (very rare).

Pleural
- Pneumothorax, particularly during labour
- Small asymptomatic effusions post-partum
- Ovarian hyperstimulation syndrome (very rare).

Vascular
- VTE
- Amniotic fluid embolism
- Air embolism
- Aortic dissection
- PHT.

Cardiogenic pulmonary oedema
- Exacerbation of pre-existing cardiac disease, e.g. valvular or congenital disease
- Peripartum cardiomyopathy.

Non-cardiogenic pulmonary oedema
- Iatrogenic fluid overload
- Tocolytic therapy (fl-agonists used to inhibit uterine contractions in preterm labour)
- ARDS due to pre-eclampsia, sepsis, massive haemorrhage, amniotic fluid embolism.

Other
- Anaemia
- Oesophageal rupture
- Hemidiaphragm rupture.

Investigations

Liaise with your obstetrics team, as well as with paediatricians and anaesthetists, if delivery is approaching. Management of specific conditions is discussed in the individual disease chapters in Part 2.

The following investigations may be affected by the pregnancy itself:

- *ABGs* Normal maternal pO_2 >13.3kPa and pCO_2 3.7–4.3kPa. A compensatory fall in serum bicarbonate (to 18–22mmol/L) occurs, resulting in an average pH of 7.44. During the third trimester, perform ABGs in an upright position, as pO_2 may be 2.0kPa lower when supine. A–a gradient is unaffected during pregnancy, except when supine near term
- *Blood tests* In normal pregnancy, WCC, platelets, ESR, D-dimers, and fibrinogen are usually raised, and serum creatinine levels reduced. CRP is not significantly affected. D-dimer is increased from about 6 weeks' gestation to 3 months post-partum
- *CXR* may show increased pulmonary vasculature due to normal increase in cardiac output. Required for diagnosis of pneumonia and pneumothorax. With abdominal shielding, the radiation doses to mother and baby are negligible, and CXR should be performed if clinically indicated. Lateral CXR carries a greater radiation exposure and should be avoided
- Further investigation to exclude PE should be guided by local policy. Many experts recommend bilateral *leg vein ultrasound (US)* first; if an asymptomatic deep vein thrombosis (DVT) is confirmed in the setting of clinical features, suggestive of PE, then treatment may be started without the need for radiation exposure from further imaging. *V/Q scans* are associated with a higher radiation dose to the foetus and, as such, a slightly higher risk of childhood cancer, whereas *CTPA* carries a greater maternal radiation dose and, in the setting of the hormonal changes within the breast during pregnancy, leads to an increased risk of breast cancer in the mother. The ventilation component of a V/Q scan can often be omitted during pregnancy, reducing the radiation dose. CTPA can identify other pathology, e.g. aortic dissection.

Chapter 11

Preoperative assessment

Introduction

The respiratory physician may be asked to assess a patient prior to elective or emergency surgery. These patients are usually those with pre-existing respiratory disease such as COPD.
- The usual functional status of the patient should be determined
- Their respiratory function should be optimized, if possible, with medication changes where appropriate.

These patients may require ventilatory support post-operatively. Ultimately, the decisions regarding fitness for surgery rest with the surgeon and the anaesthetist.

Preoperative assessment

- Usual functional state and exercise tolerance (those with an exercise tolerance of <5m will not come off a ventilator)
- O_2 saturations on air and after exertion such as walking or climbing up and down a step for 2min. Cardiopulmonary exercise test (CPET) may be necessary (see ➲ p. 880)
- ABG on air, if saturations <94%. *Risk of surgery increases as the CO_2 increases*
- Spirometry, with bronchodilator reversibility testing. *Risk of surgery increased if FEV_1 <0.8L*
- CXR—if 65+ and no CXR in last year, or if acute respiratory symptoms
- History of snoring or OSA
- ECG
- Echo, if cardiac function compromised.

Management options

- Regular inhaled or nebulized bronchodilators, if airflow obstruction
- Regular inhaled steroid, if evidence of steroid reversibility
- Preoperative course of oral steroids, if evidence of steroid reversibility
- Preoperative course of antibiotics, if evidence of infection
- Consider pulmonary rehabilitation
- Consider chest physiotherapy with deep breathing exercises
- Referral for CPAP, if OSA present
- Optimize nutrition
- Lose weight
- Advise to stop smoking—ideally 8 weeks prior to surgery; reduces post-operative complication rate.

Risk factors for perioperative complications

- Thoracic or upper abdominal surgery
- Anaesthetic length >3.5h
- Smoker
- Chronic lung disease
- Raised $PaCO_2$
- Current respiratory symptoms
- Poor performance status
- Concurrent cardiac disease
- Obesity
- Older age.

Chapter 12

Pulmonary disease in the immunocompromised (non-HIV)

Clinical assessment

Pulmonary disease is a significant cause of morbidity and mortality in the immunocompromised, and its diagnosis and management are challenging. In the UK, this is encountered most commonly in the setting of immuno-compromise 2° to cytotoxic chemotherapy, haematological malignancy, immunosuppression post-transplant (particularly renal and haematopoietic stem cell transplant (HSCT, including bone marrow, foetal cord blood, and growth factor-stimulated peripheral blood transplantation)), prolonged corticosteroid use, and AIDS (see ➜ p. 83).

Most pulmonary diseases present in a similar manner in the setting of immunocompromise, with fever, dyspnoea, dry cough, chest pain, and often hypoxia. This non-specific clinical presentation, combined with the large number of possible causes, makes reaching a precise diagnosis difficult; the diagnosis remains unclear in up to 10% of cases, even at autopsy. There is limited evidence to demonstrate that obtaining a definitive diagnosis leads to an overall improvement in mortality, although, in subgroups such as patients with respiratory infection, early identification and treatment of pathogens have been shown to improve outcome.

Causes of pulmonary infiltrates in the non-HIV-infected immunocompromised are presented on ➜ pp. 78–9, and treatment on ➜ p. 82. Specific conditions are described separately (e.g. invasive aspergillosis, see ➜ pp. 466–7; PCP, see ➜ pp. 472–3).

Key steps in the management of these patients are as follows.

Clinical assessment In the history, the underlying cause of immuno-compromise and the timing and location of respiratory disease onset may provide clues to the diagnosis. The rate of disease onset may also suggest possible causes:

• *Acute onset* (<24h) Bacterial pneumonia, viral pneumonitis (e.g. CMV), pulmonary oedema or haemorrhage, PE, ARDS
• *Subacute onset* (days) Fungi (e.g. *Pneumocystis*, *Aspergillus*), bacteria (e.g. *Nocardia*, *Legionella*), viral (e.g. CMV), drug-induced pneumonitis
• *Chronic onset* (weeks) Malignancy, mycobacteria, fungi.

Chest *examination* may suggest the extent of pulmonary involvement, although this can be misleading and there are often no abnormal signs (e.g. in PCP, or bacterial pneumonia in the setting of neutropenia). Assess fluid status; pulmonary oedema is common following transplantation. Extrapulmonary involvement may be helpful in suggesting a pathogen, e.g. cutaneous lesions (herpes simplex and varicella-zoster; necrotic lesions from *Pseudomonas* and other Gram-negative bacteria, mycobacteria, and fungi; subcutaneous abscesses in *Staphylococcus aureus* and *Nocardia*), CNS involvement (*Pseudomonas*, *Aspergillus*, *Cryptococcus*, *Nocardia*, mycobacteria, *Streptococcus pneumoniae*, *Haemophilus influenzae*, varicella-zoster).

Initial investigations

- *CXR* appearance is very variable; may be normal or show consolidation, nodular infiltrate, or diffuse shadowing. CXR is of limited diagnostic value, as appearances are non-specific and atypical presentations are common; the 'first-choice' diagnosis based on CXR is correct in only a third of cases. CXR may, however, be helpful in monitoring disease progression and response to treatment
- *Blood and pleural fluid* (if available) sampling for microscopy andculture. Consider viral serology (e.g. CMV following transplantation), urinary *Legionella* antigen
- *Sputum examination* is often of little diagnostic value in immunocompromised patients, with the possible exceptions of invasive aspergillosis and TB. Send sputum for acid-fast stain and mycobacterial culture, fungal stain, and culture. Induced sputum has a low yield for PCP in non-HIV patients
- *The degree of hypoxia* is often not appreciated; measure O_2 saturations, and consider ABGs. Severe hypoxia tends to be more commonly associated with infection due to bacteria, viruses, or *Pneumocystis* than with mycobacteria or fungi.

Is immediate antibiotic treatment required? Immediate empirical treatment with broad-spectrum antibiotics prior to further investigation should be considered, depending on the nature of immunological defect and local hospital policy. In general, neutropenic patients with fever are at significant risk of developing overwhelming sepsis and should receive prompt antibiotic cover, irrespective of the CXR appearance and presence or absence of respiratory symptoms/signs. More invasive diagnostic procedures can then be reserved for patients who deteriorate or fail to improve within a period of observation (e.g. 2–3 days). In non-neutropenic patients, depending on the clinical circumstances, it is often possible to withhold treatment until definitive investigations have taken place.

Further investigations

More invasive diagnostic techniques are usually required for a definitive diagnosis.

CT chest
- Specific indications not yet defined. May not be needed in typical cases of bacterial pneumonia or PCP
- Useful in identifying the location and extent of pulmonary disease, and aiding invasive sampling procedures
- Often detects pulmonary disease in the presence of a normal CXR—consider if respiratory symptoms or unexplained fever, but normal CXR
- May be diagnostic, e.g. PE (CTPA), lymphangitis carcinomatosis, invasive aspergillosis ('halo' and 'air crescent' signs).

Bronchoscopy with BAL
- First-line investigation; consider early in management. Diagnostic inabout 60% of patients overall; up to 70% of patients with infection. Results in change to treatment in ~50% of cases overall. Complications are rare
- Useful in the diagnosis of bacterial pneumonia, PCP (sensitivity 80–90%), CMV (sensitivity 85–90%), aspergillosis (sensitivity 50%), TB, malignant disease, diffuse alveolar haemorrhage, and alveolar proteinosis
- BAL fluid analysis: routine microscopy and culture for bacteria; additional stains and culture for fungi, mycobacteria, *Nocardia*; silver or immunofluorescence stain for *Pneumocystis*; cytology, including flow cytometry, for malignant cells; viral serology; haemosiderin-laden macrophages if alveolar haemorrhage suspected
- Consider additional tests on BAL fluid such as *Cryptococcus* antigen detection or CMV PCR. *Aspergillus* antigen detection or PCR and *Toxoplasma gondii* PCR are less well validated
- TBB has a slightly higher sensitivity than BAL for the diagnosis of infection but carries a risk of bleeding and pneumothorax, which can be serious complications in this patient group; it is not usually performed at initial bronchoscopy although may be considered, e.g. if lymphangitis is suspected.

Lung biopsy Consider as a second-line investigation if BAL is non-diagnostic. Options include:
- *Repeat bronchoscopy with transbronchial lung biopsy* is useful in the diagnosis of malignancy, mycobacteria, fungi, OP, and drug-induced lung disease
- *VATS or open lung biopsy* has a greater diagnostic yield than TBB, although it is unclear if this can be directly translated into an improved survival. Results in change to treatment in <50% of patients, and complications may be serious
- *Percutaneous image-guided fine-needle aspiration (FNA) or biopsy* for investigation of peripheral nodules.

Causes

Causes of pulmonary disease in the immunocompromised can be broadly divided into infectious and non-infectious; multiple disease processes are common. The nature of immunosuppression may provide clues to the cause(s) of pulmonary disease—solid organ (kidney and liver) transplants are further discussed on ➜ p. 80, lung transplantation on ➜ p. 319, HSCT on ➜ pp. 80–1, and HIV on ➜ p. 83.

Infectious causes (*>75% of cases*) Infection is the commonest cause of respiratory disease in the immunocompromised. The nature of immunological defect may provide clues to the likely infectious agent:

- *Neutropenia or impaired neutrophil function (e.g. 2° to leukaemia or cytotoxic treatment)* Bacteria (*P. aeruginosa, S. aureus, S. pneumoniae, E. coli, Klebsiella, H. influenzae, Nocardia*), fungi (*Aspergillus, Candida,* mucormycosis)
- *Impaired T-lymphocyte function (e.g. 2° to transplantation, cytotoxic treatment, high-dose steroids, lymphoma, AIDS)* Fungi (PCP, *Cryptococcus neoformans, Candida,* endemic mycoses), viruses (CMV, herpes simplex, varicella-zoster), bacteria (mycobacteria, *Listeria, Legionella, Nocardia*), parasites (*Toxoplasma gondii*)
- *Hypogammaglobulinaemia or impaired B-lymphocyte function (e.g. 2° to myeloma, acute and chronic lymphocytic leukaemia, lymphoma)* Encapsulated bacteria (*S. pneumoniae, H. influenzae*).

It should be noted, however, that considerable overlap exists between immune deficiencies, and the pattern of infection will be further modified by prophylactic treatment, e.g. CMV and PCP prophylaxis.

Non-infectious causes (*<25% of cases*) Often present with similar, if not identical, clinical and radiological features to infection, and signs, such as fever, do not reliably differentiate between them. Causes include:

- *Pulmonary oedema Particularly following renal transplant or HSCT*
- *ARDS,* e.g. 2° to sepsis, drugs (e.g. cytarabine, gemcitabine, OKT3 antilymphocyte antibodies, interleukin-2), massive blood trans-fusion, transfusion-related acute lung injury, aspiration, 'engraftment syndrome' (coinciding with neutrophil engraftment) following HSCT
- *Drug-induced disease* Causes include all-trans retinoic acid (ATRA), antithymocyte globulin, azathioprine, bleomycin, busulfan, carmustine, chlorambucil, cyclophosphamide, cytosine arabinoside, hydroxycarbamide, liposomal amphotericin B, melphalan, mitomycin, methotrexate, sirolimus
- *Respiratory involvement from the underlying disease,* e.g. lymphoma, leukaemic infiltration, lymphangitis carcinomatosis, connective tissue disease, leucostasis with very high leucocyte counts in leukaemia
- *PE* Often complicated by 2° infection; clinical/radiological features may be confused with invasive aspergillosis; may be more common after kidney transplant
- *Radiation-induced pulmonary disease* Pneumonitis (dyspnoea; clear margins on CT; typically follows lung radiotherapy; may be delayed and triggered by subsequent chemotherapy treatment, so-called 'radiation

recall pneumonitis') or OP (cough; extends beyond radiation field on CT; typically follows breast radiotherapy).

- *Diffuse alveolar haemorrhage* is not an uncommon complication of leukaemia and allogeneic or autologous HSCT; similar clinical presentation to that of pneumonia; haemoptysis is rare; multilobar CXR/CT infiltrates; proposed diagnostic criteria include exclusion of infection, progressively bloodier returns from BAL of three different subsegmental bronchi (although limited sensitivity and specificity), and ≥20% of alveolar macrophages haemosiderin-filled (although may require several days to appear); reported mortality ranges 30–100%
- *'Idiopathic pneumonia syndrome'* following allogeneic or autologous HSCT; breathlessness with hypoxia and multilobar CXR/CT infiltrates; infection excluded with BAL and ideally a second later investigation (e.g. repeat BAL or lung biopsy); diffuse alveolar damage or interstitial pneumonitis on biopsy; mortality >70%
- *Engraftment syndrome* comprises fever, ARDS, and erythematous rash during marrow recovery post-HSCT
- *Bronchiolitis obliterans syndrome (BOS)* following allogeneic HSCT (from non-identical sibling or unrelated individual; occurs only extremely rarely following autologous procedure); typically associated with other forms of chronic graft-versus-host disease (GVHD), e.g. cutaneous; gradual onset of dry cough, dyspnoea; CXR often normal; fixed obstructive spirometry with FEV_1 <75% predicted, FEV_1/FVC ratio <0.7, and RV >120% predicted; air trapping and bronchial dilatation on HRCT (request expiratory images); superimposed airways infection is common
- *Post-transplant lymphoproliferative disease* may complicate allogeneic HSCT or solid organ transplant, most commonly lung (see ➲ p. 319)
- *Pulmonary alveolar proteinosis* (see ➲ pp. 632–3)
- *Pulmonary veno-occlusive disease*
- *Pulmonary metastatic calcification* may complicate chronic renal failure and rarely progress after transplantation; usually asymptomatic, rarely causes restrictive ventilatory defect; CXR shows single or multiple nodules or patches of consolidation, may not appear calcified; CT typically diagnostic, although biopsy occasionally needed
- *Right hemidiaphragm dysfunction* is common after liver transplant and usually not relevant clinically.

Multiple disease processes About 30% of patients have two or more disease processes accounting for their respiratory involvement. 2° infection with a different infectious agent (commonly *Aspergillus* or Gram-negative bacteria such as *P. aeruginosa*) may complicate either a 1° respiratory infection or a non-infectious process such as PE. 2° infection is associated with a poor prognosis; consider particularly in patients who deteriorate after an initial response to treatment and in patients who are neutropenic.

Pleural effusion Causes in non-HIV immunocompromised patients include cardiac failure and fluid overload, PE, drug-related, parapneumonic (bacterial, including *Nocardia*; fungal, e.g. PCP), or related to underlying disease (e.g. leukaemic infiltrates, lymphoma, chylothorax, myeloma). Pleural effusions are common after liver transplant: usually right-sided or bilateral transudates and resolve by third week; may require drainage if symptomatic.

Differential diagnosis of pulmonary complications based on time course after transplantation

Solid organ transplantation

First month post-transplant (recent surgery ± ICU)
- Nosocomial bacterial infection (Gram-negative, *S. aureus*—including MRSA, *Legionella*)
- ARDS
- Pulmonary oedema
- Drug-induced
- PE
- Pleural effusion (especially after liver transplant)
- Right hemidiaphragm dysfunction (after liver transplant).

Months 1–6 (maximal immunosuppression)
- Opportunistic infection (CMV, PCP, *Nocardia*, *Aspergillus*, *Scedosporium apiospermum*)
- Drug-induced
- Post-transplant lymphoproliferative disease.

Months >6 (reduction in immunosuppression, unless rejection)
- Common community-acquired pathogens (*H. influenzae*, *S. pneumoniae*, *Legionella*, TB, non-tuberculous mycobacteria (NTM), PCP, endemic mycoses, e.g. *Histoplasma*, viruses, e.g. influenza, parainfluenza, adenovirus, RSV)
- Opportunistic infection (see under Months 1–6)
- Post-transplant lymphoproliferative disease
- Pulmonary metastatic calcification.

HSCT

First month post-transplant (prolonged neutropenia pre-engraftment)
- Infection (bacteria, e.g. *P. aeruginosa*, *E. coli*, *Klebsiella pneumoniae*, *H. influenzae*, *S. aureus*, *Legionella* species; fungi, e.g. *Aspergillus*; viruses, e.g. herpes simplex, adenovirus)
- Pulmonary oedema
- ARDS
- Transfusion-related acute lung injury
- Drug-induced
- Diffuse alveolar haemorrhage
- Idiopathic pneumonia syndrome.

Months 1–3 (impaired cellular immunity post-engraftment, related in part to immunosuppressive drugs and GVHD)
- Opportunistic infection (Gram-negative bacteria, *Nocardia*, CMV, herpes simplex, PCP)
- Drug-induced
- Diffuse alveolar haemorrhage

- Idiopathic pneumonia syndrome
- Engraftment syndrome
- Post-transplant lymphoproliferative disease
- Pulmonary veno-occlusive disease.

Months >3 (poor lymphocyte function, particularly following allogeneic HSCT)
- Infection (Gram-positive bacteria, CMV, herpes, varicella-zoster, TB, NTM, PCP, *Aspergillus*, endemic mycoses, e.g. *Histoplasma*)
- BOS (pulmonary GVHD; may occur up to 5y post-allogeneic HSCT, typically within 2y)
- Post-transplant lymphoproliferative disease
- Pulmonary veno-occlusive disease.

Treatment

Antimicrobials Depending on the clinical circumstances, antimicrobials may need to be started prior to definitive investigations (see ➲ p. 75), although blood cultures should always precede antibiotic treatment. Choice of antimicrobial depends on the underlying condition and local hospital policy.

* In general, most neutropenic patients are treated with broad-spectrum antibiotics providing both Gram-positive and Gram-negative cover, e.g. piperacillin (4.5g IV qds); antifungals are considered if slow response to treatment or subsequent deterioration. Consider vancomycin if MRSA is a possibility
* Treatment for CMV and PCP is associated with significant side effects and ideally should be based on a definitive diagnosis. In unwell patients who are strongly suspected to have PCP, treatment (see ➲ pp. 474–5) can be started immediately, as BAL *Pneumocystis jirovecii* stains remain positive for up to 2 weeks
* Antituberculous treatment should only rarely be administered in the absence of a microbiological diagnosis.

Diuretics Fluid overload and pulmonary oedema are common following renal transplantation and HSCT, and typical clinical and radiological signs may be disguised; consider a trial of diuretics.

Steroids Despite a lack of RCTs, prednisolone (1mg/kg/day PO or methylprednisolone 1g IV daily for 3 days) is often considered in the treatment of drug- or radiation-induced lung disease, engraftment syndrome, diffuse alveolar haemorrhage, and idiopathic pneumonia syndrome following HSCT. Ideally, exclude underlying infection prior to starting steroids. Prednisolone (40–80mg daily PO) is recommended for the treatment of PCP in patients with respiratory failure. BOS, following allogeneic HSCT, is usually treated with increased immunosuppression (after exclusion/treatment of airways infection), typically oral prednisolone 1mg/kg/day, and there may also be roles for inhaled steroids, azithromycin, and anti-reflux therapy in this condition.

Supportive treatment Administer O_2 to maintain saturations 94–98%. Respiratory failure in immunocompromised patients is associated with a poor outcome; mortality following intubation and mechanical ventilation ranges 60–100%. Early intermittent use of NIV in immunocompromised patients with pulmonary infiltrates and hypoxia has been shown to reduce the need for intubation and improve mortality. Before NIV is commenced, a decision regarding suitability for intubation and mechanical ventilation should be made.

Surgery Surgical wedge resection or lobectomy may be considered in the treatment of invasive aspergillosis, either acutely for lesions adjacent to pulmonary vessels that are judged to have a significant risk of massive haemoptysis, or at a later date for residual lesions at risk of reactivation with further chemotherapy.

Chapter 13

Pulmonary disease in the immunocompromised (HIV)

Clinical assessment

Widespread use of antiretroviral therapy (ART) and antimicrobial prophy-laxis in HIV has resulted in a longer survival, as well as changes in the nature of respiratory involvement. Respiratory disease remains common in the setting of HIV, and patients should be managed in consultation with an HIV specialist.

Major causes of respiratory disease in the HIV-infected patient are listed on ➲ p. 86. Specific conditions are described separately (e.g. PCP, see ➲ pp. 472–3; TB, see ➲ p. 485). Key management steps are as follows:

Clinical assessment

- As with other causes of immunocompromise, clinical features of respiratory disease in HIV-infected patients are non-specific: breathlessness, cough, fever, weight loss, and fatigue are common, although chest symptoms are not always present
- Ask about treatment and compliance with ART and PCP prophylaxis
- Source of HIV infection may be relevant: Kaposi's sarcoma occurs particularly in homosexual men and in African men and women; TB and bacterial pneumonia are more common in IV drug users (IVDUs)
- Travel history may be useful: infection with 'endemic mycoses' (histoplasmosis, blastomycosis, coccidioidomycosis) is well recognized in the USA but rare in the UK
- Careful examination may provide clues to the respiratory condition. Pulmonary Kaposi's sarcoma is unusual in the absence of disease elsewhere; palatal Kaposi's sarcoma, in particular, is predictive of pulmonary involvement. Extrapulmonary mycobacterial disease is common and may involve the liver, lymph nodes, pericardium, and meninges.

Investigations

CXR

- CXR changes are relatively non-specific. Appearances of bacterial pneumonia may be atypical, e.g. diffuse bilateral infiltrates mimicking PCP, and TB may present with focal or diffuse CXR consolidation
- PCP classically appears as bilateral perihilar infiltrates that progress to alveolar shadowing; more specific patterns include small nodular infiltrates or focal consolidation; CXR is normal in 10% of cases. Pneumothorax is suggestive of PCP although may also occur with TB
- Pleural effusion or hilar/mediastinal lymphadenopathy are unusual in PCP and are more suggestive of mycobacterial infection or Kaposi's sarcoma
- Common causes of CXR cavitation are PCP, TB (with high CD4 count), *P. aeruginosa*, fungi, *R. equi*, *Nocardia*. Cavitation is relatively unusual in TB occurring late in the course of HIV
- Common causes of pleural effusion in HIV infection are Kaposi's sarcoma, parapneumonic effusion, TB, cardiac failure, and lymphoma (including 1° effusion lymphoma).

CD4 count may be useful in narrowing the differential diagnosis: bacterial infection, including TB, occurs at any stage of disease, although infection is more severe at lower CD4 counts; PCP and atypical presentations of TB occur most commonly at CD4 $<200 \times 10^6/L$; NTM, Kaposi's sarcoma, *P. aeruginosa* pneumonia, and lymphoma occur late in the disease (CD4 $<50 \times 10^6/L$). A recent increase in CD4 count (following the introduction of ART) may suggest an immune reconstitution inflammatory syndrome (IRIS, see Box 13.1).

Blood cultures should be taken prior to antimicrobial treatment. Bacteraemia is relatively common with bacterial pneumonia in HIV, particularly with *S. pneumoniae* infection. Bacteraemic TB may occur in advanced disease.

Other blood tests Raised inflammatory markers are a non-specific finding.

Sputum Induced sputum may assist the diagnosis of PCP and mycobacterial disease. Induced sputum has a sensitivity of about 60% for the diagnosis of PCP. TB is more likely to be smear-negative in the setting of HIV, as cavitation in these patients is less common. Induced sputum should ideally be obtained in a negative-pressure room.

Other cultures Consider sampling urine, stool, lymph node, or bone marrow in suspected mycobacterial disease, as extrapulmonary disease is common.

CT chest is useful in looking for evidence of respiratory disease in patients with symptoms, but a normal CXR, and may be helpful in directing invasive diagnostic procedures. CT is also of benefit in the diagnosis and staging of Kaposi's sarcoma and lymphoma.

Box 13.1 IRIS

IRIS (immune restoration disease or paradoxical reaction) is a clinical syndrome resulting from restored immunity to infectious or non-infectious antigens, following the introduction of ART. The *mechanism* is uncertain but probably includes partial recovery of the immune system or an exuberant host-antigen response with host genetic susceptibility. It is more likely in the context of current infection due to mycobacteria, herpes, varicella, and CMV. The *clinical features* are variable and diverse and depend on the underlying infectious or non-infectious agent. A clinically silent infection may be 'unmasked', as the CD4 count rises, and may be associated with an excessive inflammatory response. The commonest clinical features are fever, lymphadenopathy, and worsening respiratory symptoms. New pulmonary infiltrates and pleural effusions are common. TB-IRIS tends to develop within 2 months of the start of ART, and CNS TB-IRIS is reported up to 10 months after ART initiation. *Treatment* with corticosteroids appears to be effective, although no RCT data exist. Various regimes are suggested, including methylprednisolone 40mg bd and prednisolone 20–70mg od for up to 7 weeks. Infectious agents must also be treated, and, in the very unwell, this may mean empirical treatment for PCP and TB and high-dose steroids, whilst awaiting confirmatory microbiology.

Causes of respiratory disease in HIV infection

(commoner causes in bold)

Infectious

Bacteria
- *Streptococcus pneumoniae*
- *Haemophilus influenzae*
- *Staphylococcus aureus*
- **Gram-negative bacteria**, especially *Pseudomonas aeruginosa*
- *Nocardia asteroides*
- *Rhodococcus equi.*

Mycobacteria
- *Mycobacterium tuberculosis*
- *Mycobacterium avium-intracellulare*
- *Mycobacterium kansasii.*

Viruses
- Influenza
- Parainfluenza
- RSV
- Herpes simplex
- Adenovirus
- CMV.

Fungi
- *Pneumocystis jirovecii* (PCP)
- *Aspergillus* spp.
- *Cryptococcus neoformans*
- Endemic mycoses.

Parasites
- *Strongyloides stercoralis* (hyperinfection syndrome).

Non-infectious
- Malignancy
  - **Kaposi's sarcoma**
  - **Lung cancer**
  - Non-Hodgkin's lymphoma
- IRIS
- Drug-induced lung disease
- Cardiogenic pulmonary oedema (e.g. 2° to cardiomyopathy)
- HIV-associated PAH
- Interstitial pneumonitis
  - Non-specific interstitial pneumonitis
  - Lymphocytic interstitial pneumonitis.

Further investigations and treatment

Bronchoscopy and BAL

- Bronchoscopy and BAL are safe and frequently diagnostic in this patient group and should be considered early in management, particularly in the presence of a diffuse CXR abnormality or following non-diagnostic induced sputum analysis. BAL should also be considered in patients with a localized CXR abnormality that has not responded to a trial of broad-spectrum antibiotics
- BAL fluid analysis: routine microscopy and culture for bacteria; additional stains and culture for fungi, mycobacteria, *Nocardia*; silver or immunofluorescence stain for *Pneumocystis*; cytology, including flow cytometry for malignant cells; respiratory viral serology. Consider additional tests such as *Cryptococcus* antigen detection or CMV PCR
- Both *Nocardia* and *Rhodococcus equi* stain weakly acid-fast and so may be confused with mycobacteria
- Kaposi's sarcoma appears as 'raised bruises' in the trachea or bronchi on bronchoscopy; routine biopsy is not usually recommended, as diagnostic yield is low and significant haemorrhage may occur
- Lung cancer is more common in the setting of HIV, typically affecting relatively young patients with mild to moderate immunocompromise.

Lung biopsy If bronchoscopy and BAL are non-diagnostic, consider repeat bronchoscopy with TBB or surgical lung biopsy. TBB has a greater sensitivity than BAL, but potentially serious complications (such as pneumothorax or haemorrhage) are significantly more common.

Treatment

- Consider broad-spectrum antibiotics and empirical treatment for PCP (high-dose co-trimoxazole, and steroids if the patient is in respiratory failure; see ➔ pp. 474–5). BAL *Pneumocystis* stains remain positive for up to 2 weeks despite treatment, and so empirical treatment for PCP should not be delayed, pending bronchoscopic confirmation, if the patient is unwell and this diagnosis is suspected
- In the absence of another identifiable cause, consider empirical treatment directed at TB, pending sputum and BAL culture results
- Further antimicrobial treatment can be directed at specific pathogens isolated from BAL or biopsy
- Although isolation of *Aspergillus* spp. from respiratory samples may reflect contamination or colonization, consider treatment with voriconazole or amphotericin B if isolated from BAL in setting of severe immunocompromise (CD4 <30 x 10^6/L)
- Supportive therapy with O_2; consider NIV. PCP is the commonest cause of respiratory failure requiring ICU admission in HIV-positive patients and was historically considered to carry a very high mortality rate, although recent studies have reported more favourable outcomes and ICU admission for invasive ventilation may be appropriate for selected patients.

Chapter 14

Sleep and ventilation

History

The problem Sleep apnoea and related problems are now a common reason for referral to many respiratory units. This is due to much better recognition of the syndromes and the increasing prevalence of obesity in the general population. Respiratory units with sleep services are seeing increasing numbers of patients, primarily for possible OSA, and, therefore, most patients tend to be sleepy, and referrals for insomnia are not usually encouraged.

Patients arrive at a respiratory sleep unit for several different reasons. They are commonly:
• Concerns that the patient may have sleep apnoea, with or without a full house of symptoms
• Concerns that an obese individual may have obesity hypoventilation
• Loud snoring, with the patient or spouse seeking advice about noise reduction
• Referrals from the ENT department who may be considering offering surgery for snoring and wish to exclude OSA first
• Excessive daytime sleepiness, diagnosis unclear, might just be OSA, might be narcolepsy, etc.
• Assessment pre-bariatric surgery, as prevalence of OSA very high
• Other nocturnal symptoms such as sleepwalking, panic arousals, etc.

Thus, in sleep outpatients, the issues revolve around making the correct diagnosis of the excessive daytime sleepiness or nocturnal symptoms (and referring on, if appropriate), offering simple advice for snoring, or putting the patient through the CPAP induction programme.

Some units perform a sleep study first, on the basis of an appropriate referral letter, as it is more efficient; others see the patient first and then book a sleep study if indicated (usually >95% are studied). For the purposes of this account, it is assumed that the patient is seen first.

History A clear history of the exact presenting complaint is obviously necessary, concentrating on the following points when OSA is suspected (a full discussion is available in the section on OSA; see ➲ p. 569).
• Sleepiness: how severe, what does it interfere with, over how long has it been coming on, and does it reduce QoL? The Epworth sleepiness scale (ESS) is useful as part of the assessment of this (see Fig. 14.1); scored out of 24: 0–9 is considered normal, and >9 excessively sleepy. It is only a guide and should be interpreted with the overall history
• Important to differentiate sleepiness (tendency to nod off, due to inadequate sleep) from tiredness (feelings of exhaustion due to many causes, often without a tendency to nod off). OSA usually causes sleepiness more than tiredness, although this is not always so clear-cut, especially in women
• Snoring and apnoeas. Best assessed from a witness: how loud, continuous, intermittent, and are there recognized 'stopping breathing' or choking episodes during sleep?
• Other OSA symptoms such as nocturia and restless sleep
• History of weight and neck size increases over the last 5–10y (recent weight gains common)

- History of nasal or other ENT surgery (previous palate surgery increases discomfort of CPAP)
- Previous medical history (certain risk factors such as mandibular surgery, hypothyroidism, acromegaly, Down's, Prader–Willi, etc.)
- Previous cardiovascular/cerebrovascular history (especially atrial fibrillation (AF)) and hypertension history (may influence decision to treat)
- Alcohol and smoking history (both worsen OSA, especially alcohol)
- Occupation (is it vigilance-critical?)
- Shift working (may exacerbate the sleepiness from OSA)
- Driving issues: such as sleepiness while driving and 'near misses' or actual sleep-related accidents (sensitive issue requiring careful handling)
- Does the patient drive for a living and what kind of vehicle or licence?

If OSA seems unlikely, then other causes of sleepiness need to be considered more carefully, concentrating on the commonest (see Box 14.1).

Box 14.1 Alternative diagnoses for excessive daytime sleepiness

- Depression, often missed
- Lifestyle issues—alcohol, late night working, shift work, caffeine abuse, family circumstances, etc.
- Drugs—some of the antihypertensives (e.g. β-blockers) and psychoactive drugs (e.g. antidepressants, sedatives, opiates, and anxiolytics) can provoke sleepiness
- Narcolepsy—e.g. associated with cataplexy (sudden loss of muscle tone in response to excitement or anticipation), sleep paralysis (frightening paralysis on wakening for a few seconds or minutes), and prolific vivid dreaming, often at sleep onset or during daytime naps
- Periodic limb movements during sleep (associated with restless legs during the day, especially in renal failure, low iron levels)
- Post-severe head injury or cranial irradiation (hypothalamic damage)
- Post-infectious (e.g. Epstein–Barr virus)
- Idiopathic (sometimes hereditary)
- Certain neurological disorders such as myotonic dystrophy, Parkinson's, and previous stroke
- Simply being at the sleepier end of the normal spectrum
- The symptom may really be tiredness such as in 'ME' or insomnia, when the ESS is usually low
- Blind insomnia/sleepiness—circadian problem when 24h cycle not linked with the real world through blue light exposure and melatonin production.

Examination and investigations

Examination of these patients is often relatively unhelpful.

In OSA, the main features to look for are:
- Neck circumference (best measure of the obesity contribution to the cause of OSA, >17in) and body mass index (BMI)
- Oropharynx, often crowded with boggy mucosa, enlarged tonsils (Mallampati score can be used; see ➲ p. 595)
- Teeth, crowding suggests retrognathia/micrognathia (and mandibular advancement devices require sound teeth)
- Nasal patency (how easy will CPAP be?).

Also (see Box14.2)
- Assessment of respiratory function, signs of cor pulmonale, FEV_1/VC ratio, and SaO_2 (associated COPD increases likelihood of being in type II ventilatory failure, so-called 'overlap syndrome')
- BP (may influence decision to treat OSA)
- Endocrinology: hypothyroidism, acromegaly, Cushing's, diabetes.

It may also be appropriate to look for:
- Evidence of a neuromuscular disorder including a previous stroke
- Evidence of heart failure (central sleep apnoea (CSA), or Cheyne–Stokes respiration, which can produce overnight oximetry tracings similar to those of OSA).

Box 14.2 Clinic tests to perform
- Blood gas estimation if respiratory failure suspected (these OSA patients will require more urgent treatment)
- Thyroid function (hypothyroidism not always clinically obvious) plus other hormones, if indicated
- Routine haematology and biochemistry (prevalence of type II diabetes will be high in this overweight population)
- Some would recommend a fuller cardiovascular risk assessment, including cholesterol, fasting triglycerides, glucose, and folate, since these patients are often in a high-risk group (untreated 10y cardiovascular event risk typically predicted to be about 35%).

Other scenarios If it is known already that the patient has OSA, then a joint decision between the doctor and the patient needs to be made as to whether to undergo a trial of treatment (usually CPAP). This will depend mainly on the symptom severity vs the perceived inconvenience of the treatment. Recent evidence suggests that even relatively asymptomatic patients with OSA, presenting to a sleep clinic, may benefit from a trial of CPAP, thus to quote, 'if in doubt, blow up the snout'. However, an abnormal sleep study is rarely a reason in its own right for CPAP. Weight loss works but is rarely achievable. Other causes must not be missed (e.g. hypothyroidism, tonsillar hypertrophy) simply because CPAP is available.

EPWORTH SLEEPINESS SCALE

Name:......................Hospital number.................. Date:....................

Your age (Y)...........Your sex (Male = M/Female = F)..................

- How likely are you to doze off or fall asleep in the situations described in the box below, in contrast to feeling just tired?
- This refers to your usual way of life in recent times.
- Even if you haven't done some of these things recently try to work out how they would have affected you.
- Use the following scale to choose the *most appropriate number* for each situation:-

0 = Would *never* doze   2 = *Moderate* chance of dozing
1 = *Slight* chance of dozing   3 = *High* chance of dozing

Situation	Chance of dozing
Sitting and reading	❏
Watching TV	❏
Sitting, inactive in a public place (e.g. a theatre or a meeting)	❏
As a passenger in a car for an hour without a break	❏
Lying down to rest in the afternoon when circumstances permit	❏
Sitting and talking to someone	❏
Sitting quietly after a lunch without alcohol	❏
In a car, while stopped for a few minutes in the traffic	❏
Thank you for your cooperation	Total score = ❏

Fig. 14.1 Epworth Sleepiness Scale questionnaire. Reproduced from Murray W. Johns - A New Method For Measuring Daytime Sleepiness: The Epworth Sleepiness Scale - Sleep 1991;**14**:540–5, with permission from Associated Professional Sleep Societies, LLC.

If the patient has come via ENT and is being considered for pharyngeal surgery, then the respiratory physician's role is to dissuade the patient from this route, as the objective success rate is poor and the hazards significant. The presence of significant OSA is a contraindication to surgery. All other approaches to snoring, such as the use of mandibular advancement devices, should be considered first and pharyngeal surgery regarded as the last resort of the totally desperate.

Chapter 15

Unexplained ventilatory failure

Causes

Definition Ventilatory failure is conventionally divided into type I (hypoxia only, PaO_2 <8kPa) and type II (hypoxia and hypercapnia, $PaCO_2$ >6kPa): they are conceptually quite different. Type I is an increased A–a O_2 gradient (implying increased V/Q mismatch), with adequately increased alveolar ventilation maintaining a normal $PaCO_2$. The causes are numerous, including most of respiratory medicine, and requires the usual 'history, examination, and investigations'.

A more difficult, less common clinical scenario is an unexplained rise in $PaCO_2$ (>6kPa, type II), with no obvious cause following a standard assessment. This may occur in the outpatient, ward, A&E, or ICU setting.

Pathophysiology A rise in $PaCO_2$ can be due to V/Q mismatch with inadequate compensatory hyperventilation, e.g. overwhelming asthma, when there will also be a large A–a gradient indicating this increased V/Q mismatch. However, it can also be due to inadequate ventilatory drive or primary ventilatory pump failure where the A–a gradient will usually be normal. The following list contains mainly the causes that might not have been suspected from the initial assessment but, for completeness, also includes some more obvious causes. The conditions with asterisks are the ones most commonly discovered when the cause is not immediately obvious.

Failure of drive

Brainstem abnormality
- Polio and post-polio syndrome* (exact mechanism unclear)
- Brainstem stroke (involvement of respiratory centres bilaterally)
- Arnold–Chiari malformation—herniation of cerebellum into foramen magnum, compressing the brainstem
- Syringobulbia—expansion of a fluid compartment in the middle of the spinal cord extending up into the medulla (can be associated with Arnold–Chiari malformation)
- Surgical damage during operations for Arnold–Chiari and syringobulbia
- Encephalitis
- Brainstem tumour
- Congenital hypoventilation syndrome—usually presents soon after birth, can be later; abnormalities of neural crest development due to increased number of 'alanine repeats' in one of the homeobox genes (*PHOX2B*).

Suppression
- Sedative drugs, including alcohol, opiates, etc.*
- Metabolic alkalosis (hypokalaemic alkalosis, diuretic-induced, prolonged vomiting).

Pump failure

Neurological (particularly if diaphragm involved)
- Myopathies
  - Acid maltase deficiency (Pompe's), diaphragm paralysis commonly occurs early on*
  - Duchenne muscular dystrophy

- Myotonic dystrophy
- Several other very rare primary or secondary myopathies, e.g. limb girdle, hypothyroid, drugs (hydroxychloroquine)
- Neuropathy
  - MND* can affect diaphragm early on
  - Bilateral diaphragm paralysis*, e.g. trauma, bilateral neuralgic amyotrophy (also known as 'brachial neuritis', inflammatory damage to nerves of lower brachial plexus—cause unknown)
  - Guillain–Barré
  - Spinal muscular atrophy, autosomal recessive, spinal cord motor neurones
  - High cord transection
- Neuromuscular junction abnormalities
  - Myasthenia gravis*
  - Lambert–Eaton myasthenic syndrome (LEMS)
- Anti-acetylcholine esterase poisoning (usually from organophosphate insecticides)
- Mixed
  - Post-ITU ('critical care neuropathy'), post-muscle relaxants*.

Chest wall
- Obesity, especially abdominal (obesity hypoventilation syndrome)*
- Raised abdominal pressure, 'abdominal compartment (or hypertension) syndrome', e.g. ascites, or gut and mesentery oedema
- Scoliosis*
- Post-thoracoplasty (usually 'three stage', many ribs caved in, starting from the top down—done for TB prior to effective chemotherapy)
- Flail chest
- Pneumothorax/large pleural effusion
- Severe ankylosing spondilitis.

Airways obstruction/mixed
- Unrecognized COPD/severe asthma*
- OSA and additional COPD/obesity/muscle weakness*, sometimes called 'overlap syndrome'.

The ventilatory loading effects of obesity, COPD, and OSA commonly summate to produce ventilatory failure when each on their own would not be regarded as of sufficient severity. Estimating the contribution each is making to an individual's ventilatory failure can influence therapy and expectations of success, e.g. if OSA dominant (>30, >4% SaO_2 dips/h), the ventilatory failure is likely to respond to CPAP; dominant COPD (FEV1 <25% predicted) will need maximal lower airways dilator therapy (thresholds only for general guidance), but the likely poor response of the lower airways obstruction will mean that even limited additional weight reduction and/or treatment of milder OSA may be useful in this situation.

*The conditions most commonly discovered when the cause is not immediately obvious.

Clinical presentation

Slow onset

In several of the conditions listed previously, e.g. acid maltase deficiency, MND, and scoliosis, the onset of ventilatory failure can be insidious and include:

- General fatigue and/or hypersomnolence
- Headaches on awakening
- Morning confusion
- Morning cyanosis
- Ankle oedema (fluid retention, cor pulmonale, from the hypoxia)
- Orthopnoea, particularly if diaphragmatic weakness
- Dyspnoea standing in the swimming pool (this usually indicates diaphragm paralysis, as the pressure of water, even at 1m depth, pushes the unopposed diaphragm further up into the chest)
- Swallowing difficulties (often MND) or other evidence of a more generalized proximal neuromuscular problem.

Apparent rapid onset

Sometimes, the significance of these symptoms is missed for a while, and a relatively trivial respiratory tract infection, a general anaesthetic, or the prescription of a ventilatory depressant tips the balance and the patient goes into severe ventilatory failure, with impaired conscious level or coma. These individuals will end up ventilated on ICU and may be difficult to wean, or present again with ventilatory failure a few weeks after discharge.

Further information

Chuen-Im P et al. Heterozygous 24-polyalanine repeats in the PHOX2B gene with different manifestations across three generations. *Pediatr Pulmonol* 2014;**49**:E13–6.

Hedestierna G, Larsson A. Influence of abdominal pressure on respiratory and abdominal organ function. *Curr Opin Crit Care* 2012;**18**:80–5.

Resta O et al. Sleep-related breathing disorders, loud snoring and excessive daytime sleepiness in obese subjects. *Int J Obes Relat Metab Disord* 2001;**25**:669–75.

Clinical assessment and management

History, examination, and investigations

History Carefully taken history, e.g. symptoms of subtle weakness prior to presentation, episode of shoulder pain (neuralgic amyotrophy), past history of polio, orthopnoea (diaphragm weakness), drug history. Often this is not available, as the patient may present unconscious.

Examination Thorough examination, particularly neurological, e.g. fasciculation, diaphragm weakness (when supine, inward drawing of abdomen on inspiration or sniffing—masked if on positive pressure ventilation), myotonia, as well as rarer signs seen in some of the conditions listed previously.

Blood gases taken breathing air (following >20min off extra O_2)
- Degree of CO_2 retention
- Presence of a base excess indicating chronicity of CO_2 retention
- Calculate A–a gradient to detect any V/Q mismatch (see ➔ p. 825)
- In pure hypoventilation, there should be no significant A–a gradient (<2kPa), unless there is 2° basal atelectasis from poor lung expansion and/or obesity.

PFTs
(See ➔ p. 867.)
- Presence of unexpected severe airways obstruction
- Reduced VC (neurological or chest wall)
- Further fall of VC on lying down (>20% change, definitely abnormal)— indicative of diaphragm paralysis. When supine, VC is <25% predicted, very likely to be the main cause of the raised $PaCO_2$
- Mouth pressures, sniff pressures, or transdiaphragmatic pressures; not much more helpful than the % fall in VC on lying down.

Specific tests—for some of the conditions listed previously such as:
- EMG studies—MND, myotonia
- MRI (gadolinium-enhanced)—Arnold–Chiari, brainstem lesion, syrinx
- CPK—some myopathies
- Sleep study—e.g. (i) REM hypoxia (early marker of ventilatory failure, when supine VC has usually dropped below 60% predicted normal), (ii) continuous nocturnal hypoventilation (when supine VC has dropped below 40% predicted), and (iii) additional OSA
- Blood film for abnormal lymphocyte cytoplasmic vacuolation (mainly acid maltase deficiency)
- Muscle biopsy—acid maltase deficiency (glycogen-containing vacuoles and low enzyme levels).

Management of the underlying condition, if possible, is paramount. Weak expiratory muscles and weak laryngeal adduction prevent effective coughing, with an increased incidence of serious chest infections. Clearing retained secretions can be a major problem. Physiotherapists can help teach patients and their carers sputum clearance techniques. Increasing the lung volume, prior to coughing, with positive pressure devices (e.g. using the patient's own ventilator, the Bird device, or simple bag and face mask) and 'breath stacking' techniques generate a higher expiratory flow with improved sputum clearance. Mechanical insufflator/exsufflator devices are available that both increase inspiratory volume and speed expiratory flows. Their acute and prophylactic role is still being evaluated.

Lying down and sleeping with the *whole bed tipped head up* by about 15–20° greatly improves ventilation in the presence of bilateral diaphragm paralysis or major abdominal obesity. Just elevating the top half of the bed and bending the patient in the middle, leaving the abdomen and legs horizontal, does not work. The abdominal contents have to descend into the pelvis to effectively 'offload' the diaphragm. This posture will also improve the ability to wean from assisted ventilation.

When the underlying condition is irreversible, the decision will need to be taken as to whether long-term NIV is appropriate (see ➔ pp. 700–1).

Part 2

Clinical conditions

Acute respiratory distress syndrome

Pathophysiology and diagnosis

Definition and epidemiology ARDS (previously 'shock lung') is not a single entity but represents the severe end of a spectrum of acute lung injury due to many different insults. Manifests as acute and persistent lung inflammation with increased vascular permeability. Most commonly seen on the ITU where about 10–20% of such patients will have ARDS depending on the definition. The 2012 'Berlin Definition' of ARDS requires:

- Respiratory symptoms within 1 week of known clinical insult
- Bilateral opacities consistent with pulmonary oedema on CXR or CT
- Respiratory failure must not be fully explained by cardiac failure or fluid overload. Echo may be required to exclude hydrostatic pulmonary oedema
- Oxygenation impairment, defined by PaO_2/FiO_2 ratio at least <300mmHg (40kPa) despite positive end-expiratory pressure (PEEP) ≥5cmH$_2$O:
  - Mild ARDS—PaO_2/FiO_2 >200mmHg (27kPa)
  - Moderate ARDS—PaO_2/FiO_2 >100mmHg (13kPa)
  - Severe ARDS—PaO_2/FiO_2 ≤100mmHg (13kPa).

Other ARDS grading scores exist, e.g. Murray lung injury score (based on plain CXR findings, oxygenation, PEEP level, and respiratory system compliance; see ➔ p. 109).

Pathophysiology Inflammatory damage to the alveoli, either by locally produced pro-inflammatory mediators or remotely produced and arriving via the pulmonary artery. Changes in pulmonary capillary permeability allow fluid and protein leakage into the alveolar spaces with pulmonary infiltrates. The alveolar surfactant is diluted with loss of its stabilizing effect, resulting in diffuse alveolar collapse and stiff lungs. This leads to:

- Gross impairment of V/Q matching with shunting, causing arterial hypoxia and very large A–a gradients. There are usually enough remaining functioning alveoli such that hyperventilation maintains CO_2 clearance; thus, hypercapnia is infrequently a problem
- PHT will develop 2° to the hypoxia, but this may be helpful (aids V/Q matching), rather than deleterious
- Reduced compliance (stiff lungs) due to loss of functioning alveoli (alveolar collapse, filled with fluid and protein) and hyperinflation of remaining alveoli to their limits of distension.

There are many causes of pro-inflammatory mediator release sufficient to cause ARDS, and there may be more than one present. Common causes, in order of prevalence:

- Sepsis/pneumonia (2° risk factors for developing ARDS, when septic, alcoholism, and cigarette smoking)
- Gastric aspiration (even if on a PPI, indicating that a low pH is not the only damaging component)
- Trauma/burns (via sepsis, lung trauma, smoke inhalation, fat emboli, and possibly direct effects of large amounts of necrotic tissue).

Less common causes
- Acute pancreatitis
- Transfusion-related acute lung injury (TRALI), caused by any blood product (possibly due to HLA/white blood cell antibodies, commoner with older blood products, >6U); usually occurs within a few hours of transfusion. No specific therapy or evidence of steroid response
- Transplanted lung—worse if the lung poorly preserved
- Post-bone marrow transplant as bone marrow recovers
- Drug overdose, e.g. tricyclic antidepressants, opiates, cocaine, aspirin
- Near drowning
- Following upper airway obstruction; mechanism unclear.

The course of ARDS is fairly characteristic. *Phase 1* is the early period of diffuse alveolar damage and hypoxaemia with pulmonary infiltration. *Phase 2* develops after a week or so as the pulmonary infiltrates resolve and, on histology, seems to be associated with an increase in type II pneumocytes (surfactant producers), myofibroblasts, and early collagen formation. *Phase 3* occurs in some. This is a fibrotic stage that leaves the lung with cysts, deranged micro-architecture, and much fibrosis on histology.

Clinical features ARDS should be considered in any patient with a predisposing risk factor who develops severe hypoxaemia, stiff lungs, and a widespread diffuse pulmonary infiltrate. Approximately 1–2 days following the clinical presentation of the precipitating cause (sepsis, aspiration, etc.), there is rapidly worsening dyspnoea (± a dry cough) and hypoxaemia, requiring rapidly escalating amounts of supplemental O_2 up to 100% via a non-rebreathe system (see ➌ pp. 704–6). Coarse crackles in the chest. Intubation and ventilation are nearly always required, although initiating CPAP via a face mask at 5–10cmH$_2$O with 100% O_2 can improve oxygenation temporarily.

Diagnosis There are no specific tests that allow a confident diagnosis, and exclusion of other more specifically treatable diagnoses is required. The cause for the ARDS needs to be established and prevented from continuing or recurring, if possible. The CXR or CT shows diffuse alveolar infiltrates and air bronchograms, similar in appearance to cardiogenic pulmonary oedema or diffuse pulmonary haemorrhage.
  Differential diagnoses include:
- *LVF* (may be excluded on clinical grounds, echo, or, less commonly, checking pulmonary capillary wedge pressure <18mmHg)
- *Diffuse alveolar haemorrhage* (e.g. Goodpasture's, Wegener's, and SLE; clues will include a drop in Hb, blood in the airways and pulmonary secretions, and other clinical features of one of these disorders)
- *ILD* (e.g. AIP or fulminant OP; see ➌ pp. 276–7 and p. 278)
- *Idiopathic acute eosinophilic pneumonia*
- *Cancer and lymphangitis carcinomatosis.*

Some centres advocate lung biopsy to exclude alternatives, although most reserve biopsy for cases when the differential diagnosis includes conditions for which management would be changed (e.g. fungal infection, vasculitis, COP).

Management and complications

Management The essential aspects of management are to treat the precipitating cause, provide best supportive care with adequate oxygenation, and avoid further damage from barotrauma, hyperoxia, and nosocomial infections. Mechanical ventilation with PEEP and high inflation pressures are almost always required to maintain oxygenation (SaO_2 values in the low 90s are entirely adequate). There is evidence that high inflation pressures may worsen ARDS directly (micro-barotrauma); therefore, try to maintain plateau pressures $\leq 30cmH_2O$.

Many ventilation strategies have been tried to reduce the high inflation pressures that result from the stiff lungs (low compliance). For example, using low tidal volume ventilation to reduce inflation pressures (6mL/kg ideal body weight, compared with 12mL/kg) reduces mortality by 9% and increases ventilator-free days. Use of high PEEP (attempt to open collapsed alveoli) has been shown in a meta-analysis to improve oxygenation and decrease time on a ventilator, and is associated with a lower ITU mortality for patients with PaO_2/FiO_2 $\leq 200mmHg$ (27kPa). Reducing the minute ventilation and allowing the $PaCO_2$ to rise (permissive hypercapnia) also reduces the inflation pressures.

Prone ventilation has been tried in an attempt to improve V/Q matching, and initial increases in PaO_2 are observed. A meta-analysis suggested a possible survival advantage for those with severe hypoxia, and a recent RCT has shown a significant reduction in both 28- and 90-day mortality for patients with severe ARDS.

Several different artificial surfactants have been tried to try and improve lung compliance, although good delivery to the abnormal areas is unlikely. Although effective in animal models, the RCTs have been negative in humans.

Haemodynamic monitoring, guided by central venous catheters, has a similar efficacy to pulmonary artery catheters but are associated with a 2× reduction in catheter-related complications (mostly, arrhythmias).

Different degrees of hydration have been compared, with reduced fluid balances improving gas exchange and shortening duration of mechanical ventilation. Secondary analysis of a cohort study suggested that a negative day 4 fluid balance is associated with decreased mortality, although this was not confirmed in a randomized study.

High-dose steroids have been used, but there is evidence of harm as well as benefit, and minimal evidence of overall improved survival. Three meta-analyses failed to demonstrate significant mortality improvements, while one showed decreased mortality. Certain subgroups may do slightly better and others worse, e.g. steroids are possibly beneficial during the first 14 days but detrimental thereafter. A 2007 RCT using prolonged methylprednisolone infusion (1mg/kg/day) for early ARDS ($\leq 72h$) showed improvement in a number of outcomes and halved mortality, but this was a small study ($n = 91$), and patient characteristics were imbalanced in the treatment arms.

Extracorporeal membrane oxygenation/CO_2 removal will buy time and allow the lung to 'rest', but these techniques are very expensive and it is difficult to demonstrate any long-term benefit.

Complications of ARDS include:
- The high ventilation pressures lead to barotrauma: pneumothorax, surgical emphysema, pneumomediastinum. Pneumothorax may be lethal but difficult to detect on a CXR in the supine patient
- Nosocomial infections occur in about half the patients, making surveillance mini-BALs important
- Myopathy associated with long-term neuromuscular blockade, high steroid doses, and poor glycaemic control
- Non-specific problems of VTE, GI haemorrhage, inadequate nutrition.

Prognosis has improved over the last 20y, probably due to improvements in supportive care and ventilator strategies, rather than an ability to modify the inflammatory process and its subsequent repair. Prognosis is worse with intra-pulmonary causes. Early deaths are usually due to the precipitating condition, and later deaths to complications. Over half of the patients will survive with varying residual lung damage, although the PFTs often show only minor restrictive abnormalities (and reduced kCO), indicating the considerable capacity of the lung to recover. A prospective cohort study showed that 6-minute walking test (6MWT) distance remained decreased (at 76% predicted), even at 5y.

Future developments
- The optimal level of PEEP in a particular patient is difficult to predict. Inadequate PEEP allows more atelectasis, but too high PEEP contributes to overdistension of remaining alveoli and further barotrauma when there are no more 'recruitable' alveoli. Ways to estimate the best PEEP are under investigation. High-frequency oscillatory ventilation (HFOV) has been around a long while, but the recent OSCILLATE and OSCAR randomized trials suggested a lack of benefit, with possible harm associated with its use. Recently, liquid ventilation with perfluorochemicals has been tried. These dense O_2-carrying liquids reduce the heterogeneity of ventilation by nullifying the requirement for surfactant, thus recruiting the collapsed alveoli. There are improvements in oxygenation but no evidence yet of clinically meaningful outcomes
- Nitric oxide (NO) has been tried, with clear improvements in oxygenation but very little effect on survival. The mode of action is not clear and may be more than just vasodilatation. Inhaled prostacyclin is similarly unconvincing. Anti-inflammatory and antioxidant therapies are still very much in the experimental phase
- 'Off the shelf' artificial lung systems are now becoming clinically useful to buy time while the lungs recover. The Novalung Interventional Lung Assist device is an example, but such therapy is very expensive.

Chapter 17

Asbestos and the lung

Asbestos

Asbestos consists of a family of naturally occurring hydrated silicate fibres that may be subdivided into two groups:
- Curly *serpentine* fibres, of which chrysotile (white) is the only fibre currently in commercial use
- Straight needle-like *amphiboles*, which comprise crocidolite (blue), amosite (brown), anthophyllite, tremolite, and actinolite.

Fibres have a predisposition to localize to the pleura. They differ in their lung clearance kinetics and pathogenic potential; amphibole fibres clear more slowly from the lung and are more carcinogenic than chrysotile. Whilst asbestos usage in developed countries is restricted, the use of chrysotile asbestos in developing economies continues to rise.

Mechanisms of exposure

Occupational exposure accounts for the majority of cases of asbestos-related disease and includes:
- Mining, milling, and transport of asbestos
- Use of asbestos products, e.g. in construction and demolition, floor tiling, insulation, fireproofing, textiles, friction materials (brake linings), ship building, pipefitting, electrical repair, boiler fitting and lagging, carpentry, plumbing, and welding.

Domestic exposure may include:
- Relatives of asbestos workers exposed to 'carry home' asbestos in hair or clothes
- Following remodelling or renovation in contaminated buildings
- Local geological exposure from natural deposits, e.g. areas of central and south-east Turkey, north-west Greece, and Corsica
- Urban environment (although undisturbed and non-friable asbestos building insulation is not considered hazardous).

A complete occupational history is essential if asbestos-related disease is suspected and should include the method of exposure, with dates and names of employers. This information may be of medicolegal importance and ideally should be elicited during the first consultation.

Asbestos-related lung disease comprises:
- Benign asbestos-related pleural disease
  - Pleural plaques
  - Benign asbestos-related pleural effusion
  - Diffuse pleural thickening
  - Rounded atelectasis
- Asbestosis
- Mesothelioma
- Lung cancer (multiplicative risk from smoking).

Other diseases linked to asbestos exposure include pericarditis and perhaps head and neck and GI cancers. Whether asbestos exposure truly leads to an increased risk of lung cancer in the absence of asbestosis remains controversial.

Asbestos-related disease typically exhibits a long latency period of 20–40y from exposure. Peak industrial asbestos use in the UK occurred in the early 1970s, and asbestos-related disease is likely to remain common for at least the next 20y. The incidence of mesothelioma is forecast to peak in 2015–2020 in Europe.

All deaths should be notified to the coroner if asbestos-related disease is suspected or proven.

Benign asbestos-related pleural disease

Pleural plaques

- Most common manifestation of asbestos exposure
- Discrete areas of white or yellow thickening on the parietal pleura; may calcify. Histologically, these are acellular, avascular areas of hyaline collagen fibrosis
- Bilateral and occur particularly on the posterolateral chest wall (particularly adjacent to ribs), over the mediastinal pleura, and on the dome of the diaphragm but are absent in the costophrenic angles
- Develop 20–30y after exposure; incidence (but not the extent of plaques) increases with longer duration of exposure; found in up to 50% of asbestos-exposed workers and may also occur after low-dose exposures
- Usually asymptomatic although, if extensive, may be associated with mild breathlessness due to pleural restriction
- Effect on pulmonary function is uncertain: most studies have failed to demonstrate abnormal lung function, although otherwise unexplained mild airways obstruction or restriction has been described in some populations of asbestos workers with pleural plaques—the mechanism of this is unclear, although it may reflect asbestos-induced small airway disease or early interstitial fibrosis, respectively
- HRCT is more sensitive than CXR in detecting pleural plaques
- There is no evidence that plaques are pre-malignant
- Asymptomatic plaques are no longer eligible for compensation in England and Wales but are in Scotland and Northern Ireland (see ➲ pp. 122–3)
- TB, trauma, and haemothorax may each cause single pleural plaques; multiple plaques are highly suggestive of asbestos exposure.

Benign asbestos-related pleural effusions

- Relatively early manifestation of asbestos pleural disease; usually occurs within 10y of exposure
- Development is considered to be dose-dependent although can occur after minimal exposure
- Typically small and unilateral and may be asymptomatic or occasionally associated with pleuritic pain, fever, and dyspnoea
- Usually resolve spontaneously over a few months, although some recur
- The pleural effusion is an exudate, often bloodstained, with no characteristic findings on pleural fluid analysis
- Diagnosis depends on a history of asbestos exposure and the exclusion of other causes, including mesothelioma
- Benign asbestos pleurisy may precede the development of diffuse pleural thickening; there is no clear association with mesothelioma
- Treat symptomatically, with pleural aspiration for breathlessness and NSAIDs for pain.

Diffuse pleural thickening (DPT)

- Consists of extensive fibrosis of the visceral pleura, with areas of adhesion with the parietal pleura and consequent obliteration of the pleural space
- Unlike pleural plaques, its margins are ill-defined, and it may involve the costophrenic angles, apices, and interlobar fissures
- Development appears to be dose-related and may follow recurrent asbestos pleurisy
- On CXR, it may be defined as a smooth, uninterrupted pleural opacity, extending over at least a quarter of the chest wall, with or without obliteration of the costophrenic angles; on CT, the pleural density extends >8cm craniocaudally, 5cm laterally, and is >3mm thick
- Symptoms are relatively common and comprise exertional breathlessness and chest pain, which can be chronic and severe
- May lead to significant restrictive pulmonary function impairment, especially if the costophrenic angle is obliterated; hypercapnic respiratory failure has been described
- Pleural biopsy may be required to distinguish it from mesothelioma
- Treatment is difficult; decortication often fails to result in clinical or functional improvement
- Patient may be eligible for compensation (see ⮕ pp. 122–3).

Rounded atelectasis

(Also known as folded lung, Blesovsky syndrome, or shrinking pleuritis with atelectasis.)

- Develops as contracting visceral pleural fibrosis; ensnares and then twists the underlying lung, resulting in the distinctive radiological appearance of a rounded or oval pleural-based mass of 2.5–5cm in diameter
- Asbestos exposure is the most common cause, although any cause of pleural inflammation may result in rounded atelectasis
- CT is often diagnostic, demonstrating a 'comet tail' of vessels and bronchi converging toward the lesion, adjacent thickened pleura, and volume loss in the affected lobe
- An atypical appearance may require biopsy to exclude malignant disease
- Typically asymptomatic, although breathlessness or dry cough may occur
- Usually stable or slowly progressive, and no specific treatment is required
- Surgical decortication may improve symptoms but frequently results in reduced lung volumes and is not generally recommended.

Further information

American Thoracic Society Statement. Diagnosis and initial management of non-malignant diseases related to asbestos. *Am J Respir Crit Care Med* 2004;**170**:691–715.

Asbestosis

Definition Chronic interstitial fibrosis resulting from asbestos inhalation.

Causes Factors affecting disease development include:
- *Degree and length of asbestos exposure* A clear dose-response relationship exists; usually seen in workers with many years of high exposure although may follow a very high exposure of short duration, resulting in a shorter latency period
- *Fibre type* Amphibole fibres are probably more fibrogenic than chrysotile, although most exposures are mixed fibre types
- *Cigarette smoking* increases the severity and rate of progression of asbestosis.

Latency period from first exposure to clinical disease is usually at least 15–20y and may be >40y.

Clinical features Insidious onset of breathlessness, dry cough. Bibasal late-inspiratory crackles, clubbing in 40% of cases. May progress to respiratory failure, cor pulmonale.

Differential diagnosis includes other causes of interstitial fibrosis, particularly UIP.

Investigations

- *CXR* Bilateral symmetrical reticulonodular pattern, primarily affecting the lower lobes peripherally, which may extend upwards to involve the mid- and upper zones; may progress to honeycomb lung. Massive bilateral upper lobe fibrosis (without lower lobe involvement) is rare but well described. Associated pleural thickening or plaques may be seen and suggest a diagnosis of asbestosis, rather than UIP. Classification is based on size, thickness, and profusion of opacities. CXR insensitive to early disease; may be normal in 15–20% of symptomatic biopsy-proven asbestosis
- *HRCT* is more sensitive than CXR and is abnormal in 10–30% of cases with a normal CXR. Features include basal 'ground-glass' opacities (seen early in the disease), parenchymal bands, subpleural curvilinear lines and opacities, interlobular septal thickening, and signs of fibrosis (traction bronchiectasis, loss of lobular architecture, honeycombing in advanced disease)
- *PFTs* are classically restrictive with reduced lung volumes and transfer factor, although obstructive or mixed patterns may also occur (perhaps reflecting asbestos-induced small airway disease)
- Positive *gallium scan* may be seen with normal CXR; correlates poorly with lung function
- Analysis of *sputum* or *BAL* may demonstrate asbestos bodies, although sensitivity is limited. The finding of interstitial fibrosis, in the absence of asbestos bodies, on *lung biopsy* makes asbestosis unlikely. Analysis of material for asbestos bodies is only very rarely indicated, usually for research or litigation purposes.

In general, CXR and HRCT show only limited correlation with physiological disease severity.

Diagnosis Gold standard is pathological demonstration of fibrosis with mineralogical quantification of asbestos bodies. The College of American Pathologists and Pulmonary Pathology Society have defined a 5-point scheme for grading asbestosis:

- Grade 0—fibrosis confined to bronchiolar walls
- Grade 1—fibrosis extends only to first-tier alveoli
- Grade 2—fibrosis involves alveolar ducts and second-tier alveoli
- Grade 3—fibrosis of all alveoli between respiratory bronchioles
- Grade 4—honeycombing.

In practice, histology is rarely required, and a diagnosis can be made on the basis of a history of significant asbestos exposure, with appropriate delay between exposure and disease, and radiographic evidence of fibrosis (particularly when seen with pleural plaques).

Treatment
- No pharmacological treatment is of proven benefit
- Supportive management, including supplementary O_2, as required, influenza and pneumococcal immunization, smoking cessation, compensation if exposure was occupational (see ➲ pp. 122–3).

Prognosis varies widely. After removal from exposure, progression occurs in 5–40% of patients over 10y; progression is faster following greater exposure, although rapid progression over 1–2y is unusual and more in keeping with UIP. Fewer CXR opacities after exposure are associated with better prognosis. Increased risk of developing lung cancer.

Mesothelioma: diagnosis

Definition Malignant tumour of mesothelial surfaces (most commonly the pleura), usually resulting from asbestos exposure.

Causes Asbestos is the major single cause, and there is a history of occupational asbestos exposure in up to 90% of cases. All types of asbestos can cause mesothelioma—amphibole is the most potent, but also evidence for chrysotile. Mean latent interval between first exposure and death is around 40y; cases with latency <15y are rare. Not dose-related (unlike asbestosis or bronchogenic cancers) and no evidence for a threshold asbestos dose below which there is no risk, although the risk at low exposure levels is small. No significant association with smoking. The mechanism through which asbestos fibres result in mesothelioma is unclear; possibilities include direct irritation of the parietal pleura, disruption of mitosis, generation of toxic O_2 radicals, and stimulation of mitogen-activated kinases leading to proto-oncogene activation.

Other causes of mesothelioma include non-asbestos fibres, such as erionite, which is found in rocks in Cappadocia, Turkey—mesothelioma accounts for up to a quarter of all adult deaths in local villages. Evidence for Simian Virus 40 (contaminated polio vaccine in 1950s/60s) is limited. Rare cases of mesothelioma caused by ionizing radiation or chest injury are described. 'Spontaneous' mesothelioma in children is also documented.

Clinical features of pleural mesothelioma:
- Chest pain (typically dull ache, 'boring', diffuse, occasionally pleuritic), breathlessness; a small proportion are asymptomatic. Profuse sweating may occur
- Consider in any patient with a pleural effusion or pleural thickening, particularly if chest pain is present
- Rarely may present with persistent chest pain and a normal CXR
- Weight loss and fatigue uncommon at presentation (<30% of cases)
- Clubbing is very rare (<1%)
- Chest wall invasion may be seen (especially at thoracentesis sites)
- Bilateral pleural involvement is unusual at presentation
- Paraneoplastic syndromes are described, e.g. DIC.

Differential diagnosis includes benign asbestos pleural effusion, DPT, and adenocarcinoma involving the pleura.

Investigations

Pleural fluid aspiration typically reveals an exudative straw-coloured or bloody effusion. Cytological analysis may provide the diagnosis (sensitivity range 32–84%) and is often useful in excluding other pathology, e.g. adenocarcinoma. Poor at diagnosing sarcomatoid mesothelioma. Pleural fluid glucose and pH may be low in extensive tumours. Mesothelioma may track through the chest wall along thoracentesis sites; avoid repeated pleural aspiration if the diagnosis is suspected.

Imaging CXR and CT features include:
- Moderate to large unilateral pleural effusion, usually with pleural nodularity and enhancement following pleural contrast, and involvement of mediastinal pleura
- Localized pleural mass or thickening without free fluid
- Uniform encasement of lung, resulting in small hemithorax
- Local invasion of chest wall, ribs, heart, mediastinum, hilar nodes, and diaphragm; transdiaphragmatic spread and invasion of contralateral pleura
- Associated pleural plaques or interstitial fibrosis in a minority of cases.

The role of MRI is unclear—it may provide additional information in some cases, e.g. chest wall invasion, although is rarely required. PET-CT may have a role in distinguishing benign and malignant pleural disease, as well as identifying lymph node spread for staging, and can help to select sites for image-guided biopsy.

Biopsy Diagnosis usually requires histological confirmation, except when the patient is too unwell or too frail for biopsy. US- or CT-guided cutting needle biopsy and thoracoscopic biopsy of pleural masses have a high diagnostic yield and should be used in preference to blind (Abrams') biopsy techniques. Early use of thoracoscopy may both provide a diagnosis and enable treatment of large effusions with talc pleurodesis, thereby avoiding repeated non-diagnostic procedures with attendant problems of needle-track spread.

Histological subtypes
- Epithelioid (50% of cases; may be confused with adenocarcinoma; better prognosis)
- Sarcomatoid (or fibrous; includes lymphohistiocytoid and desmoplastic patterns)
- Mixed (biphasic; contains both subtypes).

Immunohistochemistry is key to making the diagnosis. Stains which are positive for mesothelioma include calretinin, EMA (CA15-3/mucin-1– dense peripheral staining pattern), keratin CK5/6, WT-1, and podoplanin. Stains that are usually negative for mesothelioma include CEA, TTF-1, B72.3, CD15 (usually positive for lung adenocarcinoma), ER (usually positive for breast carcinoma), and p63 (squamous cell carcinoma). Electron microscopy of histopathological specimens may also help to distinguish mesothelioma from adenocarcinoma.

Staging No widely accepted staging system. The International Mesothelioma Interest Group (IMIG) system is commonly used and gives stages I–IV, based on TNM classification. Imaging may underestimate extent of disease, and accurate staging would require surgical exploration. Poor prognostic features include transdiaphragmatic muscle invasion and involvement of mediastinal lymph nodes, ♂ gender, age >75, chest pain, poor performance status, high WCC, thrombocytosis, and non-epithelioid histology. A low standardized uptake value (SUV) on PET may also be prognostically beneficial.

Mesothelioma: treatment and outcome

Treatment

Management of pleural effusions Early definitive treatment is key; repeated pleural aspirations should be avoided. Talc pleurodesis can be achieved either using a chest drain or at thoracoscopy, depending on local resources. Pleurodesis is not possible if the lung does not re-expand following drainage of pleural fluid ('trapped lung') and the resulting recurrent pleural effusions are difficult to manage; indwelling pleural catheters (IPCs) allow fluid drainage without needle aspiration and are useful in this situation. A recent RCT suggested that 1° use of IPCs was reasonable, dependent on patient preference (see ⦾ p. 767).

Radiotherapy Prophylactic radiotherapy appears to reduce chest wall invasion by tumour following large-bore chest drain insertion or biopsy: three fractions reduced the risk of tracking from 40% to 0 in a randomized study of 40 patients, although a subsequent study failed to demonstrate a benefit. Recurrence may follow delayed prophylactic radiotherapy, so it is usually administered within 4 weeks. Palliative radiotherapy provides pain relief in a proportion of patients with chest wall pain but is less useful in the treatment of breathlessness or SVCO.

Surgery Four types of surgery have been used—extrapleural pneumonectomy (EPP), pleurectomy with decortication (PD; lung-sparing, may help with re-expansion of trapped lung), limited pleurectomy, and thoracoscopy with pleurodesis, but their roles require further investigation. Trimodal therapy (chemotherapy, followed by EPP and radiotherapy) was evaluated in the MARS randomized feasibility study for 'resectable disease', finding the EPP group to have a shortened survival without any gain in QoL, although the study has been controversial. Operative mortality is ± 7–16% for EPP and ± 4% for PD. Results are awaited from a further study comparing talc pleurodesis vs VATS pleurectomy (MesoVATS).

Chemotherapy Patients with good performance status should be considered for chemotherapy. Pemetrexed (an inhibitor of DNA synthesis proteins, e.g. thymidylate synthase) plus cisplatin has an objective response rate (tumour shrinkage of >50%) of 41% and appears to convey a survival advantage of just under 3 months when compared with cisplatin alone. Since the National Institute for Health and Clinical Excellence (NICE) approval of pemetrexed in 2008, cisplatin/pemetrexed combination is a frequently used combination, although carboplatin may be substituted for cisplatin in those at increased risk of toxicity. Ongoing treatment of an individual may be guided by objective metabolic responses based on PET-CT. Other studies have shown that addition of raltitrexed to cisplatin improves surival by 2.5 months, and gemcitabine plus cisplatin led to objective response rates of 33 and 48% in two trials, with QoL benefits. Trials are ongoing.

General management Early involvement of a pain relief and palliative care service is required. Ensure adequate analgesia: opiates and non-steroidal anti-inflammatory drugs (NSAIDs) for chest wall pain; consider amitriptyline, pregabalin, or gabapentin for neuropathic pain (from intercostal nerve or vertebral involvement); nerve blocks or cordotomy may be required. Breathlessness may be multifactorial, e.g. pleural effusion, lung compression, chest wall restriction, pericardial involvement, anaemia, pain, anxiety, and fear. Discuss compensation issues (see ➲ pp. 122–3). Liaise with GP, specialist nurse, palliative care teams. Remind GP that all deaths have to be reported to the coroner. The Coroners' Society of England and Wales and the British Thoracic Society (BTS) have encouraged coroners to avoid post-mortems where biopsy has already confirmed mesothelioma. A coronial inquest is opened and adjourned soon after death but may take ± 3 months for the full inquest to complete.

Clinical course Median survival is 4–12 months from diagnosis. Typically progresses by local extension, sometimes leading to involvement of the contralateral lung or peritoneum, SVCO, cardiac tamponade, or spinal cord compression. Distant metastases are common (50% at autopsy), although occur late and are rarely clinically apparent.

Peritoneal mesothelioma is rarer than pleural mesothelioma and may be associated with more prolonged asbestos exposure. Remains intra-abdominal in most cases. Clinical features include abdominal discomfort, weight loss, ascites, and, in some cases, organ involvement (e.g. intestinal obstruction). FNA of omental masses may provide a diagnosis, although laparoscopy is often required. Prognosis is worse than for pleural mesothelioma, with median survival 7.4 months. No treatment is of proven benefit.

Mesothelioma has also been described affecting *other serosal surfaces* such as pericardium and tunica vaginalis.

Future developments
- Several biomarkers have shown promise in mesothelioma diagnosis, but none are recommended as sole diagnostic tests. Mesothelin (expressed on the surface of mesothelial cells) is an FDA-approved diagnostic and prognostic marker for mesothelioma, with a sensitivity of 48–84% and specificity of 70–100%. Other malignancies can raise levels (including ovarian, pancreatic, and lung carcinomas, lymphoma). Other potential markers include megakaryocyte-potentiating factor (MPF) and osteopontin
- Microarray studies of gene expression in tumour samples may prove to be useful in both distinguishing mesothelioma from adenocarcinoma and in predicting prognosis
- Novel therapeutic strategies using immunotherapy (e.g. antimesothelin monoclonal antibodies), gene therapy, anti-angiogenic agents, and photodynamic therapy are in development. Combinations of immunotherapy with chemotherapy appear particularly promising.

Further information

BTS statement on malignant mesothelioma in the United Kingdom. *Thorax* 2007;**62**:ii1–ii19.
Scherpereel A *et al.* Guidelines of the European Respiratory Society and the European Society of Thoracic Surgeons for the management of malignant pleural mesothelioma. *Eur Respir J* 2010;**35**:479–95.

Compensation for asbestos-related diseases

Identification of asbestos exposure is essential for the patient to be able to claim compensation. Patients are not eligible for compensation if their exposure occurred whilst they were self-employed. There are two principal sources of support and compensation.

From the government Apply to the Department for Work and Pensions for Industrial Injuries Disablement Benefit, using form BI100PD (health care team fill in form BI100PN(A)). Available for the following diseases:
- DPT
- Asbestosis
- Lung cancer associated with DPT or asbestosis or some asbestos exposure.
- Mesothelioma.

There must be a clear history of asbestos exposure at work. Compensation is not available for pleural plaques alone. If successful and employer is no longer in business, may apply for a single payment from the government under the *Pneumoconiosis, etc. (Worker's Compensation) Act 1979*. The value of compensation reflects the degree of disability from which the patient is considered to suffer and their age at diagnosis. Next of kin may also claim within 6 months posthumously. Other benefits may be available, including *Diffuse Mesothelioma Payment* (for patients who have had secondary asbestos exposure from their partner, and the self-employed), *Constant Attendance Allowance*, *Exceptionally Severe Disablement Allowance*, and *Reduced Earnings Allowance*. The War Disablement Pension scheme may provide compensation for disease resulting from asbestos exposure with HM forces.

From the courts: Civil law compensation directly from a previous employer. Can be claimed from the employer's insurer, even if the employer is now out of existence. Advise patient to seek advice as soon as possible from a solicitor with relevant experience. Claims must be initiated within 3y of the individual's first awareness that they have an asbestos-related disease; attempts to initiate claims after 3y may be statute-barred. Inform the patient of this, and document the conversation in the medical notes. In England and Wales, a Court of Appeal ruling in 2006 concluded that pleural plaques alone should now no longer be considered an indication for compensation, and a subsequent 2007 appeal failed to overturn this ruling in the House of Lords. Subsequent 2011 legislation in Scotland and Northern Ireland has made plaques compensable in these countries. Awards for asbestosis range from £15,000 to £50,000, depending on symptoms and the degree of disability; such patients may accept an interim settlement, allowing further claims to be made, or may wish to take a greater 'once and for all' award and forego their right to further claims in the event of mesothelioma developing. Typical awards for mesothelioma are £45,000–£50,000, with additional amounts awarded for care and future loss of wages and pension; total compensation may be ± £100,000 (or significantly more for younger patients). Successful claims have also been made for mesothelioma occurring in relatives who had 2° exposure to asbestos whilst washing work clothes.

Further information

Benefits Enquiry Line ☎ 0800 882200. Advice on available benefits and completing claim applications. Guide to Industrial Injuries Disablement Benefits (DB1) gives guidance on IIDB, Pneumoconiosis, etc. (Worker's Compensation) Act 1979 and other benefits: ℘ http://www.dwp.gov.uk/publications/specialist-guides/technical-guidance/db1-a-guide-to-industrial-injuries/;℘ http://www.gov.uk/industrial-injuries-disablement-benefit.

℘ http://www.mesothelioma.uk.com.

Chapter 18

Asthma

Definition, epidemiology, pathophysiology, aetiology

Definition There is no universally agreed definition. Asthma is a chronic inflammatory disorder of the airway characterized by bronchial hyperreactivity to a variety of stimuli, leading to a variable degree of airway obstruction, some of which may become irreversible over many years.

It is a clinical diagnosis based on:
- A history of recurrent episodes of wheeze, chest tightness, breathlessness, and/or cough, particularly at night
- Evidence of generalized and variable airflow obstruction, which may be detected as intermittent wheeze on examination or via tests such as peak expiratory flow (PEF) measurement.

Epidemiology It is the commonest chronic respiratory disease in the UK, with a prevalence of 10–15%. There is a wide variation in disease prevalence, with highest levels seen in English-speaking countries (where there is also a high prevalence of sensitization to common aeroallergens). The reason for the increasing worldwide prevalence over the last few decades is unclear.

Pathophysiology Best described as chronic eosinophilic bronchitis/bronchiolitis. Airway inflammation is seen, with cellular infiltration by T helper 2 (Th2) cells, lymphocytes, eosinophils, and mast cells. There is large and small airway involvement, and cytokine production (e.g. platelet-activating factor (PAF), IL5, and leukotrienes).

Airway obstruction occurs due to a combination of:
- Inflammatory cell infiltration
- Mucus hypersecretion with mucus plug formation
- Smooth muscle contraction.

This may become irreversible over time due to:
- Basement membrane thickening, collagen deposition, and epithelial desquamation
- Airway remodelling occurs in chronic disease, with smooth muscle hypertrophy and hyperplasia. This is now recognized as increasingly important in the pathophysiology of the most difficult to treat chronic asthma.

Aetiology This is due to a combination of genetic and environmental factors, with many different genes identified.

Immunological mechanisms A subgroup of asthmatics are atopic and therefore react to antigen challenge by producing specific IgE from B-lymphocytes. This leads to the formation of IgE-antigen complexes that bind to mast cells, basophils, and macrophages, leading to the release of preformed mediators, e.g. histamine, IL5, and other eosinophil chemotactic factors. These factors cause bronchoconstriction and airway oedema.

Prostaglandins, leukotrienes, kinins, and PAF are all important 2° messengers involved in the inflammatory response.

A subgroup of asthmatics (up to 25%) are now recognized to have non-eosinophilic disease, which may be associated with a poorer short-term response to inhaled corticosteroids and is associated with neutrophilic airway inflammation and innate immunity. This subgroup may turn out to need a different treatment strategy.

Genetic factors A hereditary component to asthma and atopy is well established, and a number of chromosomes and linkages are implicated. The multiple mechanisms and 2° messengers involved in asthma make the contribution of the effects of specific genes difficult to determine. Established susceptibility loci include the genes *ADAM33, GPRA* (G protein-related receptor for asthma), and *ORMDL3*, a member of a gene family that encodes transmembrane endoplasmic reticulum proteins. The latter was very recently identified by a genome-wide screen, and its function and role in the pathogenesis of asthma are not yet clear.

Hygiene hypothesis This suggests that asthma may be a by-product of modern 'first world' cleanliness. Early life exposure to bacterial endotoxin switches off the allergic response (by reducing Th2-mediated pathways), and, when this exposure is lost, the likelihood of developing allergic diseases, such as asthma, increases considerably. Large epidemiological studies support this hypothesis.

Environmental factors The increasing prevalence of asthma appears to be associated with a rising standard of living worldwide, and not just in westernized societies. This has implicated a number of environmental factors. A number of explanations are speculated (but not proven), including dietary changes, a reduction in childhood infections, increased immunization, or a combination of all three.

Phenotypic differences It is increasingly recognized that 'asthma' is likely to represent a number of different 'diseases' or subphenotypes, rather than one disease with a unifying pathological mechanism. Subphenotypes may differ in underlying pathophysiology, clinical features, and disease course, and research aimed at clearly identifying such disease subgroups (e.g. through the use of biomarkers, such as blood eosinophilia, or the host genetic profile) is ongoing.

Further information

McGrath KW et al. A large subgroup of mild-to-moderate asthma is persistently noneosinophilic. *Am J Respir Crit Care Med* 2012;**185**:612–19.

Clinical features

- Cough
- SOB
- Wheeze
- Chest tightness.

Classically, these are variable, intermittent, worse at night, associated with specific triggers, e.g. pollens, cat and dog dander, and non-specific triggers, e.g. cold air, perfumes, and bleaches, due to airway hypersensitivity. Asthma may be labelled 'cough variant' or 'cough predominant' when cough is the major symptom (see Box 18.1).

Examination

- May be entirely normal
- Classically, expiratory wheeze is heard
- Chest deformity/hyperinflation—long-standing/poorly controlled asthma
- Severe life-threatening asthma may have no wheeze and a silent chest.

Diagnosis

This is often a clinical diagnosis but should be supported by objective measurements. Important to:

- Identify provoking factors, e.g. cold air, bleach, perfume, and environmental aeroallergens (grasses, pollen, hay), and any occupational exposures
- Assess disease severity. Longitudinal studies show greater decline in lung function in asthmatics than non-asthmatics—greater still in asthmatics who smoke.

Don't forget to look for/ask about:

- Nasal symptoms—obstruction, rhinorrhoea, hyposmia
- Atopic dermatitis/eczema/hay fever
- Allergies, including food allergy (see Box 18.2)
- Reflux/GORD disease (treating reflux may improve symptoms which have been wrongly attributed to asthma, particularly cough)
- Laryngo/pharyngeal reflux (hoarse voice, throat clearing, acid in throat)
- Triggers, including exercise, menstruation
- Social situation/stresses
- Aspirin sensitivity (associated with later-onset asthma and nasal polyps; see Box 18.3)
- Family history.

Box 18.1 The diagnosis is based on the presence of:

- Symptoms (cough, wheeze, breathlessness)
- Day-to-day peak flow variability (>15% variability or reversibility to inhaled β_2 agonist)
- Airway hyperresponsiveness.

Consider the diagnosis of asthma in:

- Recurrent cough, episodic breathlessness, and wheeze
- Chest tightness
- Isolated or nocturnal cough
- Exercised-induced cough or breathlessness
- Hyperventilation syndrome (see ➜ p. 259).

Box 18.2 Oral allergy syndrome

A subset of patients sensitized to aeroallergens, such as tree and grass pollens, develop localized lip angio-oedema after ingestion of specific fruits that share cross-reactive epitopes with pollen allergens. The reaction occurs immediately after ingesting the fruit. Cooked fruit is usually tolerated, presumably because the culpable proteins are denatured with cooking. Birch pollens cross-react with apples, hazelnuts, and potato. Ragwort shares epitopes with melon and bananas.

Box 18.3 Aspirin-induced asthma (AIA)

- Defined as chronic rhinoconjunctivitis, nasal polyps, and asthma
- Asthma is precipitated by ingestion of aspirin or other NSAIDs
- Occurs in up to 20% of asthmatics and is commoner in women
- The mechanism is thought to be via aspirin inhibition of the cyclo-oxygenase pathway, with excess leukotriene production via the lipo-oxygenase pathway
- BAL and urine in AIA patients show excess leukotrienes post-aspirin exposure
- Loss of anti-inflammatory prostaglandin E2 may also be important.

Investigations

The number of investigations required depends on the certainty of the diagnosis from the history, simple spirometry, and peak flow recordings. Most patients referred for a respiratory opinion will already have completed home peak flow recordings and have had a CXR. Repeating PEFs may still be of benefit. Objective evidence of asthma is important before starting long-term therapy with potentially harmful drugs such as inhaled steroids. For differential diagnoses, see Box 18.4.

Essential investigations (on which the diagnosis is based)

- *Peak flow recording/simple spirometry* looking for variability and response to treatment. Airway obstruction leads to decreased peak expiratory flow rate (PEFR) and forced expiratory volume in 1s (FEV_1); may be normal between episodes of bronchospasm. If persistently normal, the diagnosis must be in doubt. The diagnosis is highly likely if:
  - 20% diurnal PEF variation on >3 days/week, in a week of peak flow diary measures
  - FEV_1 >15% decrease after 6min exercise
  - FEV_1 >15% (and 200mL) increase after 2-week trial of oral steroid (30mg prednisolone od)
- *Bronchodilator reversibility testing* FEV_1 >15% (and 200mL) increase after a single dose of a short-acting β_2 agonist therapy (e.g. salbutamol 400 micrograms by metered dose inhaler (MDI) with spacer or 2.5mg by nebulizer) or 200 micrograms bd of inhaled beclometasone or equivalent for 6–8 weeks. A 400mL improvement is strongly suggestive of asthma; smaller improvements are less sensitive and need careful interpretation.

Non-essential/optional investigations

- *Blood tests*
  - FBC (eosinophilia is common in asthma, but, if the total eosinophil count is unusually high, consider eosinophilic granulomatosis with polyangiitis (EGPA; Churg–Strauss syndrome))
  - IgE (associated atopy, i.e. positive skin prick tests to common allergens, often with associated allergic rhinitis and eczema)
- Specific IgE if other environmental triggers suspected
- *CXR* if atypical symptoms. May show hyperinflation or evidence of localized abnormality simulating wheeze, e.g. adenoma (rare)
- *Skin tests* to define atopic constitution or identify potential triggers
- *Methacholine/histamine challenge* measures bronchial hyperresponsiveness (BHR) as a PC_{20}, the dose (provocative concentration) of agent (histamine or methacholine) causing a 20% fall in FEV_1.
- Asthma is suggested by a PC_{20} <8mg/mL (the lower the PC_{20}, the more likely the diagnosis is asthma). Normal subjects have a PC_{20} >16mg/mL. The absence of BHR virtually excludes the diagnosis of asthma; however, the presence of BHR does not prove asthma.

- *Bronchial provocation tests* aim to demonstrate bronchospasm to an inhaled agent, usually occupational. The response to an aerosolized sample of a suspected agent may be useful if the diagnosis of occupational asthma is suspected, but PEF recordings at home, work, and on holiday may be more useful. Should only be carried out in a tertiary referral centre, under expert supervision
- *Sputum analysis* Sputum eosinophilia may help confirm the diagnosis
- *Aspergillus* Specific IgE to *Aspergillus* or skin tests may be useful if *Aspergillus* sensitivity is a concern. See ➲ p. 463
- *Laryngoscopy/ENT examination* Useful if concerns about nasal symptoms or obstruction, e.g. from polyps, or to exclude upper airway obstruction, or a vocal cord abnormality
- *Bronchoscopy* Rarely needed. Its main use is to exclude an obstructing airway tumour, e.g. carcinoid
- *Lung biopsy* is very occasionally needed in those in whom no adequate explanation for persistent and minimally reversible airflow obstruction is seen, to exclude another cause, e.g. bronchiolitis obliterans
- *Biomarker* studies support the measurement of exhaled nitric oxide concentration (feNO) to determine optimum inhaled corticosteroid dose in moderate asthma. This may also be useful in diagnosis (but is not a very specific measure), along with measures of induced sputum and blood eosinophils.

Box 18.4 Important differential diagnoses in asthma

Consider especially if unusual features in the history, or poor correlation between objective measures and symptoms, or poor treatment response:
- Upper airway obstruction (breathlessness, noisy, stridulous breathing, low peak flows out of proportion to FEV_1)
- Foreign body aspiration
- Tumour, especially tracheal (but can respond to steroids)
- Congestive cardiac failure (CCF) (young patient with a murmur)
- Vocal cord dysfunction (VCD)
- Hyperventilation syndrome
- Chronic thromboembolic disease or primary pulmonary hypertension (PPH)
- ILD
- EGPA (Churg–Strauss syndrome) and other eosinophilic lung diseases
- Bronchiolitis (see ➲ p. 164)
- GORD.

Acute severe asthma (in adults)

Most asthma deaths occur outside hospital and are:
- In patients with chronic severe disease
- In those receiving inadequate medical treatment
- In those who have been symptomatically deteriorating and may have already sought medical help
- Associated with adverse behavioural and psychosocial factors
- See Box 18.5 for hospital management of acute asthma.

Fatality in asthma is due to cardiac arrest 2° to hypoxia and acidosis—reversal of hypoxia is paramount.

Give high-flow O_2.

Risk factors for fatal or near-fatal asthma
- Previous near-fatal asthma, e.g. previous ventilation or respiratory acidosis
- Three or more classes of asthma medication
- Repeated A&E attendances
- High β_2 agonist use
- Adverse psychosocial features
- Background difficult asthma.

Severity of acute asthma
Moderate
- Increasing symptoms
- PEFR ≥50–75% predicted or best
- No features of acute severe asthma
- 1h following treatment in A&E, patients with PEF >75% predicted or best may be discharged home with appropriate changes to their asthma medication in the absence of concerns, e.g.:
  - Significant ongoing symptoms
  - Compliance concerns
  - Living alone
  - Psychological problems or learning difficulties
  - Previous near-fatal or brittle asthma
  - Nocturnal presentation
  - Pregnant
  - Exacerbation despite adequate oral steroid pre-presentation.

Severe asthma

Defined as any of:
- PEFR 33–50% predicted or best
- RR ≥25
- HR ≥110
- Inability to complete sentence in one breath.

Life-threatening asthma

Any one of:
- PEFR <33%
- SaO_2 <92% (NB needs ABG)
- *PaO_2 <8kPa*
- Normal CO_2 (4.6–6kPa)
- Silent chest
- Cyanosis
- Poor respiratory effort
- Bradycardia/arrhythmia/hypotension
- Exhaustion
- Confusion
- Coma.

Near-fatal asthma
- Raised $PaCO_2$, and/or
- Needing mechanical ventilation with raised inflation pressures.

▶▶ **Box 18.5 Hospital treatment of acute asthma**
- Airway—ensure no upper airway obstruction
- Breathing—give high-flow O_2
- Circulation—gain IV access.

Monitoring
- Record PEF on arrival in A&E, 15–30min after starting treatment, and regularly thereafter, according to response
- Record O_2 saturation, and maintain 94–98%
- ABG for pH and $PaCO_2$ (if saturation <92% or other severe features)
- Record and document HR and RR
- Measure glucose and potassium
- O_2—high concentration (40–60%) and high-flow mask, e.g. Hudson
- CXR to exclude infection/pneumothorax.

NB CO_2 retention, following administration of high-flow O_2, is not a problem in acute asthma. *A high CO2 indicates a life-threatening attack and should precipitate urgent ITU review for invasive ventilatory support, not controlled O2 therapy or NIV.* CO_2 is often low (due to hyperventilation), thus a normal CO_2 may indicate a tiring patient.

(Continued)

Box 18.5 (Continued)

Treatment

- β_2 *agonist*—inhaled or nebulized, e.g. nebulized salbutamol 2.5–5mg, driven by O_2
  - Give repeated doses or continuous, e.g. 5–10mg/h
  - Use IV only if inhaled therapy cannot be used reliably (rarely the case)
  - Note: risk of hypokalaemia with β_2 agonist and steroids. Repeated use of β_2 agonists may lead to lactic acidosis
- *Anticholinergic*—nebulized ipratropium bromide added to β_2 agonist therapy may improve bronchodilatation in acute severe asthma, if poor initial β_2 agonist response
- *Steroids*—the earlier given in an attack, the better the outcome
  - Oral is as effective as IV
  - Dose 40–50mg PO prednisolone, continuing for at least 5 days or until recovery. There is no agreed definition of recovery, but sensible to continue oral steroids until peak flow is maintained for 5–7 days. The dose can be stopped abruptly (assuming the patient continues on inhaled steroid). This does not apply to patients on repeated doses or long-term steroids where a longer course may be appropriate
  - Inhaled corticosteroids should be continued (or started as soon as possible) as part of the chronic disease management plan
- *IV magnesium sulfate*—immediately if very severe and if poor response to above therapies, 1.2–2g IV infusion over 20min. The safety and efficacy of repeated doses have not been assessed. Recent data suggest nebulized magnesium may also be of benefit though must be adequately diluted. Further data are awaited
- *IV aminophylline*—some patients may respond; give if poor response to initial therapy, in acute severe or life-threatening disease
  - Dose—5mg/kg loading dose over 20min, followed by continuous infusion of 0.5–0.7mg/kg (500mg in 500mL normal saline or 0.5% glucose at 0.5 × body weight in kg/mL/h). If on maintenance therapy, do not give loading dose, but start continuous infusion
  - Note: needs therapeutic drug monitoring. Side effects: nausea, arrhythmias, palpitations
- *Antibiotics*—only give if definite infective element to the exacerbation. Most exacerbations are due to viruses, especially the common cold. *C. pneumoniae* and *M. pneumoniae* are also implicated
- *IV fluids*—patients are often dehydrated. Hypokalaemia (due to β_2 agonists) must be corrected
- *IM adrenaline*—may be useful if near arrest, whilst awaiting ICU support.

ICU referral

Liaise with ICU early! Better to discuss early a patient who does not subsequently need ICU input, than to find you and your patient in difficulty, with no ICU bed. See Box 18.6.

There is no evidence to support the use of NIV in the management of asthma. Hypercapnic respiratory failure in acute severe asthma is an urgent indication for endotracheal intubation.

Box 18.6 When to discuss with ITU
- Worsening PEF despite treatment
- Worsening hypoxia
- Hypercapnia (or rising CO_2 even if not yet >6kPa)
- Falling pH
- Exhaustion/poor respiratory effort
- Drowsiness/confusion
- Respiratory arrest.

Discharge
Consider discharge when:
- Reduced β_2 agonist dose
- Off nebulized drugs and on inhalers ≥24h
- PEF ≥75% predicted or best
- Minimal PEF diurnal variation
- Appropriate education has been given.

Prior to discharge, consider:
- Reason for the exacerbation. Could it have been avoided?
- Check patient's self-management plan/asthma action plan
- Check inhaler technique (see ➜ p. 685)
- Book an appointment with GP or practice nurse for within 2 days
- Book chest clinic appointment.

Chronic asthma: management (adults)

Aim to minimize symptoms and prevent exacerbations, prevent the potential consequences of long-standing airway inflammation leading to airway remodelling and chronic unresponsive airway obstruction, and improve QoL (see Box 18.7).

The emphasis should be on education, self-management, and personal asthma action plans. Aim for:

- Minimal day and night symptoms
- No exacerbations
- Normal lung function and prevention of lung function decline with the development of fixed airflow obstruction
- No limit to physical activity
- Minimum steroid dose.

Treatment is based on disease severity, using a step-up/step-down approach, starting treatment at the level appropriate to disease severity, based on the history, spirometry, and medication usage.

> **Box 18.7 The main aims during outpatient review are:**
> - Ensure the diagnosis is correct and that symptoms are due to asthma and not coexistent/alternative pathology (e.g. reflux, hyperventilation syndrome, etc.)
> - Aim for no symptoms/normal lung function on minimal treatment
> - Ensure an action plan is in place for exacerbations
> - Identify patients at risk of an adverse outcome.

Pharmacological management

BTS guidelines for the management of asthma

Step 1—mild intermittent asthma

- Short-acting β_2 agonist
- Check compliance, inhaler technique (including with spacer, if used), and eliminate potential triggers
- Ten puffs/day (two or more canisters/month) is a marker of poorly controlled disease.

Step 2—regular preventer therapy

- Start at 400 micrograms/day beclometasone (BDP) or equivalent in a twice-daily dose
- Titrate steroid dose to symptoms, aiming for lowest effective dose
- Local steroid side effects only (oral *Candida*, dysphonia) from BDP ≤800 micrograms/day
- Possible dose-related bone density effects at this dose or above
- Fluticasone provides equal clinical activity to budesonide at half dosage. Mometasone is an alternative inhaled steroid; the current limited evidence suggests it is equivalent to twice the dose of BDP. Ciclesonide

is a pro-drug, and the available evidence suggests it may have fewer local oropharyngeal side effects and less systemic activity than conventional inhaled steroids. The clinical benefit and efficacy to safety ratio data have not been fully established

- Qvar® (beclometasone dipropionate) has a smaller particle size and may be of benefit in some; 400 micrograms bd is comparable to fluticasone 500 micrograms bd and budesonide 800 micrograms bd.

Step 3—add-on therapy
- If taking 200–800 micrograms/day inhaled steroid, consider adding a long-acting β_2 agonist (LABA). A combination preparation may be appropriate
- If there is no response to a LABA, stop it and increase the inhaled steroid
- The combination of an inhaled corticosteroid and LABA is licensed as maintenance *and* reliever therapy, if a rapid-onset LABA, e.g. formoterol, is used in the context of a personal asthma action plan.

Step 4—poor control on moderate-dose inhaled steroid and add-on therapy: addition of fourth drug
- Ensure definite benefit is obtained from any of these subsequent drugs before continuing
- Leukotriene receptor antagonist—about a third of patients respond. May be useful if atopic or for exercise-induced asthma. Trial for 1 month, and stop if there is no response. Also indicated in allergic rhinitis—so consider if this is present as well
- Theophylline (has side effects, e.g. nausea, and needs therapeutic drug monitoring)
- Slow-release oral β_2 agonist, e.g. bambuterol 10–20mg nocte
- If control is inadequate on 800 micrograms BDP equivalent with a LABA, can increase inhaled steroid dose to 2,000 micrograms BDP equivalent in a combination inhaler
- Consider the use of tiotropium or equivalent.

Step 5—continuous or frequent use of oral steroids
- NB Risk of side effects if on oral steroids for >3 months or 3–4 courses/year
- Warn patient of potential side effects (hypertension, diabetes, cataracts, and gastric erosions), and ask GP to monitor. Start osteoporosis prophylaxis with calcium and vitamin D, or a bisphosphonate. Document baseline bone densitometry in those receiving prednisolone for >3 months (see ➲ p. 676). See ℘ http://www.rcplondon.ac.uk/publications/glucocorticoid-induced-osteoporosis
- Aim for the lowest possible dose of steroid.

Additional points
- **Regular review**—to ensure patients are on appropriate treatment for their disease severity and are maintained on the lowest possible inhaled steroid dose. This may include adherence/prescription reviews. Step down treatment if patient stable for 3 months or more. Step down

inhaled steroid by reducing dose by 25% at 3-monthly intervals. The Royal College of Physicians (RCP) has suggested three routine questions for monitoring (see Box 18.8)
- *Asthma action plan*—all patients with severe asthma should have an agreed written asthma action plan (self-management plan), their own peak flow meter, and regular checks on compliance and inhaler technique. A self-management plan should include specific advice about recognizing loss of asthma control and action to take if asthma deteriorates. Patients on low-dose inhaled steroids (200 micrograms) should have their dose increased 5-fold at the start of an exacerbation. This should not be extrapolated to higher inhaled steroid doses. The previous recommendation of doubling the dose of inhaled steroid at the start of an exacerbation is unproven.

Box 18.8 Monitoring morbidity—the three RCP questions

In the last week or month:
- Have you had difficulty sleeping because of your asthma symptoms (including cough)?
- Have you had your usual asthma symptoms during the day (cough, wheeze, chest tightness, or breathlessness)?
- Has your asthma interfered with your usual activities (e.g. work, housework)?

Chronic asthma: additional treatment options

Steroid-sparing drugs, e.g. methotrexate, oral gold, and ciclosporin—may be useful if other treatments are unsuccessful. They may reduce long-term steroid requirements, but all have side effects and need haematological surveillance. There are very few data to support their use, and significant variability in response. Guidelines suggest a 3-month trial, once other drugs have proven unsuccessful, with treatment in a centre with experience of their use.

Continuous subcutaneous terbutaline infusion via a portable syringe driver may be useful. Standard dose is 5mg over 24h, but up to 15mg/24h may be given. Use terbutaline nebulizer solution (2.5mg/mL), e.g. for 10mg/24h, use 4mL of nebulizer solution, with 6mL of saline and infuse the 10mL over 24h. Beneficial effects have been reported in severe asthma, but safety and efficacy have not been assessed in RCTs. Best responders may be those with marked PEF variability ('type 1 brittle asthmatics') to allow steroid reduction.

Omalizumab Recombinant humanized monoclonal antibody against IgE has been shown to reduce early and late asthmatic responses after allergen challenge and is licensed for atopic individuals with difficult-to-control disease, in combination with other standard treatments. The drug removes circulating and tissue IgE by promoting loss of high-affinity IgE receptors on mast cells, basophils, and dendritic cells, leading to reduced airway inflammation. Compared with placebo, it has been shown to reduce exacerbation rates, with improvement in asthma symptoms and QoL scores, but with no overall change in lung function. Meta-analyses suggest a reduction of around 100 micrograms of inhaled corticosteroid is achieved per day, compared with placebo.

Omalizumab is given as a subcutaneous injection every 2–4 weeks. The dose depends on the patient's weight and serum IgE concentration; the peak response is at 12–16 weeks, and two-thirds of patients respond. The serum IgE should be 30–700IU/mL, with higher IgE levels acceptable at higher body weights. There is a high risk of anaphylaxis at higher IgE levels.

There is some debate as to whether the high cost of the drug can be justified. The 2013 NICE guideline suggest its use for severe persistent allergic asthma, which is unstable despite optimized standard therapy (continuous oral steroid or >4 courses/year), and it should be used for a trial period of a maximum of 16 weeks, ceasing if there is no clinical response.

Mepolizumab A not yet licensed, humanized monoclonal antibody against IL5 (a growth and differentiation factor for eosinophils) has been shown in a recent RCT to approximately halve the exacerbation rate in those prone to exacerbations with evidence of eosinophilic inflammation (i.e. one or more of: sputum eosinophils ≥3%, feNO ≥50ppb, blood eosinophils ≥0.3 × 10^9, prompt asthma deterioration following ≤25% reduction in inhaled or oral steroid therapy).

Macrolides Early evidence suggests azithromycin may reduce the rate of severe exacerbations in non-eosinophilic asthma (blood eosinophils ≤200/mL).

Further information

Walker S. Anti-IgE for chronic asthma. *Cochrane Database Syst Rev* 2003;**3**:CD003559.

Holgate ST. Efficacy and safety of anti-immunoglobulin-E antibody (omalizumab) in severe allergic asthma. *Clin Exp Allergy* 2004;**34**:632.

Pavord ID et al. Mepolizumab for severe eosinophilic asthma (DREAM): a multicenter, double-blind, placebo-controlled trial. *Lancet* 2012;**380**:651–9.

Brusselle GG et al. Azithromycin for prevention of exacerbations in severe asthma (AZISAST): a multicenter randomized double-blind placebo-controlled trial. *Thorax* 2013;**68**:322–9.

Non-pharmacological management

Allergen avoidance may reduce severity of disease in sensitized individual; however, despite theoretical benefits, it is generally hard to demonstrate the benefit of allergen avoidance in clinical trials. House dust mite control measures need to be comprehensive—there is no current evidence to support it, although trials are ongoing. Pet removal may be useful, if the history is suggestive and sensitivity has been demonstrated by skin prick testing or raised specific IgE levels.

Smoking cessation may reduce asthma severity. Current and previous smoking reduces the effect of inhaled steroid; these individuals may need higher steroid doses.

Complementary therapies No consistent evidence of benefit.

Dietary manipulation No consistent evidence and none supported by interventional trials. Low magnesium intake is associated with increased asthma prevalence. Fish oils may be beneficial.

Weight reduction in obese asthmatics leads to improved control.

Immunotherapy Desensitization using allergen-specific immunotherapy may be beneficial in a small subgroup of patients.

Buteyko breathing technique is a series of breathing exercises involving breathing control. One study showed a reduction in the use of inhaled bronchodilator and steroid use in asthmatics carrying out these exercises, with no change in lung function or BHR. A Cochrane review of breathing exercises concluded that there was no evidence of improvement in lung function but improved QoL scores.

Future developments

New steroids Research for 'dissociated steroids' is ongoing. These are steroids in which the useful anti-inflammatory effects (mediated by transcription factor inhibition) are dissociated from the side effects (mediated via glucocorticoid DNA binding). Safer steroids, e.g. ciclesonide, a new once-a-day inhaled steroid, appear to have an improved side effect profile. Ciclesonide is a pro-drug, activated by airway esterases, with fewer side effects due to high degrees of protein binding.

Eosinophil inhibitors A variety of approaches to inhibit eosinophil recruitment are under investigation, including adhesion molecule inhibition and eosinophil chemotactic receptor inhibition, and IL5 inhibition (e.g. mepolizumab).

Phosphodiesterase-4 inhibitors New-generation phosphodiesterase (PDE)-4 inhibitors, e.g. roflumilast, are being investigated in clinical trials. These drugs have a broad anti-inflammatory action, with neutrophil inhibitory effects. Early clinical trial data looks promising.

Cytokine modulators Tumour necrosis factor (TNF)-α plays an important role in the pathogenesis of asthma. Anti-TNF antibodies have been beneficial in the treatment of inflammatory bowel disease (IBD) and RA.

Anti-TNF may be useful in the treatment of severe asthma, as it may block other important leukotrienes, e.g. IL13.

Bronchial thermoplasty This is the application of controlled radiofrequency energy to the airway wall, using a specialized catheter at bronchoscopy. It heats the tissue to about 65°C, reducing muscle mass in the small and medium-sized airways, with several airways treated under direct vision at each session. Three separate sessions are required to treat all accessible airways. This has only been assessed in a small trial and is well tolerated. Improved asthma QoL scores, reduced airway hyperresponsiveness, and reduced oral steroid doses are reported, with small reductions in hospital admissions. The mechanism of action is unlikely to be improved airway contractility alone, and neurohumoral effects are postulated. A small placebo-controlled trial in 32 patients has shown significantly worse initial symptoms and side effects, but a small longer-term improvement at 22 and 52 weeks. This procedure should only be used with special arrangements for clinical governance, consent, and audit or research.

Further information

BTS/SIGN Asthma Guidelines. ℘ http://www.brit-thoracic.org.uk/Portals/0/Guidelines/AsthmaGuidelines/sign101%20Jan%202012.pdf.

NICE guidance on bronchial thermoplasty. ℘ http://guidance.nice.org.uk/IPG419.

Wu Q et al. Meta-analysis of the efficacy and safety of bronchial thermoplasty in patients with moderate-to-severe persistent asthma. *J Int Med Res* 2011;**39**:10–22.

℘ http://www.brit-thoracic.org.uk/guidelines/asthma-guidelines.aspx—a good site from which to download copies of the asthma guidelines in various formats and to obtain training information.

℘ http://www.occupationalasthma.com.

℘ http://www.ginasthma.com.

Difficult/refractory asthma

Patients with refractory asthma are a small subgroup of asthma patients (5–10%). They have disease that is difficult to treat, evidenced by high maintenance medication requirements or persistent symptoms and airflow obstruction, with multiple exacerbations, despite high medication use. They have high numbers of admissions and cause significant anxiety to their families and medical staff. There is a wide range of disease severity, including those with highly labile disease and those with severe, more chronic airflow obstruction. No consensus definition.

The disease is usually 'defined' on the basis of:

- Medication requirements (continuous or near continuous oral steroids)
- Asthma symptoms
- Frequency of exacerbations
- Severity of airflow limitation.

Patients exhibit the features of asthma, and it is thought that the airflow obstruction, airway hyperresponsiveness, and PEF diurnal variability are more severe in refractory disease, though the physiological reasons for this remain unclear.

These patients typically fail to completely reverse their airflow obstruction following a 2-week course of oral prednisolone and demonstrate a poor bronchodilator response to inhaled β_2 agonists.

The pathological mechanism is likely to be ongoing airway inflammation, with increasing airway fibrosis, but this is not proven. Other possibilities include steroid resistance (see ➔ p. 145), β_2 receptor down-regulation, or a different disease process altogether. They may represent the non-eosinophilic end of the spectrum of asthma. Treatment non-adherence is overrepresented in patients with difficult asthma.

Diagnosis of refractory asthma

- Confirm the diagnosis is correct—this will mean going back through the notes and retaking a thorough history
- Confirm reversible airflow limitation now or in the past (as for non-refractory asthma; see ➔ p. 130)
- Consider other diagnoses for cough, breathlessness, and wheeze, and investigate for potential exacerbating diseases:
  - COPD/smoking/α1-AT deficiency
  - Bronchiectasis/CF
  - Sinus disease—consider ENT review
  - EGPA (Churg–Strauss syndrome)/eosinophilic syndromes—consider ANCA
  - Systemic disease—thyroid disease or vasculitis
  - ABPA—consider *Aspergillus* precipitins/skin tests/IgE
  - VCD—consider laryngoscopy
  - Hyperventilation syndrome/dysfunctional breathing
  - Gastro-oesophageal reflux—consider OGD/24h pH
  - Upper airway obstruction—consider CT or bronchoscopy
  - OSA—consider sleep study

- Obesity
- Cardiac dysfunction—consider echo and/or cardiological opinion
- Psychiatric/emotional issues/depression/2° gain—consider psychiatry or psychology review
- Functional wheeze by breathing near residual volume.

Refractory asthma

Before labelling a patient as 'refractory', compliance must be confirmed. This may be by checking pharmacy prescription records, using inhaler devices monitoring medication usage, or by measurement of plasma prednisolone or early morning cortisol levels.

Treatment is that of non-refractory asthma, with inhaled LABA and high-dose inhaled corticosteroids (see ➲ pp. 136–8). Ensure treatment trials are adequate and adhered to.

- In patients unable to tolerate a prednisolone dose <20mg/day, corticosteroid pharmacokinetic studies may be useful. However, <25% of patients with severe asthma show clinically significantly increased prednisolone clearance (usually a specific reason can be identified such as concomitant use of enzyme-inducing medication). IM steroid, e.g. triamcinolone 120mg, may be useful if compliance is a major problem
- Nebulized budesonide (Respules®, 1–2mg bd) may be of benefit
- Inflammatory markers, e.g. sputum or plasma eosinophil counts or feNO, may be useful to assess medication response, although no trials have demonstrated their use clinically in this group of patients
- Anti-inflammatory and immunomodulating drugs (specialized centre only). Include methotrexate, ciclosporin, oral gold, and IV gammaglobulin. None of these have been studied in an RCT in this group of patients, and none have demonstrated improvement in airway hyperresponsiveness
- Macrolide antibiotics have anti-inflammatory and immune modulatory effects, reducing airway reactivity and inflammation, and have been shown to reduce oral steroid requirements and reduce exacerbation rate in non-eosinophilic asthma. Persistence of airway infection by *C. pneumoniae* and *Mycoplasma* is increasingly recognized as a contributory factor in persistent airflow obstruction and recurrent exacerbations, and macrolide antibiotics may act in this situation to clear persistent infection. Use, e.g. azithromycin 250mg, on alternate days or 3 times a week, or 500mg twice weekly. 6-weekly LFT monitoring is required. Risk of hearing loss.

'Steroid-resistant' asthma This subgroup of patients represents a very small proportion of refractory asthma patients. They are likely to be the non-eosinophilic end of the spectrum. Middle-aged obese women, often with other additional diagnoses, are overrepresented in this group. They require supportive treatment, without high doses of glucocorticoids. Diagnoses other than asthma are likely, and investigation should be directed towards these. Whether they represent a further 'asthma phenotype' is not clear.

Further information
Robinson DS *et al*. Systematic assessment of difficult-to-treat asthma. *Eur Respir J* 2003;22:478–83.
Thomas PS *et al*. Pseudo-steroid resistant asthma. *Thorax* 1999;54:352–6.

Asthma in pregnancy

- Pregnancy can affect asthma
- Asthma can affect the outcome of pregnancy
- Prognosis—1/3 worsen, 1/3 improve, 1/3 no change
- Asthma course is likely to be similar in successive pregnancies
- Severe asthma is more likely to deteriorate than mild asthma
- Most exacerbations occur late, in the second and third trimester, and are due to viral infections and non-adherence to inhaled corticosteroid.

Pre-pregnancy counselling

- Asthmatics must continue normal asthma medication
- Give smoking cessation advice
- Monitor the pregnant asthmatic closely
- Severe exacerbations in pregnancy are associated with low birthweight infants, an effect similar to maternal smoking in pregnancy.

Acute asthma in pregnancy

- Risk to foetus of uncontrolled asthma outweighs any small risk of drugs
- Asthma medications are generally safe in pregnancy
- Steroids should be continued.

- Drug therapy as for non-asthmatics, including inhaled and oral corticosteroids
- Maintain O_2 saturation >94–98%
- Continuous foetal monitoring for acute severe asthma
- Liaise with obstetrician if acute severe asthma

Leukotriene receptor antagonists

Limited safety data available for use in pregnancy, and it is recommended not to start using whilst pregnant. Continue in women who have previously demonstrated significant improvement in disease control prior to pregnancy.

Management during labour

- Acute asthma is rare in labour (probably due to high sympathetic drive)
- Close liaison between the respiratory and obstetric teams is paramount, with close foetal monitoring
- Management should be as for non-pregnant individuals (see ➌ pp. 136–8), maintaining the O_2 saturation >94–98%. There is no RCT data for magnesium sulfate, although it is used in eclampsia
- Regional anaesthetic blockade is preferable to general anaesthesia
- Prostaglandin E_2 may be safely used for induction of labour
- Prostaglandin $F_2\alpha$ (for post-partum bleeding) may cause bronchospasm
- Give parenteral hydrocortisone, 100mg 6–8-hourly, during labour if on oral prednisolone at >7.5mg daily for >2 weeks prior to delivery.

Breastfeeding
- An asthmatic mother may reduce the chance of atopy in her child by breastfeeding; current opinion is divided
- Prednisolone is secreted in breast milk, but the infant is exposed to only tiny, and clinically irrelevant, doses.

Occupational asthma

- This is asthma due to specific workplace sensitizers and may account for 10% of adult-onset asthma
- The diagnosis is often difficult to make
- Early diagnosis is important, as earlier removal from the workplace in affected individuals leads to a better outcome
- It is different to asthma exacerbated by irritants in the workplace and can occur in individuals with or without prior asthma.

- Agents induce asthma through immunological and non-immunological mechanisms. Immunological disease appears after a latency period of exposure; thus, it is necessary for the worker to be sensitized to the causal agent. Non-immunological disease is characterized by the absence of a latent period and occurs after accidental exposure to high concentrations of a workplace irritant. This is irritant-induced asthma (previously named reactive airways dysfunction syndrome), usually caused by exposure to, e.g. smoke, vapours, or fumes, with a strong temporal relationship between irritant exposure and the development of asthma-type symptoms
- The latency between first exposure and symptom onset can be long and depends on the sensitizing agent—an accurate history therefore includes current and past exposures
- Once sensitized, re-exposure to very low concentrations can provoke symptoms
- May be associated with rhinitis and urticaria
- Improves away from work but can take several days to settle.

Risk factors
- Atopy
- HLA type (e.g. HLA-DQB1*0503 associated with isocyanate allergy)
- Smoking (especially for high molecular weight agents).

Diagnosis
- Confirm the diagnosis of asthma
- Confirm the relationship between asthma and work exposures
- Find the specific cause
- There are two useful screening questions:
  - Is your asthma worse when at work?
  - Does your asthma improve when away from work or on holiday?

Document lung function deterioration in the workplace, usually by serial peak flow recording at work, at home, and on holiday.

Bronchial provocation/challenge testing using suspected agent—only in specialized centres, but difficulties with testing and producing a valid test substance mean that a negative specific bronchial challenge in a worker with otherwise good evidence of occupational asthma is not sufficient to exclude the diagnosis.

Skin prick testing/specific IgE for certain sensitizers (although a positive test only indicates sensitization which can occur with or without disease).

Document
- The range of chemicals used, and look up the literature on their propensity to cause asthma (see Table 18.1)
- Working practices
- Use of personal protective equipment.

Serial PEF recording in occupational asthma
- Record every 2h from waking to sleep
- For 4 weeks, whilst no changes to treatment
- Document home/work periods and any holidays
- Analysis is best made by experts, usually using a criterion-based analysis system, e.g. OASYS (a computer program that plots and interprets serial peak flow recordings; see ℬ http://www.occupationalasthma.com)
- Patients may be sensitized to >1 agent, and >300 agents have been identified.

Table 18.1 Causes of occupational asthma

Sensitizing agent	Occupational exposure
Low molecular weight agents (act as haptens)	
Isocyanates	Paint spraying, adhesives, polyurethane foams
Acid anhydrides	Epoxy paint, varnish, resins, baking
Metals	Welding, plating, metal refining
Glutaraldehyde and other disinfectants	Health care workers
Drugs	Pharmaceutical industry
High molecular weight agents	
Amine dyes	Cosmetics, hair dyes, rubber workers
Wood dusts, bark	Textile workers, joiners, carpenters
Animal-derived antigens	Vets, laboratory workers (20% affected)
Biological enzymes	Detergent industry, pharmaceuticals
Plant products	Bakers, hairdressers
Fluxes, colophony	Solderers, electronics industry

Management of occupational asthma

- Identify the cause
- Remove the worker from exposure
- Support continued employment away from the cause, if at all possible
- Early diagnosis and removal from exposure are important factors for a good outcome
- Improvement in FEV_1 may be maintained for 1y following last exposure, and for up to 2y for non-specific responsiveness
- The decision to remove the patient from the workplace should not be taken lightly and should be made by a consultant with experience of occupational lung disease
- The employee may be eligible for *Disablement Benefit* (no proof of negligence is required).

Latex allergy is seen in up to 18% of health care workers and is the leading cause of occupational asthma in this group due to the widespread use of latex gloves. It is potentially serious, with avocado, bananas, kiwi, and chestnuts cross-reacting to give a similar clinical picture. Treatment is absolute avoidance; those affected should wear a MedicAlert bracelet and always use non-latex gloves.

Vocal cord dysfunction

A proportion of patients labelled as having severe asthma will have symptoms originating from the upper airway. This can be due to VCD and/or so-called 'upper airway hyperresponsiveness'; these are different but overlap. VCD is likely to arise from interrelationships between laryngeal hyperresponsiveness and autonomic imbalance, with inputs from potential aetiological/aggravating factors such as reflux, psychological stress, hypocapnia (hyperventilation). Increased laryngeal hyperresponsiveness can occur following respiratory tract infections and possibly asthma itself. Upper airway hyperresponsiveness may include more than just the larynx, but this is not clear.

Patients will typically present with asthma symptoms, with associated triggers, e.g. odours, cold air. They typically have no reduction in peak flow or response to asthma medications (though this is possible).

A careful history will reveal shortness of breath that is of short duration, worse on inspiration, and extremely sudden in onset, with symptom-free periods.

Pathogenesis

- Recent URTI, may take months to settle
- Post-nasal drip/chronic sinusitis
- GORD with micro-aspiration
- Chronic laryngitis
- Hyperventilation in association with anxiety/panic
- It is postulated that the origin of the vocal cord closure may stem from a reflex airway protective mechanism.

Diagnosis is based on excluding other causes of cough and breathlessness. It may be suggested by hearing a more stridulous noise and lack of basal wheeze. The gold standard is visualization of abnormal vocal cord movement at laryngoscopy, where there is excessive adduction of the anterior two-thirds of cords with the creation of a posterior 'glottic chink', although this finding may not always be present at the time of study. The flow–volume loop should show inspiratory flow limitation, with 'stuttering' of the flow.

Treatment (for which there are no RCTs)
- Speech therapy
- Panting (autopeep)
- Coughing and cough suppression techniques
- Inspiratory resistance devices
- HELIOX/nebulized saline/lidocaine spray
- Sedatives
- Exercise.

Further information

Newman KB et al. Clinical features of vocal cord dysfunction. Am J Respir Crit Care Med 1995;**152**:1382–6.

Stanton AE, Bucknall CE. Vocal cord dysfunction. A review. Breathe 2005;**2**:31–7 (ℛ http://www.ers-education.org/publications/breathe/archive/september-2005.aspx).

Allergic rhinitis (hay fever)

This is the syndrome of nasal discharge or blockage, with nasal and/or eye itching and sneezing. It is often associated with post-nasal drip, cough, fatigue, and with significant morbidity. Allergic rhinitis is defined as perennial if the symptoms occur year round, and seasonal if occurring at a particular time of year. The prevalence is increasing and affects up to 15% of the UK population. Up to 30% of patients with persistent allergic rhinitis have asthma.

Aetiology The lining of the nose is in continuum with the lower respiratory tract, and inflammation of the upper and lower airways often coexists. Common aeroallergens provoking seasonal allergic rhinitis are tree pollen in the spring and grass pollen in the summer months. Perennial rhinitis usually reflects allergy to indoor allergens such as house dust mite (the provoking allergen is a digestive enzyme that is shed in the faeces), cat salivary protein, cockroaches, or animal dander.

Pathophysiology Symptoms occur following the inhalation of allergen to which the subject is sensitized and against which they have IgE antibodies. These antibodies bind to mast cell IgE receptors, with the release of mediators, including tryptase and histamine, causing symptoms immediately after exposure.

Diagnosis is usually made from the history, which should identify the triggers to the disease. The main differential diagnosis is with sinusitis due to bacterial infection and upper airway involvement due to vasculitis. Asthma is common in association with rhinitis, and treatment of rhino-sinusitis in association with asthma leads to improved asthma control. Up to 50% of asthma patients will have allergic rhinitis.

Treatment

- Allergen avoidance This may be easier said than done. It can take up to 20 weeks to remove cat allergen from a house. Keeping car and house windows shut may help avoid pollen. Pollen counts are highest in the afternoon and early evening. Wearing sunglasses may reduce the ill-understood 'photic-sneeze' reflex, commoner in allergic rhinitis sufferers.
- Desensitization with increasing doses of the subcutaneous allergen (see ➲ p. 142), debatable value, small risk of anaphylaxis during such therapy
- Non-sedating antihistamines improve sneezing and itching but have less effect on nasal blockage
- Topical intranasal steroid, e.g. budesonide, triamcinolone
- Topical anticholinergics, e.g. ipratropium, may be useful for rhinorrhoea, if uncontrolled with topical nasal steroids
- Topical sodium cromoglicate may be beneficial, particularly for allergic conjunctivitis
- Decongestants, e.g. oxymetazoline, may help, but rebound nasal blockage and tachyphylaxis are a potential problem if used regularly
- Leukotriene receptor antagonists (e.g. montelukast) may be beneficial.

Chapter 19

Bronchiectasis

Epidemiology, pathophysiology, and causes

Definition Irreversible abnormal dilatation of one or more bronchi, with chronic airway inflammation. Associated chronic sputum production, recurrent chest infections, and airflow obstruction.

Epidemiology Prevalence of bronchiectasis is unknown but is probably falling due to vaccinations and the improved and earlier treatment of childhood infections. However, the advent of HRCT scanning may now lead to the diagnosis of more subtle (and possibly subclinical) disease.

Pathophysiology An initial (usually infectious) insult is needed to damage the airways. Disordered anatomy leads to 2° bacterial colonization, perpetuating inflammatory change and damaging the mucociliary escalator. This prevents bacterial clearance and leads to further airway damage. Major airways and bronchioles are involved, with mucosal oedema, inflammation, and ulceration. Terminal bronchioles become obstructed with secretions, leading to volume loss. A chronic host inflammatory response ensues, with free radical formation and production of neutrophil elastase, further contributing to inflammation. Bronchial neovascularization, with hypertrophy and tortuosity of the bronchial arteries (which are at systemic pressure), may lead to intermittent haemoptyses.

Aetiology The causes of bronchiectasis are many and varied (see Table 19.1). In general, the aetiology is either a one-off infectious insult or an underlying immune deficiency. Determining the aetiology of the condition may lead to different management if, for example, the underlying cause is found to be CF, rather than an immune deficiency. The cause is idiopathic in around 50% of cases, and these are likely to be due to an (as yet unidentified) impairment in host defence.

The most important cause to exclude is CF (see ➲ p. 209). Even relatively mild bronchiectasis diagnosed in middle age can be due to CF; this diagnosis will alter management, with:
- Involvement of the multidisciplinary CF team
- Attention to other potential problems, e.g. GI disease, diabetes
- Inheritance (relevant to the rest of the family)
- Fertility issues.

Consider investigations for CF (CFTR mutation screen and sweat test; see ➲ pp. 210–1) if:
- Predominantly upper lobe disease
- Persistent *S. aureus* infection or *Haemophilus influenzae* or *Pseudomonas aeruginosa* colonization
- Malnutrition ± malabsorption, diabetes
- Family history of CF or bronchiectasis
- Associated subfertility or infertility
- Age <40 at presentation and no other cause for bronchiectasis identified.

Table 19.1 Causes of bronchiectasis

Genetic	CF
Congenital	Pulmonary sequestration
Post-infective	TB
	Whooping cough (if infection in a localized area)
	Severe pneumonia
	NTM (see → p. 518–9)—there is some debate as to whether the bronchiectasis seen in association with NTM (classically in elderly ♀) is caused or secondarily infected by NTM
Immune deficiency	1°
	2°—HIV, CLL, nephrotic syndrome
	(Excessive immune response—ABPA) (see → pp. 464–5)
Mucociliary clearance abnormalities	
	CF
	1° ciliary dyskinesia (see → pp. 630–1)
	Kartagener's syndrome
	Young's syndrome (bronchiectasis, sinusitis, and azoospermia, i.e. clinical features similar to those of CF)
Toxic insults	Aspiration
	Inhalation (toxic gases, chemicals)
Mechanical insults	Foreign body aspiration
	Extrinsic lymph node compression
	Intrinsic (intraluminal) obstructing tumour
Associations	Bronchiectasis is associated with a number of systemic diseases, so cough and sputum production in these conditions should trigger referral to determine the cause:
	RA (up to 35% of RA patients have bronchiectasis) (see → pp. 192–3)
	Connective tissue diseases, e.g. Sjögren's syndrome, SLE (see → p. 200)
	Ulcerative colitis and Crohn's disease (see → p. 251)
	Chronic sinusitis
	Yellow nail syndrome
	Marfan's syndrome

Clinical features and diagnosis

Suspect bronchiectasis in a patient with recurrent episodes of 'bronchitis' over several years prior to presentation.

Diagnosis is usually made clinically, with HRCT chest for confirmation.

Investigations are aimed at:

- Confirming the diagnosis
- Identifying a treatable underlying cause for the bronchiectasis (possible in about 50%)
- Optimizing management to prevent exacerbations and lung damage.

Essential investigations

- *CXR* sensitivity is only 50%, classically shows 'ring shadows' and 'tramlines'—indicating thickened airways, and the 'gloved finger' appearance. Consolidation around thickened and dilated airways
- *HRCT* chest is 97% sensitive in detecting disease. Typically shows airway dilatation to the lung periphery, bronchial wall thickening, and the airway appearing larger than its accompanying vessel (signet ring sign). Expiratory scans may be useful to demonstrate post-obstructive air trapping, indicative of small airways disease. If the bronchiectasis is localized to a single lobe, CT is useful to determine whether a central obstructing lesion is present. Contiguous 3mm slices are needed to exclude a central airway lesion if there is associated haemoptysis. Symptoms correlate with wall thickening and mucous plugging on CT scan. The radiological term 'traction bronchiectasis' refers to airway dilatation 2° to airway distortion, seen with chronic severe interstitial fibrosis. These patients rarely have clinical features of bronchiectasis
- *Lung function* FEV$_1$/FVC and flow-volume loop
- *Sputum microbiology* Standard M, C, & S (including for atypical organisms), AFB, and *Aspergillus*
- *PFTs* with reversibility testing
- *Immunoglobulins A, M, G*
- *Aspergillus* precipitins, *Aspergillus*-specific RAST, total IgE (see ➲ p. 464–5).

Additional investigations

- *CFTR mutation screen and sweat test* (see ➲ pp. 210–1)
- *Autoantibodies* (ANA, RhF, dsDNA) if associated arthritis/connective tissue disease
- *Vaccination response* to tetanus, *H. influenzae*, and pneumococcal antibodies if underlying immunosuppression suspected. If pneumoccoccal antibodies are low, arrange vaccination with Pneumovax, and repeat antibody testing 6 weeks later; failure to generate adequate pneumococcal antibody levels is suggestive of an immunodeficiency (e.g. IgG subclass deficiency), and referral to an immunologist may be required
- *Detailed immunological investigation* (including neutrophil and lymphocyte function studies)

- *Skin tests/RAST* to identify specific sensitizers (usually *Aspergillus*)
- *Bronchoscopy* to exclude a foreign body if suggested by CT; obtain microbiological samples if unusual clinical presentation or failure to respond to standard antibiotics
- *Nasal brushings/biopsy* (in tertiary centre) to assess ciliary beat frequency with video microscopy
- *Saccharin test* The time for saccharin to be tasted in the mouth after deposition of a 0.5mm particle on the inferior turbinate of the nose. Normal is <30min. A poor man's cilial function test
- α*1-AT levels* if deficiency is suspected
- *Barium swallow/oesophageal imaging* if recurrent aspiration suspected.

General management

The main aims of management of non-CF bronchiectasis are:
- Treatment of any underlying medical condition
- Prevention of exacerbations and progression of underlying disease by daily physiotherapy. The options for airway clearance include:
  - Active cycle of breathing technique—this involves breathing control with forced expiration (huffing) using variable thoracic expansion
  - Postural or autogenic drainage
  - Cough augmentation—using flutter valves/cough insufflator/ high-frequency oscillation/positive pressure devices
  - Exercise regimes—important to prevent general deconditioning
  - The physiotherapist is also vital during admission for exacerbations to help clear tenacious sputum
  - Nebulized hypertonic saline may improve airway clearance, although there is no RCT data to support its use in non-CF disease
- Reduction of bacterial load and prevention of 2° airway inflammation and damage with antimicrobial chemotherapy
- Supportive treatment—treatment of associated airflow obstruction
- Optimize nutrition
- Refer for pulmonary rehabilitation if breathlessness limits activities of daily living
- Refer for surgery if necessary—localized resection of affected area
- Refer for transplantation if indicated.

Antimicrobial chemotherapy
- This may be intermittent for exacerbations only (for mild disease) or long term for more severe disease. Antibiotics may be oral, nebulized, or IV
- Regular sputum surveillance will ensure the likely colonizing organism is known
- *In vivo* sensitivity may be different to *in vitro* sensitivity
- Patients need a higher antibiotic dose and for a longer time period (usually 2 weeks) than people without bronchiectasis
- Antibiotic treatment choice depends on the severity of the underlying disease
- Treatment response is usually assessed by a fall in sputum volume and change to mucoid from purulent or mucopurulent sputum, with an improvement in systemic symptoms, spirometry, and CRP
- *Pseudomonas*-colonized patients have more frequent exacerbations, worse CT scan appearances, and a faster decline in lung function.

Exacerbation treatment An exacerbation is usually a clinical diagnosis, with an increase in sputum volume and tenacity and with discoloration. It may be associated with chest pain, haemoptysis and wheeze, and systemic upset—fevers, lethargy, and anorexia. The CRP is not always elevated. Treatment depends on the potential pathogens and resident flora. Nebulized bronchodilators and regular physiotherapy (as an inpatient or outpatient) may also be needed.

Exacerbation of mild bronchiectasis
- Antibiotics for exacerbations only (tailored to the colonizing organism—review previous sputum microbiology)
- Sputum samples should be sent for M, C, & S prior to starting antibiotics, but empirical treatment can be started whilst awaiting culture results
- In the absence of prior positive microbiology, amoxicillin 500mg tds or clarithromycin 500mg bd for 14 days
- Use a higher-dose oral regime, e.g. amoxicillin 1g tds for 2 weeks, especially if colonized with *H. influenzae*
- A 2-week course of oral ciprofloxacin at 750mg bd if *Pseudomonas aeruginosa* colonized
- If early relapse, with a return to purulent sputum within 6–8 weeks, consider a longer course of oral antibiotics, e.g. amoxicillin 500mg bd or doxycycline 100mg od. If treatment failure, change to appropriate IV antibiotics until clinical improvement.

Exacerbation of more severe bronchiectasis
Chronic suppressive antibiotics aim to prevent progression of disease by reducing bacterial load and preventing ongoing inflammation, thereby reducing morbidity and improving QoL.
- Antibiotics are usually given for at least 2 days after the sputum has cleared—often for 2 weeks
- If oral antibiotics fail, IV treatment is required. This may mean inpatient admission or could involve long-line insertion, patient education in self-administration of IV antibiotics, and involvement of a home care team.

First isolate of Pseudomonas aeruginosa
(See ⏵ pp. 214–5.)
- Initial treatment is a 4–6-week course of oral ciprofloxacin 500–750mg bd and concurrent nebulized colistin 1–2MU bd
- If this fails and the patient still has *Pseudomonas* on sputum culture, there are several options—IV antibiotics, usually an anti-pseudomonal penicillin (minimum 2 weeks), a further 4 weeks of ciprofloxacin 750mg bd with nebulized colistin 2MU bd or 3 months nebulized colistin 2MU bd
- Combination IV antibiotics are only needed if there is resistance to one or more anti-pseudomonal antibiotics. Aminoglycoside antibiotic drug levels need careful monitoring
- Consider long-term therapy with daily nebulized colistin or gentamicin to reduce levels of *Pseudomonas* in colonized patients with frequent exacerbations.

Macrolide antibiotics have both antibacterial and immunomodulatory properties and decrease mucous production, alter inflammatory mediator release, and inhibit *Pseudomonas* virulence factors and biofilm formation. Five small trials have reported beneficial effects of macrolides in bronchiectasis, with reduced sputum volume and improved lung function and symptoms. The drugs are well tolerated, though concerns have been raised about NTM resistance with long-term use (see ⏵ pp. 520–1). Azithromycin 250mg 3 times weekly or 500mg twice weekly (with LFT monitoring) are possible regimes. Warn patient about possible side effects of hearing loss and tinnitus.

Further management

- *Self-management plan* Patients need an individual plan for exacerbations, which usually involves having a supply of home antibiotics
- Treatment of associated *airflow obstruction/wheeze* with inhaled steroids and/or bronchodilators
- There is no specific treatment for abnormalities of mucociliary function, although β_2 agonists may enhance airway clearance
- *Nebulized hypertonic saline* (7%) may aid sputum clearance
- *Acetylcysteine* may reduce sputum viscosity
- *Annual influenza and pneumococcal vaccinations*
- *Osteoporosis prophylaxis* (if on long-term steroids)
- *Reflux* treatment if aspiration
- *Immunoglobulin replacement therapy* Patients found to have immunoglobulin deficiency should be referred to an immunologist for further assessment. IV immunoglobulin replacement therapy is usually given once or twice monthly, as a day case or weekly subcutaneous at home
- *NIV* Hypercapnic ventilatory failure due to end-stage disease may need long-term nocturnal NIV. This can also be used as a bridge to transplantation
- *Surgery* This is the only potential curative treatment, with resection of a single chronically infected lobe occasionally being of benefit. It is less commonly needed now, as the incidence of single lobe disease related to previous severe childhood pneumonia is falling.
- *Transplant* is most commonly performed for CF bronchiectasis, but referral may be warranted for severe non-CF-related disease (see ➔ pp. 320–1)
- *Nebulized DNase* (dornase alfa)—no evidence for the use of this in non-CF bronchiectasis; it is not recommended.

Complications of bronchiectasis

- Infective exacerbation
- Haemoptysis—small-volume haemoptysis (increasing during exacerbations) is common. Massive haemoptysis (usually from tortuous bronchial arteries around damaged lung) is a life-threatening emergency (see ➔ p. 47)
- Pneumothorax
- Respiratory failure
- Opportunistic mycobacterial colonization
- ABPA
- Brain abscess (now very rare)
- Amyloidosis.

Bronchiectasis and *Aspergillus*

- ABPA—excessive immune response to environmental fungus *Aspergillus* (most commonly *fumigatus species*); may be the cause of bronchiectasis (suspect particularly if upper lobe disease), as mucus plugs become impacted in distal airways, causing airway damage and subsequent dilatation (see ➲ pp. 464–5)
- Aspergilloma—*Aspergillus* may colonize a previously formed cavity. This is extremely difficult to treat. Most commonly, it causes systemic upset and haemoptysis (see ➲ pp. 470–1).

Further information

Evans DJ, Bara A. Prolonged antibiotics for purulent bronchiectasis in children and adults. *Cochrane Database Syst Rev* 2009;**2**:CD001392. ℗ http://onlinelibrary.wiley.com/doi/10.1002/14651858. CD001392.pub2/abstract.

Guideline for non-CF bronchiectasis. *Thorax* 2010;**65**(Suppl. 1). ℗ http://www.brit-thoracic.org.uk/ Portals/0/Guidelines/Bronchiectasis/non-CF-Bronchiectasis-guideline.pdf.

Chapter 20

Bronchiolitis

Pathophysiology and causes

Definition and epidemiology Bronchioles are small airways of <2mm diameter, lined by bronchial epithelium and with no cartilage in their walls. Terminal bronchioles lead to alveoli. Many bronchioles need to be affected by disease before a patient becomes symptomatic, when there will be increased airway resistance unresponsive to β2 stimulants. Bronchiolitis is poorly understood and is a mixture of conditions.

Disease seems to affect bronchioles in two main ways:
- Affecting the bronchioles in isolation, with non-specific injury causing subsequent epithelial damage and inflammation, e.g. viral bronchiolitis
- As a bronchiolitis associated with other airway disease where the bronchiolitis may be more of an incidental finding, along with other pathologies, e.g. COP, HP, RB-ILD, LCH.

Pathophysiology is unclear. There is probably an initial injury to the epithelium of the bronchioles with subsequent inflammation. Adjacent alveoli are often also involved. There are two main pathological patterns of bronchiolitis. Both can exist in the same patient.
- *Proliferative bronchiolitis* More common of the two patterns. Non-specific reaction to bronchiolar injury, with organizing exudate within the bronchiolar lumen. Proliferation of intraluminal fibrotic buds, called Masson bodies, seen in bronchioles, alveoli, and alveolar ducts. Associated alveolar wall inflammation and foamy macrophages in alveolar spaces. May completely or partially resolve. Tends to be more responsive to steroids. The pathology merges with that of COP (see ➔ pp. 276–7)
- *Constrictive bronchiolitis* Less common. Concentric narrowing of the bronchiolar wall due to cellular infiltrates ± smooth muscle hyperplasia, which may cause extrinsic compression, obliteration, distortion, mucus collection, peribronchiolar fibrosis, and scarring. Patchy in distribution. Typically progressive and unresponsive to steroid therapy. Usually leads to respiratory failure and death.

In practice, these are the commonest situations in which a diagnosis of bronchiolitis is useful:
- Viral bronchiolitis (e.g. RSV)
- Post-lung transplant (bronchiolitis obliterans syndrome, BOS)
- Post-bone marrow transplant
- Connective tissue disease (usually RA)
- In association with ILD and airways disease
- Diffuse pan-bronchiolitis (including Japanese pan-bronchiolitis).

Clinical features Insidious onset of cough and dyspnoea over weeks to months. There may be an associated medical history, such as recent viral illness, transplant, connective tissue disease, or vasculitis, or a history of mineral dust or drug exposure.

Causes of bronchiolitis

Proliferative bronchiolitis (associated with OP)

Commoner causes
- COP (see ➲ pp. 276–7)
- HP (see ➲ p. 253)
- Chronic eosinophilic pneumonia (see ➲ p. 236)
- Connective tissue disease—RA, polymyositis, dermatomyositis (see ➲ p. 189)
- Post-bone marrow, heart, and lung transplant
- Organizing acute infection—mycoplasma, *Legionella*, influenza, CMV, HIV, PCP.

Rarer causes
- ARDS (see ➲ p. 105)
- Vasculitides, including GPA (formerly Wegener's) (see ➲ pp. 656–7)
- Drug-induced reactions such as L-tryptophan, busulfan, cocaine
- Chronic thyroiditis
- Ulcerative colitis
- Radiation or aspiration pneumonitis
- Distal to bronchial obstruction
- Common variable immunodeficiency syndrome.

Constrictive bronchiolitis

Commoner causes
- Connective tissue disease, particularly RA, especially women in their 50s and 60s, with long-standing RA. May be related to penicillamine or gold therapy. May improve with TNF-α inhibitor therapy
- Infection—viral (adenovirus, RSV, influenza, parainfluenza), mycoplasma.

Rarer causes
- 'Chronic rejection phenomenon' in heart, lung, bone marrow transplants—affects up to 65% of lung transplant patients after 5y post-transplant and is the 1° cause of late death, BOS (see ➲ pp. 328–9). Patients taking statins post-transplant have a lower incidence of this; reasons unclear
- Diffuse pan-bronchiolitis (including Japanese pan-bronchiolitis)
- Following inhalation injury: mineral dusts, such as asbestos, silica, iron oxide, aluminium oxide, talc, mica, coal, sulfur dioxide, nitrogen oxide, ammonia, chlorine, phosgene—may develop cough days to weeks after exposure
- Drug reaction
- Hypersensitivity reactions
- Ulcerative colitis
- Cryptogenic. Rare, mostly women >40. Cough and dyspnoea. PFT: progressive airflow obstruction and air trapping. TLCO decreased, no bronchodilator response.

Management

Investigations

- *PFTs* Obstructive defect may be found, with air trapping and no bronchodilator reversibility, in constrictive bronchiolitis. Proliferative bronchiolitis can cause a restrictive or mixed defect. Impaired TLCO in both
- *CXR* can be normal or may show hyperinflation, especially with constrictive bronchiolitis, diffuse infiltrates with proliferative bronchiolitis, which may be migratory
- *HRCT* is helpful and may be performed prone in full expiration. (Prone CT is used to minimize any gravity-dependent changes.) Normal bronchioles are too small to be seen; indirect signs of disease may be hyperinflation, air trapping, causing a mosaic pattern and subsegmental atelectasis. Bronchioles with thickened walls due to inflammation and dilatation may be seen. CT is also useful to assess for signs of associated ILD
- *Open or thoracoscopic lung biopsy* may be required to make the diagnosis, as TBBs are usually inadequate. The small airways need particularly careful examination.

Management

- Treat any underlying disorder
- Cough suppressants
- Long-term macrolide antibiotics, such as erythromycin 200–600mg/day, may improve symptoms, lung function, and mortality, especially in those with *diffuse pan-bronchiolitis* and *cryptogenic bronchiolitis*. Erythromycin lowers the neutrophil count by an unknown mechanism and reduces the number of lymphocytes
- Steroids are effective in cases of proliferative bronchiolitis and can treat the associated OP, e.g. 0.5–1mg/kg prednisolone/day, maximum 60mg/day. They may also be beneficial in bronchiolitis due to inhalation injury, both in early and later stages. Relapses of the bronchiolitis may occur on stopping the steroids.

Bronchiolitis: specific conditions

Diffuse pan-bronchiolitis This is a distinct condition and used to be thought of as rare outside Japan. Described 30y ago in Japan as a condition involving both the upper and lower respiratory tracts, with bronchiolar inflammation and chronic sinusitis. An infectious aetiology was postulated as the cause of this disease, but no particular organism has been consistently found. It can be familial and is associated with HLA-B54 (specific to East Asians) and A11 (Korea). Rarely seen in people of Asian descent living abroad. More prevalent in men, mean age at presentation 45, occurs particularly in non-smokers. Chronic sinusitis can precede the chest symptoms often by years. Most patients have a productive cough with copious purulent sputum, exertional dyspnoea, wheeze, and weight loss. There may be progressive respiratory failure with signs of cor pulmonale and crackles and wheezes on auscultation. More recently, a very similar clinical condition has been increasingly described outside Japan in which sinusitis is less commonly found. This diffuse version is also an idiopathic inflammatory and suppurative disorder of the respiratory bronchioles, causing progressive and severe airways obstruction. It is presumably very similar to the Japanese variety and probably under-recognized.

- *PFTs* are obstructive although may show a mixed pattern, with minimal airway hyperresponsiveness. TLCO is reduced
- *CXR and CT may show diffuse ill-defined nodules (sometimes 'tree-in-bud'), bronchiectasis*, and air trapping
- *Sputum cultures* may repeatedly show growths of *Haemophilus influenzae, Pseudomonas aeruginosa*, and less commonly *Streptococcus pneumoniae, Klebsiella pneumoniae*, or *Staphylococcus aureus*. These should be treated but can be hard to eradicate
- *Cold agglutinins* may be positive; mycoplasma tests are negative
- *BAL* shows marked neutrophilia, along with mild blood neutrophilia
- *Open or thoracoscopic lung biopsy*, although this may not be considered necessary in areas where pan-bronchiolitis is prevalent. Bronchiolar histology is characteristic, although not pathognomonic, with transmural infiltrate of lymphocytes, plasma cells, and foamy macrophages. The intraluminal exudates may be organized to form a polypoid plug.

Treatment with low-dose erythromycin 400–600mg/day for 6 months, and, in some Japanese studies, over 2y, confers a significant survival benefit, most likely related to its anti-inflammatory and immunomodulatory effects (inhibits many cytokines), as well as reducing mucin secretion, rather than through its antibacterial effects. Untreated, 50% 5y mortality. With treatment, >90% 10y survival. Azithromycin 250mg three times a week may be a suitable alternative but less experience. Relapses occur but usually respond to macrolides again.

Acute bronchiolitis This is a seasonal epidemic viral infective illness, common in infants <2y, who present with coryza, low-grade fever, cough, wheezing, tachypnoea, respiratory distress, hyperinflation, and tachycardia. It is most commonly caused by RSV, but also adenovirus, influenza, parainfluenza, rhinovirus, human metapneumovirus, coronavirus, and human bocavirus. *Mycoplasma* and *Chlamydophila* cause a similar picture of wheeze and lower respiratory tract infection. In adults, acute bronchiolitis is caused by the same organisms but is less severe.

- *CXR* may be normal or show hyperinflation, occasionally with patchy opacities, consolidation, and collapse
- *Histologically*, there is acute and chronic inflammation of bronchioles, with necrosis, sloughing, oedema, and inflammatory exudates in the bronchiolar lumen.

Treatment is supportive, with O_2 and fluids. Steroids and bronchodilators may be given if severe, but systematic reviews in children show no significant outcome benefit.

Further information

Ryu JH et al. Bronchiolar disorders. *Am J Respir Crit Care Med* 2003;**168**:1277–92.

Smyth RL, Openshaw PJ. Bronchiolitis. *Lancet* 2006;**368**:312–22.

Poletti V et al. Diffuse panbronchiolitis. *Eur Respir J* 2006;**28**:862–71.

Koyama H, Geddes DM. Erythromycin and diffuse panbronchiolitis. *Thorax* 1997;**52**:915–18.

Chapter 21

Chronic obstructive pulmonary disease (COPD)

Definition, aetiology, pathology, and clinical features

COPD is common and is mostly due to smoking. Patients with COPD represent a large proportion of inpatient (~12% of all general medical admissions) and outpatient work for the chest physician.

Definition
- Fixed airflow obstruction
- Minimal or no reversibility with bronchodilators
- Minimal variability in day-to-day symptoms
- Slowly progressive and irreversible deterioration in lung function, leading to progressively worsening symptoms.

Aetiology
95% of cases are smoking-related, typically >20 pack years. COPD occurs in 10–20% of smokers, indicating that there is probable genetic susceptibility. COPD is increasing in frequency worldwide, particularly in some developing countries, due to high levels of smoking, but also because of biomass fuel exposure. Smoking tobacco with marijuana increases COPD risk. It can also be caused by environmental and occupational factors such as dusts, chemicals, and air pollution.

Pathology
- *Mucous gland hyperplasia*, particularly in the large airways, with mucous hypersecretion and therefore a chronic productive cough. Other mucosal damage from smoke:
  - *Squamous metaplasia* Replacement of the normal ciliated columnar epithelium by a squamous epithelium
  - *Loss of cilial function* This leads to impairment of the normal functioning of the mucociliary escalator, another reason for the chronic productive cough
- *Chronic inflammation and fibrosis* of small airways, characterized by CD8 lymphocyte, macrophage, and neutrophil infiltration, with release of pro-inflammatory cytokines. Recurrent infections may perpetuate airway inflammation
- *Emphysema* due to alveolar wall destruction, causing irreversible enlargement of airspaces distal to the terminal bronchiole (the acinus), with subsequent loss of elastic recoil and hyperinflated lungs
  - Panacinar emphysema can occur with dilated airspaces evenly distributed across acini
  - Centriacinar or proximal emphysema can occur with dilated air spaces found in association with the respiratory bronchioles
  - Periacinar or paraseptal emphysema can occur with dilated air spaces at the edge of the acinar unit and abutting a fixed structure such as the pleura or a vessel
- *Thickened pulmonary arteriolar wall and remodelling* occur with hypoxia. Leads to increased pulmonary vascular resistance, PHT, and impaired gas exchange.

The cause of the increase in airways resistance, and hence expiratory flow limitation, is multifactorial. Small airway inflammation reduces the airway lumen. Emphysema destroys the radial attachments to the small airways, which normally hold them open and resist dynamic compression.

COPD is increasingly being recognized as having features not only of pulmonary, but also systemic, inflammation, and this may be the cause of the comorbidities found in patients with COPD. Daily activities are often modified to avoid dyspnoea, which can lead to deconditioning, muscle weakness, and wasting, meaning standing and walking become even harder. This leads to a vicious cycle of inactivity.

Clinical features
- Dyspnoea
- Chronic cough, may be productive
- Decreased exercise tolerance
- Wheeze.

Significant airflow obstruction may be present before the patient is aware of it. Symptoms are rare below age 35 and should prompt consideration of alternate diagnoses.

Signs depend on the severity of the underlying disease.
- Raised RR
- Hyperexpanded/barrel chest
- Prolonged expiratory time >5s, with pursed lip breathing
- Use of accessory muscles of respiration
- Quiet breath sounds (especially in the lung apices) ± wheeze
- Quiet heart sounds (due to overlying hyperinflated lung)
- Possible basal crepitations
- Signs of cor pulmonale and CO_2 retention (ankle oedema, raised JVP, warm peripheries, plethoric conjunctivae, bounding pulse, polycythaemia. Flapping tremor if CO_2 acutely raised).

Further information
NICE clinical guideline 101. Management of COPD in adults in primary and secondary care (partial update), June 2010. ℜ http://www.nice.org.uk/cg101.

ERS Consensus Statement—optimal assessment and management of COPD. *Eur Respir J* 1995;**8**:1398–420.

MacNee W, Calverley PMA. Management of COPD. *Thorax* 2003;**58**:261–5.

Patient information websites. ℜ http://www.copd-international.com; ℜ http://www.lunguk.org/copd.

Investigations

PFTs

- Obstructive spirometry and flow–volume loops
- Reduced FEV_1 to <80% predicted or FEV_1 >80% with other respiratory symptoms such as cough or breathlessness. COPD severity scale is shown in Table 21.1 and MRC dyspnoea scale in Box 21.1). FEV_1 is the measurement of choice to assess progression of COPD, but it correlates weakly with the degree of dyspnoea. Changes in FEV_1 do not reflect the decline in a patient's health
- FEV_1/FVC <0.7 (post-bronchodilation)
- Minimal bronchodilator reversibility (<15%, usually <10%) and minimal steroid reversibility (how to perform these, see ➲ p. 179). It is not necessary to test these in most patients but is useful if there is diagnostic uncertainty or if the patient is thought to have both COPD and asthma
- Raised total lung volume, FRC, and RV because of emphysema, air trapping, and loss of elastic recoil
- Decreased TLCO and kCO because presence of emphysema decreases surface area available for gas diffusion.

CXR is not required for diagnosis, and repeated CXR is unnecessary, unless other diagnoses are being considered (most importantly, lung cancer or bronchiectasis).

- Hyperinflated lung fields, with attenuation of peripheral vasculature— 'black lung sign'; >7 posterior ribs seen
- Flattened diaphragms (best CXR correlate of post-mortem degree of emphysema)
- More horizontal ribs
- May see bullae, especially in lung apices, which, if large, can be mistaken for a pneumothorax due to loss of lung markings (CT can differentiate).

Consider checking α1-AT levels (see ➲ pp. 186–7), FBC to ensure not anaemic or polycythaemic (suggesting persistent hypoxia), TFT if unduly breathless. CRP is slightly increased in COPD but decreases after steroid treatment. It may be related to the presence of comorbidities and may aid the assessment of the systemic effects of COPD, particularly in the research setting. ECG and echo to assess cardiac status if features of cor pulmonale.

Diagnosis is based on the history of smoking and progressive dyspnoea, with evidence of irreversible airflow obstruction on spirometry. Asthma is the most important differential diagnosis. Asthma is steroid- and bronchodilator-responsive. Nearly all patients with COPD will have a smoking history; this is not universal in asthma. Symptoms are common under the age of 35 in asthma; rare in COPD. Chronic productive cough is common is COPD and uncommon in asthma. Breathlessness is progressive and persistent in COPD but variable in asthma. In asthma, there is significant diurnal or day-to-day variability of symptoms, and night-time waking with SOB or wheeze is common; these symptoms are uncommon in COPD. Some patients have both.

Table 21.1 COPD severity according to NICE guidelines 2004 (which differ slightly from the GOLD guidelines)

Mild	FEV_1 50–80% predicted. May or may not be symptomatic with cough or sputum
Moderate	FEV_1 30–49% predicted. Increased FRC, reduced TLCO. Likely to be symptomatic (cough, sputum, dyspnoea), often managed by patient's GP
Severe	FEV_1 <30% predicted. Marked hyperinflation, TLCO usually low. Usually hypoxic, with signs of cor pulmonale. Symptomatic, often needing hospital admissions

Box 21.1 MRC dyspnoea scale

1 Not troubled by breathlessness except on strenuous exercise
2 Short of breath when hurrying or walking up a slight hill
3 Walks slower than contemporaries on level ground because of breathlessness or has to stop for breath when walking at own pace
4 Stops for breath after walking about 100m or after a few minutes on level ground
5 Too breathless to leave the house, or breathless when dressing or undressing.

Table 21.2 BODE index

Variable	Points on BODE index			
	0	1	2	3
FEV_1 (% predicted)	≥65	50–64	36–49	≤35
Distance walked in 6min (m)	≥350	250–349	150–249	≤149
MRC dyspnoea scale	0–1	2	3	4
BMI	>21	≤21		

BODE index (see Table 21.2) is a simple multidimensional grading system for COPD, using **B**MI, airflow **O**bstruction, **D**yspnoea, and **E**xercise capacity as its scoring variables. It has been shown to be better than FEV_1 at predicting risk of hospitalization and death in patients with COPD, as it is multidimensional. Patients are scored as having a BODE index of between 0 and 10, with higher scores indicating a higher risk of death. It is being increasingly used, with recommendations to calculate it in the clinical setting to give prognostic information (Celli BR *et al. New Engl J Med* 2004; **350**: 1005–12).

Non-pharmacological management of stable COPD

Aims of COPD management should include:
- Ensuring the diagnosis is correct
- Stopping smoking
- Optimizing treatment by minimizing symptoms where possible
- Helping the patient maintain their QoL.

Management should be delivered by a multidisciplinary team (MDT).

No treatment has yet been shown to modify disease progression in the long term, except for stopping smoking.

Smoking cessation is the only intervention that is proven to decrease the smoking-related decline in lung function. All patients with COPD who smoke should be encouraged to stop at every opportunity. Fig. 21.1 shows the accelerated decline in FEV_1 in susceptible smokers and the delay in this acceleration from stopping smoking; susceptible smokers, however, never regain the original curve. Nicotine replacement therapy (NRT) should be used to aid smoking cessation (see p. 733).

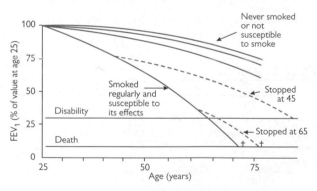

Fig. 21.1 Modification of the Fletcher–Peto diagram of FEV_1 decline in susceptible smokers.

Education can improve ability to manage illness and stop smoking.

Pulmonary rehabilitation is a multidisciplinary programme, with RCT evidence that it improves exercise tolerance, QoL, and reduces hospital admissions. Muscle mass, particularly in the lower limbs, is reduced in people with COPD, compared with age-matched healthy controls. This is an independent predictor of mortality and disability, independent of the severity of the underlying lung disease, and may reflect the systemic nature of COPD. The mainstay of rehabilitation is graded exercise to improve muscle function but also includes breathing techniques and education.

Programmes vary but are usually run on an outpatient basis over several weeks, with multidisciplinary involvement (see ➜ p. 727). Should be made available to all appropriate patients with COPD, including after hospitalization for acute exacerbation.

Diet Weight loss is recommended if the patient is obese to minimize respiratory effort. If the patient is very breathless, calorific intake may be low and a catabolic state may exist. A low BMI is associated with impaired pulmonary status, decreased diaphragm mass, lower exercise capacity, and increased mortality rate, compared with people with a normal BMI. Nutritional supplementation may therefore be necessary. Maintaining body weight and muscle mass correlates well with survival.

Self-management plan on how to respond promptly to symptoms of an exacerbation

Psychosocial support Practical support at home, day centres; car disability badge; assess for signs of anxiety and depression.

Pharmacological management of stable COPD

Pharmacological management aims to relieve symptoms and reduce exacerbations but will not modify disease. Increase treatment in a stepwise fashion. Exacerbations require additional therapeutic support (see ➲ p. 180).

Bronchodilators Simple pulmonary function testing may not show significant bronchodilator reversibility of FEV_1, but bronchodilators provide therapeutic benefit in the long term by reducing dyspnoea, perhaps by decreasing chest hyperinflation.

- Initially prescribe short-acting β_2 agonists, as required, for symptom relief
- If the patient remains symptomatic and FEV_1 >50% predicted: prescribe LABA or long-acting anticholinergic
- If symptoms and FEV_1 <50% predicted: try LABA with inhaled steroid in combination, or an anticholinergic
- If still breathless or exacerbations despite this regime (regardless of FEV_1): add long-acting anticholinergic to the LABA and inhaled steroid combination. Reduces exacerbation frequency
- Oral methylxanthines, such as theophyllines, can be used as maintenance therapy and may improve symptoms. Add after inhaled bronchodilators and trial of inhaled steroids; continue only if symptoms improve. Method of action is unclear, but they may have an anti-inflammatory effect. Care regarding therapeutic/toxic levels, especially in elderly patients
- Inhaler therapy provides adequate bronchodilator doses for most patients, especially when used with a spacer device. Check patient's inhaler technique
- Nebulizer therapy is indicated if the patient is unable to use inhalers or if they are disabled or distressed with breathlessness despite maximal inhaler therapy. Only those with a clear response, with reduction in symptoms or improvement in activities of daily living, should continue with long-term domiciliary nebulized treatment (usually with salbutamol and ipratropium), as there is a significant placebo effect.

Inhaled steroids should be prescribed to all patients with FEV_1 ≤60% predicted, who have had two or more exacerbations per year requiring treatment with antibiotics or oral steroids. Clinical trials of inhaled steroids have shown a reduction in exacerbation frequency and severity in severe COPD, but no slowing in lung function decline. Warn patients regarding side effects, and document. Use in combination with bronchodilator. Evidence of increased risk of pneumonia (without associated increase in mortality) with some inhaled steroids. Use in combination with bronchodilator.

Oral steroids are not recommended as a maintenance therapy in COPD. It may, however, be difficult to withdraw them in patients with severe COPD following an exacerbation. If so, keep the dose as low as possible, and prescribe osteoporosis prophylaxis if indicated. Warn regarding steroid side effects, and document.

O_2 can be administered via a cylinder for short-burst O_2 therapy (SBOT), as required, for symptomatic relief, such as after climbing stairs (there is little trial evidence to support this use—only continue if improvement in breathlessness documented), or as long-term O_2 therapy (LTOT) via an O_2 concentrator. The latter is for patients in respiratory failure, with a PaO_2 <7.3kPa or PaO_2 of 7.3–8kPa with any of 2° polycythaemia, peripheral oedema, or PHT present, to use for a minimum of 15h/day (including sleep). Additional ambulatory cylinders can be provided. Low-flow O_2, such as 2–4L/min via nasal prongs, is usually adequate. Small changes in CO_2 retention with O_2 administration can be tolerated if asymptomatic and no respiratory acidosis. Associated OSA is a risk factor for CO_2 retention (for O_2 prescribing, see ➔ p. 703).

Vaccination Influenza vaccine annually and pneumococcal vaccine. Meta-analysis showed a decrease in exacerbations occurs 3 weeks after receiving influenza vaccine, and there is no evidence of an earlier increase in exacerbations due directly to vaccination.

Antibiotics In general, not recommended prophylactically. Some prescribe low-dose rotating antibiotics, particularly over the winter in those with severe exacerbations. Mixed data. Some newer evidence for low-dose azithromycin 250mg three times per week in those with frequent exacerbations despite optimal therapy. Reduces exacerbation frequency and time to exacerbation, compared to placebo, but possible hearing impairment and nasopharyngeal colonization with more resistant organisms. Moxifloxacin 400mg PO has also been given as prophylaxis for 5 days every 8 weeks for six cycles, with beneficial effect on exacerbation rate, no increased resistance, but some GI side effects. Azithromycin favoured.

Mucolytics (carbocisteine, mecysteine hydrochloride) may benefit some patients with chronic productive cough to facilitate expectoration by reducing sputum viscosity. Prescribe for a 4-week trial period, and only continue if there is evidence of improvement. Meta-analyses show mucolytics cause a significant decrease in the number of COPD exacerbations and decrease the number of days of disability, although the benefit may only apply if the patient is not taking inhaled steroids. Worth trying in those with moderate to severe COPD, with frequent or prolonged exacerbations, or those repeatedly in hospital with COPD exacerbations. Caution if known peptic ulcer disease.

Palliative care/respiratory sedation Use of low-dose sedatives, such as morphine sulfate solution 10mg prn or diazepam 2mg bd, can be used as a palliative measure (see ➔ pp. 724–5), aiming to relieve the sensation of dyspnoea and associated anxiety, in those with severe COPD. Dose may need to be titrated against any rise in CO_2 (surprisingly uncommon).

Newer anti-inflammatory drugs

Erdosteine is a thiol compound with effects on bacterial adhesiveness as well as antioxidant and mucoactive properties. RCT in moderate COPD showed decreased exacerbations vs placebo over 8 months, no loss of lung function, and improved health-related QoL.

Roflumilast and cilomilast are PDE-4 inhibitors, which elicit anti-inflammatory effects. RCT of roflumilast in moderate to severe COPD showed a significant improvement in FEV_1 over 24h vs placebo and a reduction in the rate of mild exacerbations. Long-term studies are required to evaluate its efficacy and role further. Cilomilast has shown similar results.

Statins have anti-inflammatory properties which suggest improvements in COPD, but prospective studies are needed.

An approach to COPD in the outpatient clinic

- Establish diagnosis and severity—PFTs, CXR
- Ensure there are no other causes for symptoms, e.g. anaemia, PE, heart failure, ILD, thyroid dysfunction, pneumothorax, large bulla, arrhythmia, depression
- Consider chest CT only if CXR abnormalities require clarification or symptoms disproportionate to spirometry or if surgery being considered
- Encourage the patient to stop smoking
- Review current treatment—optimize bronchodilatation and inhaled steroids
- Assess whether there is any need for a nebulizer
- Check O_2 saturation, and perform blood gas if <92%. Consider LTOT
- Consider pulmonary rehabilitation
- Consider sputum culture if persistent purulent sputum
- Check vaccinations are up to date
- Involve respiratory nurse specialist for input in the community, if appropriate
- Follow-up in clinic if ongoing medical issues, including whether patient may be a lung transplant candidate (see → p. 319). Otherwise, discharge back to GP
- Inform GP of all the above decisions.

Further information

Poole PJ et al. Influenza vaccination for patients with COPD. *Cochrane Database Syst Rev* 2006;1:CD002733.

Poole PJ, Black PN. Mucolytic agents for chronic bronchitis or COPD. *Cochrane Database Syst Rev* 2006;3:CD001287.

Black P et al. Prophylactic antibiotic therapy for chronic bronchitis. *Cochrane Database Syst Rev* 2003;1:CD004105.

Crosbie PAJ, Woodhead M. Long-term macrolide therapy in chronic inflammatory airway diseases. *Eur Respir J* 2004;24:822–33.

How to perform a steroid trial to help distinguish asthma from COPD (if diagnosis unclear)

Measure FEV_1 and slow VC before and after:
- Either a high-dose inhaled steroid for 6–8 weeks, or
- A 2-week course of oral prednisolone 30mg/day.

Over 15% increase in FEV_1 implies steroid reversibility, and patient is likely to have asthma.

Over 15% increase in slow VC suggests significantly reduced air trapping and may indicate significant asthma. May occur with a significantly smaller change in FEV_1.

Document results of trial clearly in notes.

Testing for bronchodilator reversibility to help distinguish asthma from COPD

- Check FEV_1. Give patient a short-acting β_2 agonist, either nebulized or inhaled via spacer; 15–30min after this, recheck the FEV_1.
- Subtract the pre-test value from the post-test value; divide the difference by the pre-test value, and express as a % increase from baseline; >15% increase or >200mL indicates bronchodilator reversibility
- Avoid short-acting bronchodilator in the preceding 6h, a long-acting bronchodilator in the preceding 12h, or a long-acting anticholinergic or slow-release theophylline in the preceding 24h.

COPD exacerbations

Exacerbations may cause mild symptoms in those with relatively preserved lung function but can cause considerable morbidity in those with limited respiratory reserve. It has been increasingly recognized that significant numbers of patients do not regain their premorbid lung function or QoL following an exacerbation, and those with frequent exacerbations experience a more rapid FEV_1 decline than those with fewer exacerbations. Exacerbation frequency increases with COPD severity. Exacerbations are 50% more likely in winter (possibly viruses survive better in the cold, and people crowd together indoors). An exacerbation is essentially a clinical diagnosis of an acute increase in symptoms beyond normal daily variation.

Causes may be infective organisms, either viral or bacterial, or non-infective causes such as pollution or temperature fall. Common bacterial pathogens are *Haemophilus influenzae, Streptococcus pneumoniae,* and *Moraxella catarrhalis*, and the commonest viral pathogens are rhinovirus, RSV, influenza, parainfluenza, coronavirus, human metapneumovirus, and adenovirus. Consider the possibility of PE or pneumothorax.

Symptoms include increased cough, increased sputum volume and/or purulence, increasing dyspnoea or wheeze, chest tightness, fluid retention.

Pathophysiology There is increased airway resistance due to bronchospasm, mucosal oedema, and increased sputum. This worsens expiratory flow limitation, and expiration takes longer. Shallow rapid breathing further limits the time for expiration. This promotes dynamic hyperinflation, and this itself causes mechanical compromise within the lung and the airway. Maximal recruitment of the accessory muscles is required, and thoraco-abdominal dysynchrony is often present.

▶▶ **Management summary: acute exacerbation of COPD**

- Assess the severity of the exacerbation by measuring RR, O_2 saturations, degree of air entry, tachycardia, BP, peripheral perfusion, conscious level, mental state
- Exclude a pneumothorax clinically
- If hypoxic, give controlled 24–35% O_2 via Venturi face mask to aim for SaO_2 88–92%, salbutamol nebulizer; establish venous access
- Check blood gas
- Request a CXR
- Perform ECG
- Check bloods for WCC, CRP, potassium, etc.
- Optimize volume status
- Take a brief history, if possible. Important to know what patient's normal functional status is like such as exercise tolerance and the need for help with activities of daily living. Old hospital notes are helpful regarding severity of disease and whether previous decisions have been made regarding ventilation or resuscitation
- Nebulized bronchodilators—salbutamol 2.5–5mg and ipratropium 500 micrograms on arrival and 4–6-hourly. Run nebulizer with air, not O_2
- Continued O_2 therapy, aiming to maintain saturations between 80% and 90%. Repeat blood gases after 60min to ensure improvement if hypoxic or acidotic. Repeat if clinical deterioration
- Consider antibiotics
- Oral steroids
- Consider IV aminophylline if not improving with nebulizers
- Consider intensive care—ideally, consultant-led decision with the patient, their family, and ITU regarding invasive mechanical ventilation. Document in the medical notes. Consider resuscitation status
- Consider NIV—pH 7.3 or less, hypoxia, hypercapnia, conscious level. Decide if this is the ceiling of therapy
- Consider doxapram if NIV not available or not tolerated
- DVT prophylaxis
- Early mobilization
- Nutrition.

Further information

Intermediate care hospital-at-home in COPD: BTS guideline. *Thorax* 2007;**62**:200–10.

Ram FSF *et al.* Hospital at home for patients with acute exacerbations of COPD: systematic review of the evidence. *BMJ* 2004;**329**:315–18.

Review series: COPD exacerbations. *Thorax* 2006;**61**:164–8, 250–8, 440–7, 535–44, 354–61.

Management of exacerbations

- Assess the severity of the exacerbation: increase in dyspnoea, tachypnoea, use of accessory muscles, new cyanosis, pedal oedema, or confusion
- Exclude alternative diagnoses such as pneumothorax, PE, pulmonary oedema
- Can the patient self-care and self-medicate? In the presence of severe symptoms, with possible comorbid disease and decreased functional activities, the patient is likely to need hospital management
- Investigate with CXR, ABGs, ECG, FBC, and U&Es. *Admission arterial pH is the best predictor of survival.* A pH <7.25 is associated with a rapidly rising mortality. A *raised* pH may imply an alternative diagnosis, not associated with worsening airways obstruction. Check theophylline level if patient is taking regularly; consider sending sputum for culture if it is purulent.

Treatment

- *Antibiotics* if sputum purulent, pyrexial, high CRP, new changes on CXR. Recently published study found increased risk of cardiovascular events in people with COPD exacerbation treated with clarithromycin (hazard ratio 1.7, *BMJ* 2013;346:f1235). Effect not seen with β-lactams or doxycycline—further data set studies required
- *Systemic steroids* for all patients with exacerbations of COPD who are admitted to hospital or are significantly more breathless than usual. Give prednisolone 30mg/day for 1–2 weeks, unless there are specific contraindications. Optimum dose and length of steroids not established. This improves FEV_1 and symptoms, and shortens recovery time. Avoid long-term steroid treatment due to side effects. If the patient has a longer course of steroids, or repeated courses due to repeated exacerbations, the dose will need to be tailed off slowly. Frequent short courses of steroids may merit long-term bone protection
- *Inhaled or nebulized bronchodilators* Breathless unwell patients may benefit from nebulizer therapy in the acute period to reduce symptoms and improve airflow obstruction
- *Controlled O_2 therapy* 24–35% via Venturi face mask, with oximetry, ABGs, or capillary gas monitoring. Guidelines suggest maintaining saturations between 88% and 92%, balancing hypoxia, hypercapnia, and pH (see ➲ pp. 704–6). Too little O_2 causes anaerobic metabolism and metabolic acidosis (probably SaO_2 >80% would prevent this); too much O_2 (SaO_2 >92%) can cause hypercapnia and a respiratory acidosis. A deteriorating pH to below 7.25 has a much poorer prognosis. Make sure your instructions to the ward staff are clear as to the need to keep the SaO_2 within this window by changing the % O_2 delivered as necessary. Falling conscious level is the best clinical marker of significant CO_2 retention and acidosis
- *IV aminophylline* Evidence is lacking, but it may be beneficial, particularly if the patient is wheezy and has not improved with nebulizers alone. Give a loading dose, unless the patient is on regular oral aminophylline,

followed by a maintenance infusion. Monitor aminophylline levels daily. Main side effects are tachycardia and nausea

- *NIV* Effective in supporting patients during an exacerbation when maximal medical treatment has not been effective. Appropriate for conscious patients with ongoing respiratory acidosis (pH 7.35 or less), hypoxia, and hypercapnia. May avoid intubation. Ceiling of treatment should be determined *before* its use (see ➲ p. 692)
- *Doxapram* IV respiratory stimulant. Can be used to drive RR (if <20/min) and depth in COPD exacerbation and hence improve hypoxia, hypercapnia, and respiratory acidosis, particularly when induced by O_2 therapy. It can overdrive breathing to the point of respiratory muscle fatigue, collapse, and death and causes metabolic acidosis, agitation, and cardiac arrhythmias. It should only be used at the lowest possible dose (0.5–3mg/min) in the short term (usually 24–36h), aiming to reduce $PaCO_2$ (and raise pH) by only a small amount. Its use has largely been replaced by NIV but may be used if NIV is not available or not tolerated
- *Acetazolamide* generates a metabolic acidosis by reducing the kidney's ability to secrete [H^+] into urine (blocks carbonic anhydrase that interconverts CO_2 and H^+/HCO_3^-). There is only one situation in which provoking a metabolic acidosis might be appropriate: following a transient period of hypoventilation (perhaps due to pump failure/increased airways obstruction) or after permissive hypercapnia on the ICU, the previous appropriate compensatory rise in blood [HCO_3^-] can now be too high for the improving $PaCO_2$. This generates a blood alkalosis (pH >7.4), which itself depresses ventilation, and delays the return of PaO_2 and $PaCO_2$ to normal. The judicious use of a few doses of acetazolamide (250mg od), but only safe when the pH is alkaline, can hasten the recovery
- *Intubation/intensive care* If the patient is not responding to medical therapy, a decision regarding invasive mechanical ventilation needs to be made. This may be considered to be appropriate if the patient usually has a good functional status, with minimal other comorbidity. These decisions should ideally be discussed with the patient, their family, their consultant, and the ITU consultant and documented in the medical notes. Resuscitation decisions should also be made
- *Early rehabilitation* to prevent muscle wasting and deconditioning
- *Nutrition*
- *Acute respiratory assessment service (ARAS)/'hospital at home'* Respiratory nurse-led service supporting early discharge of COPD patients after hospital assessment and providing ongoing respiratory care at home. CXR, SaO_2, and baseline spirometry (if this is first presentation) should be performed prior to discharge. Reduces length of inpatient stay and hence is an economic alternative. Unsuitable patients are those with impaired GCS, acute confusion, pH <7.35, acute changes on CXR, concomitant medical problems requiring inpatient stay, insufficient social support (including living far from the hospital and not having a telephone), new hypoxia with SaO_2 <90%, and unable to provide O_2 at home.

Surgical treatment

Lung transplant In young patients (below 60–65) with severe disease, often due to α1-AT deficiency, lung transplant may be an option. Local transplant teams will advise regarding local criteria (see ➜ pp. 320–1).

Bullectomy Suitable for selected patients who are breathless, have FEV$_1$ <50% predicted, and isolated large bulla seen on CT. Improves chest hyperinflation.

Lung volume reduction surgery (LVRS) Resection of areas of bullous emphysema to reduce chest hyperinflation and improve diaphragmatic function, elastic recoil, physiology of the lungs, and hence functional status of the patient. Patients who may be considered are those with FEV$_1$ 20–30% predicted, with symptomatic dyspnoea despite maximal medical therapy, and with upper lobe-predominant emphysema on CT, giving target areas to resect. PaCO$_2$ should be <7.3kPa and TLCO >20% predicted. Patients should have completed pulmonary rehabilitation and have stopped smoking. Preoperative assessment: PFTs, 6MWT, QoL and dyspnoea indicators. Surgery is performed in specialist centres via median sternotomy or by thoracoscopy. Usually, the upper lobe is stapled below the level of the emphysema and then removed. Improvements are seen in FEV$_1$ and RV, dyspnoea, and QoL scores. These effects are maximal between 2 and 6 months post-surgery. Symptomatic improvement is sustained for about 2–4y. Post-operative complications: persistent air leak >7 days in 30–40%, pneumonia in up to 22%, respiratory failure in up to 13%. Reported post-operative mortality 2.4–17%.

The National Emphysema Treatment Trial (NETT, Michigan, USA) randomized 1,218 patients to receive medical treatment or LVRS. Mean airflow limitation of the subjects was 27% predicted. The most recent analysis, published after 4y of follow-up, has shown LVRS demonstrating an overall survival advantage, compared with medical therapy alone. Improvements in maximal exercise and health-related QoL were also found over 3y and 4y, respectively. The greatest survival benefits, improved exercise and symptoms over 5y, were in those with both low exercise capacity and upper lobe-predominant emphysema. Those with high exercise capacity and upper lobe-predominant emphysema obtained no survival advantage, but exercise and health-related QoL improved. Interim analysis had shown increased mortality from LVRS for patients with FEV$_1$ or TLCO <20% predicted, or with homogeneous emphysema. Surgery is not therefore recommended for these groups.

Bronchoscopic lung volume reduction surgery (bLVR) refers to techniques to reduce emphysematous hyperinflation via a flexible bronchoscope and thus avoid potential mortality and morbidity associated with surgery. Now this mainly refers to one-way valves, placed within the segmental and sub-segmental bronchi that supply the hyperinflated lobes. They allow mucus to leave the bronchus but no air to enter. Two sizes are currently available and are inserted under direct bronchoscopic vision. It is a minimally invasive variation on LVRS, with the aim of improving lung function and QoL. Pilot studies in end-stage emphysema (mean FEV$_1$ 30% predicted) have shown the procedure to be safe, although a small subset of patients developed pneumothorax and one death (in 98 patients) has been reported. Significant improvements in RV, FEV_1, FVC, and 6MWT were found at 30 and 90 days. Inclusion and exclusion criteria were similar to the NETT protocol, with patients with FEV_1 <20% predicted, hypercapnia, PHT, or DLCO <25% predicted excluded. A multicentre RCT (the VENT trial) has been completed of best medical care (including pulmonary rehabilitation) vs best medical care plus unilateral endoscopic bronchial valve, with CT determination of lobe to target. There were 321 patients randomized, FEV_1 15–45% predicted. There were small, but significant, improvements in FEV_1 and 6MWT in the valve group, with those with intact interlobar fissures on CT having a much greater improvement than those with incomplete fissures (which allow collateral ventilation, and thus occluding the segmental bronchi with valves does not isolate the lobe). Lobar occlusion appears to be essential for clinically significant improved outcomes. Intrabronchial valves, coils, biological sealants, and thermal airway (steam to cause inflammation, and subsequent fibrosis and contraction) have also been used in small studies. Knowledge and skill are improving in this area, and more programmes are developing. Clearly, there are different COPD phenotypes, and those with a greater degree of CT heterogeneity are more likely to have intact fissures with areas of worse emphysema which may be more amenable to these therapies.

Airway bypass aims to improve respiratory mechanics by creating new exit pathways for air trapped in emphysematous lungs. The wall of a segmental bronchus is punctured under bronchoscopic guidance, and a drug-eluting stent is inserted, creating an internal bronchopulmonary communication for expiration. Hence, hyperinflation decreases and lung mechanics are improved. Multicentre Exhale Airway Stents for Emphysema (EASE) trial randomized 208 people to bypass or sham bronchoscopy. There was no difference between groups at 12 months.

Further information

Herth FJF et al. Efficacy predictors of lung volume reduction with Zephyr valves in a European cohort. *Eur Respir J* 2012;**39**:1334–42.

Sciurba FC et al. A randomized study of *endobronchial* valves for advanced emphysema. *N Engl J Med* 2010;**363**:1233–44.

Shah PL et al. Bronchoscopic lung-volume reduction with Exhale airway stents for emphysema (EASE trial): randomized, sham-controlled, multicentre trial. *Lancet* 2011;**378**:997–1005.

Naunheim KS et al. Long term follow-up of patients receiving LVRS vs. medical therapy for severe emphysema by the NETT research group. *Ann Thoracic Surg* 2006;**82**:431–43.

Fishman A et al. A randomized trial comparing lung-volume-reduction surgery with medical therapy for severe emphysema. *N Engl J Med* 2003;**22**:2059–73.

Criner GJ et al. Prospective randomised trial comparing bilateral LVRS to pulmonary rehabilitation in severe COPD. *Am Respir Crit Care Med* 1999;**160**:2018–27.

Geddes D et al. Effect of LVRS in patients with severe emphysema. *N Engl J Med* 2000;**343**:239–45.

Toma TP et al. Bronchoscopic volume reduction with valve implants in patients with severe emphysema. *Lancet* 2003;**361**:931–3.

Benditt JO. Surgical therapies for COPD. *Respir Care* 2004;**49**:53–63.

α1-antitrypsin (α1-AT) deficiency

This is an inherited condition that is associated with the early development of emphysema. It is common (estimated 1 in 2,000–5,000 individuals) and is probably under-diagnosed, as it is often asymptomatic in non-smokers.

Pathophysiology α1-AT is a glycoprotein protease inhibitor produced by the liver. It is secreted via the bloodstream into the lungs and opposes neutrophil elastase, which destroys alveolar wall connective tissue. Elastase is produced in increased levels by pulmonary neutrophils and macrophages in response to smoking and lung infections. If α1-AT is deficient, the elastase cannot be opposed, and subsequently basal emphysema develops. The disease is worse in smokers and can cause COPD at a young age (40s and 50s). There may also be associated liver dysfunction, chronic hepatitis, cirrhosis, and hepatoma, as abnormal protein secretion accumulates in the liver. Predisposition also to skin disease (panniculitis) and vasculitis (especially ANCA +ve).

Genetics α1-AT deficiency is inherited as an autosomal co-dominant disorder. So far, >100 different alleles have been identified for this gene (*SERPINA 1*) on the long arm of chromosome (Chr) 14. The commonest alleles are the M allele (normal), the partially defective S allele, and the almost fully defective Z allele (lysine is substituted for glutamic acid at position 342, leading to abnormal folding, preventing post-translational processing with retention within cells), commonest in Scandinavia.
- MM, the normal phenotype. Background population risk of emphysema
- MS, MZ have 50–70% of normal α1-protease inhibitor (Pi) levels. Background risk of emphysema
- SZ, SS have 35–50% of normal levels. 20–50% risk of emphysema
- Homozygous ZZ has only 10–20% of normal levels. 80–100% risk of emphysema.

Screening for the defect should be carried out, especially in patients <40 with COPD or minimal smoking history or family history. Also patients with unexplained liver disease should be screened. Send blood for α1-AT concentrations and genotyping if levels are low. Siblings should be screened and the particular importance of not smoking and avoiding passive smoking emphasized. Non-smokers are usually asymptomatic.

Treatment includes usual therapy for COPD. Specialist centre involvement recommended. Specific treatment is known as augmentation therapy, with ideally weekly, but also 2-weekly or monthly infusions, of purified α1-AT from pooled human plasma. This raises concentrations in serum and epithelial lining fluid above the protective threshold. It appears to be safe, with minimal side effects, and is well tolerated. A large cohort study showed reduced mortality amongst infusion recipients, with a slowing of lung function decline (by 27mL/y, $p = 0.03$) in a subgroup with moderate emphysema. An RCT showed no significant differences between augmentation and control groups, although there was a trend towards slower loss of lung tissue on CT scan in the augmentation group ($p = 0.07$). It has, however, been recommended as a treatment by groups, including the American

Thoracic Society (ATS) and European Respiratory Society (ERS), for those with moderate (FEV_1 35–60% predicted) emphysema due to α1-AT deficiency, who are non-/ex-smokers, but not those with mild disease (optimal therapy unclear) or severe disease (less clinical efficacy) or those post-lung transplant for α1-AT deficiency, except during episodes of acute rejection and infection (when inflammation causes free elastase activity). It is expensive, and its cost effectiveness in terms of cost per year of life saved is high. It is, however, the only specific therapy available at present.

Future developments Inhaled α1-AT may provide a way of delivering the enzyme to the lower respiratory tract to have its action locally and potentially reduce inflammation. Gene therapy is under development, finding ways of delivering the α1-AT gene into the cell. Other strategies include inhibition of hepatic polymerization of α1-AT, promotion of hepatic secretion, inhibition of neutrophil elastase by synthetic inhibitors to avoid the use of human plasma, and pegylation of α1-AT to prolong its serum half-life.

Further information

Stoller JK, Aboussouan LS. α1-antitrypsin deficiency. *Lancet* 2005;**365**:2225–36.

Review series: α1-antitrypsin deficiency. *Thorax* 2004;**59**:64–9, 259–64, 441–5,529–35, 708–12, 904–9.

UK α1-antitrypsin deficiency UK support group. ℛ http://www.alpha1.org.uk.

Chapter 22

Connective tissue disease and the lung

Differential diagnosis and standard tests

Patients with connective tissue diseases often develop pulmonary complications, for which they should be referred to a chest physician. Patients typically present with symptoms of dyspnoea, cough, fever, or chest pain. They may often already be on immunosuppressive drugs.

Differential diagnosis

In practice, a few tests (see Box 22.1) will help distinguish the main differential diagnoses.

Opportunistic pulmonary infection

- May be in those on immunosuppressive drugs or functionally immunosuppressed from underlying disease
- Any usual organism, but also TB, NTM, PCP, fungi, CMV
- Often acute onset, with non-specific features of low-grade fever, productive cough, raised inflammatory markers
- Can be very unwell and need full supportive treatment with ICU.

Original connective tissue disease now affecting the lung

- Often inflammation or fibrosis
- Usually more indolent presentation, with dry cough and dyspnoea, but can become acutely unwell on background of chronic lung disease
- Fine inspiratory crackles on auscultation
- Consider development of PHT in patients with systemic sclerosis.

New pathology

- Unrelated to the original condition, including pulmonary thromboembolic disease, heart failure.

Drug side effects

- Methotrexate—pneumonitis occurs in 5% of patients receiving methotrexate. Potentially life-threatening. Mortality 15–20%. Cough, fever, dyspnoea, widespread crackles, restrictive defect, and pulmonary infiltrates on CXR and CT. Peripheral eosinophilia in 50%. BAL lymphocytosis. Usually subacute onset but may be sudden. Usually within 4 months of starting methotrexate. Non-specific histological findings. No more common in those with pre-existing lung disease. Treatment: stop the drug; commence steroids (high-dose methylprednisolone is often used), and avoid methotrexate in the future. Can be reversible. Can get mild intractable cough with methotrexate
- Leflunomide—pneumonitis may occur although appears to be rare; consider this diagnosis, and discontinue the drug if new or worsening respiratory symptoms. Avoid leflunomide in patients with pre-existing ILD
- Anti-TNF-α therapy—includes infliximab (a monoclonal antibody), etanercept (a receptor fusion protein), and adalimumab (a humanized IgG1 antibody). All may predispose to severe infection (viral, bacterial, and fungal), particularly when used in association with other immunosuppressants. Opportunistic infection is common, including PCP

and mycobacterial disease (both tuberculous, see ➨ pp. 510–1, and non-tuberculous, see ➨ pp. 518–9). The risk of mycobacterial disease appears to be less with etanercept than with infliximab and adalimumab. All patients should be screened for latent TB prior to starting anti-TNF-α drugs (see ➨ pp. 508–9). Concern has also been raised that these drugs may lead to increased rates of malignancy, and a recent meta-analysis has shown a dose-dependent increase in cancer diagnoses in RA patients treated with infliximab. ILD may worsen on these drugs; consider stopping anti-TNF-α if pre-existing ILD worsens

- Penicillamine—causes obliterative bronchiolitis in RA. Can also cause HP and a pulmonary-renal syndrome causing alveolar haemorrhage. May respond to stopping the drug
- Gold—alveolar opacities seen on HRCT, with associated fever and skin rash. BAL lymphocytosis. Treatment: stop the drug, and commence steroids. Usually reversible.

Box 22.1 Standard tests to consider for the investigation of these patients

- O_2 saturations and blood gas
- CXR ± HRCT
- Culture of respiratory secretions
- PFTs, including kCO
- Autoantibody (see ➨ p. 203) and inflammatory marker levels
- Bronchoscopy and BAL
- Transbronchial or open lung biopsies.

For an approach to:
- Diffuse lung disease, see ➨ p. 31
- Diffuse alveolar haemorrhage, see ➨ p. 27
- Pulmonary disease in the immunocompromised host (non-HIV), see ➨ p. 73.

Further information

British Society for Rheumatology. Rheumatoid arthritis guidelines on safety of anti-TNF therapies. *Rheumatology* 2010;49:2217–19.

Rheumatoid arthritis (RA)

- Persistent deforming symmetrical peripheral arthropathy with non-articular manifestations, including vasculitis
- Pulmonary/pleural disease is commoner in men and occasionally occurs before the development of joint problems
- Pneumonia is a common terminal event, causing 15–20% of RA deaths.

Pleuritis Frequent, occurring in >30% of patients and usually mild. Pleuritic pain, with no obvious other cause.

Pleural effusion Usually asymptomatic. Fluid is typically exudative, with a low glucose, low pH, and usually a lymphocytosis, may be pseudochylous (see ➲ p. 58). Often in association with other lung manifestations. Need to exclude other causes for effusion such as empyema or malignancy. If problematic, may require drainage and steroids (see ➲ p. 358).

Pulmonary fibrosis Similar to the IIPs (see ➲ p. 265), minor pulmonary fibrosis found in up to 60% of patients in lung biopsy studies, but CXR changes only seen in 1–5%. Hence symptomatic disease is unusual. Tends to occur in patients who have multi-system disease, including vasculitis, and those with nodules, seropositive disease, and high ANA titres. More common in men, and smoking is a risk factor for fibrosis development.
- *Presents* with progressive dyspnoea
- *Examination* Clubbing and bilateral basal crepitations
- *PFTs* Low kCO, restrictive pattern
- Radiologically and histologically similar to UIP, with subpleural basal reticular pattern, but can be like NSIP
- *Treatment* Steroids or immunosuppressants do little to change the course but should be tried.

Acute pneumonitis also recognized, which presents with rapidly deteriorating dyspnoea and development of respiratory failure, or acute deterioration on a background of chronic fibrosis. Acute pneumonitis tends to be more steroid-responsive.

Pulmonary nodules Occur in <5% of patients with RA. Usually found incidentally on CXR. Only occur in seropositive disease, and patients may have other nodules elsewhere such as elbows and fingers. Single or multiple; may measure up to 7cm, mainly subpleural or along interlobular septa. May cavitate and rarely cause haemoptysis or pneumothorax. Mostly asymptomatic. Main differential diagnosis is lung cancer. Usually followed on CT to ensure they are of stable size. They typically show mild uptake on PET, consistent with other benign lesions. May need biopsy to exclude malignancy.

Organizing pneumonia The clinical syndrome of pneumonia, with fever, dyspnoea, cough and weight loss, and multifocal consolidation, which do not respond to antibiotics. Can be disease- or drug-induced (gold) or have no obvious cause, i.e. cryptogenic (COP, see ➲ pp. 276–7). Confirmed by transbronchial or open lung biopsy showing acini filled with loose connective tissue and a variable inflammatory infiltrate. Often a dramatic response to steroids. May need long-term immunosuppression.

Small airways disease and obliterative bronchiolitis Evidence of mild small airways disease found in about a third when looked for on HRCT, but often asymptomatic, variable histology. Obliterative bronchiolitis is a rarer problem, with lymphocytic infiltration of terminal bronchioles progressively obliterated by inflammatory connective tissue.

- May present with dyspnoea, dry cough, and hyperinflated chest, with basal crepitations and mid-inspiratory 'squeak or squawk'
- *PFTs* Irreversible obstructive pattern, hypoxia
- *CXR* Hyperinflation, no infiltrates
- *HRCT* Mosaic pattern
- *Biopsy* shows destruction of terminal bronchiolar wall by granulation tissue, effacement of the lumen, and replacement of the bronchiole by fibrous tissue. Irreversible pathology, usually unresponsive to treatment
- May be rapidly progressive
- Can give trial of oral steroids, continuing with high-dose inhaled steroids if any response. Penicillamine was thought to be a causative factor, but the evidence for this is now weaker. Consider transplant.

Vasculitis rarely involves the lung and very rarely causes pulmonary haemorrhage. Rare cause of PHT.

Cricoarytenoid arthritis Seen in studies in up to 75% of patients with RA by fibre-optic laryngoscopy and HRCT, but rarely symptomatic (commoner in women). Unrelated to lung fibrosis. Can cause sore throat, hoarse voice, upper airways obstruction with stridor, or OSA. Flow–volume loop may be abnormal. This may need tracheostomy and steroids—oral and joint injection.

Bronchiectasis is often subtle with minimal clinical features but may be found in 30%. Traction bronchial dilation may be seen in association with pulmonary fibrosis. Diagnosis made on HRCT.

Sjögren's syndrome causing mucosal drying, often in association with ILD, produces dry cough and increased airway infections (see ➔ p. 200)

Caplan's syndrome RA, single or multiple chest nodules, and coal-worker's pneumoconiosis, see ➔ pp. 364–5 (now rare).

Further information

Amital A et al. The lung in rheumatoid arthritis. *Press Med* 2011;**40**:e31–48.

Systemic lupus erythematosus (SLE)

- Multi-organ autoimmune disease, mainly affecting women
- dsDNA antibodies present in high titres, and these may be the causative agent
- Can also get a drug-induced lupus syndrome (see Box 22.2), improves on stopping drug
- Pulmonary disease (lung, vasculature, pleura, diaphragm) often seen and may be a presenting feature of the disease
- American College of Rheumatology classification—see Box 22.3.

Pleural disease Most common manifestation of pulmonary disease. Often asymptomatic but may have pleuritic pain due to pleuritis with a pleural rub. ('Pleuritic' pain may also be due to musculoskeletal causes.) Pleural effusions found in 50% of patients, which may cause breathlessness. These are often bilateral and exudative, with a neutrophilia, or a lymphocytosis if the effusion is chronic. Can be haemorrhagic. Rarely develops into fibrothorax. Pleural biopsy findings are non-specific. Need to exclude other causes for effusion such as empyema or malignancy. If symptomatic, may need treatment with NSAIDs or steroids.

Atelectasis Associated with pleurisy or effusion.

Diffuse ILD Occurs in up to 70% of patients, but usually mild and asymptomatic. Radiologically similar to rheumatoid lung fibrosis. Only 5% develop clinical disease similar to UIP, with dyspnoea, cough, and basal crackles. May be associated with pleuritic pain. PFTs show restrictive defect with reduced kCO. Rarely, progressive and severe.

Acute lupus pneumonitis In <2%, severe illness with mortality rate >50%. Cough, dyspnoea, fever, pleuritic pain, hypoxia. Widespread crackles. CXR shows infiltrates, which may be widespread. Histologically, non-specific acute alveolar wall injury. Need to exclude infection, pulmonary oedema. Treatment: steroids and cytotoxic drugs may be necessary, may have good response. Can progress to chronic interstitial pneumonitis.

PHT due to pulmonary vasoconstriction, rather than pulmonary vasculitis. Commoner in those with Raynaud's phenomenon. Associated with poorer prognosis: 50% 2y mortality. Diagnosed on echo. Need to exclude PE as a cause, especially in those with antiphospholipid antibodies. Treatment as for idiopathic PHT (see ➜ pp. 392–3).

PE Commoner in the 20–30% with antiphospholipid antibodies.

'Shrinking lung syndrome' Dyspnoea (± episodic pleurisy) caused by reduced lung volumes and poor respiratory reserve, probably due to diaphragmatic muscle weakness. Small lungs on CXR. Normal lung parenchyma on CT. Restrictive lung function tests, with normal/high kCO. May improve with steroids.

Alveolar haemorrhage Rare. May be life-threatening. Can have associated glomerulonephritis. Acute dyspnoea, with infiltrates on CXR. Raised kCO. Treat with high-dose steroids + cyclophosphamide.

Chronic organizing pneumonia (COP or bronchiolitis obliterans) See ➔ pp. 276–7.

Box 22.2 Drug-induced lupus—causative drugs include:

- Isoniazid
- Procainamide
- Hydralazine
- Minocycline
- Penicillamine
- Anticonvulsants.

Box 22.3 Criteria of the American College of Rheumatology for the classification of SLE

SLE if four or more criteria present, serially or simultaneously, during any interval:

- Malar rash
- Discoid rash
- Photosensitivity
- Oral ulcers
- Arthritis
- Serositis
- Pleuritis or pericarditis
- Renal disorder: proteinuria >0.5g/24h or 3+ persistently, or cellular casts
- Neurological disorder: seizures or psychosis (having excluded drugs or other causes)
- Haematological disorder: haemolytic anaemia or leucopenia ($<4.0 \times 10^9$/L on two or more occasions), lymphopenia (1.5×10^9/L on two or more occasions), thrombocytopenia ($<100 \times 10^9$/L)
- Immunological disorder: raised anti-dsDNA antibody, anti-Sm antibody, positive finding of antiphospholipid antibodies
- ANA in raised titre (in the absence of drugs known to be associated with drug-induced lupus).

Further information

Keane M, Lynch J. Pleuropulmonary manifestations of SLE. Rare diseases 7. *Thorax* 2000;**55**:159–66.

Polymyositis and dermatomyositis

These are two separate idiopathic inflammatory myopathies:
• Polymyositis (PM) causes symmetrical proximal muscle weakness
• Dermatomyositis (DM) has a characteristic rash
• Diagnostic criteria in Box 22.4.

CK levels raised up to 50 times normal. ANA and myositis-specific antibodies positive. DM is frequently associated with underlying malignancy, including lung, oesophagus, breast, colon, and ovary, so therefore needs thorough investigation. Pulmonary complications are a common and frequent cause of death, occuring in both conditions. As with other connective tissue diseases, differentiation of the pulmonary problems from those due to drugs and infection is important.

ILD in 20–30% (commoner when CK levels normal and/or antisynthetase +ve (see further text); less common when DM is associated with malignancy). Patients present with dyspnoea, cough, arthralgia, and fevers, with fine bibasal crackles.
• *HRCT* shows patchy consolidation and peripheral reticular pattern
• *Histology* Wide variation, with UIP, NSIP, COP, and diffuse alveolar haemorrhage all reported, related to steroid response
• Lung involvement frequently associated with antisynthetase antibodies
• May require treatment with steroids or cyclophosphamide.

Ventilatory failure Due to intercostal and diaphragm muscle weakness. Restrictive defect on PFTs.

Chronic organizing pneumonia Poorer prognosis if associated with features of fibrosis.

PHT 2° to lung disease.

Pulmonary vasculitis Causing haemoptysis (rarely alveolar haemorrhage).

Aspiration pneumonia In 20%, associated with marked increase in mortality. Caused by dysphagia and pharyngeal muscle weakness and regurgitation.

Antisynthetase syndrome A subset with polyarthritis, fever, and Raynaud's, in addition to myositis, that have serum antibodies to one or more of the aminoacyl-transfer RNA synthetases, a family of intracytoplasmic enzymes involved in protein synthesis. Antibodies to Jo-1, PL-7, PL-12, OJ, and EJ are the ones that have been recognized and for which specific tests are available.

Spontaneous pneumomediastinum Occurs rarely (acute retrosternal pain, neck and face subcutaneous emphysema), usually in association with ILD, in DM more often than PM.

Box 22.4 Criteria for diagnosis of poly/dermatomyositis

- Symmetrical proximal muscle weakness, developing over weeks or months
- Elevated serum muscle enzymes, CK, and aldolase
- Typical EMG findings:
  - Myopathic potentials (low amplitude, short duration, polyphasic)
  - Fibrillation
  - Complex repetitive discharges
  - Typical muscle biopsy findings—endomysial inflammation
- Dermatological features of DM:
  - Gottron's papules, involving fingers, elbows, knees, and medial malleoli
  - Heliotrope sign around the eyes
  - Erythematous rash around back, shoulders, upper chest, and face.

Further information

Tzioufas AG. Antisynthetase syndrome. ℘ https://www.orpha.net/data/patho/Pro/en/Antisynthetase-FRenPro8611.pdf.

Systemic sclerosis

This disease affects women more than men (4:1), has HLA associations, and often presents in the fifth decade. It is largely a clinical diagnosis, and there are several types:

- *Limited cutaneous* (many have CREST syndrome). 60% of systemic sclerosis cases. Patients often have long-standing Raynaud's, developing non-pitting oedema of the fingers, which become 'sausage-shaped'. Develop thick, shiny skin after a few weeks to months. Later, they can develop skin changes on the hands, face, and neck, microstomia, digital and facial telangiectasia, intra- and subcutaneous calcification, and oesophageal dysmotility (74%). Patients can also develop pulmonary fibrosis (26%), PHT (21%), and cardiac (9%), oesophageal (90%), and renal disease (8%), but less common than in diffuse cutaneous disease
- *Diffuse cutaneous* Abrupt-onset disease, with widespread symmetrical itchy, painful swelling of fingers, arms, feet, legs, and face, and associated constitutional symptoms. There is oedema, which is replaced by tight, shiny skin, bound to underlying structures extending proximal to the wrists, within a few months. There is cutaneous thickening, as well as hypo- or hyperpigmentation. Raynaud's phenomenon is present, as well as skin sclerosis on the trunk and upper arms, arthropathy, renal disease (18%), pulmonary fibrosis (41%), PHT (17%), cardiac (12%) and GI disease (90%)
- *Overlap syndromes*, or mixed connective tissue diseases, have features of systemic sclerosis, together with those of at least one other autoimmune rheumatic disease such as SLE, RA, PM. Over time, other organ involvement may develop and evolve into a more defined disease
- *Systemic sclerosis sine scleroderma* Vascular or fibrotic visceral features without skin scleroderma. May or may not have Raynaud's phenomenon. May develop ILD, oesophagitis, arrhythmias, malabsorption, pseudo-obstruction, renal failure (>2% of cases)
- *Environmentally induced* Contentious but may result from exposure to vinyl chloride, pesticides, or epoxy resins.

Pulmonary complications are the most common cause of death.

Pulmonary fibrosis is seen at post-mortem in up to 80% of patients. ANA is positive in 60% and of speckled or nucleolar type. Pulmonary involvement is seen, particularly if Scl-70 antibody is present. Anti-centromere antibodies, however, are associated with reduced risk. Micro-aspiration from oesophageal dysmotility may be contributory.

- *Present* with dyspnoea and a history of Raynaud's
- *Examination* Signs of systemic sclerosis, fine bibasal crackles
- *PFTs* show restrictive defect and reduced kCO. Rapidly falling kCO is a poor prognostic sign. HRCT shows mostly NSIP pattern but can be UIP pattern. May need open lung biopsy to confirm diagnosis
- *Treatment* with steroids and cyclophosphamide. An RCT of oral cyclophosphamide vs placebo in patients with active alveolitis and scleroderma-related ILD showed a modest, but significant, effect on FVC, dyspnoea, and QoL (Taskin DP *et al. N Engl J Med* 2006;**354**:2655–66)

- *Prognosis* Systemic sclerosis-associated ILD has a better prognosis than pure UIP. This may be related to slower disease progression, rather than any greater response to immunosuppressive treatment; 15% of patients have progressive and severe disease. Associated increased risk of lung cancer.

PHT May be isolated or 2° to ILD. Isolated PHT is characteristic of limited cutaneous disease, especially in those with cutaneous telangiectasias and anti-centromere antibodies. Pathologically similar to PPH. Subintimal cell proliferation, endothelial hyperplasia, and the obliteration of small intrapulmonary vessels.
- *Presents* with dyspnoea, RV hypertrophy, and right heart failure
- *Diagnosis* by echo
- *Treatment* as for PPH (see ➔ pp. 392–3). May respond to prostacyclin infusions or may need transplant
- *Prognosis* Better than for those with PPH.

Chest wall limitation by skin scleroderma over chest ('hide-bound chest'), very rare.

Chronic organizing pneumonia See ➔ pp. 276–7.

Aspiration pneumonia Uncommon and due to oesophageal dysmotility.

Bronchiectasis Often seen on HRCT, but much less commonly of clinical significance.

Further information
McMahan ZH, Hummers LK. Systemic sclerosis—challenges for clinical practice. *Nat Rev Rheumatol* 2013;9:90–100.

Sjögren's syndrome

- Inflammation, lymphocytic infiltration, and destruction of primarily the salivary and lachrymal glands
- Keratoconjunctivitis sicca or xerostomia (dry eyes and dry mouth) is usually evidence of 1° disease but, when associated with connective tissue disease, especially RA, is 2° Sjögren's
- Classical sicca syndrome includes dry eyes and mouth, with parotid or salivary gland enlargement
- Pulmonary involvement occurs in about 25%, commoner in women and in their 60s.

Pleuritic chest pain.

Airways inflammation BHR, chronic bronchitis, and small airways disease. Mild abnormalities on PFTs, rarely significant.

Dry cough Atrophy of mucus gland in trachea and bronchi and lymphoplasmocytic infiltrate (xerotrachea). Possibly a higher incidence of chest infections. Treatment: nebulized saline, physiotherapy, inhaled steroids.

Diffuse lung disease Develops later, often asymptomatic, but may have cough, dyspnoea, and crackles on examination. PFTs show a restrictive defect and NSIP, LIP, or UIP pattern on CT.

Lymphoma Unusual but is 40 times more common in Sjögren's syndrome, especially in patients with high levels of immunoglobulins, autoantibodies, and cryoglobulins. Usually non-Hodgkin's B-cell lymphoma. Can mimic OP.

OP

Pleural thickening/effusion Rare.

PHT, thromboembolism Rare.

Ankylosing spondylitis

- Chronic inflammatory disease causing spinal ankylosis with sacroiliac joint involvement
- 90% of Caucasian patients are HLA-B27 +ve.

Pulmonary fibrosis occurs in 5–15%, especially those with advanced disease. Typically bilateral in the upper lobes. May develop cysts/cavities and become colonized with *Aspergillus*.

Pleural involvement Pleuritis and apical pleural thickening.

Restrictive defect Due to costovertebral rigidity causing fixed restrictive deformity of the thorax, rarely leading to respiratory failure with nocturnal hypoventilation. Nocturnal NIV may be indicated.

Behçet's syndrome

- Systemic vessel vasculitis involving arteries and veins of all sizes, with recurrent painful oral ± genital ulceration, skin lesions, arthritis, and chronic relapsing uveitis, which can cause blindness
- Marked geographical distribution, with greatest prevalence in Turkey, Iran, and Japan. Mainly young adults
- Musculoskeletal, skin, neurological, GI, and major artery and vein involvement.

Pulmonary arterial aneurysms, arterial and venous thrombosis, and pulmonary infarcts in <5%. Recurrent haemoptysis is the main manifestation. This can be massive and fatal. Pulmonary aneurysms are seen as non-cavitating shadows on CXR and confirmed by CT. These are associated with DVT, therefore making anticoagulation difficult due to possible haemoptysis from the aneurysm.

Pleural effusion, eosinophilic pneumonia Both rare.

Autoantibodies: disease associations

Antinuclear antibody (ANA)	+ve in
SLE	99%
RA	32%
Juvenile RA	76%
Chronic active hepatitis	75%
Sjögren's syndrome	68%
Systemic sclerosis	64%
Polymyositis	
Polyarteritis nodosa	
Myasthenia gravis	
Autoimmune thyroid disease	
Extensive burns	
Normal controls	0–2%

Extractable nuclear antigen (ENA)	(done by lab if ANA +ve)

Anti-dsDNA—SLE
Anti-Sm—SLE
Anti-topoisomerase-1—diffuse scleroderma
Anti-centromere—limited scleroderma
Anti-Scl-70—lung fibrosis in scleroderma
Anti-Jo-1 and other synthetases—myositis
Anti-Ro—Sjögren's, SLE, foetal heart block
Anti-RNP—SLE, scleroderma, myositis, mixed connective tissue disease, and RA
PR3(c)-ANCA (proteinase 3)—GPA (Wegener's)
MPO(p)-ANCA (myeloperoxidase)—microscopic polyangiitis

RhF	+ve in
RA	70–80%
Sjögren's syndrome	<100%
Felty's syndrome	<100%
Systemic sclerosis	30%
Still's disease	Rarely +ve
Infective endocarditis	<50%
SLE	<40%
Normal controls	5–10%
Also: Neoplasms, after radio- or chemotherapy	
Hyperglobulinaemic states	
Dermatomyositis	

Cor pulmonale

Definition, causes, and pathophysiology

Cor pulmonale is the traditional term for changes in the cardiovascular system resulting from the chronic hypoxia (and usually hypercapnia) of chronic lung disease, mainly PHT and fluid retention. It does not include similar changes seen in some left-sided disorders such as mitral incompetence.

Cor pulmonale can occur in most situations where there is chronic hypoxia (see Box 23.1):

- Most often in the setting of hypoxic and hypercapnic COPD
- Hypoventilation syndromes (scoliosis, neuromuscular diseases, obesity)
- Much less common when there is no associated rise in $PaCO_2$ (e.g. with ILDs, altitude, right-to-left shunts)

Cor pulmonale is often also referred to as 'right heart failure', which is misleading as the cardiac output in cor pulmonale is usually *normal or high* with *increased* peripheral perfusion (hence, the 'bounding pulse' and warm peripheries of type II ventilatory failure). If allowed time to adapt, the right ventricle (RV) can generate much higher pressures (e.g. in idiopathic pulmonary arterial hypertension (IPAH)) than are usually seen in cor pulmonale in response to the hypoxia. In true right heart failure, the RV acutely fails to develop an adequate cardiac output, e.g. following right-sided MI or PEs that occlude a large proportion of the pulmonary vascular bed. This also produces a raised JVP, as occurs in the fluid overload of cor pulmonale, but, in contrast, there will of course be a low cardiac output and poor peripheral perfusion.

Box 23.1 Cor pulmonale results from the following sequence of events

- Lung disease causes hypoxia, cyanosis, and sometimes polycythaemia
- Hypoxia is sensed both within the kidney and via the carotid body, generating increases in sympathetic activity and renal vasoconstriction
- Increased sympathetic activity (and other mechanisms) leads to renal retention of salt and water
- This extra salt and water is mainly held in the capacitance vessels (the large veins), often with a raised JVP
- If vascular permeability rises (particularly when the $PaCO_2$ rises, producing peripheral vasodilatation and an increase in capillary pressure), extra fluid accumulates in dependent tissues, mainly the ankles
- A raised JVP and ankle oedema in this setting are NOT due to impaired RV function, but to fluid overload and increased vascular permeability.

Patients often present with their first episode of ankle swelling during an exacerbation of their COPD when, for the first time, the $PaCO_2$ rises and the PaO_2 falls, far enough to provoke the above events. Body weight may not actually rise very much with the onset of ankle oedema; however, the extra salt and water, retained in the capacitance vessels leading up to the exacerbation, move into the subcutaneous tissues, probably due to the CO_2-induced vasodilatation, raising mean capillary hydrostatic pressure.

Loss of pulmonary vascular bed from emphysema also contributes to the raised PAP, and the ECG often shows RV hypertrophy. During an exacerbation, extra hypoxia will produce further rises in PAP, with which the hypertrophied RV usually copes, helped by the raised JVP providing a larger pre-load to increase RV filling. Excessive diuresis can lead to a true fall in right-sided output due to inadequate filling of the RV.

Clinical features and investigations

- The underlying disease causing the hypoxia, e.g. COPD/bronchiectasis
- Easily visible veins and a raised JVP
- Cyanosis and a suffused conjunctiva (polycythaemia and vessel dilatation from the raised CO_2)
- Sometimes marked polycythaemia, very rare consequences due to hyperviscosity
- Peripheral vasodilatation, with a 'bounding' pulse and warm peripheries
- Ankle swelling and pitting oedema
- RV hypertrophy (sternal heave uncommon, masked by hyperinflated lung between heart and chest wall; more often seen with the higher pressures of IPAH
- Tricuspid incompetence (not usually severe)
- CXR—enlarged pulmonary arteries/underlying lung disease
- FBC—may have associated polycythaemia
- Oximetry—cor pulmonale is unlikely if awake SaO_2 >92%
- Blood gases—cor pulmonale progressively more likely as PaO_2 drops below 8kPa (equivalent $SaO_2 \approx 91\%$) and $PaCO_2$ rises above 6kPa
- ECG—may indicate right axis deviation (RAD), p pulmonale (right atrial hypertrophy), and right bundle branch block (RBBB)
- Echo—dilated or hypertrophied RV, tricuspid regurgitation (TR), providing estimate of PAP, and exclude other diagnoses such as a patent atrial septal defect (ASD)
- Overnight oximetry—to reveal unexpected degrees of hypoxia, e.g. from OSA, obesity, neuromuscular disease.

Management

Minimal ankle oedema needs no treatment. 'Trimming' the ankles to normal is unnecessary and may reduce RV output by reducing RV filling. If the oedema is more substantial, then the following may help:
- Treat underlying condition to raise PaO_2 and lower $PaCO_2$
- Raise PaO_2 through added O_2; provide long-term O_2 at home
- In hypoventilation syndromes, home overnight NIV likely to be the correct management
- Promote a limited diuresis with judicious use of diuretics
- Always elevate legs when sitting
- Some will venesect if haematocrit exceeds 0.6, but no RCT evidence of physiological benefit or a reduction in hyperviscosity complications.

In general, 'cor pulmonale' is overtreated. It is often a relatively harmless by-product of hypoxia, rather than a problem in its own right. Treating the blood gas disturbance and making it easier for the patient to get his shoes on are the main therapeutic aims. The long-term O_2 trials showed that improving the PaO_2 was useful, not that lowering the PAP was important.

Further information

Stewart AG et al. Hormonal, renal, and autonomic nerve factors involved in the excretion of sodium and water during dynamic salt and water loading in hypoxaemic chronic obstructive pulmonary disease. Thorax 1995;50:838–45.

Chapter 24

Cystic fibrosis

General principles

Definition and pathophysiology
- CF is a multi-system disease due to mutations in the gene encoding the CF transmembrane conductance regulator (CFTR), a complex chloride channel
- CFTR is essential for regulating chloride permeability across epithelial tissues and, in addition, has other complex cellular roles (e.g. CFTR downregulates transepithelial sodium transport, in particular the epithelial sodium channel, and influences expression of other genes, including those involved in inflammatory responses, ion transport, and cell signalling)
- Loss of CFTR function or quantity causes inadequate hydration of mucous secretions. In the lungs, this results in defective mucociliary clearance, mucus obstruction of the luminal space, and colonization with pathogenic bacteria. Recurrent cycles of infection and inflammation contribute to lung damage and subsequent development of bronchiectasis
- In the pancreas, the exocrine ducts become blocked by secretions, leading to pancreatic destruction, pancreatic enzyme insufficiency, and CF-related diabetes.

Genetics
- CF is an autosomal recessive disease, with a carrier frequency of 1 in 25 in Caucasians; 1 in 2,500 UK live births have CF. CF is rare in Afro-Caribbeans but is seen in patients of Asian origin in the UK and USA
- Heterozygote advantage through resistance to diarrhoeal disease may have led to persistence of *CFTR* mutations at relatively high population frequencies, despite the lethal homozygous form
- >1,800 different mutations in the *CFTR* gene are recognized and can be classified on the basis of the mechanism by which they cause disease (see Table 24.1)
- The most common mutation is F508del (previously termed DeltaF508; a deletion of three nucleotides, causing the loss of a phenylalanine at residue 508), which accounts for ~70% of defective *CFTR* alleles in patients, with a decreasing prevalence from north-west to south-east Europe
- Thirteen other mutations have a frequency >1% (e.g. G542X (3.4%), G551D (2.4%), W1282X (2.1%), 3905insT (2.1%)), accounting for 85% of CF alleles altogether. These can be effectively screened for
- CF is characterized by wide variation between patients in disease severity, rate of progression, and, to an extent, organ involvement. This phenotypic variation is caused, at least in part, by (i) class of *CFTR* mutation (correlates highly with pancreatic status but not with severity of lung disease), (ii) polymorphism in non-*CFTR* 'modifier' genes (e.g. *IFRD1*, which regulates neutrophil function), and (iii) environmental factors (e.g. compliance, socio-economic status, access to care, smoke exposure, pathogen-specific factors).

Screening In the UK, neonatal heel-prick for immunoreactive trypsinogen measurement is offered routinely as part of a national screening programme. Positive samples are tested for common *CFTR* mutations and, if needed, a second immunoreactive trypsinogen screen, followed by sweat testing.

Diagnosis Patients are usually diagnosed with CF as neonates or children (genetic screening, family history, failure to thrive, meconium ileus, rectal prolapse, cough, recurrent chest infections). Diagnosis is based on the presence of two disease-causing *CFTR* mutations, along with a positive sweat test (sweat chloride concentration >60mmol/L, usually 90–110mmol/L) and compatible clinical features. Sweat chloride levels are usually lower in CF that presents in adulthood (borderline is 40–60mmol/L; <40 is considered normal although can occur in CF).

CFTR-related disease refers to patients with mild manifestations of CFTR dysfunction such as single organ involvement (e.g. late-onset bronchiectasis, congenital bilateral absence of the vas deferens, or idiopathic pancreatitis). These typically occur with 'milder' *CFTR* mutations (classes IV or V; see Table 24.1) that result in residual CFTR function, and patients tend to be pancreatic-sufficient. A grey area exists between CF and CFTR-related disease, and, in some cases, a firm diagnosis is not possible on initial investigation but becomes apparent during follow-up; note that CF remains a clinical diagnosis.

Management The ongoing care of CF patients moves to the adult CF centre around the age of 16–18 (often when the patient leaves school), although a period of transitional care may occur between ages 14–16. An MDT approach is essential, comprising respiratory physician, specialist nurse, physiotherapist, pharmacist, dietician, and psychologist, with regular additional input from gastroenterology and endocrine teams.

Improved treatment of CF has led to an increase in median survival to around 40y, and >55% of UK CF patients are adults. The predicted lifespan for a baby born with CF now is at least 50y.

Table 24.1 Classes of CFTR mutation

Class I	Defective protein synthesis, e.g. G542X
Class II	Defective protein maturation and trafficking, e.g. F508del
Class III	Impaired chloride channel opening (gating), e.g. G551D
Class IV	Defective channel ion transport (conductance), e.g. R117H
Class V	Defective splicing
Class VI	Accelerated turnover at cell surface

Further information

UK CF Trust. ♪ http://www.cysticfibrosis.org.uk.

CF Trust consensus documents on aspects of cystic fibrosis care. ♪ http://www.cysticfibrosis.org.uk/about-cf/publications/consensus-documents.aspx.

CF mutation database. ♪ http://www.genet.sickkids.on.ca.

CF microbiology: overview

Chronic pulmonary sepsis and its complications account for much of the morbidity and mortality in CF. The airways of a CF patient are chronically colonized by pathogenic bacteria from an early age. Bronchiectasis is usually established by a young age (around 5y).

- Patients commonly expectorate variable volumes of purulent sputum, even when well
- When organism levels are high, patients may feel generally unwell or more tired, or have anorexia, weight loss, temperature >38°C
- They may have symptoms of dyspnoea, increased volume of more purulent sputum, haemoptysis, wheeze, and chest ache
- Examination and CXR can be unchanged from normal
- With effective antibiotic treatment, FEV_1 levels should rise to the pre-infection normal. If they do not, further antibiotics may be necessary, and other diagnoses or unusual organisms should be considered
- In practice, the FEV_1 is the most reliable marker of disease progression and can be used to assess overall decline, as well as to determine an exacerbation and response to treatment (as PEFR would be used in asthma).

Organisms Airway colonization changes over time, with increasing age, and organisms become more resistant to antibiotics. Typical progression of organism colonization with time is *Staphylococcus aureus*, followed by *Haemophilus influenzae*, and then *Pseudomonas aeruginosa* (see Fig. 24.1). Goals of management should be initially to prevent infection, then to eradicate it, and finally to control the infection. Material for culture should be collected; most commonly sputum, but BAL if necessary. Polymicrobial infection is common.

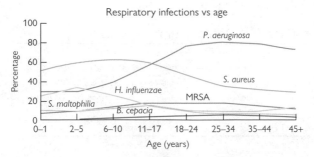

Fig. 24.1 Prevalence of selected respiratory pathogens in patients with CF over time. Reproduced from Goss C., *Thorax* (2007) 62: 360–7 with the kind permission of BMJ

CF antibiotics 1

Antibiotic courses in patients with CF need to be longer and at higher doses than in non-CF patients. Indications for treatment in adults include any new isolate from sputum (even if asymptomatic) or features of an exacerbation (see ⟳ pp. 218–9). Treatment should be for 14 days with either oral or IV antibiotics. IV antibiotics are indicated for severe infection or failure to eradicate organisms with oral antibiotics. Choice of antibiotics is based on clinical response more than *in vitro* resistance patterns, but recent sputum culture results will also guide therapy.

- In practice, it is usually appropriate to give the patient the same regime they had during their last exacerbation, provided there was a good clinical response, taking into account the patient's antibiotic allergies (desensitization may be required; see ⟳ pp. 220–1)
- Recent sputum culture results can be helpful, although note that sputum cultures lack sensitivity. Have a low threshold for including anti-pseudomonal cover if *P. aeruginosa* has previously been isolated (even if assumed to have been eradicated). Results of *in vitro* antibiotic susceptibility testing do not always correlate with clinical response to antibiotics
- All CF centres will have written management protocols which should be followed. Seek expert advice from your local CF centre if unsure.

Pseudomonas aeruginosa is associated with a more rapid decline in lung function. Most CF patients are chronically infected with P. aeruginosa by their early teens: non-mucoid species colonize initially, which may be asymptomatic or intermittent and can be eradicated, and mucoid species then follow and permanent eradication is rare. The aims of treatment are prompt eradication of new isolates and maintenance therapy to reduce the bacterial load in colonized patients.

- *First isolates of P. aeruginosa* in patients who were previously *Pseudomonas*-free or who have never had *P. aeruginosa* should lead to prompt treatment with an eradication regimen (even if asymptomatic). Failure to treat may lead to the development of chronic airway infection. There is no clear evidence favouring a specific eradication regimen. An initial treatment protocol combining nebulized colistin 2MU bd for 3 months with oral ciprofloxacin 750mg bd (avoid in epilepsy; reduce dose in severe renal impairment; warn patient to stop if ankle pain, as risk of Achilles tendon rupture) for 3 months is widely used. Consider a 2-week course of IV anti-pseudomonal antibiotics (see Box 24.1) before starting treatment with nebulized colistin and oral ciprofloxacin in patients with a new *P. aeruginosa* isolate in the context of a respiratory exacerbation. Failure of eradication with oral and nebulized antibiotics should also prompt IV therapy
- *Maintenance treatment for chronic P. aeruginosa infection* comprises long-term nebulized anti-pseudomonal therapy, typically either nebulized colistin 1–2MU bd or alternate months of nebulized tobramycin 300mg bd (the alternate month can either be medication-free or the patient may nebulize colistin). Alternative, recently approved maintenance

anti-pseudomonals include dry powder inhaler forms of colistin and tobramycin and nebulized aztreonam

- *Treatment of exacerbations in patients with chronic P. aeruginosa infection* Mild exacerbations (e.g. following a viral URTI) should be treated with a 2-week course of oral ciprofloxacin, alongside usual maintenance nebulized antibiotics. IV anti-pseudomonal antibiotics (see Box 24.1) for a minimum of 2 weeks are indicated for moderate and severe exacerbations as well as for first *P. aeruginosa* isolates not cleared by ciprofloxacin and colistin.

Box 24.1 2-week course of IV antibiotic treatment of *Pseudomonas aeruginosa* in CF

Combinations of two drugs are typically used to achieve a synergistic effect—select one drug from the left-hand column alongside one drug from the right-hand column:

Ceftazidime 2–3g tds	Tobramycin 7mg/kg/day
Piperacillin/tazobactam 4.5g tds	Amikacin 15mg/kg/day
Aztreonam 2g tds	Colistin 2MU tds
Meropenem 2g tds	

Notes:

- IV tobramycin, amikacin, and colistin all require *therapeutic drug monitoring*; follow local policy. Use previous treatment doses (if available) as a guide to starting doses in individual patients, adjusted for current weight. Ensure adequate hydration and normal renal function at the start of therapy. Reduce dosage in renal impairment
- Symptoms of dizziness, hearing loss, or tinnitus during IV aminoglycosides (tobramycin, amikacin) suggest *oto- or vestibulo-toxicity*. The aminoglycoside should be stopped and ENT referral made for pure tone audiogram. Previous oto- or vestibulo-toxicity is an absolute contraindication to further IV aminoglycosides
- Note that IV gentamicin is no longer recommended in CF patients, and once-daily aminoglycoside dosing (rather than tds) is recommended
- Use of *nebulized* antibiotics in conjunction with IV administration of the same antibiotic may result in toxic drug levels, and many clinicians will stop nebulized antibiotics whilst the patient is receiving IV antibiotics
- IV fosfomycin may also be useful in the treatment of resistant *P. aeruginosa* infections.

CF antibiotics 2

Staphylococcus aureus is a significant pathogen causing exacerbations. Prevention and eradication are important, even if the patient is asymptomatic. In adults, a minimum of 2 weeks of treatment should be given when S. aureus is cultured, with flucloxacillin, or erythromycin or clindamycin if penicillin-allergic. Note that macrolide resistance is increasingly common in MRSA. If S. aureus continues to grow, despite treatment with flucloxacillin, check that the S. aureus isolate is not MRSA, and add in a second anti-staphylococcal antibiotic (e.g. sodium fusidate or rifampicin) for 2 weeks. More prolonged oral antibiotics (e.g. further 4 weeks) or a course of IV antibiotics may be required. There is some evidence to support long-term flucloxacillin prophylaxis in colonized children, but this is not widely practised in adults, reflecting a lack of evidence of benefit in this age group as well as concerns regarding the development of MRSA.

Haemophilus influenzae should be treated with, e.g. co-amoxiclav or doxycycline, even if the patient is asymptomatic. More prolonged oral antibiotics or a course of IV antibiotics (e.g. co-amoxiclav or ceftriaxone) may be required. Resistance to amoxicillin and macrolides is common.

Burkholderia cepacia complex comprises at least ten different subspecies (genomovars) of B. cepacia. These organisms are often resistant to many antibiotics and display inherent resistance to colistin. Some genomovars are highly transmissible, and patients colonized with B. cepacia should be segregated (including separate clinics and spirometers, and side rooms on a different ward) from non-colonized patients. Clinical consequences of infection are highly variable, ranging from asymptomatic to severe worsening of pulmonary infection with septicaemia ('cepacia syndrome'), which can be rapidly fatal. B. cenocepacia (genomovar III) is particularly associated with cepacia syndrome and is usually considered an absolute contraindication for lung transplant due to poor outcomes. Treat exacerbations with combination antibiotic therapy, directed by *in vitro* sensitivities where available. Meropenem appears to be a particularly useful antibiotic, and other options often include ceftazidime, piperacillin-tazobactam, aminoglycosides, and temocillin. Mild exacerbations may respond to oral ciprofloxacin, doxycycline, or co-trimoxazole.

MRSA has been associated with increased mortality in CF and leads to difficulties in antibiotic choice and delivery of care. Follow local guidelines for topical eradication in patients with MRSA skin carriage. 4-week long courses of oral rifampicin with sodium fusidate are useful for sputum eradication; other options include linezolid or nebulized vancomycin. IV teicoplanin or vancomycin are required for MRSA pulmonary exacerbations.

NTM *Mycobacterium avium* complex (MAC) and *Mycobacterium abscessus* are the most frequently encountered NTM in CF (see ➲ pp. 518–9 for diagnosis and treatment). In general, consider and treat other causes of deterioration (e.g. *P. aeruginosa*) prior to initiating anti-mycobacterial therapy. The clinical and radiological features of NTM may be difficult to distinguish from other infections, particularly *P. aeruginosa*, and both long-term antibiotics (e.g. macrolides, tobramycin) and bacterial overgrowth may inhibit NTM culture. Recent studies have suggested that the *M. abscessus* subspecies *massiliense* may be spread between patients within CF centres, although the transmission route and infection control measures required to control this organism are currently unknown. Furthermore, isolation of *M. abscessus* pre-transplant appears to be a risk factor for the development of post-transplant NTM disease and a poor outcome, and active *M. abscessus* infection is considered an absolute contraindication to transplant in many units.

Stenotrophomonas maltophilia The clinical significance of *S. maltophilia* colonization in CF remains unclear. Address other causes of clinical deterioration in colonized patients prior to considering antibiotic treatment directed at *S. maltophilia*. *S. maltophilia* is inherently resistant to carbapenems, and most strains are also resistant to anti-pseudomonal drugs. Co-trimoxazole is the usual antibiotic of choice; other options include doxycycline, ticarcillin-clavulanic acid, or tigecycline.

Achromobacter xylosoxidans The clinical significance of *A. xylosoxidans* infection is uncertain; consider treatment in chronically colonized patients with evidence of clinical deterioration in the absence of other causes. *A. xylosoxidans* is often multi-resistant, and antibiotic choice should be on the basis of susceptibility testing results; useful agents often include minocycline, meropenem, piperacillin-tazobactam, and chloramphenicol.

Further information

CF Trust consensus document on antibiotic treatment for cystic fibrosis, 3rd edn, 2009. ℜ http://www.cysticfibrosis.org.uk/about-cf/publications/consensus-documents.aspx.

Management of exacerbations

Pulmonary exacerbations are the most common reason for hospital admission of CF patients. Patients are usually adept at recognizing a deterioration in their condition requiring treatment, and treatment is *usually* required if they present acutely, even if they appear fit and healthy.

Signs and symptoms of an exacerbation include:

- Increase in productive cough or dyspnoea
- Change in appearance or volume of sputum
- New signs on auscultation (often absent)
- New CXR changes (often absent)
- Weight loss >1kg or 5% of body weight, associated with anorexia
- Fall in FEV_1 >10%
- Fever.

Persistent, low-grade symptoms, such as cough alone, are an indication for IV antibiotics if oral antibiotics have failed to bring about an improvement. IV antibiotics should also be considered if a new positive sputum culture fails to clear with appropriate oral antibiotics.

Investigations

- Baseline spirometry for FEV_1
- Weight
- O_2 saturation and, if <92%, blood gas
- CXR (exclude pneumothorax)
- Sputum (M, C, & S, including specific testing for *P. aeruginosa* and *B. cepacia*, and AFBs)
- Bloods, including CRP (note that not all patients exhibit high inflammatory markers, even during severe exacerbations)
- Monitor blood sugars.

Treatment is with appropriate antibiotics (see ➜ p. 214–5), O_2 therapy, increased physiotherapy and nutritional support, and control of hyperglycaemia. Many patients will self-administer IV antibiotics at home (see ➜ pp. 220–1). Indications for inpatient treatment include: too unwell for home therapy; significant weight loss; poor response to recent home IVs; poor compliance or unable to self-administer IV therapy; patient preference; other complications (e.g. significant haemoptysis or pneumothorax; see ➜ pp. 224–5).

If *failing to improve* with empirical antibiotics:

- Review microbiology; repeat sputum M, C, & S and AFBs, and consider empirical change in antibiotics, including anti-pseudomonal cover (see ➜ pp. 214–5)
- Consider hospital admission if failing to improve with home-based treatment
- Optimize airway clearance with intensive physiotherapy, and review mucolytics (see ➜ pp. 222–3)
- Optimize nutritional support and glycaemic control (see ➜ pp. 226–7)

- Assess adherence to treatment
- Exclude ABPA (see ➲ pp. 224–5)
- Review and repeat CXR imaging, and consider CT chest, followed by bronchoscopic lavage targeted to area of nodularity/consolidation on imaging (?NTM or fungal infection); stopping all antibiotics (including long-term macrolides and nebulized anti-pseudomonals) may increase the yield from bronchoscopy
- Consider empirical oral prednisolone in severely unwell patients who are failing to improve with appropriate antibiotics.

NIV may assist with airways clearance, in addition to providing ventilatory support. Consider the appropriateness of ICU admission as well as resuscitation status in severe exacerbations—liaise with CF consultant.

IV antibiotic administration

- The majority of IV antibiotic courses can be administered at home, after an initial assessment and with home support from nursing staff. Many patients are relatively well during courses of IV antibiotics and are able to continue attending work or college, although it can take them considerable extra time to administer the antibiotics
- Most antibiotic regimes involve 14 days of IV antibiotics. This may require the siting of an IV cannula with a microbiological filter (to make it last longer), or preferably a long line
- Many patients have an indwelling venous access device (see following section) that can be accessed when required
- Prior to starting IV antibiotics, clinical assessment, including spirometry, should be made. Patients should be reviewed at day 7 to ensure satisfactory clinical progress (and to consider changing antibiotics if little or no improvement) and at end of the course in outpatients to ensure clinical improvement
- Courses of IV antibiotics are often administered prophylactically before surgery, and regular elective courses of IV antibiotics may be useful for patients who have experienced a rapid and progressive increase in the decline of their lung function or who suffer frequent exacerbations.

Implantable venous access devices (IVADs)

(e.g. Port-A-Cath®)

- Inserted in patients with difficult IV access or those needing frequent courses of IV antibiotics
- Usually accessed by a trained nurse, patient, or family member. Access only with a Huber point needle of the appropriate length; do not use standard needles, which may damage the IVAD
- Flush with 5–10mL of 100U/mL heparin monthly and with 5mL of 10U/mL heparin at the end of each IV dose
- Avoid taking blood from IVAD, if possible, as this increases the risk of blockage and infection. Other complications include venous obstruction (including SVC obstruction), thrombosis, tip dislocation, and leakage
- If pain or swelling around IVAD site, arrange a portagram/linogram to look for occlusion or damaged catheter. If IVAD blocks: injection of 20–50mL heparinized saline, gently alternating between irrigation and aspiration, may clear small occlusions. If this fails, consider urokinase 25,000U in 3mL 0.9% saline instilled into IVAD
- Infected or fractured lines need surgical removal.

Antibiotic desensitization Antibiotic sensitivity is a major problem in CF, as repeated antibiotic courses are associated with the development of allergic reactions, especially to β-lactams. Rashes are common, but anaphylaxis (see ➔ pp. 644–5) can occur. Always give first doses of a new antibiotic in hospital with resuscitation facilities at hand. Desensitization regimes can enable treatment with antibiotics that have previously caused an allergic reaction. Such regimes need to be given at the start of the antibiotic course each time it is used and during the course if doses are missed for >1 day. Depending on local policy, give a dilute antibiotic dose over 20min, followed by slightly stronger concentration, and repeat for seven concentration strengths until full antibiotic strength is given. Takes 3–4h. Stop infusion if any side effects develop.

Other pulmonary interventions

Physiotherapy Specialized CF physiotherapists teach effective airway clearance with the aim that patients perform this themselves twice daily on a long-term basis. This improves secretion clearance, decreases airflow obstruction, and improves ventilation. Several techniques are used: active cycle of breathing control (tidal volume breathing, then deep inspiration, and passive expiration, followed by forced expiration to mobilize secretions prior to coughing/huffing), autogenic drainage, Acapella or flutter devices, high-frequency oscillatory (vest) therapy, positive expiratory pressure mask, and use of NIV for airway clearance. More intensive physiotherapy is administered during exacerbations. Physiotherapists also have key role in assessment of functional ability with exercise testing, evaluating treatments, and encouraging aerobic exercise.

Recombinant DNase (dornase alfa) is a nebulized mucolytic that cleaves DNA from dead neutrophils, decreasing sputum viscosity and aiding its clearance. Recommended in patients with FVC >40% predicted to improve pulmonary function. Used once daily 2500U nebulized and should be taken at least 30min prior to doing airway clearance. Only continue in patients with clear benefit, e.g. 10% improvement in spirometry and shuttle walk test (SWT). It is expensive and only effective in 30–40%.

Hypertonic saline Use of regular nebulized hypertonic (7%) saline appears to increase mucociliary clearance and improves QoL and reduces exacerbations in trials. Consider if secretions are thick, tenacious, and difficult to expectorate. It is used immediately before or during usual airway clearance regime. Bronchospasm is a relatively common side effect: patients should receive a test dose, and pre-dosing with bronchodilators is usually required.

Inhaled mannitol has recently been approved for use in CF patients with rapidly declining lung function (defined as fall in FEV_1 >2%/y) who cannot use DNase (because of ineligibility, intolerance, or inadequate response) or other osmotic drugs.

Macrolides have anti-inflammatory and immunomodulatory effects, in addition to their antimicrobial activity, and seem to improve FEV_1 and decrease exacerbations in a subset of CF patients. They do not exhibit intrinsic anti-pseudomonal activity, but there is *in vitro* synergy between macrolides and anti-pseudomonal antibiotics, and the macrolide azithromycin decreases sputum viscoelasticity and disrupts *P. aeruginosa* biofilms. Consider a 6-month trial of oral azithromycin (250mg taken three times per week if <40kg, or 500mg three times per week if >40kg) in patients who are deteriorating on conventional therapy. Checklist when considering macrolide therapy:

• Check LFTs after 1 month; use with caution if pre-existing liver disease
• Warn patient to stop immediately if symptoms of ototoxicity (hearing loss, disequilibrium, tinnitus), and omit macrolide whilst receiving IV aminoglycosides
• Macrolides may prolong QT interval—check baseline corrected QT interval is <430ms (♂) or <450ms (♀) on ECG, and use with caution

alongside other QT-prolonging drugs (e.g. citalopram, domperidone, moxifloxacin, antifungals, etc.)
- Care with drug interactions, e.g. warfarin, itraconazole
- Avoid in patients with evidence of NTM infection and screen sputum for NTM prior to starting macrolides and whilst on treatment.

Ivacaftor is a mutation-specific, small molecule CFTR potentiator that is the first treatment to effectively target the basic CFTR defect: oral treatment resulted in significant improvements in lung function, exacerbation rate, weight gain, and QoL, and notably a halving of sweat chloride, in patients with a G551D mutation. Very high cost but recently approved for UK use in the 5% of CF patients with this mutation. It is widely believed that ivacaftor is likely to transform the prognosis for these patients, although long-term outcome data are awaited.

Respiratory support Respiratory failure and cor pulmonale can occur with later stage disease. Home O_2 may be required. Nocturnal NIV may be necessary as a 'bridge to transplant' in chronic respiratory failure and may also be useful in the palliation of symptoms of hypercapnia.

Steroids Short oral courses may improve lung function, but side effects, such as growth impairment, osteoporosis, and diabetes, are significant. They are used in ABPA, severe unresponsive exacerbations, and occasionally in terminal care.

Immunization Annual influenza as well as pneumococcal vaccination.

Lung transplantation (see p. 319) has a well-established role in CF, and patients should be considered for referral when their risk of death within 2–3y is high. Predicting prognosis in CF is difficult; historically, an FEV_1 ≤30% predicted was associated with a poor prognosis and used as a trigger to consider transplantation, but, in the modern treatment era, this low level of lung function is associated with a median survival of 5.3y and should not constitute the sole criterion for referral. Additional factors should be considered alongside absolute FEV_1 such as evidence of rapid progressive deterioration (e.g. increasing number of admissions/exacerbations, rapid fall in FEV_1), recurrent major haemoptysis not controlled by embolization, and recurrent or refractory pneumothorax; hypoxia (PaO_2 <7.3kPa) and hypercapnia ($PaCO_2$ >6.7kPa) are associated with <50% survival at 2y and remain useful guidelines for transplantation. Young female patients with rapid deterioration have a poor prognosis and should be considered for early referral.

Active *M. abscessus* or *B. cenocepacia* infection is considered an absolute contraindication to transplant in most UK centres. Whilst on the transplant waiting list, the patient should have optimal nutrition and physical care, including treatment of low bone mineral density and gastro-oesophageal reflux, and maintenance of good diabetes control and BMI >17. Average waits are around 1y in the UK, and approximately one in three CF patients die whilst on the waiting list. Following transplantation, the main immediate problems are infection and acute rejection, with bronchiolitis obliterans the predominant late complication (see pp. 328–9). 1y survival following transplant is ~85%.

Other pulmonary disease

Pneumothorax is more common in patients with advanced lung disease and is associated with a poor prognosis (48% 2y mortality rate). Presentation is typically with breathlessness and chest pain and interestingly often also haemoptysis. Manage according to standard pneumothorax guidelines (see ➲ p. 378). Consider IV antibiotics and physiotherapy (with modification of airway clearance, as necessary). Withhold positive pressure techniques if the pneumothorax is undrained. Avoid spirometry. The collapsed lung can be stiff and take longer to reinflate and require prolonged drainage and suction. Persistent air leaks may require surgical input, ideally with a limited procedure such as local abrasion. Pleurodesis is no longer considered a contraindication to later lung transplantation. Liaise with transplant centre if surgery is required.

Haemoptysis Small-volume haemoptysis is common, especially with concurrent infection and advanced disease. Massive haemoptysis (see ➲ p. 47) typically reflects bronchial artery bleeding and can be fatal. Management of haemoptysis: correct clotting (e.g. vitamin K 10mg od) and platelets; stop NSAIDs; low threshold for IV antibiotics; oral or IV tranexamic acid 1g every 6–8h (contraindications include renal failure, ischaemic arterial disease). For massive haemoptysis, anaesthetist may be required for airway management; sit patient upright, and give an ice-cold drink (reduces pulmonary pressures and vasoconstricts bronchial arteries); cross-match blood; consider nebulized adrenaline (1mL of 1:1,000 made up to 5mL with NaCl 0.9%); consider IV terlipressin (vasopressin analogue, increases systemic arterial pressure and reduces PAP; follow local guidelines for administration, typically 2mg IV and then 1–2mg every 4–6h if continued bleeding). Physiotherapy review: airway clearance is usually stopped during active bleeding and then modified and recommenced as bleeding subsides. Many clinicians temporarily stop NIV in patients with massive haemoptysis; nebulized drugs may also provoke further bleeding (particularly hypertonic saline); we recommend weighing their benefit against risk on an individual patient basis. Bronchoscopy is rarely of value, instead perform CTPA to look for bronchial artery hypertrophy; *bronchial artery embolization* is the gold standard treatment of massive haemoptysis or recurrent bleeding; discuss with interventional radiology.

ABPA (see also ➲ pp. 464–5) May be difficult to diagnose in CF, as hypersensitivity (with positive *Aspergillus* skin prick tests and precipitins) and sputum culture of *Aspergillus* are both common. ABPA is screened for annually and should be considered when exacerbations respond poorly to appropriate antibiotics. Guidelines define a 'classic case' of ABPA in CF as:
- Acute or subacute clinical deterioration (cough, wheeze, exercise intolerance, exercise-induced asthma, decline in pulmonary function, increased sputum) not attributable to another cause
- Serum total IgE concentration >1,000IU/mL (unless receiving systemic corticosteroids, which will suppress IgE)
- Presence of serum IgE antibody (RAST) to *A. fumigatus*

- Precipitating antibodies to *A. fumigatus*
- Infiltrates or mucus plugging on CXR or chest CT that have not cleared with antibiotics and physiotherapy.

Blood eosinophilia is also a common finding, and ABPA may occur with intermediate serum IgE concentrations of 500–1,000IU/mL.

Treatment is with oral **prednisolone** 0.5–1.0mg/kg (non-enteric-coated; maximum dose 60mg) for 2 weeks, and, if there is a clinical improvement, these should be continued at decreasing doses for 2–3 months. Intensive physiotherapy is also an important part of the treatment regime, and hypertonic saline may be useful. Add antifungal therapy with **itraconazole** for 3–6 months if there is a slow or poor response to corticosteroids, relapse of ABPA, and in corticosteroid-dependent cases. Itraconazole checklist:

- Initial itraconazole dose is 5mg/kg/day; give od, unless dose exceeds 200mg/day, in which case it should be given bd; maximum daily dose 400mg/day
- H_2 antagonists and PPIs reduce absorption of itraconazole—take itraconazole with an acidic drink (e.g. orange juice or cola) if also taking antacids
- Check LFTs at baseline, after 1 month, and then every 3 months if therapy continues
- Review concomitant medications to avoid a drug-drug interaction.

In addition to ABPA, other forms of *Aspergillus*-related lung disease described in CF include aspergillomas (see ➋ pp. 470–1) and '*Aspergillus* bronchitis' (a newly proposed entity of positive respiratory cultures for *A. fumigatus* and radiological infiltrates in symptomatic patients who do not fulfil the above diagnostic criteria for ABPA but respond to antifungal therapy).

CF 'asthma' Some CF patients have coexisting asthma, and some have asthma-like symptoms of prolonged exhalation, wheeze, and crackles due to underlying lung inflammation. This is difficult to diagnose, as these symptoms and a variable PEFR are found in many CF patients due to airway hyperresponsiveness. There may be bronchodilator responsiveness or bronchoconstriction after exercise or nebulized hypertonic saline. Treat with the standard asthma stepwise treatment: short-acting bronchodilator, inhaled corticosteroid, LABA, theophyllines (which may aid mucociliary clearance), leukotriene receptor antagonist (limited evidence in CF but may decrease eosinophilic inflammation), oral steroids.

Extrapulmonary disease

Nutritional management The maintenance of good nutrition correlates with survival in CF, and dietician input is crucial. Nutrition is more problematic as respiratory disease progresses (raised basal metabolic rate, increased work of breathing, ongoing infection, and inflammation). High-calorie, high-protein diets are encouraged. Patients may need nutritional supplements ± supplemental overnight enteral (nasogastric (NG) or gastrostomy) tube feeding. Weigh patients at every review, and aim for BMI >19.

- *Pancreatic enzyme supplementation* to avoid high faecal fat/energy loss is essential if pancreatic-insufficient (85% of patients). Use the smallest dose of pancreatin-containing lipase, required to control steatorrhoea. Typical preparations are Creon® (contains lipase, protease, and amylase) 10,000, 25,000, or 40,000, taken pre-meals. Typically, patients take 10–20 tablets/day and are educated to adjust the dosage, according to the fat and protein content of each meal. High-strength pancreatic enzyme preparations have been linked to fibrosing colonopathy; maximum lipase levels of 10,000U/kg/day are recommended
- Fat-soluble *vitamins* are poorly absorbed in most patients with CF (particularly if pancreatic-insufficient) and require supplementation—a widely used combined preparation is AquaDEKs®, two capsules daily.

GI disease

- *Distal intestinal obstructive syndrome* (DIOS, previously termed meconium ileus equivalent) comprises bloating, abdominal pain, possible palpable right lower quadrant mass, and complete or incomplete intestinal obstruction by viscid faecal material in terminal ileum and proximal colon. Abdominal X-ray characteristically shows 'foamy' gas pattern in the right flank ± dilated small bowel loops/fluid levels. Can occur spontaneously or secondary to dehydration or intercurrent infection. *Treatment* is medical. Mild cases may respond to high doses of regular polyethylene glycol (Movicol®). Correct hydration using IV fluids, if necessary. More severe cases may be relieved by oral Gastrografin® (50mL mixed with 200mL of water or cordial tds for up to 5 days) or Klean-Prep® (can be given orally but usually via NG, and not nocturnally as risk of aspiration). If this is unsuccessful, patients will require a Gastrografin® enema (under radiological guidance) to determine the site of obstruction and for therapeutic benefit. Treatment is complete when clear fluid is passed from the rectum and symptoms have resolved. If not resolving, consider further imaging and surgical opinion (differential diagnosis includes acute small bowel obstruction, e.g. 2° to adhesions, and intussusception)
- *Gastro-oesophageal reflux* is common and may worsen lung disease. Combinations of PPIs, H_2 receptor antagonists, and prokinetics (e.g. domperidone 10–20mg tds) are usually required
- *Coeliac disease* appears to be more common in CF
- *Pancreatitis* occurs in pancreatic-sufficient patients, presenting as acute attack or chronic recurrent abdominal pain. Treat with bowel rest, PPI, IV rehydration
- *GI and pancreatic cancer* is more common in CF.

Liver and biliary disease

- *Focal biliary cirrhosis* affects 5–10% of CF patients and leads to portal tract fibrosis, often with preserved hepatic architecture. Cirrhosis is frequently asymptomatic and develops insidiously in childhood. Annual screening liver USS is performed, as blood tests can be unhelpful (although ALP most sensitive). Biopsy unhelpful as patchy disease. Treatment with ursodeoxycholic acid improves biochemical indices of liver function, although its long-term benefits are unproven. Established cirrhosis can lead to portal hypertension and variceal bleeding; annual screening endoscopies are performed in patients with cirrhosis.

Metabolic disease

- *CF-related diabetes (CFRD)* is becoming increasingly common (e.g. affects ~50% of patients >40y) and is associated with a higher mortality. Pancreatic damage in CF (due to fibrosis) causes decreased insulin secretion. CFRD is a distinct type of diabetes but shares certain clinical features of both type I and type II diabetes. Unlike type I diabetes, onset of CFRD is usually insidious, and patients may be asymptomatic at diagnosis or present with a decline in pulmonary function or weight; ketoacidosis is very rare in CFRD. CFRD differs from type II diabetes in that weight loss is often an early feature and reactive hypoglycaemia is not unusual. Some patients exhibit overt diabetes during an infective exacerbation but return to normal glucose tolerance later. Early identification and treatment of CFRD improves health status, even in the absence of fasting hyperglycaemia; screening oral glucose tolerance test should be performed annually. Management is with insulin (usually as basal bolus regimen), with blood glucose targets of 4–7mmol/L; there is no role for oral hypoglycaemics or a hypoglycaemic diet. Microvascular complications can occur after 5–10y of CFRD
- *Low bone mineral density* and increased fracture risk is common in CF. Risk factors include malabsorption of vitamin D and calcium, low BMI, decreased physical activity, delayed puberty, steroid use, diabetes. Screen with DEXA scans from age 18y. Treatment is with calcium and vitamin D supplements to ensure vitamin D-sufficient, bisphosphonates.

Other organ systems

- *Arthropathy and CF vasculitis* Acute or subacute arthritis occurs in around 5% of patients and often responds to NSAIDs. Sometimes arthritis is associated with skin lesions such as purpura or erythema nodosum
- *Chronic rhinosinusitis* is often troublesome and may worsen lung disease. Consider sinus CT. Treatment with topical steroids and decongestants is often unhelpful, and surgery may be required
- *Acute kidney injury* is more common in CF and associated with IV aminoglycosides, NSAIDs, dehydration, and pulmonary exacerbations
- *Electrolyte abnormalities* include hyponatraemia, hypokalaemia, hypochloraemia, and metabolic alkalosis. Salt tablets are required in hot weather due to excessive losses in sweat
- *Stress incontinence* is very common in women; treat with pelvic floor exercises.

Other issues

Fertility

Women with CF may be subfertile but should always be offered contraception if of reproductive age. If planning a pregnancy, their physical state should be optimized with antibiotics and nutrition. The outcome of pregnancy is improved by optimizing and maintaining pulmonary function and weight gain during the pregnancy, and close monitoring is required. Women with CF are also at risk of developing diabetes during pregnancy. Pregnancy does not affect survival when compared with the entire adult ♀ CF population, but impaired pulmonary function with FEV_1 <60% predicted and BMI <18 are likely to be the main predictors of worse maternal and foetal outcome, and some patients do experience an accelerated decline after pregnancy. PHT is considered an absolute contraindication to pregnancy. Breastfeeding is possible but intensifies the nutritional strain put on the mother. Many CF antibiotics are safe to use in pregnancy, but avoid ciprofloxacin, chloramphenicol, metronidazole, and IV colistin, and, if possible, avoid IV aminoglycosides. Ceftazidime at a reduced dose of 2g tds is a safe first-line choice for patients infected with *P. aeruginosa*.

Men are usually infertile due to failure of the normal development or blockage of the vas deferens, seminal vesicle, ejaculatory duct, and body and tail of epididymis. Testicular histology is normal, and hence one option is surgical sperm retrieval for intracytoplasmic sperm injection (ICSI) into an egg, performed by fertility clinics.

Genetic counselling and screening should be offered to patients with CF and their partners.

Psychosocial support Trained psychologists offer personal and family support regarding education, employment, financial benefits, burden of treatment, and adapting to progressive disease. Pre-transplant psychological assessment is carried out, as well as terminal care and bereavement counselling. Consider and treat depression, anxiety, and emotional difficulties, with referral to psychiatric services, if necessary. Social worker involvement may help with benefit entitlements, travel insurance, disabled car badge.

Care of the dying CF patient When all acknowledge that there are no further active treatment options, the focus of care should adjust to being palliative, with an emphasis on symptom relief, at home or in hospital or a hospice. The transition from active treatment to palliative care is often difficult in CF, as many end-of-life events begin as an exacerbation, and it may be difficult to predict or define when patients are entering a terminal phase. There is often an overlap between active and palliative care, e.g. some 'active' treatments (such as gentle physiotherapy and even NIV) may have a palliative role in symptom control, and, for this reason, most deaths occur in hospital. A particular challenge is palliative care of patients on an active transplant waiting list when unrealistic hopes about the availability of a last-minute transplant may delay discussion of end of life and compromise symptom control. Open and sensitive discussion about end-of-life care is encouraged, but approaches should be dynamic and tailored to the needs of individual patients. Effective communication amongst the CF team and ward staff is essential.

Future developments

Small molecule CFTR modulators (correctors and potentiators) The example of ivacaftor treatment for patients with a G551D mutation has proven that small molecule-based approaches to correcting the basic CFTR defect by targeting specific mutations can provide clinical benefit in CF. Long-term clinical outcome data for ivacaftor is still awaited, however. Many other orally bioavailable compounds targeting specific CFTR mutations are in clinical trials, including VX-809 and VX-661 which target the F508del mutation. Combinations of these compounds (e.g. with ivacaftor) may prove to be particularly effective in restoring CFTR function.

Gene therapy aims to restore CFTR function by inserting a normal copy of the *CFTR* gene into epithelial cells to prevent progressive airways disease. This will theoretically be of benefit to patients with any mutation class, in contrast to mutation-specific small molecule-based therapies. A major challenge has been finding a suitable vector for delivery, with recent interest in adeno-associated viruses and liposomes. A multi-dose trial of a nebulized CFTR-expressing plasmid complexed with a (non-viral) cationic lipid is currently underway, run by the UK Gene Therapy Consortium.

Chapter 25

Eosinophilic lung disease

Eosinophilic lung disease

Definition Pulmonary eosinophilias are disorders classically associated with CXR infiltrates and a raised blood eosinophil count, although eosinophilic infiltration of the lung can occur *without* blood eosinophilia. Eosinophilia is found on lung biopsy or BAL.

- Eosinophils are phagocytes that are produced in bone marrow and circulate for up to 10h before localizing in tissues
- Their blood levels are usually tightly regulated
- In health, they accumulate in the GI tract mucosa, but they may be attracted to other tissues by chemoattractant mechanisms, including mast cell activation and complement activation
- Eosinophils can survive in the tissues for weeks if appropriate cytokines are present
- Normal eosinophil counts are below 0.4×10^9/L (1–3% of peripheral WCC)
- Counts of 0.4×10^9/L upwards can be seen in pulmonary eosinophilia
- Persisting high eosinophil levels ('hypereosinophilia') cause tissue damage, due to their pro-inflammatory effects, whatever the cause
- Eosinophils accumulate in allergic or hypersensitivity disease, parasitic infections, and cancer
- Steroids and severe sepsis both decrease eosinophil levels
- Asthma can cause a raised eosinophil count, especially if there is associated eczema, but an absolute eosinophil count of $>1 \times 10^9$/L is very unusual and raises the possibility of an alternative diagnosis such as Churg–Strauss syndrome (now known as eosinophilic granulomatosis with polyangiitis, EGPA)
- Blood eosinophilia can occur in a variety of conditions. 1° eosinophilia occurs in haematological malignancies; 2° eosinophilia is a response to a stimulus, such as a parasite or allergy, and third, idiopathic eosinophilia, with no identifiable cause, is also known as the hypereosinophilic syndrome
- Possible causes of CXR infiltrates ± blood eosinophilia are shown in Table 25.1.

Table 25.1 Causes of CXR infiltrates ± blood eosinophilia

Condition	Characteristic points
Asthma with ABPA	Known asthma, with worsening symptoms, over weeks to months. Associated systemic symptoms. Raised blood eosinophil count, positive *Aspergillus* skin test, raised IgE, raised *Aspergillus* precipitins
Simple pulmonary eosinophilia (Löffler's syndrome)	Foreign travel. Symptoms for days to weeks. Cough, malaise, anorexia, rhinitis, night sweats, fever, dyspnoea, wheeze. Sputum contains eosinophils and larvae. Low-level blood eosinophilia. Occurs due to an allergic response to the passage of larvae through the lungs
Tropical pulmonary eosinophilia	Foreign travel. Symptoms for weeks to months, with remissions and relapses. Cough, wheeze, sputum, dyspnoea, chest pain, fever, weight loss, fatigue. Sputum contains eosinophils. Raised blood eosinophil count, high IgE. Occurs in response to filaria in blood and lymphatics
Chronic eosinophilic pneumonia	Symptoms for weeks to months, with associated systemic symptoms. Cough, sputum, haemoptysis, dyspnoea, recent-onset asthma, fever, weight loss, night sweats. Sputum eosinophilia, but blood levels can be normal
Acute eosinophilic pneumonia	Short duration of symptoms, <5 days. Fever, cough, dyspnoea, and myalgia. Unwell, hypoxic. High BAL eosinophil count, no blood eosinophilia
Hypereosinophilic syndrome	Symptoms for weeks to months. Associated systemic symptoms and other organ involvement. Fever, weight loss, cough, night sweats, pruritus. High blood eosinophil count
Churg–Strauss syndrome/EGPA	Rhinitis, past history of asthma. Other organ involvement. Associated systemic symptoms. Longer duration of symptoms, weeks to months. Blood eosinophilia and eosinophilic tissue infiltration
Drug-induced pulmonary eosinophilia	Recent new drug. Possible associated skin reaction. Symptoms within hours to days. Spectrum of illness, from mild to severely unwell, with cough, dyspnoea, fever, and hypoxia. Eosinophilic tissue infiltration, but blood eosinophilia not universal

Causes of eosinophilic lung disease 1

Asthma and ABPA

(See ➔ pp. 464–5.)
- Fever or worsening asthma symptoms may be caused by types I and II hypersensitivity reactions to airway colonization by *Aspergillus fumigatus*
- Untreated, can cause central bronchiectasis
- *CXR* shows fleeting shadows
- *Blood* eosinophilia
- *Aspergillus skin prick test* is positive, and serum *Aspergillus* IgG precipitins are positive. IgE levels are raised
- *Treatment* is with steroids, and antifungal agents may be necessary.

Simple pulmonary eosinophilia (Löffler's syndrome)

- Caused by parasitic infection, usually *Ascaris lumbricoides*, but also *Strongyloides* and hookworm (e.g. *Ancylostoma*)
- Occurs worldwide, especially in SE Asia, Africa, Central and South America
- The eggs of the parasite are found in the soil and are ingested. After 10–14 days, larvae migrate from the intestine via lymph and blood to the liver and lung. From the lung, they pass up the bronchial tree to be swallowed, to develop into roundworms in the gut
- The passage of larvae through the lung causes an allergic reaction. This may be asymptomatic but may cause cough, malaise, anorexia, rhinitis, night sweats, low-grade fever, occasional wheezing, and dyspnoea. The illness lasts around 2 weeks
- *CXR* shows transient bilateral shadows that are discrete and perihilar. They disappear usually between 6 and 12 days but can take up to 1 month
- *Sputum* also contains eosinophils and larvae
- *Blood* eosinophilia at a low level
- *Stool examination* reveals parasites, but only 2–3 months later when the adult worms are passed
- *Treatment* is with an antihelminth agent, such as albendazole or mebendazole, for 3 days. Steroids may be necessary if the pulmonary manifestations are severe.

Tropical pulmonary eosinophilia

- Hypersensitivity to migrating larvae of filarial worms *Wucheria bancrofti*, *Brugia malayi*, and *Brugia timori*, similar to Löffler's syndrome
- Occurs in the Indian subcontinent, SE Asia, and the South Pacific islands
- Insidious onset of cough, wheeze, sputum, dyspnoea, and chest pain, with associated fever, weight loss, and fatigue. Symptoms last for weeks to months, with remissions and relapses
- *Examination* reveals crepitations
- *CXR* shows bilateral uniform mottling of the lung fields, especially in the middle and lower zones. There may be cavitation and pleural effusion
- *Sputum and BAL* contain eosinophils

- *PFTs* may be obstructive initially but can become restrictive in long-standing untreated cases
- *Histology* shows eosinophilic bronchopneumonia and eosinophilic abscesses
- *Blood eosinophil count* is raised. IgE is raised
- *Filarial complement test* is positive
- *Treatment* is with a filaricide diethylcarbamazine for 3 weeks. This rapidly improves symptoms.

Drug-induced pulmonary eosinophilia

- Pulmonary shadowing develops within hours to days of starting the drug and resolves usually within 1 week of stopping it
- It is due to an allergic reaction in the pulmonary vessel wall, caused by the drug, and occurs again on drug re-challenge
- There may be an associated skin reaction
- The drug should be avoided in the future and steroids given if necessary
- Severity of illness varies from mild to severely unwell, with cough, dyspnoea, fever, hypoxia. May occur in those with concomitant asthma
- Tissue eosinophilia, but may not have blood eosinophilia
- Possible drugs include ampicillin, carbamazepine, chlorpropamide, cocaine (inhaled), daptomycin, inorganic chemicals such as nickel, methotrexate, minocycline, NSAIDs, nitrofurantoin, penicillin, phenytoin, sodium aminosalicylate, sulfonamides, tetracycline. There are case reports of others (⌖ http://www.pneumotox.com).

Causes of eosinophilic lung disease 2

Chronic eosinophilic pneumonia
- Unknown cause
- ♀:♂ = 2:1. Occurs in middle age, non-smokers
- Insidious onset over weeks to months, with cough, sputum, possibly haemoptysis, dyspnoea, recent-onset asthma, weight loss, night sweats, and high fever. Differential diagnosis includes TB
- *Diagnosis* is usually clinical and radiological but may need BAL or open lung biopsy
- *CXR* shows peripheral dense opacities with ill-defined margins (photographic negative of pulmonary oedema)
- *CT* shows peripheral airspace infiltrates
- *Sputum* eosinophilia
- *BAL* eosinophil count high
- *Blood* eosinophilia may not occur. ESR is raised
- *Treatment* is with steroids, such as prednisolone 30–40mg/day, and improvement is usually rapid, with the CXR clearing within 2–3 days and normal in 2 weeks. Decrease steroid dose once stable, but continue for 6 months
- Relapses common when steroids stopped, and they may need further courses.

Acute eosinophilic pneumonia Unknown cause, occurs in any age or sex. Presents with fever, dry cough, dyspnoea, and myalgia.
Diagnostic criteria:
- Acute febrile illness of <7 days' duration
- Hypoxic respiratory failure
- Interstitial or alveolar CXR infiltrates
- BAL eosinophils >25%
- No parasitic, fungal, or other infection
- Prompt and complete response to steroids (oral prednisolone or IV methylprednisolone if respiratory failure)
- Failure to relapse after stopping steroids.

May be unwell and hypoxic, requiring ventilatory support. No peripheral blood eosinophilia. High-dose steroids should be given until the respiratory failure resolves, and then the dose can be tapered over 2–4 weeks. It possibly represents an acute hypersensitivity reaction to an unidentified inhaled antigen; case series of recent-onset smoking in some.

Hypereosinophilic syndrome
- Unknown cause. Rare
- Most common in men aged 30–40
- Present with fever, weight loss, night sweats, cough, and pruritus
- *Diagnosis* based on:
  - Marked blood eosinophilia of $>1.5 \times 10^9/L$ for 6 months or more
  - Signs and symptoms of eosinophilic tissue infiltration on histology
  - No evidence of another cause of eosinophilia

- Pulmonary involvement with interstitial infiltrates and pleural effusions on CXR. Cardiovascular involvement also occurs, with myocarditis, endocardial fibrosis, restrictive cardiomyopathy, valvular damage, and mural thrombus formation. These may cause considerable morbidity and mortality. Skin may be involved with urticaria and angio-oedema; CNS involved with encephalopathy, arterial and venous embolism, peripheral neuropathy, or mononeuritis multiplex; GI tract with gastritis, nausea, diarrhoea, alcohol intolerance, and hepato- or splenomegaly; joints with effusions and Raynaud's. Kidney and muscles can also be infiltrated by eosinophils. Can be fatal
- *Blood* eosinophil levels may be as high as 70%. IgE levels are high
- *Treatment* is with high-dose steroids (e.g. 60mg prednisolone), which improves about 50% of cases. May need to use other immunosuppressants such as cyclophosphamide, hydroxycarbamide, azathioprine, or interferon-alfa. Treatment should be tapered, according to falling eosinophil counts and end-organ improvement.

Churg–Strauss syndrome/EGPA

(See ➲ pp. 660–1.)
- Severe asthma, blood eosinophilia, and pulmonary infiltrates occur as part of a small- and medium-vessel vasculitis
- Also can affect GI tract, CNS, skin, and cardiovascular system
- There may be eosinophilic tissue infiltration
- ANCA usually, but not always, positive
- Treatment with steroids and immunosuppression.

Chapter 26

Extreme environments— flying, altitude, diving

Lung disease and flying

Problems Flying presents problems for three reasons:
• Extra hypoxia
• Volume changes in gas compartments
• Closed environment and disease transmission.

Extra hypoxia Some more recent airplanes may be pressurized to the equivalent of about 5,000ft (1,500m). This gives an atmospheric pressure of about 85kPa and an FiO_2 of about 18kPa, compared with 21kPa at sea level. In normal subjects, this causes inconsequential falls in PaO_2 and SaO_2. However, many companies pressurize to the minimum allowed 8,000ft (e.g. Boeing 767—7,900ft or 2,400 m, the same as some of the lower ski resorts in Colorado), equivalent to an FiO_2 of 16kPa (equivalent to breathing 15% O_2 at sea level), and, even in normal subjects, the SaO_2 may fall to 90% or so. The new Airbus 380 is pressurized to 5,000ft (1,500m), and the new Boeing 787 to 6,000ft (1,800 m).

Patients with lung disease and a degree of hypoxia will be nearer the steep part of the Hb dissociation curve and will experience bigger proportional falls in O_2 carriage by the blood. The estimated PaO_2 at 8,000ft (2,400m) (the lowest cabin pressurization likely to be encountered) is empirically estimated by the formula:

$$\text{Estimated } PaO_2 \text{ at 8,000ft (2,400m)} = (0.24 \times PaO_2 \text{ at sea level}) + (2.7 \times FEV_1/VC) + 3$$

For example, if sea level PaO_2 = 8kPa, FEV_1/VC = 0.40, estimated PaO_2 = 6kPa.

This is a rough approximation and will vary considerably from patient to patient, particularly due to differences in hypoxic drive. An alternative is to give the patient a hypoxic challenge for 15min minimum, and measure the PaO_2/SaO_2. This is most easily achieved by feeding a 40% Venturi mask with 100% nitrogen, which simulates a little under 8,000ft (2,400m) (equivalent to 16% O_2). There is no evidence this predicts whether a patient will, or will not, run into trouble. Recently, Edvardsen et al. confirmed that the result of a hypoxic challenge test in patients with moderate to severe COPD did not predict whether they developed symptoms during a flight, although the pre-flight MRC dyspnoea score did predict symptoms. Those that had supplemental O_2 had fewer symptoms, regardless of the simulated hypoxia testing.

Empirically, O_2 is often prescribed if the in-flight PaO_2 at 8,000ft (2,400m), estimated from the above equation or by experimentation, is <6.6kPa or 85% SaO_2. Others have used SaO_2 during a 6MWT to try and improve the ability to predict SaO_2 during 15% hypoxia testing. None of this is *evidence-based*, so a simple recommendation based on sea level oximetry measurements is likely to be as valid, in conjunction with further information such as how disabled the patient is already by shortness of breath, their previous flight experience, length of proposed flight, time since last exacerbation, and importance of the trip to the patient, etc.

Box 26.1 Simple recommendations for O₂ when flying

Sea level SaO₂

>92%	No O₂ required
90–92%	Perform challenge test
<90%	Recommend O₂

The suggestions in Box 26.1 are similar to BTS guidelines, which are a little more complex and consider comorbidities. 2L/min via nasal cannulae, or 28% Venturi mask, is usually sufficient to raise SaO_2 to sea level equivalent. Airlines vary over charging for this; allow at least a month to arrange it (see British Lung Foundation (BLF) reference under Further information for each airline's procedure). A MEDIF form or equivalent will require completion by the GP or specialist. Occasionally, patients are allowed to bring their own O₂ on board as hand luggage. Some airlines prohibit using O₂ during take-off and landing.

Volume changes in gas compartments Ascent to the equivalent of 5,000ft (1,500m) increases gas trapped in compartments by 20%, ascent to 8,000ft (2,400m) by nearly 40%. A pneumothorax or non-communicating bullae therefore increases by this amount; patients with current pneumothoraces should not fly. It used to be advised not to fly within 6 weeks of a pneumothorax (slightly higher chance of recurrence and lack of adequate emergency treatment on board). This has recently been changed to 1 week after full radiographic resolution, or 2 weeks in the case of a traumatic pneumothorax. Patients having had recent thoracic surgery (for whatever reason) are now advised they can fly once recovered from the surgery itself (previously advised to wait 2 weeks). None of this is evidence-based, and the true risks of ignoring these guidelines are not known. It is probable that the risk of a second pneumothorax, in the absence of definitive management (pleurodesis, etc.), is only high enough to worry about in patients with pre-existing lung disease who should be made aware of this higher risk.

Closed environment Patients with infectious diseases, such as TB, should not fly. There seems to be a significant risk of infecting others.

Further information

Edvardsen A et al. COPD and air travel: does hypoxia-altitude simulation testing predict in flight respiratory symptoms? Eur Respir J 2013;42:1216–23.

Edvardsen A et al. High prevalence of respiratory symptoms during air travel in patients with COPD. Respir Med 2011;105:50–6.

Cottrell JJ. Aircraft cabin pressures. Chest 1988;98:81.

British Thoracic Society guidelines: ℘ http://www.brit-thoracic.org.uk/Guidelines/ Air-Travel-Guideline.aspx. Editorial: ℘ http://thorax.bmj.com/content/66/9/831.abstract.

BTS patient advice leaflet. ℘ http://www.brit-thoracic.org.uk/Portals/0/Patient_and_carer_ Information/AirTravel_patient_information.pdf.

Coker R et al. Is air travel safe for those with lung disease? Eur Respir J 2007;30:1057–63.

BLF patient advice. ℘ http://www.blf.org.uk/Page/Air-travel-with-a-lung-condition.

BLF information on oxygen and airlines. ℘ http://www.blf.org.uk/Page/Airline-oxygen-policies.

Altitude sickness

Definitions of acute mountain or high altitude sickness are not precise but include several symptoms provoked by the hypoxia.

Pathophysiology Some of the pathophysiology is well understood and explains some of the symptoms and signs. These largely fall into two categories, minor and major.

Minor Due to hyperventilation/hypocapnia/alkalosis/cerebral vasoconstriction provoked by the hypoxia, and include:

• Light-headedness/fatigue
• Numbness/tingling of extremities
• Nausea/vomiting and anorexia
• Headache
• Insomnia/sleep disturbance
• Periodic ventilation during sleep.

These symptoms are common, develop over 6–12h after arrival, and affect at least a quarter of those flying to Colorado for a skiing holiday (altitude 2,400–3,400m, ~10,000ft, barometric pressure 70kPa, inspired O_2 tension 14.5kPa, average SaO_2 on arrival 89–90%). Most of the symptoms are due to a respiratory hypocapnic alkalosis and resolve as the kidney retains $[H^+]$ and excretes $[HCO_3^-]$, returning pH towards normal. This allows further hyperventilation, and the rise in SaO_2 helps resolve any of the symptoms due to the hypoxia itself. This scenario tends to be common in those with a higher hypoxic drive (measured at sea level, as it encourages greater hypocapnia and alkalosis). Confusingly, these symptoms may also indicate the early development of the more major category.

Major Those due to the hypoxia itself. These are more serious, can develop rapidly, and tend to occur more in those with a lower hypoxic drive. There is also a genetic component influencing susceptibility, related to the *ACE* gene. In *high altitude pulmonary oedema (HAPE)*, the hypoxia provokes a non-uniform pulmonary vasoconstriction, raising PAP; hence some pulmonary capillaries are unprotected and receive the full rise in PAP. Fluid leakage into alveoli, pulmonary oedema, and capillary damage (with pulmonary haemorrhage) produce clinically apparent disease. The dominant symptoms/signs are:

• Extra breathlessness/cough
• Cyanosis
• Blood-tinged frothy sputum
• Crackles on auscultation/raised JVP.

In *high altitude cerebral oedema (HACE)*, hypoxia also causes increased cerebral blood flow, cerebral oedema, retinal haemorrhages, cerebral thrombosis, and petechial haemorrhages. The dominant symptoms are:

• Ataxia (may be the first sign)
• Confusion/disorientation/hallucinations/behavioural change
• Severe headache/reduced conscious level
• Papilloedema.

Both HAPE and HACE are potentially fatal.

Management Risk factors are mainly the rate and degree of altitude attained. Keep ascent to ≤300m (1,000 ft)/day, and rest every third day. The minor form of altitude sickness is likely to resolve spontaneously over a few days with simple symptomatic treatment, analgesics, and plenty of hydration. However, prophylaxis, or early treatment on symptom appearance, with *acetazolamide* is very effective, as are limiting further ascent and encouraging descent. Acetazolamide provokes a mild metabolic acidosis (by reducing [H+] availability for excretion in the distal tubule) and 'pre-acclimatizes' the subject to allow greater hyperventilation in response to hypoxia without the usual alkalosis. It is recommended when rapid ascent to altitudes ≥2,500m (8,200ft) is unavoidable (such as a package ski trip to Aspen). 500mg/day (slow release) for the 2 days prior to ascent is probably adequate for most subjects (or as treatment after symptoms develop). The commonest side effect is a harmless and reversible tingling of the extremities.

Temazepam has been shown to reduce the periodic breathing at night (by reducing the arousals that help maintain the periodicity) and does not appear to worsen the hypoxia or reduce vigilance levels the following day.

The best predictor of severe altitude sickness is a prior episode. It may be possible to predict likely severe problems, based on sea level estimates of a poor hypoxic response, but this has not been fully validated.

The management of the more severe forms of altitude sickness that tend to occur with rapid ascent to over 4,000m (13,000ft), pulmonary and cerebral oedema, is urgent.

Management of severe altitude sickness

- Increase inspired O_2 tension by rapid descent, extra inspired O_2, or a local pressurized environment (e.g. a portable hyperbaric chamber such as the Gamow bag, ℗ https://www.youtube.com/watch?v=sJAzu2ZHUuE).

HAPE

- Sit upright, and keep warm
- Nifedipine (20mg bd up to qds + loading dose, 10mg sublingually) to reduce PAP
- Acetazolamide may help by also reducing PAP as well as increasing the effective ventilatory response to altitude hypoxia.

HACE

- Dexamethasone (4mg qds + loading dose, 8mg) to reduce cerebral oedema.

Improvement is usually rapid once inspiratory O_2 tension is raised. Prophylaxis for this severe form of altitude sickness is controversial, but graded ascent is important; acetazolamide probably helps, and nifedipine is used by some, particularly if there is a history of a previous episode.

Further information

Information for doctors/patients. ℗ http://www.thebmc.co.uk/downloads/Mountaineering/International.

Information for patients. ℗ http://familydoctor.org/familydoctor/en/diseases-conditions/high-altitude-illness.html.

Information for patients and doctors. ℗ http://www.high-altitude-medicine.com.

Luks AM et al. Wilderness Medical Society consensus guidelines for the prevention and treatment of acute altitude illness. *Wilderness Environ Med*. 2010;21:146–55.

Diving

Problems Increased recreational diving has raised the awareness of respiratory problems at depth. These can essentially be divided into five:
• Barotrauma, e.g. ruptured bullae and pneumothorax
• Worsening of pre-existing disorder whilst at depth, e.g. asthma
• Nitrogen gas evolved from solution in body fluids (the 'bends')
• Breath-hold diving and ascent hypoxia
• Pulmonary oedema.

Pathophysiology

Barotrauma (second commonest cause of death in SCUBA divers after drowning) During descent, any air-containing cavity in the body will be compressed by the rise in external pressure. If there is any communication with the airways (e.g. middle ear, lung bullae), then gas will slowly move into the airspace. On ascent, the airspace will expand and, if air cannot escape quickly enough, may lead to rupture of the eardrum or the bullae. *A tension pneumothorax can be rapidly fatal in this situation.* Obstructive lung diseases in general can predispose to ruptured alveoli. In addition to pneumothoraces, the escaped air can produce a pneumomediastinum, causing chest pain, and a radiolucent band (air in the pericardium) along the cardiac border on CXR. Breathing 100% O_2 will clear this air more quickly. Air emboli can also occur and produce a wide range of symptoms; hyperbaric O_2 may be required.

Pre-existing lung disease The onset of asthma during a dive can be disastrous and may be provoked by the dry gases breathed from SCUBA gear (self-contained underwater breathing apparatus). See *British Sub-Aqua Club (BSAC) recommendations on asthma and diving* (see Box 26.2). Many lung diseases, such as CF, COPD (FEV_1 <80% predicted), fibrotic lung disease, previous pneumothorax (with no pleurodesis), and lung bullae, are considered contraindications to diving. However, recently, BSAC has adopted the pragmatic approach of accepting that, in individuals with a history of spontaneous pneumothorax, who have had no pneumothorax for 5y, the risk of pulmonary barotrauma is small and not significantly greater than for many in the general population, e.g. smokers. Such individuals may dive, provided that a CT scan of the chest and lung function tests (including flow–volume loops) show no reason to suggest that there is significant residual lung disease.

The bends or caisson disease (caisson is an underwater air chamber in which people work) During periods of high pressure, extra nitrogen dissolves into the blood and other tissue fluids. This takes many minutes. On ascent, this nitrogen literally bubbles off. If the amount coming out of solution is too great, nitrogen bubbles act as emboli and limit blood flow. This produces micro-infarction, with activation of inflammatory and clotting cascades and damage to several organs, e.g. joints, spinal cord, brain. Limited diving times and slow ascents reduce this problem, as do breathing mixtures containing helium, rather than nitrogen. Severe cases require treatment in hyperbaric chambers.

Breath-hold diving During breath-hold diving, increased pressure on the chest elevates alveolar and arterial PO_2. This extends breath-hold time, particularly with prior hyperventilation to reduce $PaCO_2$. During the dive, O_2 is used and PO_2 falls. On ascent, with rarefaction of the thoracic gas, PO_2 falls quickly, with possible loss of consciousness and drowning.

Pulmonary oedema has been reported whilst SCUBA diving in cold water, but the mechanism is not clear.

Box 26.2 BSAC recommendations on asthma

- Asthma may predispose to air trapping, leading to pulmonary barotrauma and air embolism, which may be fatal. An acute asthma attack can also cause severe dyspnoea that may be hazardous or fatal during diving
- These theoretical risks should be explained fully to the asthmatic diver. There is little, if any, evidence that the mildly controlled asthmatic that follows the guidelines below is at more risk
- Asthmatics may dive if they have allergic asthma, but not if they have cold-, exercise-, or emotion-induced asthma
- All asthmatics should be managed in accordance with BTS guidelines
- Only well-controlled asthmatics may dive
- Asthmatics should not dive if needed a *therapeutic* bronchodilator in the last 48h or have had any other chest symptoms.

Control of asthma
- The asthmatic should not need more than occasional bronchodilators, i.e. daily usage would be a disqualifying factor, but inhaled steroids/cromoglicate/nedocromil are permissible
- During the diving season, he/she should take bd peak flows. A deviation of 10% from best values should exclude diving until within 10% of best values for at least 48h before diving
- The medical examiner should perform an exercise test such as the 18in (43cm) step test for 3min or running outside (not a bicycle ergometer) to increase the heart rate to 80% (210 minus age). A decrease in PEFR of 15% at 3min post-exercise should be taken as evidence of exercise-induced bronchoconstriction and hence disbars. The patient should be off all bronchodilators for 24h before the test
- A β_2 agonist may be taken pre-diving as a *preventative*, but not to relieve bronchospasm at the time.

Further information

Aberdeen emergency number for hyperbaric chambers. ☎ 07831 151523 (☎ 0845 4086008 in Scotland). ✍ http://www.hyperchamber.com and ✍ http://www.ukdiving.co.uk/information/hyperbaric.htm.

Plymouth Diving Disease Research Centre. ✍ http://www.ddrc.org/ (24h helpline and register of hyperbaric chambers). ☎ 01752 209999. Email info@ddrc.org

BTS guidelines (2003). ✍ http://www.brit-thoracic.org.uk/guidelines/diving-guideline.aspx.

Diving and medical conditions. ✍ http://www.bsac.com/page.asp?section=1480&sectionTitle=Medical+Matters.

Diving and asthma/pneumothorax. ✍ http://www.bsac.com/page.asp?section=1533&sectionTitle=Respiratory+conditions.

Cochard G *et al.* Pulmonary oedema in scuba divers. *Undersea Hyperb Med* 2005;32:39–44.

Chapter 27

Gastrointestinal disease and the lung

Hepatic hydrothorax and hepatopulmonary syndrome

Hepatic hydrothorax Predominantly right-sided pleural effusion occurring in patients with liver disease and no cardiorespiratory disease, often with minimal ascites. The ascitic fluid accumulates in the chest as a result of diaphragmatic defects. Occurs in 5–12% of patients with cirrhosis and portal hypertension. Spontaneous bacterial empyema can occur and is associated with mortality of 20%. Diuretics are rarely effective. The definitive treatment is liver transplantation.

Hepatopulmonary syndrome (HPS) is the triad of:
- Chronic liver disease and portal hypertension
- Arteriovenous (AV) shunting in the lungs, predominantly at the bases and subsequent ventilation-perfusion abnormalities
- Arterial hypoxia.

It occurs in 4–29% of patients with chronic liver disease. Enhanced pulmonary production of NO is the key priming factor for pulmonary vasodilatation. Although levels of NO are increased in exhaled air, consistent with lung origin, levels normalize after *liver* transplantation. The mechanism is thought to be related to the release of *vasoactive mediators from portal hypertension causing altered bowel perfusion, which, in turn, leads to pulmonary vascular dilatation*, with decreased pulmonary vascular resistance (right-to-left shunt). *Patients with cirrhosis who develop HPS have a worse prognosis.*

Presentation is with progressive dyspnoea and cyanosis. Examination reveals clubbing and telangiectasia, with associated stigmata of chronic liver disease.

Diagnosis
- *Hypoxia* on blood gases: <8.6kPa on air, at rest, and upright. Platypnoea and orthodeoxia are present, i.e. breathlessness and desaturation on sitting upright, caused by preferential perfusion of basal pulmonary vasculature where the AVMs will be, and AV shunting is therefore increased. Lying flat relieves this. These changes may be seen in other lung diseases but, in the presence of liver disease, is suggestive of HPS. Hypoxia is only partially corrected by 100% O_2 due to the pulmonary shunting
- *Contrast-enhanced echo* is positive. Contrast/saline bubbles are injected peripherally and are normally seen only in the right heart and are then filtered by the pulmonary bed. In the presence of intrapulmonary shunts, these are seen in the left atrium within 3–6 cardiac cycles after opacification in the right atrium. (False positive results occur if right-to-left cardiac shunt present, which can be excluded during echo.) This is the most practical method of detecting pulmonary vascular dilatation. This qualitative method is more sensitive and less invasive than technetium-labelled albumin scan

- *Pulmonary technetium-99 perfusion scan* assesses the shunt fraction. Normally, the radiolabelled albumin is trapped in the pulmonary capillary bed. In the presence of intrapulmonary or cardiac shunts, there is significant uptake of radiolabelled albumin in the brain or spleen. A shunt index fraction of >20% indicates severe HPS (normal uptake <6%)
- *CT chest* is performed to rule out other pulmonary comorbid disease
- *Single breath diffusion capacity for CO* is consistently abnormal in HPS. This is not specific and may not normalize after transplant.

Treatment
- O_2 if PaO_2 <8kPa
- Avoid vasodilators. There is minimal evidence for pharmacological intervention
- Mainstay of treatment is liver transplantation, which cures the condition in 80%. Hypoxia may take up to 14 months to improve. Severe hypoxia (PaO_2 <6kPa) is associated with increased mortality post-transplant, as there is increased risk of hepatic ischaemia
- Transjugular intrahepatic portosystemic shunt (TIPS) is ineffective
- Coil embolization can be tried in selected cases with AV communications.

Prognosis is poor, with a mortality of 40% in 2.5y.

Porto-pulmonary hypertension

Porto-pulmonary hypertension (POPH) is PAH occurring in association with liver cirrhosis and portal hypertension. It occurs in an estimated 2–5% of patients with cirrhosis and is present in around 16% of those referred for liver transplant. The mechanism is unclear but probably relates to a hyperdynamic circulation, high cardiac output, cytokine release, and possible PEs.

Defined as:

- Elevated PAP (>25mmHg at rest, >30mmHg during exercise)
- Increased pulmonary vascular resistance due to pulmonary vasoconstriction and obliterative vascular remodelling (>120dyn·s/cm^5)
- Abnormal LV end diastolic/wedge pressure (<15mmHg)
- In the setting of portal hypertension (portal pressure >10mmHg).

Presentation Dyspnoea on exertion, possibly syncope, chest pain, fatigue, palpitations, haemoptysis, and orthopnoea. There may be signs of volume overload with raised JVP and pedal oedema. P2 may be loud, with pulmonary and tricuspid regurgitation, as well as stigmata of chronic liver disease. It is usually diagnosed 4–7y after the diagnosis of portal hypertension.

Diagnosis
- *Hypoxia* on blood gases, but less so than in HPS. Worse on exertion
- *CXR* may be normal or show prominent pulmonary arteries and enlarged right heart
- *ECG* shows RVH, RBBB, RAD, and sinus tachycardia
- *kCO* may be decreased
- *Echo* is the main screening test and is diagnostic if the RV pressure is >50mmHg
- Exclude other causes of PHT
- *Right heart catheterization (RHC)* with vasodilator studies is performed
- The changes in the vessels in POPH are the same histologically as those seen in IPAH (see ⊕ pp. 388–9).

Treatment Options are the same as for patients with IPAH, with vasodilators, prostacyclin, and endothelin antagonists (see ⊕ pp. 392–3). Avoid β-blockers, so manage varices with banding. Anticoagulation is not advised due to the risk of variceal bleeding. LTOT if PaO$_2$ <8kPa. If mean PAP <40mmHg, can undergo liver transplantation, which may reverse mild to moderate POPH, although symptoms may take weeks to months to resolve. Severe POPH is not reversed and is associated with significant intra- and post-operative morbidity and mortality. A few cases of heart-lung-liver transplants have been reported.

Prognosis is poor in severe POPH, with a median survival after diagnosis of 6 months without transplant.

Further information

Porres-Aguilar M *et al.* Portopulmonary hypertension and hepatopulmonary syndrome: a clinician orientated overview. *Eur Respir Rev* 2012;**21**:223–33.

Rodriguez-Roisin R, Krowka MJ. Hepatopulmonary syndrome—a liver-induced lung vascular disorder. *N Engl J Med* 2008;**358**:2378–87.

Inflammatory bowel disease, coeliac disease, and pancreatitis

IBD Pulmonary involvement tends to occur after the onset of the IBD but can predate it. Pulmonary involvement is found in up to a quarter of patients, but this is usually subclinical. Patients can develop a variety of clinical syndromes, including airway inflammation, subglottic stenosis, chronic bronchitis, bronchiectasis, and chronic bronchiolitis. Bronchoscopy may reveal inflammatory tissue within the large airway walls, which, on biopsy, shows mucosal ulceration, basal cell hyperplasia, basement membrane thickening, and submucosal inflammatory cell infiltration. IBD is also associated with the development of ILD, such as COP, pulmonary infiltrates with eosinophilia, or neutrophilic necrotic parenchymal nodules. Pulmonary involvement tends to be steroid-responsive. Inhaled steroids can be tried for chronic bronchitis, but oral or IV steroids may be required for worsening lung involvement. Note that drugs used in the treatment of IBD may also cause lung disease such as sulfasalazine (alveolitis), mesalazine, or infliximab (both: pulmonary infiltrates and eosinophilia; infliximab: reactivation of latent TB).

Ulcerative colitis Pulmonary involvement is usually asymptomatic or may be associated with dry cough. Minimal interstitial change may be suggested by abnormal PFTs. Restrictive, obstructive, or reduced kCO defects may be seen. Usually normal CXR and CT. No specific treatment indicated.

Crohn's disease Pulmonary involvement less common than in ulcerative colitis, but similar changes found.

Coeliac disease
May be associated with idiopathic lung fibrosis, causing restrictive defect. Also may be at increased risk of asthma, bird fancier's lung, and haemosiderosis. Increased risk of lymphoma and malignancy in GI tract.

Pancreatitis
Acute pancreatitis is frequently associated with exudative pleural effusion. Raised amylase in the pleural fluid is suggestive (see ⮕ p. 59). ARDS may develop, which requires supportive care and mechanical ventilation (see ⮕ p. 105).

Further information
Mahadeva *et al.* Clinical and radiological characteristics of lung disease in inflammatory bowel disease. *Eur Respir J* 2000;**15**:41–8.

Hypersensitivity pneumonitis

Causes

Definition Group of lung diseases typically caused by inhalation of organic antigen to which the individual has been previously sensitized. Disease following inhalation of inorganic antigens and drug ingestion is also reported. Hypersensitivity pneumonitis (HP; previously termed extrinsic allergic alveolitis) is often divided into 'acute' and 'chronic' forms, based on the time course of presentation. Acute HP often follows a short period of exposure to a high concentration of antigen and is usually reversible. Chronic HP typically follows a period of chronic exposure to a low antigen dose and is less reversible. These two presentations may overlap, and 'subacute' forms of the disease are recognized.

Epidemiology Exact prevalence unknown. At least 8% of budgerigar and pigeon keepers and up to 5% of farmers may develop HP. HP is thought to be more common in non-smokers (mechanism unclear; may reflect inhibition of alveolar macrophage function by smoke).

Causes Many different antigens have been reported to cause HP, ranging from the relatively common (bird fancier's lung and farmer's lung in the UK; summer-house HP in Japan) to the more unusual and exotic (shell lung—proteins on mollusc shells; pituitary snuff-taker's disease; sericulturist's lung—silkworm larvae proteins; sax lung—yeast on saxophone mouthpieces). Important examples are listed in Table 28.1.

Table 28.1 Causes of HP—examples

Antigen	Sources	Diseases
Organisms		
Thermophilic actinomycetes (*Micropolyspora faeni, Thermoactinomyces vulgaris*), *Aspergillus* spp.	Mouldy hay; sugar cane; compost; mushrooms; contaminated water in humidifiers and air conditioners	Farmer's lung; bagassosis; compost lung; mushroom worker's lung; humidifier lung
Aspergillus clavatus	Mouldy barley	Malt worker's lung
Trichosporon cutaneum	House dust	Summer-house HP (Japan)
M. avium complex	Hot tub mist, ceiling mould	Hot tub lung
Animal protein		
Bird proteins	Bloom on bird feathers and droppings	Bird fancier's lung
Rat proteins	Rat droppings	Rat lung
Chemical		
Toluene diisocyanate	Paints	Isocyanate HP

Pathophysiology Pathogenesis of HP is not fully understood and may involve T-cell-mediated immunity and granuloma formation (type IV hypersensitivity) and/or antibody-antigen immune complex formation (type III hypersensitivity). It is not an atopic disease and is not characterized by a rise in tissue eosinophils or IgE (type I hypersensitivity); this may, in part, be due to the small particle size of offending antigens, which tend to be deposited more distally in the airspaces than the larger particles associated with asthma. Lung histology specimens typically reveal an interstitial inflammatory infiltrate, often with accompanying bronchiolitis and OP. Non-caseating granulomata are often present and typically are ill-defined and single (compared with sarcoidosis where granulomata are well defined and are grouped subpleurally or near bronchi). Chronic HP is characterized by fibrosis and often by the absence of granulomata and airways involvement, particularly if antigen exposure has ceased.

Diagnosis

Clinical features

Acute HP

- Breathlessness, dry cough, and systemic symptoms (fever, chills, arthralgia, myalgia, headache) occur 4–8h after exposure to antigen
- Examination: crackles and squeaks on auscultation, fever; wheeze may occur, leading to a misdiagnosis of asthma
- In the absence of ongoing exposure, symptoms settle spontaneously within 1–3 days. Episodes may be recurrent.

Chronic HP

- Slowly progressive exertional breathlessness, dry cough, sometimes systemic symptoms (weight loss) over the course of months to years. May be history of acute episodes
- Examination: crackles and squeaks on auscultation, clubbing rare; may be features of cor pulmonale.

Investigations

- Imaging: acute HP
  - *CXR* Diffuse, small (1–3mm) nodules or infiltrates, sometimes ground-glass change, apical sparing. Normal in up to 20% of cases
  - *HRCT* Patchy or diffuse ground-glass change and poorly defined micronodules. Areas of increased lucency/mosaic attenuation (enhanced on expiratory HRCT) occur due to air trapping from bronchiolar involvement
  - Both CXR and HRCT appearances may quickly normalize following removal from antigen exposure
- Imaging: chronic HP
  - *CXR* Typically upper and mid-zone reticulation, reduced lung volumes
  - *HRCT* Diffuse centrilobular nodules, ground-glass change, mosaic attenuation from air trapping, may be honeycombing and traction bronchiectasis (may mimic appearance of UIP, although upper lobe predominance is typical in HP)
- PFTs Typically restrictive pattern with reduced gas transfer and lung volumes; mild obstruction is also sometimes observed. May be normal. Hypoxia may occur
- Bloods Acute HP associated with neutrophilia but not eosinophilia. Inflammatory markers often increased
- Serum antibody (IgG) precipitin Results are presented either as an ELISA or as a number of precipitin lines, referring to the number of different epitopes an individual responds to. Precipitins to organic antigens are found in 90% of patients but are also present in up to 10% of asymptomatic farmers and 50% of pigeon breeders. Precipitin levels often fall in the absence of ongoing antigen exposure
- BAL Lymphocytosis (often >50%) is a characteristic finding, particularly in the setting of ongoing antigen exposure but is not, in itself, diagnostic and may be found in asymptomatic exposed individuals

- *Transbronchial or surgical lung biopsy* may be required in cases of diagnostic uncertainty. TBB often fails to provide sufficient tissue for adequate histological analysis
- *Inhalation antigen challenge* may be unpleasant and is not recommended routinely.

Diagnosis is based on the combination of history of antigen exposure and typical clinical and HRCT features. Atypical presentations require further investigation to support the diagnosis such as BAL lymphocytosis or characteristic histological features on lung biopsy (a bronchiolocentric granulomatous lymphocytic pneumonitis). The underlying causative antigen cannot be identified in up to 40% of cases.

Differential diagnosis
- Atypical pneumonia
- IIPs (particularly IPF, NSIP, RB-ILD)
- Sarcoidosis
- Vasculitis
- Occupational asthma (e.g. from isocyanates)
- Drug-induced lung disease (including pesticides)
- Organic dust toxic syndrome (follows very high levels of exposure to agricultural dusts; symptoms transient; benign course)
- Silo-filler's disease (variable respiratory manifestations following exposure to nitrogen dioxide in silos; ranges from mild bronchitis to fatal bronchospasm).

Management

Management centres on antigen avoidance, which is frequently difficult. If complete removal from antigen is unrealistic (e.g. farmers), measures to reduce exposure may be of benefit (such as respiratory protection with high-performance, positive-pressure masks; avoidance of particularly heavy exposure; improved ventilation and use of air filters; drying of hay prior to storage).

In acute HP, symptoms typically resolve following cessation of antigen exposure, and treatment is usually not required. Removal from exposure may also result in symptomatic and physiological improvement in chronic HP, although this is less certain and established pulmonary fibrosis is often irreversible.

When treatment is required, corticosteroids are frequently used, although there is a lack of randomized controlled evidence to support this. Steroids may hasten the resolution of impaired pulmonary function in acute HP, although their effect on long-term outcome is unclear; they appear to be of benefit in some cases of chronic HP. A typical regimen is prednisolone 0.5mg/kg until symptoms and radiological changes have resolved, and then slowly reduce dose over several months to a maintenance dose of approximately 10mg daily. Courses of 3–6 months may be sufficient in subacute HP, although more prolonged courses are usually required for progressive or chronic disease.

Prognosis is highly variable. Prognosis is usually excellent following removal from antigen exposure in acute HP, although progression to respiratory failure and death may very rarely occur after short-term exposures of very high intensity. Recurrent episodes of acute HP do not necessarily progress to chronic HP and fibrosis, and chronic HP may develop in the absence of previous acute HP episodes. Development of chronic HP with ongoing exposure may eventually lead to cor pulmonale and death, although again this is variable and many patients do not exhibit disease progression despite chronic exposure. Persistent low-dose exposure (e.g. budgerigar in the house) may be more likely to progress to the chronic fibrotic form of HP than intermittent high-dose exposure (e.g. pigeon fanciers), which predisposes more to episodes of acute HP.

Chapter 29

Hyperventilation syndrome

Definition

Poorly defined, and the term is falling into disfavour, dysfunctional breathing being the alternative. Most respiratory physicians still use hyperventilation syndrome to describe breathlessness and overbreathing associated with fear, stress, and anxiety, in the absence of any demonstrable physiological abnormality.

Usually part of a spectrum of physical symptoms (e.g. chest pain, palpitations/tachycardia, fatigue, dizziness, paraesthesiae, headache, diarrhoea, inappropriate sweating, etc.) from anxiety or panic disorder. Other specialities may have been consulted due to the mixed symptomatology.

Pathophysiology

Hyperventilation syndrome can occur *de novo* or follow a respiratory disorder that has resolved—such as an attack of mild asthma. It appears to be based on a heightened awareness of breathing and concerns as to what the SOB signifies. The $PaCO_2$ is intermittently low, with a respiratory alkalosis. Recordings of breathing pattern often show a rather chaotic pattern.

Clinical features

- Intermittent episodes of breathlessness largely unrelated to exercise, although can be worsened by exercise
- May be associated with symptoms of respiratory alkalosis, such as numbness, tingling of the extremities, feelings of impending doom, and light-headedness, occasionally to the point of losing consciousness (cerebral vasoconstriction due to the hypocapnia)
- Sensation of not being able to take a satisfactory breath
- No history suggestive of an alternative current respiratory disorder, although there may have been one previously
- History of some stressful situation in the patient's life
- Previous episodes.

Diagnosis

Is essentially one of exclusion, but with additional confirmatory findings.
- No evidence of a respiratory cause, i.e. normal lung function, normal CXR, and normal SaO_2 at rest and on exercise to the point of breathlessness (SaO_2 may even rise on exercise)
- No evidence of a cardiac cause for the breathlessness
- Irregular breathing pattern at rest and on exercise (watching the patient exercise often reveals the almost instant SOB and chaotic breathing)
- No evidence of PHT
- No evidence to support PEs
- No evidence of hyperthyroidism
- Low $PaCO_2$, raised pH on blood gases (and a normal A–a gradient)
- No metabolic acidosis on blood gases (e.g. ketoacidosis, lactacidosis)
- Unresolved psychological issues or social phobia/agoraphobia.

Differential diagnosis Important pathological causes to exclude are:
- Subtle ILD with a normal CXR: consider HRCT
- Mild asthma with normal basic PFTs at the time of testing: consider PEFR monitoring, exercise provocation, or bronchial reactivity testing
- PHT/thromboembolic disease: consider cardiac echo or CTPA
- Hyperthyroidism
- Unexpected acidosis, e.g. renal failure, lactacidosis, ketoacidosis.

Management

It is important not to dismiss the patient's symptoms, implying it is 'all in the mind'. The patient has a real symptom, which requires a real explanation. There are no controlled trials of management, but most clinicians will offer an explanation based on an 'over-awareness' of respiratory sensations (occasioned by some previous respiratory illness), heightened by anxiety. It is important to explain that the associated symptoms of tingling and light-headedness are well recognized and harmless.

Old recommendations to rebreathe into a paper bag have not stood the test of time and are rather impractical in the middle of a supermarket. Because cold peripheries often accompany an episode (vasoconstriction), placing the cold palms on to the cheeks can help suppress the desire to breathe, thought to be related to the diving reflex: again, this is an untested remedy.

Careful and convincing explanation without over investigation may be enough, stressing the normality of the investigations. A short period on an anxiolytic (e.g. diazepam 2–5mg bd) may be helpful to demonstrate that the symptoms can be controlled. Management of the psychological problem may be possible. Some experienced respiratory physiotherapists can help patients control their symptoms and divert the anxiety away from breathing.

Failure to respond should always prompt a reconsideration of whether an underlying disorder is gradually progressing to the point where an investigation becomes abnormal. On the other hand, repeated investigations will confirm the patient's concern that 'the doctors think there is something wrong.'

Prognosis

Some patients improve quickly with explanation. Some tend to relapse at times of stress. Some prove resistant to any treatment and probably should be seen in the clinic regularly, but infrequently, to reduce their likelihood of involving other medical services with another pointless round of investigations.

Nijmegen hyperventilation score

Filled in by a patient (see Table 29.1).

A score of ≥22 is highly suggestive of hyperventilation syndrome.

Table 29.1 Example of Nijmegen hyperventilation score

Before treatment	Never	Rare	Sometimes	Often	Very often
	0	1	2	3	4
Chest pain			✓		
Feeling tense				✓	
Blurred vision		✓			
Dizzy spells			✓		
Feeling confused			✓		
Faster/deeper breathing					✓
Shortness of breath				✓	
Tight feeling in the chest					✓
Bloated feeling in the stomach			✓		
Tingling fingers	✓				
Unable to breathe deeply				✓	
Stiff fingers or arms			✓		
Tight feeling around mouth	✓				
Cold hands or feet	✓				
Heart racing (palpitations)				✓	
Feeling anxious				✓	
Total score	34				

Idiopathic interstitial pneumonias

Overview

Definition The idiopathic interstitial pneumonias (IIPs) comprise a group of diffuse lung diseases of unknown aetiology that primarily involve the pulmonary interstitium—the area between the alveolar epithelium and capillary endothelium, as well as the septal and bronchovascular tissues that make up the fibrous framework of the lung. These primarily interstitial processes, however, frequently also involve the airways, vasculature, and alveolar airspaces. The underlying pathological process is one of varying degrees of inflammation and fibrosis.

The terminology used to describe the IIPs may be confusing; these conditions have been subject to much reclassification, reflecting the lack of understanding of their underlying aetiology and pathogenesis. Idiopathic pulmonary fibrosis (IPF; previously termed cryptogenic fibrosing alveolitis) is the commonest IIP and is characterized by the radiological and histological pattern of usual interstitial pneumonia (UIP). The other IIPs are distinct disease entities and are all rare. They all represent a subgroup of interstitial (or diffuse parenchymal) lung diseases.

Diagnosis Made from a multidisciplinary approach, taking into account the combination of clinical, HRCT, and histological features—distinguish from other causes of diffuse lung disease (see ➲ p. 33). Histological patterns are often considered to be the most specific but must be interpreted in the context of clinical and radiological features. Surgical lung biopsy is recommended for many cases of suspected IIP, with the exception of patients exhibiting typical clinical and HRCT features of IPF. TBBs have a very limited role due to the generally patchy distribution of the IIPs, although they may be useful in the diagnosis of acute interstitial pneumonitis (AIP) and organizing pneumonia (OP), as well as the exclusion of other causes of diffuse lung disease (e.g. sarcoidosis).

The conditions currently included within the classification of IIPs, together with their key clinical, imaging, and histological features and prognosis, are presented in Table 30.1 (see ➲ p. 267) (in order of frequency) and discussed in detail in the remainder of this chapter.

Further information
British Thoracic Society. Interstitial lung disease guideline. *Thorax* 2008;63(suppl. V):v1–58.

Table 30.1 Idiopathic interstitial pneumonias: summary of key features

Idiopathic pulmonary fibrosis (IPF) (previously cryptogenic fibrosing alveolitis (CFA))	*Onset* Over months to years *HRCT* Fibrosis, honeycombing, subpleural, basal distribution, minimal ground glass *Histology* Usual interstitial pneumonia (UIP): areas of interstitial fibrosis (made up of foci of proliferating fibroblasts) interspersed with normal lung (temporal and spatial heterogeneity), minimal inflammation *Prognosis* Poor
Non-specific interstitial pneumonia (NSIP)	*Onset* Over months to years *HRCT* Ground glass, fine reticulation, often basal distribution, minimal honeycombing *Histology* Varying degrees of inflammation and fibrosis, more uniform appearance than UIP *Prognosis* Variable, can be good
Cryptogenic organizing pneumonia (COP) (previously idiopathic bronchiolitis obliterans organizing pneumonia, BOOP)	*Onset* Over months *HRCT* Areas of consolidation, basal, subpleural, peribronchial predominance *Histology* Alveolar spaces 'plugged' with granulation tissue ± extension into bronchioles *Prognosis* Generally good
Acute interstitial pneumonia (AIP)	Many similarities to ARDS *Onset* Over days *HRCT* Diffuse ground-glass and patchy consolidation *Histology* Diffuse alveolar damage: interstitial oedema, intra-alveolar hyaline membranes, followed by fibroblast proliferation and interstitial fibrosis *Prognosis* Poor
Respiratory bronchiolitis-associated interstitial lung disease (RB-ILD)	*Onset* Over years Symptoms usually mild *HRCT* Centrilobular nodules, ground glass, thick-walled airways *Histology* Pigmented macrophages in bronchioles *Prognosis* Good
Desquamative interstitial pneumonia (DIP)	*Onset* Over weeks to months *HRCT* Ground glass *Histology* Pigmented macrophages in alveolar airspaces (perhaps a more extensive form of RB-ILD), temporally uniform appearance *Prognosis* Good
Lymphoid interstitial pneumonia (LIP)	*Onset* Over years *HRCT* Ground glass, often reticulation, cysts *Histology* Diffuse interstitial lymphoid infiltrates *Prognosis* Variable

Idiopathic pulmonary fibrosis (IPF): diagnosis

Definition Chronic interstitial pneumonia of unknown cause characterized histologically by temporal and spatial heterogeneity, with areas of fibrosis and architectural distortion interspersed with areas of normal lung. This occurs as different areas of lung are in varying stages of evolution of the pathological process. The term UIP refers to the radiological (HRCT) and histological appearance of IPF (previously known as CFA). Note that the UIP pattern is non-specific and can be seen in other conditions, e.g. connective tissue disease, asbestosis.

Epidemiology Prevalence figures vary from 6 to 14/100,000, although prevalence may be 175/100,000 in patients >75 years old. Slightly more common in ♂. Median age at presentation 66. Familial form well described but very rare.

Causes and pathophysiology The development of fibrosis was previously thought to reflect a response to chronic inflammation, although this has been questioned in light of the observations that inflammation is not a major feature of pathological specimens and that responses to 'anti-inflammatory' treatment with steroids are poor. An alternative, currently favoured theory is that repeated alveolar epithelial injury leads directly to aberrant wound healing, with activation of mesenchymal cells and the formation of fibroblastic and myofibroblastic foci that secrete excessive extracellular matrix, primarily collagens. The nature of the lung injury remains obscure; postulated triggers include inhalation of metal dust and wood dust, smoking, gastro-oesophageal reflux, or exposure to herpesviruses. Cytokine production (e.g. plasminogen activator inhibitors, matrix metalloproteinases, transforming growth factor-β) by alveolar epithelial cells may play an important role in the development of fibrosis. Host genetic factors are also likely to be important in the pathogenesis of fibrosis, e.g. *MUC5B* and *ELMOD2* gene polymorphisms and telomerase mutations.

Clinical features

- Typically presents with gradual-onset exertional breathlessness and cough; average of 9 months of symptoms prior to presentation
- 5% of patients are said to be asymptomatic, although this is likely to be an underestimate
- Fine basal late inspiratory crackles
- Clubbing in up to 50%
- Cyanosis and cor pulmonale in severe disease.

Investigations

- *Blood tests* Raised ESR and CRP and mild anaemia may occur; positive RhF and/or ANA may occur at low titres in the absence of associated connective tissue disease
- *PFTs* Typically restrictive pattern with reduced VC and transfer factor; reduced gas transfer with preserved lung volumes is suggestive of PHT or coexisting emphysema. O_2 saturations are frequently reduced, particularly on exertion; ABGs may demonstrate type I respiratory failure

- *CXR* Peripheral and basal reticular shadowing, may extend to other zones, sometimes with honeycombing; rarely may be normal
- *HRCT* Features include bilateral, peripheral, and subpleural reticulation, with honeycombing, traction bronchiectasis, architectural distortion, and minimal or no ground-glass change. Predominantly basal initially, more extensive later in disease course. Extent of disease on CT correlates with physiological impairment. Predominant ground-glass appearance suggests an IIP other than IPF—consider lung biopsy
- *BAL* is not routinely required and is rarely helpful. Typically shows neutrophilia, sometimes mild eosinophilia. Marked eosinophilia (>20%) or lymphocytosis (>50%) should raise possibility of alternative diagnosis
- *Lung biopsy* (via VATS or thoracotomy) if there is diagnostic doubt
- *Transthoracic echo* to estimate the PAP in selected patients.

Histology UIP, a fibrosing pattern characterized by temporal and spatial heterogeneity; patches of active fibroblastic foci (reflecting acute injury) are interspersed with honeycombing/architectural distortion (reflecting chronic scarring) and areas of normal lung, reflecting varying stages of evolution of the disease process in different areas of lung. Interstitial inflammation is minimal. Significant inter-observer disagreement between expert pathologists regarding the presence of a UIP pattern on lung biopsy has been reported, and an overall diagnosis taking into account clinical, radiological, and histological features is recommended.

Diagnosis can be confidently made in most cases on the basis of clinical and HRCT findings. Lung biopsy is not generally recommended in patients with typical clinical and HRCT features of IPF but should be considered in the presence of unusual features (e.g. predominant ground glass/nodules/consolidation/upper lobe involvement on HRCT, or young patient). When required, biopsies should be obtained at VATS or thoracotomy; TBBs are not recommended, as they provide smaller samples, which are rarely diagnostic.

Differential diagnosis

- LVF (a common clinical misdiagnosis in IPF, and patients are often prescribed inappropriate diuretics)
- Fibrotic NSIP and other IIPs
- Asbestosis (may mimic clinically and radiologically, with UIP pattern on histology; occupational history and presence of pleural plaques may suggest this diagnosis)
- Connective tissue disease (may mimic clinically and radiologically, with UIP pattern on histology—particularly in RA; lung involvement may precede extrapulmonary manifestations of disease)
- Chronic HP (suggested by typically upper/mid-zone predominance, micronodules, ground glass, areas of reduced attenuation, lymphocytic BAL fluid; uncommonly, it may be associated with a UIP pattern)
- Chronic sarcoidosis
- Drug-induced lung disease (refer to ℬ http://www.pneumotox.com).

IPF: management

Clinical trials of therapy in IPF are particularly challenging. Older studies were hindered by inclusion of a heterogeneous patient group, but, even within groups of patients with well-defined IPF, there remains significant heterogeneity in clinical course. Furthermore, some relatively recent large studies of IPF have been poorly designed, e.g. failing to include a placebo group. There is ongoing debate as to optimal trial design and end points, including the definition of minimally important clinical difference in FVC.

Drug treatments that are *not* recommended, based on previous studies, include: corticosteroid monotherapy, combination 'triple therapy' (with prednisolone, azathioprine, and acetylcysteine), azathioprine, cyclophosphamide, colchicine, ciclosporin, imatinib, interferon gamma-1b (INSPIRE study), bosentan (BUILD-3 study), ambrisentan, etanercept, and warfarin. Specific points of note from these studies include:

- Prior to the reclassification of IIPs, studies suggested that *corticosteroids* might improve lung function and symptoms. However, these studies almost certainly included patients with conditions other than IPF that are associated with a better treatment response and prognosis (e.g. NSIP)
- Combination of oral *prednisolone*, *azathioprine*, and *acetylcysteine* was initially reported to confer a small improvement in lung function when compared with prednisolone and azathioprine alone (IFIGENIA trial, 2005), and, despite the lack of a placebo arm, this study led to widespread use of such 'triple therapy'. Interim analysis of the PANTHER-IPF study in 2012 demonstrated that this combination was, however, associated with higher mortality and hospitalization rates than placebo, and consequently the use of azathioprine or triple therapy should be avoided
- Although a small, open-label, placebo-controlled study suggested a possible survival benefit from *anticoagulation*, a subsequent study (ACE-IPF trial, 2012) reported an increased mortality and serious adverse event rate with warfarin; anticoagulation is not recommended.

Management Treatment options should be considered in the context of the individual patient's clinical condition, comorbidity, and wishes, particularly in view of the often unpredictable disease course, unknown efficacy of treatment, and high frequency of serious side effects. Principles of treatment are as follows:

- *Supportive treatment* Consider use of home O_2 concentrator if limited by breathlessness and persistent resting PaO_2 <7.3kPa or <8kPa in the setting of clinical features of PHT. Use of ambulatory O_2 may improve exercise tolerance. Encourage pulmonary rehabilitation programme. Gastro-oesophageal reflux disease is common in IPF and may drive lung fibrosis; symptomatic patients should be treated with PPIs ± pro-motility agents (e.g. domperidone); treatment of asymptomatic GORD is recommended in the ATS 2011 guidelines, although there is currently little direct evidence to support this. Cough may be troublesome; consider oral codeine. Opioids are frequently required for palliation of severe breathlessness

- *Drugs* should be considered in a closely observed trial of therapy. Patients should be offered inclusion in clinical trials where possible. Monotherapy with oral *acetylcysteine* (an antioxidant and antifibrotic) at a dose of 600mg tds is of unproven efficacy (the final analysis of the PANTHER-IPF trial should resolve this question) but unlikely to cause significant harm, and it is widely used. Treatment with *pirfenidone* (antifibrotic, inhibits collagen synthesis, and reduces fibroblast proliferation) has been associated with a small beneficial effect on rate of FVC decline (CAPACITY trials 1 and 2) but is often limited by side effects; it has recently been approved by NICE for use in the UK for patients with FVC between 50% and 80% predicted although should be discontinued if there is evidence of ongoing disease progression (decrease in FVC by 10% or more within 12 months)
- Studies do not support treatment with *steroids* in IPF, and NICE guidance recommends that steroids should not be used in an attempt to modify disease progression (except in acute exacerbations where benefit is possible but unproven; see Box 30.1). Despite this, oral prednisolone is still sometimes used in practice, particularly when specifically requested by an informed patient, for attempted symptom control (e.g. cough), or when there is diagnostic uncertainty (may be of benefit in patients with other IIPs misdiagnosed as IPF). Significant side effects of steroid treatment (e.g. hyperglycaemia necessitating insulin, osteoporosis, myopathy, peptic ulcer disease, cataracts, raised intraocular pressure, psychosis) are very common in this patient group
- *Monitoring* Disease progression and response to treatment are best assessed by serial measurements of FVC and TLCO; document them at each clinic attendance. Absolute changes in FVC or TLCO of 10–15% or more are considered significant in terms of assessing disease progression. Note that a realistic aim of disease-modifying treatment in IPF is to slow progression, rather than improve lung function. Changes in symptoms, such as exercise tolerance and cough frequency/severity, may also be useful
- *Lung transplantation* Patients with IPF are often referred for consideration of transplantation too late, and many die whilst on the waiting list (which is around 12 months in the UK). Guidelines recommend referral of all suitable patients with histological or radiographic evidence of UIP, irrespective of VC and without delaying for trials of treatment. These are not widely applied in the UK, and, in practice, referral is often considered in symptomatic patients aged <65y, with TLCO <40% predicted, fall in FVC ≥10%, or in TLCO ≥15% over 6 months, O_2 desaturation <88% on 6min walk, and/or honeycombing on HRCT.

IPF: prognosis and future developments

Prognosis is highly variable; many patients remain stable or decline slowly over years, whilst a subgroup declines more quickly ('accelerated variant', mainly male smokers), and between 5 and 20% experience a very rapid decline after a period of relative stability ('acute exacerbation' of IPF; see Box 30.1); prognosis is difficult to predict in individual patients. Mean survival from diagnosis is 2.9–5y. Poor prognostic factors include TLCO <40% at presentation, O_2 desaturation <88% during 6min walk, and fall of ≥10% in FVC or ≥15% in TLCO in the first 6–12 months. The presence of PHT is associated with a particularly poor prognosis. More extensive fibroblastic foci on lung biopsy have also been shown to correlate with shorter survival. Death is commonly due to respiratory failure and/or infection. Increased risk of developing lung cancer, particularly in peripheral fibrotic areas of lung.

Future developments There is significant current interest in clinical trial design for IPF and specifically the development of robust outcome measures. Only relatively few trials to date have included patients with advanced disease. The development of biomarkers to identify subgroups of patients with differing responses to treatment or outcomes is another area of interest. Therapeutic agents currently under evaluation include:

- A controlled trial of *sildenafil* (a PDE-5 inhibitor) in advanced IPF (STEP-IPF trial) reported no effect on the 1° outcome of significant increase in 6min walk distance, although small, but significant, improvements in 2° outcomes (oxygenation, gas transfer, degree of dyspnoea, and QoL) were noted in the sildenafil group; trials are ongoing
- Silent *GORD* appears to be common in IPF, and episodes of micro-aspiration may drive lung fibrosis; clinical trials of treatment of asymptomatic GORD are in progress
- Treatment with the *tyrosine kinase inhibitor* BIBF 1120 (which targets growth factor receptors involved in lung fibrosis) in a phase 2 trial was associated with a reduced frequency of acute exacerbations and a trend towards a reduction in the decline of FVC; a phase 3 clinical trial is in progress
- A small single-centre study of *thalidomide* reported an improvement in cough and respiratory QoL in patients with IPF; a larger trial is awaited
- A trial of *co-trimoxazole* reported no effect on lung function but a possible mortality benefit, which may be partly explained by attenuation of increased mortality related to immunosuppression; side effects were common, particularly nausea and rash
- Trials of the *CCL2-specific monoclonal antibody* CNTO 888 are underway
- *Stem cell therapy* aimed at repairing lungs injured by fibrosis is an area of future research.

Box 30.1 Acute exacerbations of IPF

Acute exacerbations of IPF are otherwise unexplained, acute worsening of dyspnoea or new development of dyspnoea in patients with known IPF. They are usually defined as onset <30 days, although some patients experience apparent exacerbations over the course of 10–12 weeks. *HRCT* typically shows extensive ground glass and/or consolidation superimposed on a background UIP pattern of reticulation or honeycombing. Consider other exacerbants, in particular, infection (including PCP), pneumothorax, left heart failure, PE, and other causes of lung injury (e.g. drug-induced). CTPA, with HRCT slices, is usually the radiological investigation of choice, as PEs may coexist with ILD. *BAL* is helpful in excluding atypical infection (particularly PCP), but patients are often too hypoxic to safely undergo this procedure. Treatment is usually attempted with *high-dose steroids* (e.g. IV methylprednisolone 750mg–1g on 3 consecutive days, followed by maintenance therapy with 0.5–1mg/kg/day of prednisolone). In practice, infection is difficult to confidently exclude, and treatment with broad-spectrum antibiotics, alongside steroids, is usual.

Acute exacerbations are increasingly recognized as an important cause of death in mild to moderate, apparently stable, IPF, and also appear to occur in the setting of other forms of fibrotic lung disease such as connective tissue disease-associated pneumonitis, chronic HP, and fibrotic NSIP. The *mechanism* is poorly understood, although viral infection may act as a trigger and some exacerbations occur post-operatively, including after surgical lung biopsy. The *histological* pattern is of diffuse alveolar damage associated with UIP, although a minority of cases have features of OP. Inpatient *mortality* is >60%, rising to >90% within 6 months of discharge. The outcome of invasive ventilation in patients with known IPF is very poor (mortality approaching 100%), and ICU admission is not usually appropriate in the setting of underlying IPF/extensive fibrotic change.

Non-specific interstitial pneumonia (NSIP)

Definition The term NSIP is a description of a histological pattern, rather than a specific clinical entity. This form of IIP is particularly poorly understood, and the histological pattern of NSIP probably encompasses several distinct clinical/radiological conditions—indeed, a proposed sub-classification divides NSIP into three clinicoradiological syndromes: NSIP with an IPF-like profile/overlap (NSIP/IPF), NSIP with an organizing pneumonia profile (NSIP/OP), and NSIP with a hypersensitivity profile (NSIP/HP). The clinical utility of this subclassification is uncertain. Patients with NSIP on lung biopsy have a generally better prognosis and greater response to steroids when compared with patients with IPF. NSIP may be idiopathic or occur in association with other systemic conditions, most notably connective tissue diseases.

Epidemiology Typically affects younger patients than IPF, with age of onset 40–50y. May rarely affect children.

Causes/associations
- Idiopathic
- Connective tissue disease (NSIP may be the first manifestation of disease)
- Drugs
- Infection
- Immunodeficiency (including HIV, post-bone marrow transplant, chemotherapy).

Clinical features There are few specific clinical features that help distinguish NSIP from other IIPs. Described features include:
- Breathlessness, cough
- Weight loss is common
- Onset gradual or subacute; typical symptom duration before diagnosis varies 0.5–3y
- Crackles at lung bases, later more extensive
- Clubbing in a small proportion of patients.

Investigations
- *HRCT* frequently shows ground-glass change, often in a basal distribution, with or without reticulation and traction bronchiectasis. The appearance is usually more confluent and homogeneous than the patchy heterogeneous distribution seen in IPF. Honeycombing is rare
- *PFTs* Typically restrictive pattern, but impaired gas transfer in only 50%. Desaturation on exertion is common
- *BAL* Lymphocytosis common
- *Lung biopsy* is often required
- Investigations to exclude underlying disease (see under Causes/associations).

Histology Variable, ranging from a predominantly 'cellular' pattern (mild to moderate interstitial inflammation, no fibrosis) to a 'fibrotic' pattern (interstitial fibrosis, more homogeneous appearance than in UIP and lack of fibroblastic foci or honeycombing; lung architecture may be relatively preserved). NSIP may be subclassified, based on the relative proportions of inflammation and fibrosis: NSIP 1 (primarily inflammation, termed 'cellular'), NSIP 2 (inflammation and fibrosis), and NSIP 3 (primarily fibrosis). Features of both NSIP and UIP are sometimes seen on biopsies from the same individual—in such cases, the diagnosis is considered to be IPF (indicating a poor prognosis).

Diagnosis Clinical and HRCT features are non-specific, and surgical lung biopsy is often required for diagnosis. An exception is NSIP in the setting of connective tissue disease, when histological confirmation is not usually required. Biopsy evidence of NSIP should be interpreted in the context of clinical and radiological findings, using a multidisciplinary approach in order to assign to the 'best fit' NSIP syndrome (NSIP/IPF, NSIP/OP, or NSIP/HP).

Management Treatment is with corticosteroids, with a typical prednisolone dose of 0.5mg/kg. Consider routine use of bisphosphonate, PPI, and co-trimoxazole prophylaxis (960mg three times/week) against PCP. As with IPF, disease progression and response to treatment are best assessed by serial measurements of FVC and TLCO, with absolute changes of 10–15% or more considered significant. Additional immunosuppressive treatments may be considered in patients who fail to respond to corticosteroids alone.

Prognosis Variable. Most patients improve or remain stable on treatment. 'Cellular' pattern on biopsy is associated with a good prognosis. Fibrotic NSIP is associated with a markedly better prognosis than IPF (5y survival >50% in fibrotic NSIP, compared with 10–15% in IPF).

Cryptogenic organizing pneumonia (COP)

Definition COP is a disease of unknown cause, characterized by 'plugging' of alveolar spaces with granulation tissue that may also extend up into the bronchioles. In addition to the 'cryptogenic' form, OP may also occur in the context of other diseases (see under Causes of OP). Use of the term 'bronchiolitis obliterans organizing pneumonia (BOOP)' is no longer recommended, as it erroneously suggests a primarily airways disease and is easily confused with bronchiolitis obliterans, a distinct disease entity.

Epidemiology More common in non-smokers. Mean age of onset 55y although can affect any age. ♂ = ♀.

Causes of OP
- Cryptogenic (COP)
- OP 2° to:
  - Infection (including pneumonia, lung abscess, bronchiectasis)
  - Drug reaction or radiotherapy
  - Connective tissue disease (particularly myositis, RA, Sjögren's)
  - Diffuse alveolar damage
  - IBD
  - Haematological malignancy
  - Post-bone marrow transplant
  - Lung malignancy or airways obstruction
  - Pulmonary infarction.

Clinical features
- Typically short (<3 months) history of breathlessness and dry cough, often with malaise, fevers, weight loss, and myalgia. Often presents as a 'slow-to-resolve chest infection', frequently after several courses of antibiotics
- Breathlessness is usually mild, although a minority of patients experience severe breathlessness with rapid onset of respiratory failure and sometimes death ('fulminant COP')
- Examination may be normal or reveal crackles. Clubbing is absent.

Investigations
- *Blood tests* Raised CRP and ESR, neutrophilia
- *PFTs* Mild to moderate restrictive pattern is typical, although mild airways obstruction may also be seen in smokers. Mild hypoxaemia is common
- *CXR* classically shows patchy consolidation, sometimes with nodular shadowing. May present as a solitary mass on CXR
- *HRCT* Areas of consolidation with air bronchograms, sometimes with associated ground glass or small nodules. Often basal, subpleural, and peribronchial. May migrate spontaneously. Reticulation may suggest poor response to treatment. Less common appearance is as a solitary mass that may cavitate and that is often mistaken radiologically for a lung cancer. Septal thickening may occur

- *TBB* often confirms diagnosis, but there is concern that the relatively small samples may not effectively exclude associated diseases. TBB is usually adequate in patients with typical clinical and HRCT features who are subsequently followed up closely. Surgical lung biopsy (at VATS) is otherwise required
- *BAL*, if performed, shows lymphocytosis, neutrophilia, and eosinophilia.

Histology Alveolar spaces 'plugged' with granulation tissue (fibrin, collagen-containing fibroblasts, often with inflammatory cells), sometimes with extension up into the bronchiolar lumen. Patchy. Lack of architectural distortion. Examine for evidence of underlying cause, e.g. infection, vasculitis.

Diagnosis Usually made on the basis of clinical and HRCT features and TBB. Surgical lung biopsy may be required in atypical cases or if an underlying disease is suspected. Remember that the histological finding of 'OP' is non-specific, and search for 2° causes (see under Causes of OP). Lung cancers may be surrounded by patches of OP, and biopsy of these areas in patients with a solitary lung mass may give misleading results.

Differential diagnosis
- Infective consolidation
- Connective tissue disease, vasculitis
- Lymphoma, alveolar cell carcinoma
- Lung cancer (when OP presents as lung mass).

Management Steroids are the mainstay of treatment. Optimal dose and duration unknown. Typical initial dose of oral prednisolone is 1–1.5mg/kg daily for 3 months, before slowly weaning the dose over a total period of 6–12 months. In fulminant disease, use pulsed IV methylprednisolone 750mg–1g on 3 consecutive days, followed by maintenance therapy with 0.5–1mg/kg/day of prednisolone. Additional treatment with azathioprine or cyclophosphamide may be considered in patients with minimal response to steroids; IV pulses of cyclophosphamide may be tried in critically ill patients if failure to respond 5–7 days after steroid treatment.

Prognosis Generally good. Most patients respond to steroids and improve within a week of starting treatment. Consider alternative diagnosis (e.g. lymphoma) if no improvement on steroid doses >25mg/day. Relapse is common on reduction of steroid dose, and treatment courses of 6–12 months are usually required. A minority improves spontaneously. Lack of steroid response and progressive respiratory failure and death are rare but well documented.

Acute interstitial pneumonia (AIP)

Definition Rapidly progressive form of interstitial pneumonia, characterized histologically by diffuse alveolar damage. May be considered as an idiopathic form of ARDS. Formerly known as Hamman–Rich syndrome.

Epidemiology Poorly described. Mean age of onset is 50 but may occur at any age. Patients often previously healthy.

Clinical features
- Often preceded by 'viral'-type illness, with systemic symptoms, e.g. fevers, tiredness, myalgia, arthralgia
- Rapid onset (over days) of breathlessness; usually presents <3 weeks after symptom onset
- Widespread crackles on examination.

Investigations
- *CXR* Bilateral diffuse airspace shadowing with air bronchograms, progressing to widespread reticulation and ground glass; often spares costophrenic angles, heart borders, and hila
- *HRCT* Bilateral diffuse ground glass and patchy airspace consolidation in early stages; later traction bronchiectasis, cystic change, reticulation
- *PFTs* Restrictive, reduced gas transfer. Often profound hypoxia and respiratory failure
- *BAL* Increased total cells, red blood cells, and haemosiderin. Non-diagnostic but may be useful in excluding infection
- *Lung biopsy* required for diagnosis. TBB may be diagnostic; the risk of pneumothorax is higher in mechanically ventilated patients (about 10%). Surgical lung biopsy is otherwise required.

Histology Diffuse alveolar damage: hyaline membranes, oedema, interstitial inflammation, and alveolar septal thickening, progressing to organizing fibrosis and sometimes honeycombing.

Diagnosis Based on lung biopsy and exclusion of causes of ARDS.

Differential diagnosis See ➔ p. 33. Consider, in particular, the possibility of drug-induced pneumonitis or AIP occurring as a manifestation of antisynthetase syndrome (see ➔ p. 196).

Management No treatment demonstrated to be of benefit. In practice, treat infection (including consideration of unusual organisms), and consider high-dose steroids (e.g. IV methylprednisolone 750mg–1g on 3 consecutive days, followed by maintenance therapy with 0.5–1mg/kg/day of prednisolone). There is a suggestion that outcome may be better following early use of high-dose steroids, although robust evidence is lacking. Clinical and radiological features may be indistinguishable from fulminant COP, which is likely to be more steroid-responsive. High-flow O_2. ITU admission and mechanical ventilatory support usually required.

Prognosis Overall mortality at least 50%, although difficult to predict outcome in individuals. Survivors may stabilize, develop chronic progressive ILD, or experience recurrent exacerbations.

Respiratory bronchiolitis-associated interstitial lung disease (RB-ILD)

Definition 'Respiratory bronchiolitis' is a pathological term referring to the accumulation of bronchiolar pigmented macrophages in cigarette smokers and is asymptomatic in nearly all cases. A minority of smokers with respiratory bronchiolitis, however, develop a form of ILD known as RB-ILD. The exact relationship between RB-ILD and DIP is unclear—they may be considered as different forms of the same underlying disease, with DIP associated with a more extensive accumulation of macrophages throughout alveolar spaces.

Epidemiology Invariably occurs in current or previous smokers, typically >30 pack years. ♂:♀ ≈ 2:1. Usual age of onset 30–40y.

Clinical features
- Usually mild breathlessness and cough
- Small proportion have severe dyspnoea and respiratory failure
- Often crackles on examination.

Investigations
- *PFTs* Often show restrictive or combined obstructive and restrictive picture, with mildly impaired gas transfer
- *CXR* Thick-walled bronchi, reticular or ground-glass change, may be normal
- *HRCT* Centrilobular nodules, ground-glass change, thick-walled airways, often with associated centrilobular emphysema
- *BAL* Typically reveals pigmented alveolar macrophages.

Histology Accumulation of pigmented brown macrophages in terminal bronchioles. Patchy bronchiolocentric distribution. These findings are frequently incidental in healthy smokers, and the diagnosis of RB-ILD is usually made on the basis of clinical and HRCT features; BAL and lung biopsy may be of value in excluding other conditions.

Management Smoking cessation is the mainstay of treatment. Corticosteroids are occasionally used, with uncertain benefit.

Prognosis Available data are limited; prolonged survival is common, although improvements in symptoms or physiology appear to occur in only a minority of patients.

Desquamative interstitial pneumonia (DIP)

Definition ILD that occurs in smokers and is associated with the pathological finding of abundant pigmented macrophages located diffusely throughout alveolar airspaces. It may represent a more extensive form of RB-ILD, in which macrophages are restricted to peribronchiolar regions. The term DIP is misleading, as desquamation of epithelial cells is not responsible for the histological findings, as previously thought; a more accurate term is 'alveolar macrophage pneumonia', although this is not in widespread use.

Epidemiology Very rare. Majority of patients are smokers, although may also occur following inhalation of inorganic dusts, including passive inhalation of cigarette smoke. Typically occurs aged 30–50.

Clinical features Onset of breathlessness and cough over weeks to months is typical. Clubbing is common.

Investigations
- *PFTs* Mild restrictive pattern common, sometimes with reduced gas transfer
- *CXR* May be normal or may demonstrate reticular or ground-glass pattern, particularly affecting lower zones
- *HRCT* Ground glass seen in all cases, typically lower zone or peripheral predominance. Reticulation and honeycombing may be present although tend to be mild
- *BAL* Increase in pigmented macrophages.

Histology Diffuse accumulation of pigmented macrophages in alveolar airspaces. Changes are uniform.

Diagnosis Clinical and HRCT features are non-specific, and surgical lung biopsy is often required for diagnosis.

Management Smoking cessation. Corticosteroids are often used, with high response rates reported in retrospective cohorts.

Prognosis Usually good prognosis. Improvement in ground glass on HRCT may correlate with response to treatment. Survival 70% after 10y. Fluctuating course with remissions, and relapses may occur.

Lymphoid interstitial pneumonia (LIP)

Definition Interstitial pneumonia characterized by diffuse lymphoid infiltrates and often lymphoid hyperplasia. Previously considered to be a precursor to pulmonary lymphoma and difficult to distinguish from lymphoma histologically; it is now considered a distinct entity and is thought to only rarely undergo malignant transformation. Only a minority of cases are idiopathic; actively investigate for an underlying cause (see under Causes/associations).

Epidemiology Very rare. Commoner in women. May occur at any age.

Causes/associations
- Idiopathic
- Connective tissue disease—particularly Sjögren's syndrome, also RA, SLE
- Immunodeficiency, particularly HIV and common variable immunodeficiency
- Infection, e.g. PCP, hepatitis B
- Autoimmune disease, e.g. haemolytic anaemia, Hashimoto's thyroiditis, pernicious anaemia, chronic active hepatitis, primary biliary cirrhosis, myasthenia gravis
- Drugs, e.g. phenytoin.

Clinical features Gradual-onset breathlessness and cough over several years. Fever, weight loss may occur. Crackles may be heard on examination.

Investigations
- *Blood tests* Mild anaemia may occur; poly- or monoclonal increase in serum immunoglobulins is common
- *CXR* Lower zone alveolar shadowing or diffuse honeycombing
- *HRCT* Predominant ground-glass change, often with reticulation and cysts, and sometimes honeycombing and nodules
- *BAL* Non-clonal lymphocytosis
- Investigations to identify underlying cause (see under Causes/associations).

Histology Diffuse interstitial lymphoid infiltrates, predominantly involving alveolar septa, sometimes with lymphoid hyperplasia or honeycombing. Cellular NSIP, follicular bronchiolitis, and lymphoma may give similar appearances.

Management Steroids are frequently used and often appear to improve symptoms.

Prognosis Progression to extensive fibrosis occurs in around one-third of patients.

Lung cancer

Epidemiology and types

Epidemiology

- >39,000 new cases diagnosed per annum in the UK
- Commonest cause of cancer death in women in the UK
- ♂:♀ ≈ 2:1, but numbers decreasing in men, increasing in women, because of increasing smoking
- More women die from lung cancer than from any other cancer, including breast
- 90% smoking-related
- Stopping smoking decreases the risk, but the risk remains higher than in non-smokers
- Risk of lung cancer may be increased by asbestos exposure, arsenic and heavy metal exposure, pulmonary fibrosis, radiation exposure, and in patients with HIV.

Types of lung cancer See Box 31.1. In practical terms, lung cancer is divided into two groups, which influence management and treatment decisions.

Non-small cell lung cancer (NSCLC)

- Accounts for ~80% of all lung cancers
- *Squamous cell carcinoma* is the commonest histological type. Usually presents as a mass on CXR but may cavitate and look radiologically like a lung abscess. Rarely, there may be multiple cavitating lesions. Hypercalcaemia may be a feature
- *Adenocarcinoma* may not necessarily be smoking-related. Can occur in scar tissue or sites of fibrosis. Can be a lung 1° or a 2° from adenocarcinomas at other sites, especially if causing pleural infiltration and subsequent pleural effusion. Adenocarcinomas have recently been reclassified (see Box 31.2)
- *Bronchioloalveolar/bronchoalveolar cell carcinoma* (BAC) is rare and has now been reclassified (see Box 31.2). It can rarely cause copious sputum production (bronchorrhoea). Typically causes fluffy airspace shadowing on CXR and may be multifocal, sometimes in both lungs.

Small cell lung cancer (SCLC)

- Accounts for ~15% of all lung cancers
- Most aggressive of lung cancer subtypes
- Usually disseminated by the time of diagnosis (haematogenous spread)
- Frequently *metastasizes* to liver, bones, bone marrow, brain, adrenals, or elsewhere
- Syndrome of inappropriate secretion of antidiuretic hormone (SIADH) with hyponatraemia is common in SCLC
- Surgery usually not appropriate
- Chemo- and radiosensitive
- Untreated extensive stage SCLC is rapidly progressive and has a median survival of 6 weeks.

Box 31.1 WHO histological classification of lung tumours, 2004

- Squamous cell carcinoma
- Small cell carcinoma
- Adenocarcinoma
- Large cell carcinoma
- Adenosquamous carcinoma
- Sarcomatoid carcinoma
- Carcinoid tumours
- Salivary gland tumours
- Pre-invasive lesions.

Box 31.2 IASLC/ATS/ERS classification of lung adenocarcinomas, 2011

- Pre-invasive lesions
  - Atypical adenomatous hyperplasia
  - Adenocarcinoma *in situ* (previously solitary BAC)
  - Non-mucinous, mucinous, mixed
- Minimally invasive adenocarcinoma
  - Non-mucinous, mucinous, mixed
- Invasive adenocarcinoma
  - Lepidic predominant (previously non-mucinous BAC)
  - Acinar predominant
  - Papillary predominant
  - Micropapillary predominant
  - Solid predominant with mucin production
- Variants of invasive adenocarcinoma
  - Invasive mucinous (previously mucinous BAC)
  - Colloid
  - Foetal (low and high grade)
  - Enteric.

Further information

Travis WD *et al*. International Association for the Study of Lung Cancer/American Thoracic Society/ European Respiratory Society international multidisciplinary classification of lung adenocarcinoma. *J Thorac Oncol* 2011;6:244–85.

Clinical features

Smokers and ex-smokers with chest symptoms, especially those aged over 50, need investigation.

Symptoms and signs

These may be due to local tumour effects, metastatic tumour effects, or paraneoplastic manifestations. Many patients have no specific signs. In some, the lung cancer may be an incidental finding on CXR or CT performed for another reason.

Local tumour effects
- Persistent cough or change in usual cough
- Haemoptysis
- Chest pain (suggests chest wall or pleural involvement)
- Unresolving pneumonia or lobar collapse
- Unexplained dyspnoea (due to bronchial narrowing or obstruction)
- Wheeze or stridor
- Shoulder pain (due to diaphragm involvement)
- Pleural effusion (due to direct tumour extension or pleural metastases)
- Hoarse voice (tumour invasion of the left recurrent laryngeal nerve)
- Dysphagia
- Raised hemidiaphragm (phrenic nerve paralysis)
- SVCO (see ➲ pp. 302–4)
- Horner's syndrome (miosis, ptosis, enophthalmos, anhydrosis) due to apical or Pancoast's tumour damaging sympathetic chain
- Pancoast's tumours can also directly invade the rib and brachial plexus, causing C8–T1 dermatome numbness, shoulder pain, and weakness of small muscles of the hand.

Metastatic tumour effects
- Cervical/supraclavicular lymphadenopathy (common, present in 30%, and may be an easy site for diagnostic biopsy)
- Palpable liver edge
- Bone pain/pathological fracture due to bone metastases
- Neurological sequelae 2° to cerebral metastases (median survival of NSCLC with brain metastases is 2 months)
- Hypercalcaemic effects (due to bony metastases or direct tumour production of parathyroid hormone (PTH)-related peptide or PTH); see ➲ p. 305
- Dysphagia (compression from large mediastinal nodes).

Paraneoplastic syndromes
Endocrine syndromes are due to the ectopic production of hormones or hormonally active peptides. Neurological syndromes are due to antibody-mediated CNS damage.
- Cachexia and wasting
- Clubbing (up to 29% of patients; any cell type, more common in squamous and adenocarcinoma)

- Hypertrophic pulmonary osteoarthropathy (HPOA), often in association with clubbing, any cell type; more common in squamous and adenocarcinoma. Periosteal bone proliferation with symmetrical painful arthropathy (predominantly large joints, but hands and feet also affected)
- Gynaecomastia
- SIADH (mainly SCLC) in up to 10% of patients; see ➔ p. 306
- Ectopic ACTH (Cushing's syndrome, but due to rapid development; biochemical changes predominate, mainly SCLC) in 2–5% of patients
- Lambert–Eaton myasthenic syndrome (LEMS)—with SCLC. Affects proximal limbs and trunk, with autonomic involvement (dry mouth, constipation, erectile failure) and hyporeflexia (although reflexes return on exercising the affected muscle group), and only a slight response to edrophonium. Symptoms may predate diagnosis of lung cancer by up to 4y. Caused by autoantibodies against P/Q-type voltage-gated calcium channels. Decreased acetylcholine release at motor nerve terminals leads to the proximal weakness. Diagnosis made by autoantibody detection on radio-immunoprecipitation assay. EMG shows increased amplitude of muscle action with high-frequency stimulation, and repeated muscle contraction may lead to increasing strength and reflexes. Treatment of underlying SCLC may cause neurological improvement. If weakness is severe, IV immunoglobulin or plasmapheresis may give short-term benefits. 3,4-diaminopyridine may increase muscle strength in 85% of patients. Prednisolone alone or with azathioprine or ciclosporin can increase muscle strength and provide long-term control in non-responders
- Cerebellar syndrome (usually SCLC)
- Limbic encephalitis (SCLC, also breast, testicular, other cancers). Occurs within 4y of diagnosis of cancer. Personality change, seizures, depression, subacute-onset confusion, and short-term memory loss. Diagnosed by pathological or radiological involvement of limbic system. Anti-Hu antibodies positive in 50% if associated with lung cancer
- Dermatomyositis/polymyositis
- Glomerulonephritis.

Lymphangitis carcinomatosis Infiltration of pulmonary lymphatics by tumour. May be due to lung cancer or breast, prostate, stomach, or pancreatic malignancies. Causes SOB, cough, and is often associated with systemic signs of advanced malignancy. May be visible on CXR as fine linear shadowing throughout both lung fields. Septal lines present. May look like pulmonary oedema. Easily diagnosed on CT. Oral steroid treatment and diuretics can give symptomatic relief, but it is usually a short-lived response. Often part of a rapid decline.

Further information

Keogh M et al. Treatment for Lambert–Eaton myasthenic syndrome. *Cochrane Database Syst Rev* 2011;2:CD003279.

Investigations

Patients should be referred under the '2-week cancer wait' scheme and should be seen within 14 days of referral. The aim of the investigations is to reach a histological diagnosis and tumour stage in order to determine the most appropriate treatment. Current government guidelines recommend patients should receive treatment without undue delay: within 31 days of the decision to treat and within 62 days of their urgent referral.

In outpatients

- *History and examination*, including smoking and occupational histories
- *Spirometry* pre-biopsy or surgery
- *CXR* (PA and possibly lateral)—location of lesion, pleural involvement, pleural effusion, rib destruction, intrathoracic metastases, mediastinal lymphadenopathy. CXR can be normal
- *Blood tests*, including sodium, calcium, and LFTs. Check clotting if biopsy planned
- *Sputum cytology* only indicated in patients who are unfit for bronchoscopy or biopsy
- *Diagnostic pleural tap*, if effusion present
- *FNA* of enlarged supraclavicular or cervical lymph nodes.

Radiology

- *CT neck, chest, liver, adrenals (contrast-enhanced) to assess tumour site and size* Lung cancers frequently metastasize to the mediastinal lymph nodes, liver, and adrenals. CT can locate lesions amenable to biopsy (either the 1° tumour or a metastasis). Assesses size of local and regional lymph nodes. Poor at assessing whether enlarged nodes are reactive (inflammatory) or represent metastatic spread (79% sensitive, 78% specific). Can assess tumour invasion to mediastinum and chest wall
- *USS* of neck or liver may provide information about enlarged lymph nodes or metastases suitable for biopsy
- *MRI* Used to answer specific questions relating to tumour invasion/ borders. Good for assessing brachial plexus involvement. No role in nodule assessment
- *Bone scan* Indicated if any suggestion of metastatic disease such as bony pain, pathological fracture, hypercalcaemia, raised ALP. Highly suggestive of bony metastases if multiple areas of increased uptake. Solitary lesion may require further evaluation
- *CT head* Indicated if any neurological evidence of metastatic disease such as persistent vomiting, fit, focal neurological signs, headache, unexplained confusion, or personality change. Consider in patients selected for treatment with curative intent, especially stage III disease
- *Positron emission tomography (PET) scanning* Imaging technique where metabolically active tissues, such as tumours, show increased uptake of radiolabelled 18-fluorodeoxyglucose (FDG). Improves the rate of detection of local and distant metastases. Useful for assessing regional and mediastinal lymph nodes (88% sensitive, 93% specific). This is

increased if abnormal nodes are identified on CT. Now widely used and should be interpreted with the CT. Perform in:

- All patients considered for radical therapy to look for involved lymph nodes and distant metastases
- Patients with N2–3 disease on CT of uncertain significance, who are otherwise surgical candidates
- Candidates for radical radiotherapy
- Limited stage SCLC, staged by standard staging methods to identify metastases, as SCLC avidly takes up FDG.

PET-positive nodes that would exclude a patient from surgery should be confirmed as malignant with a biopsy, unless the pre-test probability of malignancy is high. PET may reveal a distant abnormality, other than the 1° lung cancer, which could be a solitary metastasis or a second cancer. It is important therefore to biopsy isolated PET abnormalities before determining that a cancer is not resectable.

False negatives occur in tumours with a low metabolic activity (such as BAC, carcinoid), small nodules, and hyperglycaemic patients. *False positives* occur in patients with benign pulmonary nodules with a high metabolic rate such as infective granulomata.

Patients fast 4h before the test, and, if they have diabetes, glucose should be within the normal range.

MDT

Should include a chest physician, radiologist, thoracic surgeon, oncologist, pathologist, lung cancer nurse, and palliative care specialist, who meet regularly in order to discuss patients and plan the most appropriate course of management.

The Department of Health and NICE in the UK have produced guidelines for performance in lung cancer care. These encourage access to the MDT in decision making for the treatment and investigation of all patients with lung cancer.

Further information

NICE lung cancer guidelines 2011. ℘ http://www.nice.org.uk.

Giving information to lung cancer patients. BTS Lung Cancer and Mesothelioma Specialist Advisory Group. April 2008. ℘ http://www.brit-thoracic.org.uk/Portals/0/Guidelines/Lung%20Cancer/WTSTPBTSfinal210408.pdf.

Diagnostic procedures

Investigations are performed to obtain a tissue diagnosis and to stage cancer in order to determine the most appropriate treatment. Aim to achieve diagnosis and staging with as few procedures as possible. Establishing diagnosis and presence of metastatic spread at a single test is desirable, if possible. Increasingly important to obtain adequate tissue to enable accurate histology ± molecular analyses (e.g. epidermal growth factor receptor (EGFR) activating mutations). Aspects of further investigation may be inappropriate if the patient has advanced disease, is frail with comorbid conditions, or does not want to pursue diagnosis. This should be documented in their notes to aid audit and cancer service evaluation.

Bronchoscopy Method of obtaining histological and cytological specimens. Suitable for central tumours. Tumours can be washed, brushed, and biopsied. Bronchoscopic samples are more likely to be histologically positive if there is:
• An ill-defined lesion on the CXR
• An endobronchial component to the tumour
• Tumour <4cm from the origin of the nearest lobar bronchus
• A segmental or larger airway leading to the mass.

Greater diagnostic yield if performed after CT scan, as radiologically abnormal areas can be targeted. Tumour position bronchoscopically may contribute to operative decisions: tumour confined to a lobar bronchus may be resectable with lobectomy; tumour <2cm from the main carina requires pneumonectomy; left vocal cord paralysis indicates inoperability due to tumour infiltration of the left recurrent laryngeal nerve; and a splayed carina occurs 2° to enlarged mediastinal nodes. Advanced bronchoscopic techniques (e.g. endobronchial ultrasound (EBUS), electromagnetic navigation guidance, or fluoroscopically guided bronchoscopy) may help obtain diagnostic samples.

Transbronchial needle aspiration (TBNA) of lymph nodes (often combined with EBUS) can be performed to obtain tissue and allow staging at the time of bronchoscopy and may reduce need for mediastinoscopy (see ➜ p. 290). May also be combined with EUS-FNA (endoscopic ultrasound-guided fine-needle aspiration).

CT/USS-guided biopsy of tumour or of an enlarged lymph node, especially in the neck, or of a metastasis (see Box 31.3). 85–90% sensitivity in lesions >2cm. Where possible, biopsy of a metastasis should be the investigation of choice, simultaneously giving staging and diagnosis.

Mediastinoscopy Biopsy of enlarged mediastinal lymph nodes to determine whether they are inflammatory or have malignant invasion. Suprasternal notch incision under general anaesthetic, blunt dissection, palpation, and endoscopic visualization and biopsy of nodes: paratracheal, prevascular, tracheobronchial, and anterior subcarinal. 93% sensitivity, 96% specificity. Technically more difficult if SVCO. Bleeding in <0.3%, left recurrent laryngeal nerve injury in 1%, pneumothorax, mediastinal emphysema, infection, oesophageal perforation (all rare). Repeat mediastinoscopies have lower positive yield and higher complication rate.

Mediastinotomy Biopsy of aorto-pulmonary, sub-aortic, phrenic, or hilar nodes. Metastatic involvement of nodes does not necessarily preclude curative surgical resection with a pneumonectomy. Also can assess direct tumour invasion of central pulmonary artery or thoracic aorta, which would preclude curative surgery. Right or left parasternal incision, blunt dissection, palpation, and endoscopic visualization and biopsy of nodes.

Thoracoscopy may be required to determine whether a pleural effusion contains malignant cells or is inflammatory, e.g. due to pneumonia caused by an obstructing lesion. Malignant effusions are evidence of M1 disease and hence are a contraindication to surgery.

Operative It is sometimes difficult to obtain definitive cytology or histology preoperatively. If there is a high suspicion of malignancy, surgery can be performed regardless. Patients undergoing surgery are given a pathological stage, which is sometimes different to the clinical stage (after histologically examining resection margins, lymph nodes, and pleura).

Box 31.3 Radiologically guided lung biopsy

Indications
- New or enlarging mass, not amenable to bronchoscopy
- Multiple chest nodules in patient not known to have malignancy
- Persistent undiagnosed single or multiple focal infiltrates
- Hilar mass.

Pre-biopsy preparation
- Discuss with MDT
- Recent spirometry, with FEV_1 >35% predicted
- Check APTT and PT ratios <1.4 and platelets >100,000/mL. If not, discuss with haematologist to determine whether it is safe to proceed
- Recent imaging available
- High-risk patients should have overnight admission following biopsy
- Written information for patient, with informed signed consent.

Biopsy preparation
- Perform without sedation, if possible
- Use USS, if possible
- Local anaesthetic to skin and subcutaneous tissue
- Perform at least two passes, may use FNA or cutting needle. FNA high diagnostic yield for malignant lesions (95%) but less for benign (10–50%). Cutting needles as good for malignancy and better for benign diagnoses. Operator decision.

Post-biopsy
- Observation by staff for 1h in case of complications
- Erect CXR 1h after biopsy and reviewed by doctor
- Manage any pneumothorax, according to BTS guidelines (see ➔ p. 380). Small pneumothoraces often resolve spontaneously but may need inpatient admission if there are concerns.

Complications
- Rates vary, but ~20% pneumothorax risk, ~3% require chest drain
- Haemoptysis 5%, death 0.15%.

Manhire A *et al*. Guidelines for radiologically guided lung biopsy. *Thorax* 2003:**58**:920–34.

Staging

Clinical and radiological tools categorize tumour size, location, regional and distant spread, and aid determination of most appropriate treatment. They can also therefore give prognostic information.

- *SCLC* is staged as limited or extensive but now also staged using the 7th edition of the TNM staging system (see Box 31.4):
  - *Limited* Confined to ipsilateral hemithorax and supraclavicular lymph nodes. Median survival with treatment, 12 months; without treatment, 12 weeks
  - *Extensive* Everything else. Median survival with treatment, 8 months; without treatment, 6 weeks
- *NSCLC* is commonly classified using TNM staging system (see Box 31.4 and Table 31.1). Frequency of patient stage at diagnosis: I and II, 42%; III, 34%; IV, 24%.

Table 31.1 Lung cancer clinical staging and survival

Stage	TNM classification	After treatment survival	
		Median (months)	5y (%)
0	Tis	?	?
IA	T1 N0 M0	60	50
IB	T2a N0 M0	43	43
IIA	T1a–2a N1 M0	34	36
	T2b N0 M0		
IIB	T2b N1 M0	18	25
	T3 N0 M0		
IIIA	T1–2 N2 M0	14	19
	T3 N1–2 M0		
	T4 N0–1 M0		
IIIB	T4 N2 M0	10	7
	Any T, N3 M0		
IV	Any T, any N, M1	6	2

Further information

Goldstraw P et al. The IASLC Lung Cancer Staging Project: Proposals for the Revision of the TNM Stage Groupings in the Forthcoming (Seventh) Edition of the TNM Classification of Malignant Tumours. J Thorac Oncol 2007;2:706–14.

Mountain CF, Dresler CM. Regional lymph node classification for lung cancer staging. Chest 1997; 111:1718–23.

Box 31.4 7th edition of the TNM staging system for lung cancer (IASLC/UICC/AJCC)

Extent of 1° tumour (T)

Tx   1° tumour cannot be assessed, or tumour proven by presence of malignant cells in sputum or bronchial washings but not visualized by imaging or bronchoscopy

T0   No evidence of 1° tumour

Tis   Carcinoma *in situ*

T1   Tumour ≤3cm, surrounded by lung or visceral pleura, without bronchoscopic evidence of invasion more proximal than the lobar bronchus

    T1a—tumour ≤2cm

    T1b—tumour >2cm but ≤3cm

T2   Tumour >3cm but ≤7cm, or in main bronchus (>2cm distal to carina) or invading visceral pleura, or associated with atelectasis or obstructive pneumonitis that extends to the hilar region, but does not involve whole lung

    T2a—tumour >3cm but ≤5cm

    T2b—tumour >5cm but ≤7cm

T3   Tumour >7cm or invading: chest wall, diaphragm, phrenic nerve, parietal pericardium, mediastinal pleura, or tumour in main bronchus (<2cm distal to carina but not involving carina) or associated atelectasis or obstructive pneumonitis of the entire lung or nodules in same lobe

T4   Tumour of any size invading: mediastinum, heart, great vessels, trachea, oesophagus, recurrent laryngeal nerve, carina, vertebral body, or separate nodules in a different ipsilateral lobe.

Regional lymph nodes (N)

Nx   Cannot be assessed

N0   No regional lymph node metastasis

N1   Ipsilateral peribronchial and/or ipsilateral hilar nodes and intrapulmonary nodes (including direct extension of tumour)

N2   Ipsilateral mediastinal and/or subcarinal nodes

N3   Contralateral mediastinal, hilar nodes, or any scalene or supraclavicular nodes.

Distant metastasis (M)

Mx   Cannot be assessed

M0   No distant metastasis

M1   Distant metastasis present

    M1a—separate tumour nodule in contralateral lobe, pleural nodules, or malignant pleural/pericardial effusion

    M1b—distant metastasis.

Also see ℛ http://www.staginglungcancer.org.

Non-small cell lung cancer (NSCLC): surgery

Much of the investigation of lung cancer is to determine whether a patient has disease that is potentially curable by surgery. Other treatment options include chemotherapy, radiotherapy, and best supportive care, i.e. symptom-based conservative management. The MDT decides the most appropriate choice of treatment which is then discussed with the patient.

Surgery

The aims of surgery for lung cancer are to completely excise the tumour and local lymphatics, with minimal removal of normal functioning lung parenchyma.
- Stages I and II NSCLC are usually amenable to surgery if the patient is fit enough (see Fitness for surgery). This has a high chance of cure in stage I (70% in IA), and a reasonable chance in stage II. 10–20% of NSCLC patients undergo resection
- In stage IIIA tumours, surgery alone is unlikely to be curative, but adjuvant chemotherapy and radiotherapy can improve survival rates
- Stages IIIB and IV are not resectable
- Stages 0/tumour *in situ* often will have no defined 1° lesion amenable to resection. The natural progression of these tumours is still unknown; they may progress or regress with time.

Resectability of a tumour implies likelihood of complete removal by surgery; this is different from patient operability, which is determined by the patient's fitness for surgery.

Fitness for surgery
- *Global risk score* May be useful for estimating risk of death (e.g. Thoracoscore)
- *Age* is not a contraindication, but increasing age is associated with an increased perioperative morbidity. Higher mortality risk if over 80 and if pneumonectomy, rather than lobectomy (14% mortality vs 7%, respectively). Right pneumonectomy has higher mortality than left pneumonectomy (more lung removed). 2y post-operative survival similar to that of other age groups
- *Lung function* Approaches vary. The 2013 American College of Chest Physicians (ACCP) guidelines suggest measurement of FEV_1 and TLCO in all, with calculation of predicted post-operative (PPO) values. PPO FEV_1 and PPO TLCO both >60% suggest low risk for death and complications and no further tests required. For values <60% but >30%, stair climb or SWT recommended. For values <30% (or SWT of <25 shuttles or <400m, or climb test <22m), full CPET recommended. If VO_2max <35% predicted (or <10 mL/kg/min) consider patient for lung-conserving procedures or non-operative treatment. LVRS may be considered if a cancer is within an area of upper lobe emphysema
- *Cardiovascular* Postpone surgery if patient has had MI within 30 days. Cardiology opinion if patient has had MI within 6 months. Echo if they have heart murmur. Preoperative ECG for all

- *CNS* If any history of transient ischaemic attacks, strokes, or carotid bruits, need carotid Doppler studies and vascular surgeon opinion, if necessary
- *Smoking* Do not delay surgery to stop smoking, but counsel patients and offer NRT
- *Nutritional* Requirements should be optimized, with advice from a dietician, if necessary. Patients presenting with a preoperative weight loss of 10% or more ± performance status ≥2 are more likely to have advanced disease or comorbidities. Therefore, require careful staging and search for evidence of comorbidity.

Types of surgery **Lobectomy** or bi-lobectomy for localized tumour, or pneu-monectomy for tumour involving >1 or 2 lobes. If hilar nodes are infiltrated by tumour, a more radical lobectomy or a pneumonectomy is required. The local lymph nodes are removed in each procedure for pathological staging. **Segmentectomy** removes part of a lobe (supplied by a segmental bronchus) along the intersegmental planes and may be performed for a localized peripheral lesion with clear regional lymph nodes, especially if the post-operative respiratory function is predicted to be borderline. **Wedge resection** is another lung-preserving operation that removes only the tumour, with minimal surrounding lung parenchyma, but there is a higher local recur-rence rate, however (up to 23%). Both segmentectomy and wedge resec-tion should have ≥2cm clear margins around a tumour. **Sleeve resections** involve a lobectomy and the removal of a section of bronchus affected by tumour, forming an anastomosis between the airway proximal and distal to it. This may avoid a pneumonectomy. Resection margins should be macro-scopically free from tumour. If there is limited local tumour invasion to the chest wall, this can be resected with a 5cm margin. Reconstruction with prosthetic material may be necessary if two or more ribs are resected, aim-ing to preserve the chest wall function.

Post-operative complications Bronchopleural fistula, respiratory failure, infection, phrenic nerve damage causing diaphragmatic paralysis, recurrent laryngeal nerve damage causing hoarse voice, prolonged chest wall pain. Mortality: 1–3.5% for wedge resection, 2–4% for lobectomy, 6–8% for pneumonectomy. Risk increases with increasing age, associated ischaemic heart disease, impaired respiratory function, and poor performance status.

Following surgery Patients are often followed up by the chest clinic on a 6–12-monthly basis for CT or CXR review for 5y (although there is no clear evidence on the necessity of such prolonged follow-up in lung cancer). This is to ensure they are radiologically clear of tumour recurrence, and there is not a second 1° tumour. They should also be advised to seek earlier review if they have symptoms of persistent haemoptysis or new cough, weight loss, new chest pain. If histology shows incomplete resection mar-gins, post-operative chemoradiotherapy would be given to try and improve local disease control.

Further information

Detterbeck FC *et al.* Executive summary. Diagnosis and management of lung cancer, 3rd edi-tion: American College of Chest Physicians Evidence-Based Clinical Practice Guidelines. *Chest* 2013;**143**:7S–37S.

NSCLC: chemotherapy

Consider in patients with stages III–IV disease, WHO performance status 0–1/2 (see ➲ p. 299), even if they are asymptomatic from their cancer (greater toxicity in those with poorer performance status). 40% respond temporarily (see Box 31.5 for criteria used to assess response). Small improvement in symptom control and QoL, compared with best supportive care, shown in RCTs. Limited survival gains, 6–7 weeks, compared with best supportive care. Median survival with chemotherapy in stage IV lung cancer: 10 months (Ps0), 7 months (Ps1), 4 months (Ps2).

- Combination chemotherapy (the use of >1 drug) is superior to single-agent chemotherapy, improving survival rates when compared with single agent at 6 and 12 months. Commonly used first-line regimens include gemcitabine (or docetaxel/paclitaxel/vinorelbine) plus a platinum-containing drug (carboplatin or cisplatin), usually for four cycles. Combination pemetrexed/cisplatin has been used as an option for first-line treatment of patients with locally advanced or metastatic adenocarcinoma/large cell tumours
- Combined chemoradiotherapy may be given with curative intent for some patients with stage III disease (or lower stages, not suitable for surgery)
- Inhibitors of EGFR, an important mediator of cell growth, differentiation, and survival, are used in selected patients. Activating mutations in EGFR (typically affecting never-smoking women ± Asian ethnicity) occur in a small proportion of NSCLC. Patients found to have this mutation with locally advanced or metastatic NSCLC may be treated by gefitinib or erlotinib
- *Side effects of chemotherapy* Nausea, myelosuppression, ototoxicity, peripheral neuropathy, nephropathy if dehydrated. Alopecia with taxanes
- Patients are monitored during chemotherapy with repeat CT, usually after two cycles, to establish whether they have partial response, stable disease, or progressive disease, despite chemotherapy. This CT influences decisions regarding further chemotherapy
- Second-line treatments (e.g. docetaxel monotherapy) can be given in patients who relapse and are of good performance status
- Recent evidence suggests benefit to the oral tyrosine kinase inhibitor crizotinib as second-line therapy for tumours with rearrangements of the anaplastic lymphoma kinase (*ALK*) gene. A phase III study showed crizotinib increased progression-free survival from 3 to 7.7 months.

Adjuvant therapy is the use of radiation or chemotherapy (or both) following complete surgical resection to improve survival. Adjuvant chemotherapy has been found to have significant survival advantages, compared with surgery alone in trials, including International Adjuvant Lung Cancer Trial and Japan Lung Cancer Research group. Those with stage IB or stage II disease had a 69% 5y survival vs 54% in those treated with surgery alone. Cisplatin-based combination treatment is now offered post-operatively to patients with good performance status (Ps0/1) and T1–3 N1–2 M0 NSCLC and should be considered in those with T2–3 N0 M0 NSCLC tumours >4cm. Adjuvant radiotherapy trials have shown no evidence of a survival benefit, except possibly in those with N2 disease.

Neo-adjuvant chemotherapy uses non-surgical therapy (radio-therapy/chemotherapy) as the initial treatment. Preoperative chemo-therapy has been shown in the multicentre LU22 trial to downstage a third of patients but with no improvement in survival vs surgery alone. Post-operative complications and QoL were no worse in the chemotherapy group. A subsequent meta-analysis suggested a 12% survival benefit when compared with surgery alone, equivalent to 5% improvement in 5y survival. It is important, however, not to delay surgery, and current practice is usually to offer surgery followed by adjuvant chemotherapy for selected patients. Chemotherapy may also be given in the context of a trial, aiming to down-stage a tumour and allow resection.

Further information

Burdett S et al. Chemotherapy and surgery vs surgery alone in NSCLC. Cochrane Database Syst Rev 2007;3:CD006157.

Gilligan D et al. Pre-operative chemotherapy in patients with resectable NSCLC. Lancet 2007; 369:1929–37.

The International Adjuvant Lung Cancer Trial Collaborative Group. Cisplatin-based adjuvant chemotherapy in patients with completely resected NSCLC. N Engl J Med 2004;350:351–60.

Box 31.5 Response evaluation criteria in solid tumours (RECIST)—method of measuring response of a tumour to treatment (particularly in chemotherapy trials), version 1.1

- Target lesion = all measurable lesions up to a maximum of two lesions per organ and five lesions in total, representative of all involved organs. Record and measure sum of their longest diameter.
- Non-target lesions = all other sites of disease, which are recorded at baseline. Measurements of these lesions are not required, but presence or absence of each is noted during follow-up.

Evaluation of target lesions
- *Complete response (CR)* Disappearance of all target lesions
- *Partial response (PR)* At least a 30% decrease in the sum of the longest diameter of target lesions
- *Progressive disease (PD)* At least a 20% increase in the sum of the longest diameter of target lesions (5mm absolute increase)
- *Stable disease (SD)* Neither sufficient shrinkage to qualify for PR nor sufficient increase to qualify for PD.

Evaluation of non-target lesions
- *Complete response (CR)* Disappearance of all non-target lesions and normalization of tumour marker level
- *Non-CR/Non-PD* Persistence of one or more non-target lesion(s) and/or maintenance of tumour marker level above the normal limits
- *Progressive disease (PD)* Appearance of one/more new lesions and/or unequivocal progression of existing non-target lesions.

NSCLC: radiotherapy

May be given for:
• Curative intent (high dose)
• Palliative control (high dose)
• Symptom relief (low dose).

Radiotherapy has no benefit following complete 1° tumour surgical resection.

Radical radiotherapy is high-dose radiotherapy given with curative intent.
• Recommended for patients with localized chest disease <5cm, stages I–III with performance status 0–1 (see Box 31.6), who are resectable but unfit for surgery or do not want surgery
• Various regimes are used in different centres. CHART (continuous hyperfractionated accelerated radiotherapy) delivers small radiation doses tds for 12 days (e.g. 54Gy in 36 fractions over 12 days; patients need to remain inpatient for their treatment; severe dysphagia more likely). Conventionally fractionated radiotherapy delivers, e.g. 66Gy in 33 fractions over 6.5 weeks or 55Gy in 20 fractions over 4 weeks
• Stereotactic ablative radiotherapy (SABR)/stereotactic body radiation therapy (SBRT) allows the delivery of very high radiation doses to small early stage lung cancers, with good local control outcomes. Increasingly used in early stage patients unfit for surgery. The treatment course is shorter (typically given in 3–5 fractions) and is usually associated with an acceptable toxicity profile
• Need PFTs, including lung volume and TLCO before radiotherapy. FEV_1 should be ≥1.5l.

High-dose palliative radiotherapy is given to patients with symptomatic disease, good performance status, no evidence of metastases, and who will be able to tolerate a high-dose regime. An example of such a regime would be 36–39Gy in 12–13 fractions over 6 weeks. Improves median survival by 2 months.

Low-dose radiotherapy is given for symptom relief in patients who would be unable to tolerate high-dose palliative radiotherapy or those with evidence of metastases. Symptoms palliated include pain, haemoptysis, breathlessness, or cough.

Urgent radiotherapy is used in combination with oral steroids for relief of SVCO by tumour, although stenting performed via CT angiography is now the treatment of choice, where possible. Radiotherapy takes ~10 days to be effective.

Prophylactic cranial irradiation is not recommended for NSCLC outside a clinical trial.

Chemoradiotherapy is used to improve tumour radiosensitization for localized disease. There may be some additional advantages with treatment of potential distant micrometastases. Should be considered for stages I–III disease in patients who are not fit for surgery.

Box 31.6 WHO/ECOG performance status

0 = Fully active, able to carry on all pre-disease performance without restriction

1 = Restricted in physically strenuous activity but ambulatory and able to carry out work of a light or sedentary nature, e.g. light house work, office work

2 = Ambulatory and capable of all self-care but unable to carry out any work activities. Up and about >50% of waking hours

3 = Capable of only limited self-care, confined to bed or chair >50% of waking hours

4 = Completely disabled. Cannot carry on any self-care. Totally confined to bed or chair.

Oken MM et al. Toxicity and response criteria of the Eastern Cooperative Oncology Group. Am J Clin Oncol 1982;5:649–55.

Small cell lung cancer (SCLC): treatment

Surgery Limited stage SCLC may be appropriate for surgical resection if there is no evidence of metastases (T1–2a N0 M0). This is rare. It requires further assessment with brain and bone scanning/PET imaging ± bone marrow biopsy if there is an unexplained abnormal FBC. The patient should also be considered for post-operative combination chemotherapy for treatment of micro-metastases, especially if histology was only determined at operation.

Chemotherapy

Combination chemotherapy is used for limited and extensive SCLC.
- Etoposide with either cisplatin or carboplatin is the standard regime
- Given 3-weekly, commonly for 4–6 cycles
- Different regimes are selected, according to performance status
- Patients with performance status 3 may benefit from less intensive outpatient chemotherapy on a 3-weekly basis
- Patients are carefully assessed, and, if there is no sign of a response to treatment, based on CXR or CT scan, they may be switched to second-line agents, although there is limited evidence of benefit
- Patients with relapsed SCLC but good Ps may be offered anthracycline-containing regimes or further platinum-based treatment for a maximum of six cycles. Oral topotecan is an option if they are unable to tolerate IV chemotherapy. Response rates to second-line chemotherapy are low (~10%)
- 80–90% response if limited disease; 60–80% if extensive disease
- Chemotherapy may increase median survival to 12 months in limited disease.

Radiotherapy

- Patients with limited stage disease (which is encompassable in a radical radiotherapy volume) with Ps0/1 should have consolidation radiotherapy to the chest disease, with the first or second cycle of chemotherapy. If unfit for combination treatment, give after chemotherapy completion if they have a response or partial response
- Prophylactic cranial radiotherapy is advised at completion of chemotherapy for those with limited disease or those with extensive disease and good prognostic factors. This improves survival by 5.4%
- In patients with extensive disease, including cerebral metastases, or poorer performance status, chemotherapy is given first. If there is a good response, palliative thoracic radiotherapy may be given
- Of benefit to symptomatic bone metastases, cord compression, SVCO.

Further information

Jackman DM, Johnson BE. Small cell lung cancer. *Lancet* 2005;**366**:1385–96.

Lung cancer: emerging areas

Radiofrequency ablation (RFA) applied via a probe inserted into a nodule/tumour under CT guidance, with sedation. Barbs/tines extrude from needle once in the tumour and cause tissue death by thermal necrosis. Lesions initially increase in size and density, and may cavitate, but then become fibrotic scar tissue. May become a tool to treat patients with 1° lung cancer unsuitable for curative surgery/radiotherapy due to comorbid disease, used with radiotherapy. The size of the cancer that can be treated is limited (maximum 5cm, best results with <3cm). Peripheral lesions are easier to access. Side effects of therapy: pleuritic chest pain, pneumothorax, empyema, haemoptysis, haemorrhage, low-grade fever. FEV_1 should ideally be >1L. Tumour follow-up with contrast-enhanced imaging, as ablated tissue does not enhance. Used currently mainly in pulmonary metastases from GI or renal cell cancers, or sarcomas, which are not suitable for surgical resection, but also some data for 1° NSCLC. In 153 patients with 1° or metastatic medically inoperable lung cancer, 78% 1y survival rate, 57% 2y, 27% 5y (Simon CJ et al. Radiology 2007;**243**:268–75). No long-term RCT reported.

Biological therapies, such as oral thalidomide, acting as an angiogenesis inhibitor are being tried. These may offer medium-term survival benefits in both SCLC and NSCLC.

Targeted molecular therapy Lung cancer is said to be at the leading edge of targeted 'personalized' molecular therapy, which may become more effective than using traditional cytotoxic agents. The presence or absence of these molecular target molecules seems to determine response to traditional treatments. The cellular targets under investigation include EGFR mutations, ALK translocations, RAS mutations, HER2 mutations, protein kinase C, vascular endothelial growth factor, and cyclo-oxygenase 2. Gene expression profiling may be used to determine the prognosis and response to therapy and to identify the mechanisms of tumour biology. In the future, lung cancer staging may also address the molecular biology of a tumour.

Further information

Dy GK, Adjei AA. Novel targets for lung cancer therapy. J Clin Oncol 2002;**20**:2881–94.

Detterbeck FC et al. Executive Summary. Diagnosis and management of lung cancer, 3rd edition: American College of Chest Physicians Evidence-Based Clinical Practice Guidelines. Chest 2013;**143**:7S–37S.

☞ http://www.cancerresearchuk.org.

☞ http://www.lungcanceronline.org

☞ http://publications.nice.org.uk/lung-cancer-cg121.

☞ http://www.roycastle.org, patient network, ☎ 0333 323 7200.

Superior vena caval obstruction (SVCO): aetiology, clinical assessment, and management

Obstruction of the flow of blood in the SVC results in the symptoms and signs of SVCO. It is caused by two different mechanisms (which may coexist): *external compression or invasion* of the SVC by tumour extending from the right lung (four times more common than the left lung), lymph nodes, or other mediastinal structure; or due to *thrombosis* within the vein.

Aetiology The commonest cause (~85%) is malignancy. Lung cancer and lymphoma together cause 95% of malignant SVCO.

Malignant causes
- *Lung cancer* Up to 4% of lung cancer patients will develop SVCO at some point during their disease. Up to 10% of SCLC present with SVCO
- *Lymphoma* Up to 4% of lymphoma patients will develop SVCO, most commonly in non-Hodgkin's lymphoma. This usually occurs due to extrinsic compression of the SVC by enlarged lymph nodes
- *Other malignant causes* Thymoma, mediastinal germ cell tumours, tumours with mediastinal metastases (commonest is breast cancer).

Benign causes include granulomatous disease, intrathoracic goitre, and central venous lines, Port-A-Cath®, and pacemaker wires (causing thrombosis). In the past, SVCO was commonly due to untreated infection, e.g. syphilitic thoracic aortic aneurysm or fibrosing mediastinitis (due to actinomycosis, TB, blastomycosis, or *Aspergillus*). These are all now rare.

Clinical features
- Facial and upper body oedema, with facial plethora, often with increased neck circumference, and a cyanotic appearance
- Venous distension of the face and upper body. SVCO due to malignancy usually develops over days to weeks, so an adequate collateral circulation does not have time to develop. Pemberton's sign—facial plethora, distress, and sometimes stridor after lifting the arms above the head for a few minutes—may suggest the diagnosis
- Breathlessness
- Headache—worse on bending forwards or lying down
- Cough/haemoptysis or other signs of an underlying lung malignancy
- Hoarse voice
- Dysphagia
- Syncope/dizziness (reduced venous return)
- Confusion.

Diagnosis is usually made clinically from the signs of facial and upper body swelling, with distension of superficial veins across the chest wall, neck, and upper arms.

Investigations The investigation and treatment of SVCO was previously considered a medical emergency. SVCO is now not considered to be immediately life-threatening, making treatment less urgent and allowing a definitive diagnosis to be made prior to treatment. The exception to this rule is the patient who presents with stridor or laryngeal oedema, which is a medical emergency.

- *CXR* Up to 85% have an abnormal CXR (as lung malignancy is the commonest underlying disorder). Mediastinal widening is common
- *CT chest with contrast* can stage the underlying malignancy and image the venous circulation and collateral blood supply
- *Histological diagnosis* Usual practice is to obtain a tissue diagnosis of the underlying disease before starting treatment, as the underlying diagnosis can alter treatment markedly. Symptomatic obstruction will have been developing for some weeks prior to presentation, and, in the clinically stable patient, a delay of 24–48h, whilst the correct underlying diagnosis is obtained, is warranted. Radiotherapy prior to biopsy can lead to problems making a subsequent histological diagnosis, and, similarly, high-dose steroids can make the diagnosis of lymphoma difficult. Diagnostic samples may be obtained using:
  - Pleural fluid cytology
  - US-guided biopsy of an extrathoracic lymph node (e.g. supraclavicular or cervical nodes—low risk)
  - Bronchoscopy, or mediastinoscopy if no endobronchial disease, may be needed, depending on CT features. There may be increased risk of bleeding post-biopsy because of venous congestion, and anaesthesia is theoretically more risky because of possible associated tracheal obstruction or pericardial effusion (potentially leading to haemodynamic compromise due to cardiac tamponade), though these can be anticipated from the CT scan
  - Sputum.

Management See Box 31.7.

▶▶ **Box 31.7 SVCO: management**

This is usually in two phases.
- Initial general treatment: O_2, analgesia, sitting the patient up (to reduce venous pressure), and steroids (in some)
- Followed by treatment of the underlying disease causing the SVCO, dependent on the tissue diagnosis. The major differential in terms of treatment is small cell carcinoma (initial chemotherapy), non-small cell carcinoma (initial radiotherapy), and lymphoma (chemotherapy). The presence of SVCO usually means that surgical resection of a NSCLC is not possible.

Steroids Limited trial data to support the use of steroids in SVCO, prior to definitive treatment, but most would start them fairly promptly (e.g. dexamethasone 8mg bd; avoid in the evening, as affects sleep). They may reduce oedema and improve symptoms. Ideally, a tissue diagnosis should

---

(Continued)

Box 31.7 (Continued)

be obtained before commencing steroids but may not always be possible. The problem arises where the underlying diagnosis is lymphoma where steroids may alter the histology, making a definitive diagnosis more difficult. In an older smoker, with an obvious CXR mass (in whom the diagnosis is likely to be lung cancer), steroids can probably be started without risk to the underlying histology.

Radiotherapy 90% of patients are oedema-free by 3–4 weeks. In those with a poor response to radiotherapy, only 25% survive 1y.

Intraluminal stents are used for malignant SVCO and may be a first-line treatment whilst radiotherapy is planned. Successful in 90% of cases, with relief of symptoms in most patients within 48h. They do not preclude subsequent radiotherapy or chemotherapy. In SCLC, however, chemotherapy will improve SVCO rapidly, so stent insertion may not be necessary. It is not clear whether post-procedure anticoagulation is required. Some centres advocate the use of low-dose warfarin anticoagulation (i.e. 1mg/day), aiming for an INR of <1.6. Thrombosis in the SVC is not a contraindication to the procedure, as clot can be dispersed mechanically or with thrombolysis at the time of the procedure.

Stent complications Stent migration is the major complication, but most patients do not live long enough for this to be a major problem.

Anticoagulation Some recommend prophylactic anticoagulation in the presence of SVCO. Small increased risk of intracerebral bleeding, but the benefits of SVCO treatment may be limited by subsequent SVC thrombus if anticoagulation is not started. This is controversial.

SVCO due to thrombosis is usually in association with central venous lines or pacemaker wires. If the clot is <5 days old (as judged by symptoms), thrombolysis is warranted. Subsequent oral anticoagulation may reduce recurrence.

Prognosis depends on the underlying disease and is unrelated to the duration of SVCO at presentation. The majority of SVCO is due to mediastinal spread of carcinoma of the lung, so the overall prognosis is generally poor but depends on the patient's performance status, stage and extent of disease, and the cell type.

Further information

Rowell NP, Gleeson FV. Steroids, radiotherapy, chemotherapy and stents for SVCO in carcinoma of the bronchus: a systematic review. *Clin Oncol (R Coll Radiol)* 2002;**14**:338–51.

Hypercalcaemia

Definition and aetiology A serum calcium level over 2.75mmol/L is considered abnormal; borderline values need repeating. In malignancy, a raised calcium is due to increased osteoclast activity, either from bony metastases or the production of PTH-related protein. A serum level over 3.25mmol/L is rare outside malignancy although can occur in sarcoidosis.

Clinical features Values over 3mmol/L are usually symptomatic. Common symptoms are confusion, weakness, nausea, reduced fluid intake, and constipation. There may be a short QT interval on ECG and renal failure.

Investigations Exclude other causes of hypercalcaemia, and identify the tumour, although, in most patients with malignant hypercalcaemia, the diagnosis of malignancy will already be known. The PTH will be suppressed in malignant hypercalcaemia but raised in hyperparathyroidism. The phosphate will tend to be low in hyperparathyroidism and hypercalcaemia due to ectopic PTH, and normal/high in sarcoidosis, metastatic bone disease, and with excess vitamin D. Check for renal failure.

Management See Box 31.8.

▶▶ Box 31.8 Management of hypercalcaemia

- Isotonic saline infusion (250mL/h initially, to reverse dehydration, but avoid fluid overload, reducing to 150mL/h), with furosemide to increase calcium excretion
- Steroids help, but less so than in sarcoid-associated hypercalcaemia, partly through reduced intestinal absorption.

In addition to this initial management:

- Reduce bone reabsorption with bisphosphonates (takes a few days for maximum effect). The bisphosphonates can also reduce the pain of 2° bony deposits and may reduce pathological fracture rate.
  - *IV preparations* Disodium pamidronate, 15–60mg infused over 2h. Works for several weeks. Zoledronic acid, 4mg over ≥15min, repeated monthly, if required
  - *Oral preparations* Sodium clodronate, one 800mg tablet bd.

Syndrome of inappropriate secretion of antidiuretic hormone (SIADH)

Definition and aetiology Excessive retention of water relative to electrolytes due to inappropriate production of antidiuretic hormone (ADH). Hence, there is hyponatraemia (<135mmol/L), hypo-osmolality, a urine osmolality >100mosmol/kg, a urine sodium concentration usually above 40mmol/L, normal acid–base (and potassium), and usually a low plasma urea concentration. Diuretic-induced hyponatraemia will be accompanied by evidence of dehydration, e.g. raised urea. Causes of SIADH include:

- Drugs, e.g. carbamazepine, fluoxetine, high-dose cyclophosphamide
- Post-major surgery
- Pneumonia
- HIV infection
- CNS disorders, e.g. stroke, infection, psychosis
- SCLC, either ectopic ADH production or stimulation of normal ADH production (poor prognostic factor).

Clinical features Lethargy and confusion often when sodium levels fall below 130mmol/L and nearly always when below 120mmol/L.

Investigations A low sodium in the presence of a low urea and an appropriate clinical setting may be adequate to make a diagnosis. If sodium depletion/water overload are a possible alternative cause of hyponatraemia, they should be accompanied by a urine osmolarity <100mosmol/kg (or a specific gravity <1.003 or a urine sodium <40mmol/L). Therefore, values increasingly above this are suggestive of SIADH (unless the patient is on loop diuretics when, of course, the urinary sodium concentration will be higher).

Management See Box 31.9.

▶▶ **Box 31.9 Management of inappropriate ADH secretion**

- Fluid restriction (0.5–1.0L/day) will help but is often unpleasant for the patient
- Drugs: demeclocycline (450mg bd, tetracycline derivative; blocks ADH action at the distal renal tubules and can be used long term) or tolvaptan (15mg od, V2 ADH receptor antagonist; monitor sodium concentration every 6h during first 2 days of treatment; watch LFTs)
- Salt tablets/extra-dietary salt
- May resolve over a few weeks following chemotherapy
- Hypertonic saline is rarely indicated and can provoke brainstem damage (demyelination) through rapid changes in osmolality.

Spinal cord compression

This is a medical emergency requiring prompt treatment within 24h to prevent irreversible paraplegia and loss of bowel and bladder function.

Definition and aetiology Spinal cord compression occurs commonly in patients with metastatic cancer (in about 5% of all cancer patients, particularly breast, lung, and prostate cancer). It may be the first presentation of cancer but often occurs in patients with a known 1° tumour. Cord compression is commonly caused by direct spread from a vertebral metastasis into the extradural space (most commonly, thoracic spine) or, less commonly, from pressure on the cord from a 1° tumour in the posterior mediastinum or the retroperitoneum, or by pressure from a mass of retroperitoneal nodes. It is unusual to have a metastasis within the cord itself, although meningeal spread can occur. Spinal cord compression causes interruption of the arterial supply to the cord and subsequent infarction.

Clinical features Patients frequently experience back pain initially, due to associated vertebral collapse. This precedes any neurological signs. Pain is not, however, universal. Neurological signs may be non-specific: weak legs, constipation, urinary incontinence. Leg weakness develops over hours to days, with associated sensory loss. Loss of bladder and bowel sensation is a late sign and usually heralds irreversible paraplegia within hours or a few days. Examination reveals bilateral upper motor neurone signs in the legs, with increased tone, weakness, brisk reflexes, and extensor plantars. There may be sensory loss in the legs, particularly with a loss of proprioception and a sensory level on the trunk. Sensory loss in the saddle area, with decreased rectal tone, suggests a cauda equina lesion. The bladder may be palpable.

Investigations
Have a low threshold for investigating a patient with known cancer with back pain.
- *MRI* of the spine is the investigation of choice to demonstrate the level of the cord compression
- *CT* is less reliable but can also be helpful, if MRI is not available
- *Plain spine X-ray* may show vertebral metastases, but this is usually unhelpful, as there is no imaging of the spinal cord. Time should not be wasted in obtaining a plain X-ray
- *Bone scan* shows vertebral metastases but again does not image the spinal cord. Earlier scans showing bony metastases may alert the physician to the possibility of future cord compression
- If patient is not known to have underlying malignant disease, a search for a 1° tumour should be performed but must not delay treatment of the spinal cord compression. Take full history (weight loss, anorexia, specific symptoms), and perform full examination, CXR, blood tests, PSA, and myeloma screen.

Management See Box 31.10.

▶▶ Box 31.10 Management of spinal cord compression

This depends on tumour type and overall prognosis. Discuss with oncologist and/or neurosurgeon to determine which definitive treatment(s) are the most appropriate for the patient.

- High-dose steroids (dexamethasone IV 4mg/6h). These should be started whilst waiting for MRI scan, if the clinical picture suggests cord compression
- Radiotherapy to the metastasis or tumour causing cord compression, particularly if there are multiple sites of cord compression or if surgery is not advised
- Surgical decompression of the cord, reconstruction, and stabilizing the spinal column
- Catheter, if in urinary retention
- Care for pressure areas
- DVT prophylaxis
- Consider chemotherapy, if appropriate, for underlying cancer causing the spinal cord compression, once the initial treatment has taken place
- Rehabilitation, ideally in unit with spinal cord expertise.

Early referral to physiotherapists and occupational therapists with oncology expertise.

A Dutch study showed 66% of patients with metastatic cord compression (from all cancers) admitted to rehabilitation centres were discharged and the average survival post-discharge was 808 days. 52% were alive at 1y.

Prognosis Patients who are mobile at presentation have the best prognosis and are likely to have preserved neurological function following treatment. If there is some preserved motor function, 25% will be able to walk post-treatment. If paraplegia is present pre-treatment, <10% will be able to walk afterwards. Loss of bladder function for >24–48h cannot be reversed.

Further information

Conway R et al. What happens to people after malignant cord compression? Survival, function, quality of life, emotional well-being and place of care 1 month after diagnosis. *Clin Oncol* 2007;**19**:56–62.

Eriks IE et al. Epidural metastatic spinal cord compression: functional outcome and survival after in-patient rehabilitation. *Spinal Cord* 2004;**42**:235–9.

Pulmonary carcinoid tumours

These are uncommon 1° lung tumours, comprising 1–2% of all lung tumours. More common in women; typical age at presentation is 40–50y. They are a form of neuroendocrine tumour and can have similar histological appearances to SCLC. Occasionally associated with multiple endocrine neoplasia type 1 (MEN 1).

Pathophysiology Although typically slow-growing benign tumours, more aggressive subtypes exist, with metastatic potential. Commonly, they are located endobronchially but can also be located peripherally in the lung parenchyma.

Clinical features

- Endobronchial carcinoids can cause isolated wheeze, dyspnoea, infection, haemoptysis, or persistent lobar collapse
- Parenchymal carcinoids are often asymptomatic, being detected on routine CXR
- Carcinoid syndrome, with flushing, tachycardia, sweats, diarrhoea, wheeze, and hypotension, occurs in 1% of pulmonary carcinoid tumours
- Carcinoid tumours can also be associated with Cushing's syndrome, due to ectopic tumour ACTH production.

Investigations

- *CXR* may reveal a well-defined tumour, which should be further characterized on CT. *Tumourlets* is the description given to multiple endobronchial or parenchymal carcinoid tumours. PET has decreased sensitivity for detecting carcinoid tumours, compared with NSCLC (75% in one study)
- *Bronchoscopy* is performed for accessible endobronchial carcinoid tumours. They typically appear to be intraluminal, cherry red, and covered with intact epithelium. Bronchial brushings may be adequate for a histological diagnosis. Bronchial biopsy had been previously thought to be associated with the risk of significant bleeding, although case series suggest the risk is likely to be low. However, some avoid biopsy altogether and proceed to surgical resection, based on a clinical diagnosis. CT-guided biopsy may be preferred for peripheral tumours
- *Histological diagnosis* can be difficult, as the appearances can be similar to those of SCLC. Special stains and immunohistochemistry are used to help differentiate between the two. Clinically, however, these tend to be quite different conditions, and clinical details can aid pathological diagnosis. Carcinoid tumours are characterized as being *typical* or *atypical*. They each have a characteristic pattern:
  - *Typical carcinoids* have no necrosis, occasional nuclear pleomorphism, and absent or late mitoses. Distant metastases are rare, and metastasis to lymph nodes occurs in 5–20% of cases. The 5y survival is 87–100%, and 10y survival is 82–87%

- *Atypical carcinoids* may show focal necrosis and often have nuclear pleomorphism. There is increased mitotic activity and increased levels of MIB-1 expression (an immunohistochemical marker of cell proliferation). They have distant metastases in ~20% and metastasize to the lymph nodes in 30–70% of cases. The 5y survival is 30–95%, and 10y survival is 35–56%.

Management

- Patients with isolated pulmonary carcinoid tumours should be considered for surgical resection. Resection is ideally limited, removing minimal amounts of normal lung parenchyma. Tumour resection is associated with resolution of any features of the carcinoid syndrome
- If the tumour is atypical or close to the resection margin, patients should be followed up with repeat CXR on an annual basis. Radiotherapy is not performed
- Endobronchial resection may be rarely possible in highly selected patients with an intraluminal polypoid tumour with no CT evidence of an extraluminal component. Careful bronchoscopic and imaging follow-up is essential
- Tumour size does not relate to the presence of lymph node metastases, and, therefore, local lymph nodes should be sampled perioperatively
- In the 1% with carcinoid syndrome, serotonin antagonists, such as octreotide or lanreotide, can be used for treatment. Isolated liver metastases can be treated with resection, arterial embolization, or RFA. Metastatic aggressive carcinoid tumours can be treated with chemotherapy, such as etoposide, cisplatin, and 5-fluorouracil, although limited trial efficacy data mean there is no standard regime. Peptide receptor radioligand therapy (e.g. therapeutic (131)I MIBG or (177) Lu-octreotate) is offered in some centres. Studies are examining the role of other drugs, such as mTOR inhibitors (e.g. everolimus) and tyrosine kinase inhibitors (e.g. sunitinib), with a possible benefit associated with addition of everolimus to long-acting octreotide therapy.

Further information

Hage R et al. Update in pulmonary carcinoid tumours: a review article. *Ann Surg Oncol* 2003;10:697–704.

Pulmonary nodules 1

Definition These are focal, round, or oval areas of increased opacity in the lung, measuring <3cm in diameter. They are detected on CXR or CT. Greater use of CT and thinner slice spiral CT scanning has led to increased detection rates. CT allows the precise localization of a nodule and reliable determination of its features. It has a high sensitivity of detecting nodules of >5mm in diameter. Volumetric analysis using CT-aided software means that a 3D nodule can be simulated to aid nodule characterization and assess whether its volume has increased over time.

Table 31.2 Causes of pulmonary nodules

Benign	Malignant
Infectious granulomata	Lung cancer
Non-infectious granulomata	Solitary metastasis
Bronchial adenoma	
Benign hamartoma (developmental abnormality, containing cartilage, epithelium, and fat. Can contain smooth muscle. Slow-growing. Can be seen at any age, especially 40+; often calcify)	

- The majority of pulmonary nodules are benign (see Table 31.2), although exact numbers depend on the characteristics of the population screened
- 20–30% of patients with lung cancer may present with a solitary pulmonary nodule
- Of the nodules detected on CT in smokers with a normal CXR, between 1% and 2.5% will be malignant
- The Early Lung Cancer Action Project screening programme in the USA used CT scans in over-60-year-olds, with at least a 10 pack year history of smoking, and found non-calcified nodules in 23%, which were seen on CXR in 7%. 11% of these nodules were malignant on biopsy
- Early detection of these malignant nodules might alter the management of the patient, with surgical resection of a stage I cancer.

Management options for patients with pulmonary nodules

Observation Baseline CT scan showing nodule >4mm, then repeat after an arbitrary time interval (guided by risk factors e.g. smoking) such as 3 and 12 months, or 3, 6, and 12 months. The Fleischner Society (and recently the ACCP) have proposed suggested follow-up protocols for solitary pulmonary nodules (solid and ground glass), dependent on patient cancer risk and nodule size. If the nodule has increased in size or shows features of malignancy, consider biopsy or proceed straight to surgical resection. PET scan may be helpful, in combination with CT (PET/CT), if the nodule is indeterminate or increasing in size but cannot be biopsied.

PET/CT scan useful in lesions >7mm. Malignancy sensitivity >95%, specificity >80%. False positives with granulomatous, infectious, and inflammatory nodules. False negatives with low metabolic activity tumours (e.g. bronchoalveolar cell carcinomas).

Biopsy Difficult on small nodules <7mm and those behind a rib or scapula.

Resection Using wedge resection/segmentectomy, if nodule has grown on serial imaging, has high clinical/radiographic likelihood of malignancy or has a positive FDG-PET scan. Nodule may need to be localized preoperatively, using a radiographically placed hook wire or injection of methylene blue.

Radiotherapy (e.g. SABR) If nodule proven to be malignant, but surgical treatment is not indicated due to performance status.

Pulmonary nodules 2

Factors that suggest a pulmonary nodule is malignant
- Size >1cm
- Smokers, older age
- Increasing volumetrically determined growth rates over time (volume doubling time 30–480 days, although bronchoalveolar cell carcinomas may have doubling time up to 900 days)
- Increased enhancement with contrast, suggesting increased vascularity (>15 Hounsfield units)
- Increased FDG uptake with PET, compared with normal tissue. Estimated sensitivity of PET is 97% for identifying a malignant process
- Occult extrathoracic disease identified on PET scanning
- Irregular or spiculated margin, with distortion of adjacent vessels—the 'corona radiata' sign
- Associated ground-glass shadowing
- Cavitation with thick irregular walls
- Pseudocavitation within nodule—bronchoalveolar cell carcinoma.

Factors that suggest a pulmonary nodule is benign
- Stable or decreasing size for 2y
- Nodule resolves during follow-up
- Non-smoker
- Lack of enhancement with contrast
- Smooth, well-defined margins (although 21% of smooth nodules may be malignant)
- Benign pattern of calcification: central, diffuse solid, laminated, or 'popcorn-like'—related to prior infections or calcification in a hamartoma
- Intranodular fat—likely hamartoma
- Cavitation with thin smooth walls
- Younger age
- Resident in histoplasmosis endemic areas such as North America.

Pulmonary nodule with extrathoracic malignancy
In a patient with pre-existing malignancy, a pulmonary nodule could be a metastasis, new lung cancer, or benign disease. The histology of the extrapulmonary neoplasm and the patient's smoking history influence this. These cases need discussion within the cancer MDT to determine whether nodule biopsy or treatment of the underlying 1° cancer would be the most appropriate management.

One study determined the likelihood of a pulmonary nodule being a new 1° or metastasis, based on the site of the original cancer.
- *New lung 1° more likely* if the 1° tumour is head and neck, bladder, breast, bile ducts, oesophagus, ovary, prostate, stomach
- *Metastasis more likely* if the 1° tumour is melanoma, sarcoma, testes
- *Either new 1° or metastasis possible* if the 1° tumour is salivary gland, adrenal, colon, parotid, kidney, thyroid, thymus, uterus.

Further information

Detterbeck FC et al. Executive summary. Diagnosis and management of lung cancer, 3rd ed: American College of Chest Physicians Evidence-Based Clinical Practice Guidelines. *Chest* 2013;**143**:7S–37S.

Naidich DP et al. Recommendations for the management of subsolid pulmonary nodules detected at CT: a statement from the Fleischner Society. *Radiology* 2013;**266**:304–17.

MacMahon H et al. Guidelines for management of small pulmonary nodules detected on CT scans: a statement from the Fleischner Society. *Radiology* 2005;**237**:395–400.

Ost D et al. The solitary pulmonary nodule. *N Engl J Med* 2003;**348**:2535–42.

Erasmus J et al. Solitary pulmonary nodules. *Radiographics* 2000;**20**:43–66.

Quint L et al. Solitary pulmonary nodule with extra pulmonary neoplasms. *Radiology* 2000;**217**:257–61.

Henschke CI et al. Early lung cancer action project: overall design and findings from baseline screening. *Lancet* 1999;**354**:99–105.

Lung cancer screening

This is an area that is currently under investigation. Screening programmes are based on the premise that the early detection of lung cancer and any subsequent intervention will improve the patient's survival. To be detectable on CXR, a lung cancer needs to be 1cm diameter and 3–4mm diameter to be detectable on CT. Low-dose CT (LDCT) have been used for screening studies, delivering an average dose of 1.5mSv, compared with 8mSv for a standard CT. LDCT finds nodules in 10–50% of those screened, and these have a significant false positive rate of 96.4% (CXR, 94.5%).

There is no evidence of reduction in lung cancer mortality from CXR or sputum cytology screening studies. A recent CT screening study demonstrated a mortality benefit, but this needs confirming in ongoing studies.

Screening studies

- Four previous CXR screening studies in the 1970s were negative, of which the *Mayo Lung Project* has been the most studied. This compared 4-monthly CXR and sputum cytology for 6y in smokers 45y old or older of 20+/day, with infrequent or no screening in a control group. 206 cancers were found in the study group and 160 in the control group, but all-cause mortality was not affected by screening, even at 20y
- More recent studies have used low-dose spiral CT scanning. The *Early Lung Cancer Action Project (ELCAP)* in New York recruited 1,000 symptom-free volunteers aged 60+ with a 10 pack year history of smoking, who would be fit for a thoracotomy. There was no control group. Baseline CXR and CT were performed. Non-calcified nodules were present in 23% of patients at baseline on CT. Repeat CT was performed for nodules <5mm; nodules >6mm were biopsied, and nodules >11mm received standard care. 2.7% of all the patients entered had malignant nodules with stage I disease in 2.3%. All but one patient had their cancer surgically resected
- *International ELCAP* screened 31,567 asymptomatic over-40-year-olds at risk for lung cancer between 1993 and 2005. The median age was 61. 13% had a positive result, requiring follow-up at baseline CT and 5% at annual CT. Lung cancer was diagnosed in 1.5% of people (85% stage I), with 411 having resection and 57 having radiotherapy ± chemotherapy. There was no non-treatment randomized control group, so it is still difficult to interpret whether the earlier diagnosis and intervention led to longer survival
- The *National Lung Screening Trial (NLST)* evaluated annual LDCT vs CXR screening in 53,454 patients aged 55–74y with a 30 pack year smoking history (including those who quit within 15y), showing a 20% reduction in lung cancer and 6.7% reduction in all-cause mortality in the CT arm. 320 patients would need to be screened to prevent one lung cancer death. Notably, the trial was delivered in specialist centres, with low complication rates, and such mortality benefits may not be reproducible in other centres
- Other randomized trials (e.g. DANTE, NELSON, and the Danish Randomized Lung Cancer CT Screening trials) are ongoing

- Given the results of NLST, the ACCP has recommended that high-risk smokers aged 55–74 should be offered annual LDCT screening, but only if provided in the same care environment as was provided in NLST. CXR and sputum cytology are not recommended. Such screening recommendations are contentious, given ongoing clinical trials, the radiation exposure associated with screening, and lack of evidence for optimal screening duration.
- The role of PET in screening also needs to be evaluated.

Further information

Detterbeck FC et al. Executive summary. Diagnosis and management of lung cancer, 3rd ed: American College of Chest Physicians Evidence-Based Clinical Practice Guidelines. *Chest* 2013;**143**:7S–37S.

National Lung Screening Trial Research Team. Reduced lung-cancer mortality with low-dose computed tomographic screening. *N Engl J Med* 2011;**365**:395–409.

International Early Lung Cancer Action Program Investigators. Survival of patients with stage I lung cancer detected on CT screening. *N Engl J Med* 2006;**355**:1763–71.

Ellis JRC et al. Lung cancer screening. *Br J Radiol* 2001;**74**:478–85.

Marcus PM. Lung cancer screening: an update. *J Clin Oncol* 2001;**19**:83s–6s.

Kawahara M. Screening for lung cancer. *Curr Opin Oncol* 2004;**16**:141–5.

Chapter 32

Lung transplantation

Patient selection

Lung transplantation was first performed successfully in the 1980s. Since then, the number of candidates for transplantation has increased significantly. However, there is a significant shortage of donor organs, and so an increasing number of patients (up to 10–15%) die on the waiting list. There are five UK transplant centres: Harefield, Papworth, Birmingham, Manchester, and Newcastle. ~175 lung transplants and five heart–lung transplants were carried out in the UK in 2011 (source: NHS Blood and Transplant). Worldwide, 3,000 lung transplants were carried out in 2009, from International Society of Heart and Lung Transplantation Registry data. Average waiting times in the UK are around 12 months for lung transplantation and 16 months for heart–lung transplantation. Matching is carried out according to patient size and major blood groups; HLA matching is not carried out.

Underlying conditions Most common diagnoses, in order:
- COPD
- IPF
- CF
- α1-AT deficiency
- IPAH
- Pulmonary fibrosis (other)
- Bronchiectasis
- PHT 2° to congenital cardiac disease (Eisenmenger's syndrome)
- Others, including sarcoidosis, LAM, LCH, collagen vascular disease-related lung disease, bronchoalveolar cell carcinoma (successful transplantation has been carried out, although tumour recurrence in the donor lung is common).

Indications Referral for transplant assessment should be considered in patients with progressive, chronic end-stage lung disease, despite maximal medical therapy, whose life expectancy is 2–3y or less (so that transplantation would be expected to prolong their survival). Candidates should be functionally disabled but still able to walk, with no significant untreatable cardiac, renal, or hepatic impairment. Suggested age limits are 55y for heart–lung, 60y for bilateral lung, and 65y for single-lung transplant.

General referral criteria for lung transplantation
- Normal renal function, with creatinine clearance >50mL/min
- Normal LV function and normal coronary arteries/coronary artery disease not amenable to intervention
- Preserved liver synthetic function
- No osteoporosis
- No systemic sepsis
- BMI >17 or <30
- No untreatable psychiatric disorder
- No history of malignancy within 5y
- Reliable social support.

Contraindications

Absolute (although occasional exceptions may occur)

- Severe, untreatable extrapulmonary organ dysfunction (including renal, hepatic, and cardiac disease)
- Active cancer or recent history (within 2y) of cancer with substantial likelihood of recurrence; a 5y disease-free interval is recommended (excluding cutaneous squamous or basal cell carcinomas)
- Severe untreatable psychiatric illness or non-compliance with treatment/follow-up
- Incurable chronic extrapulmonary infection (including HIV, active hepatitis B and C)
- Active or recent (6 months) substance addiction (cigarette smoking, alcohol, narcotics)
- Significant chest wall/spinal deformity.

Relative

- Age >65y
- Chronic medical conditions that are poorly controlled or associated with target-organ damage (hypertension, diabetes, coronary artery disease)
- Severe or symptomatic osteoporosis (risk of post-transplant fractures and poor QoL; start treatment prior to transplant)
- Severe obesity (BMI >30) or malnutrition (BMI <17)
- Poor rehabilitation potential
- Mechanical ventilation (excluding NIV) or acute critical illness
- Extensive pleural thickening (from infection or prior surgery, e.g. pleurodesis)—procedure is technically more difficult
- Active collagen vascular disease
- Preoperative colonization of the airway with pan-resistant bacteria, fungi, or *Mycobacterium* in CF; there are no clear data to support exclusion of pan-resistant *Pseudomonas*, although it remains a relative contraindication in some centres. *B. cepacia* colonization (particularly with genomovar III), however, is high risk and an absolute contraindication in many centres.

Contentious

- NTM, especially *M. chelonae*
- Aspergilloma (ABPA is not generally a contraindication, though patients would not be transplanted during an exacerbation and would be treated with prophylactic voriconazole)
- Portal hypertension (prophylactic variceal sclerotherapy may be offered).

Further information

Orens JB et al. International guidelines for the selection of lung transplant candidates: 2006 update. *J Heart Lung Transplant* 2006;**25**:745–55.

Glanville AR, Estenne M. Indications, patient selection and timing of referral for lung transplantation. *Eur Resp J* 2003;**22**:845–52.

Specific conditions

Timing of referral

This can be difficult; life expectancy should be <2–3y, but patients must be fit for the procedure during a waiting time of up to 16 months. The decision should not be based on a single factor; instead, a combination of clinical, laboratory, and functional assessments should be considered. Patients with CF and IPF have particularly high waiting list mortalities, suggesting inappropriately late referral for these conditions. Disease-specific guidelines for referral are described next:

COPD

- BODE index >5 (incorporating BMI, FEV_1, degree of dyspnoea, and 6min walk; see → p. 173)
- History of hospitalization for exacerbation associated with acute hypercapnia ($PaCO_2$ >6.7kPa; 49% 2y survival)
- PHT or cor pulmonale despite O_2 therapy
- FEV_1 <20% predicted and either TLCO <20% or homogeneous distribution of emphysema (median survival 3y with medical therapy)
- Patients should be on maximal medical therapy, have completed pulmonary rehabilitation, have stopped smoking for at least 6 months (if in doubt, check urinary cotinine levels), and ideally <60y old.

IPF

- Given the poor prognosis and high waiting list mortality associated with IPF, guidelines recommend referral of all suitable patients with histological or radiographic evidence of UIP, irrespective of VC and without delaying for trials of treatment; these are not widely applied in the UK
- TLCO <40% predicted, fall in FVC ≥10% over 6 months, O_2 desaturation <88% on 6min walk, honeycombing on HRCT (each associated with high mortality).

CF

- Defining referral criteria is especially difficult for patients with CF, due to considerable inter-individual variation in course and prognosis
- FEV_1 ≤30% predicted or FEV_1 >30%, with rapid progressive deterioration, e.g. increasing frequency of exacerbations, rapid fall in FEV_1
- History of ITU admission for pulmonary exacerbation
- O_2-dependent respiratory failure, hypercapnia, or PHT
- Severe recurrent haemoptysis despite embolization
- Refractory and/or recurrent pneumothorax
- Young (<20y) ♀ patients with rapid deterioration have a poor prognosis and should be considered for early referral
- Invasive ventilation is a contraindication in most centres.

IPAH

- New York Heart Association (NYHA) functional class III or IV, rapidly progressive disease/failing medical therapy, low (<350m) or declining 6MWT, mean right atrial pressure >15mmHg, cardiac index <2L/min/m^2.

Investigations and surgical approaches

Investigations prior to referral Consult transplant referral centre for details, and avoid repetition of investigations. Important investigations include full PFTs, tests of exercise performance (e.g. 6min walk), sputum microbiology, ECG, echo, HRCT chest, LFTs, viral serology (e.g. HIV, CMV, hepatitis B and C), 24h creatinine clearance, stress echo, and/or coronary angiography. If on waiting list, inform transplant centre of changes in clinical condition. Remember that the referring physician remains responsible for continuing regular medical care of the patient to ensure they remain optimally treated during the waiting period, with particular attention to:

- Maintenance of nutrition (may require PEG feeding)
- Avoidance of obesity
- Maintenance of mobility, continuing exercise, and rehabilitation
- Monitoring comorbid disease: heart, kidney, liver, bones. Optimize treatment of diabetes, systemic hypertension, osteoporosis, peptic ulcer disease, gastro-oesophageal reflux and sinus disease
- Early NIV, if indicated
- Avoiding intubation, if possible.

Surgical approaches for transplant

Single lung
- Technically easier, allows two recipients from one donor
- Generally now only used in ILD
- Overdistension of the compliant native lung in emphysema is uncommon but may be problematic.

Bilateral sequential
- Worldwide, 80% of lung transplants are now double
- Sequential right and left single-lung transplants at one time
- Selective lung ventilation may render cardiopulmonary bypass unnecessary.

Heart–lung
- Indicated in Eisenmenger's syndrome, or advanced lung disease with concurrent LV dysfunction or coronary disease
- Cor pulmonale is not in itself an indication, as RVH resolves rapidly following lung transplantation alone
- Certain patients without cardiac disease may undergo a 'domino' procedure where they receive a combined heart–lung transplant, because this is technically easier and their healthy heart is then used for a patient needing a heart transplant.

Living lobar transplantation
- Bilateral grafting of lower lobes from two living adult donors to replace lungs of child or small adult
- Appears to be safe for the donor, with lung volume reductions of about 15%, but potential for 300% overall mortality (two donors and one recipient)
- Not widely performed in the UK.

Follow-up

Patients are usually discharged about 1 month after transplant, following post-transplant bronchoscopy with BAL and biopsy. They will be followed up closely by their transplant centre but may also attend general respiratory clinics intermittently between transplant centre visits. Be alert to possible complications (see ➔ pp. 326–7). Spirometric values are generally very stable from 3 months after transplantation, and sustained falls ≥10–15% warrant further investigation. Remember drug interactions (particularly ciclosporin and tacrolimus) if new medications are added. Check immuno-suppressant drug blood levels, and perform routine blood tests, according to the local transplant centre policy.

Outcomes

Survival

- Survival rates: 85% 1y, 63% 3y, 50% 5y. Median survival is 5.5y from 2011 report of International Society of Heart and Lung Transplantation
- Bilateral lung transplant recipients have better median survival than single—6.8y vs 4.7y. Reason unclear: may relate to procedure or selection factors
- Compared with patients on the waiting list, lung transplant conveys a survival benefit to patients with CF and IPF, but not emphysema
- Rate of death is highest in first year (infection, 1° graft failure)
- Risk factors for early death are pre-existing PHT, ventilator dependence, recipient age >50, donor age >50
- No survival difference between single- and double-lung transplant.

Functional

- Lung function usually normalizes after bilateral transplant and markedly improves following single-lung transplant. In COPD, FEV_1 increases to 50–60% of predicted value after single-lung transplant
- Arterial oxygenation rapidly normalizes
- 6min walk distance typically doubles; most patients resume active lifestyle, although fewer than 40% of patients return to work
- Limited data on QoL; initial improvement suggested, but effects after 1y are unclear. ~85% survivors have no functional limitations after 5y.

Routine surgery after lung transplant

Routine surgery >3 months after transplant can be carried out locally, but inform the transplant centre. Routine antibiotic prophylaxis is adequate; there is no increased risk of SBE. The morning dose of calcineurin inhibitor (ciclosporin, tacrolimus) should be omitted, as there is a risk of nephrotox-icity with hypovolaemia.

Future developments are likely to address both the development of more effective treatments for chronic rejection (new immunosuppressive drugs, induction of immune tolerance) and the shortage of donor organs (e.g. living lobar transplantation, xenotransplantation, and further research in lung preservation. *Ex vivo* lung perfusion (EVLP) is now undergoing clinical trials to try to increase the number of organs available for transplant. This involves controlled perfusion and ventilation of donor lungs for a number of hours in an attempt to improve the quality of donor organs, to make previously unusable organs suitable for transplantation.

Complications 1

Early graft dysfunction

- Characterized by pulmonary infiltrates, hypoxaemia, and diffuse alveolar damage or OP on biopsy; not uncommon during first few days after transplant. Clinical severity ranges from very mild acute lung injury to ARDS
- Presumably related to preservation and ischaemia–reperfusion injury
- Exclude other causes, e.g. volume overload, pneumonia, rejection, occlusion of venous anastomosis, aspiration
- Treatment is supportive (mechanical ventilation)
- High mortality (40–60%).

Airway complications

- Anastomotic stenosis most common and typically occurs weeks to months after transplant; suggested clinically by localized wheeze, recurrent pneumonia, or suboptimal lung function. Treat with balloon dilatation (sometimes repeated) or stent placement via bronchoscopy
- Complete dehiscence of bronchial anastomosis now rare and requires immediate surgery or retransplantation
- Partial dehiscence is managed conservatively; drain pneumothorax; reduce steroid dose.

Infection

Bacteria

- May occur early (first month after transplant) or late (associated with BOS)
- Most commonly due to Gram-negative organisms, particularly *Pseudomonas aeruginosa*
- Recipients with CF are not at greater risk than other patients; an exception is *B. cepacia* colonization, which is associated with a high risk of often lethal post-operative infections.

CMV

- CMV-seronegative recipients from seropositive donors are at particular risk of severe infection, including pneumonitis; this is usually treated successfully with ganciclovir
- Increases risk of bacterial or fungal superinfection
- Ganciclovir prophylaxis probably results in later, less severe infection
- CMV infection may be a risk factor for development of BOS.

Aspergillus

- *Aspergillus* frequently colonizes the airways after lung transplant, but clinically apparent infection develops in only a minority of patients
- Peak disease incidence at 2 months after transplant
- Sites of disease include airways (may lead to mucosal oedema, ulceration, and pseudomembranes; usually responds to itraconazole, voriconazole, or amphotericin B), fresh bronchial anastomosis, lung parenchyma, and disseminated aspergillosis (associated with high mortality).

Drug-related Immunosuppressive drugs must be taken lifelong following transplantation. Agents used include ciclosporin or tacrolimus, azathioprine or mycophenolate mofetil (MMF), and prednisolone. They are associated with many drug interactions and side effects, particularly nephrotoxicity and osteoporosis. Ciclosporin and tacrolimus blood levels need to be closely monitored.

Further information

Kotloff A. Medical complications of lung transplantation. *Eur Resp J* 2004;**23**:334–42.

Knoop C et al. Immunosuppressive therapy after human lung transplantation. *Eur Resp J* 2004;**23**:159–71.

Complications 2

Acute rejection

- Very common, particularly within 3 months of transplant
- Affects approximately 60% in the first year. Rare after 12 months
- Asymptomatic or may be associated with malaise, fever, dyspnoea, cough, hypoxia. May present similarly to pneumonia or COP
- *CXR* may be normal or show non-specific infiltrates
- Common finding is fall in *spirometry* >10%, although this does not distinguish from other complications, particularly infection
- Refer back to the transplant centre if these problems develop within 3 months of the transplant
- Ideally confirm histologically: TBBs are safe and typically show perivascular lymphocytic infiltrates. Routine surveillance TBBs are increasingly used to detect acute rejection prior to falls in lung function
- *Treatment* IV methylprednisolone pulses are given within the first 3 months of transplant; after this, high-dose oral corticosteroids are used. The majority of patients respond quickly; consider switching immunosuppressive agent from ciclosporin to tacrolimus if ongoing or recurrent acute rejection
- Recurrent acute rejection is the main risk factor for the development of chronic rejection
- Acute rejection is an uncommon cause of breathlessness after 3 months, and other common causes of SOB should be considered.

Chronic rejection

- A significant problem, accounting for poor long-term prognosis following lung transplant
- Uncommon in first 6 months, but prevalence subsequently increases steadily, affecting 50–60% of patients at 5y
- *Pathogenesis* Incompletely understood, likely involves immune-mediated injury to epithelial and endothelial cells, possibly with an environmental trigger; risk factors for development include previous episodes of recurrent acute rejection, CMV pneumonitis, presence of anti-HLA antibodies pre-transplant, gastro-oesophageal reflux, community respiratory infections, and medical non-compliance
- *Clinically* Insidious onset of breathlessness and cough, and progressive airflow obstruction on spirometry
- Manifest histologically as *bronchiolitis obliterans*, a fibroproliferative process affecting small airways. Histological confirmation is difficult: TBBs have a low sensitivity, so a clinical diagnosis of 'BOS' is defined as an unexplained and sustained (≥3 weeks) fall in FEV_1 to <80% of peak value post-transplant. 'Potential BOS' is defined as FEV_1 81–90% of baseline and/or forced mid-expiratory flow ($FEV_{25-75\%}$) to ≤75% of baseline and indicates the need for close monitoring/further investigation
- *CXR* unhelpful; *HRCT* may show expiratory air trapping and peripheral bronchiectasis

- *P. aeruginosa* colonization is common, with recurrent purulent tracheobronchitis
- *Treatment* is challenging and involves either modified or increased immunosuppression (e.g. switch ciclosporin to tacrolimus; MMF to azathioprine, high-dose steroid pulses, and antilymphocyte antibodies; inhaled ciclosporin may have a role), and, if effective, this acts only to reduce the rate of disease progression. Infection is investigated and treated aggressively, sometimes with reductions in immunosuppression. Azithromycin is often used for deteriorating BOS. Gastro-oesophageal reflux is treated, sometimes with surgery. Total lymphoid irradiation is sometimes recommended when other immunomodulatory treatments have failed
- *Prognosis* is poor: mortality is 40% within 2y of diagnosis; the rate of decline is very variable between individuals
- Retransplantation is the only definitive treatment and is controversial.

Recurrence of primary disease Documented in sarcoidosis, LAM, giant cell interstitial pneumonitis, diffuse pan-bronchiolitis, and bronchoalveolar cell carcinoma.

Malignancy Increased risk of certain malignancies, e.g. lymphoma (and other EBV-related post-transplant lymphoproliferative diseases), skin, lip, vulval, and perineal carcinomas, *in situ* cervical cancer, and Kaposi's sarcoma.

- Most lymphomas appear within the first year, and the lung allograft is the most common site of involvement, with pulmonary nodule(s) ± mediastinal lymphadenopathy. Lymphocyte aggregates from acute rejection may mimic the appearance of post-transplant lymphoproliferative disease on small TBB specimens. Lymphomas presenting after the first year are more commonly disseminated or intra-abdominal (e.g. presenting with tonsillar enlargement, peripheral lymphadenopathy, skin nodules, or bowel complications such as intussusception). Patients should be referred back to the transplant centre for treatment, rather than the local haematologist. The usual treatment is a reduction in immunosuppression or rituximab (monoclonal antibody against CD20 on B cells)
- Lung cancer occurs in patients with COPD and IPF. Unclear if transplantation itself increases the risk of lung cancer. May progress unusually rapidly, mimicking infection.

Differential diagnosis of CXR nodules following lung transplant

- Post-transplant lymphoproliferative disease
- Infection (*Pseudomonas, Nocardia*, aspergilloma, TB)
- Disease recurrence
- 1° lung cancer.

Chapter 33

Mediastinal abnormalities

Introduction to mediastinal abnormalities

The mediastinum is the area within the centre of the chest containing the heart, great vessels, nerves, lymph nodes, trachea, oesophagus, and thymus. Two-thirds of mediastinal masses are benign. Age 20–40; presence of symptoms and anterior location of a mass are all associated with an increased likelihood of malignancy. Common symptoms of mediastinal disease include cough, chest pain, and dyspnoea, as well as symptoms relating to any structure being compressed such as dysphagia, stridor, or SVCO. Mediastinal disorders can also be asymptomatic. They may be found incidentally following a CXR.

Anatomy

Anterior mediastinum The area behind the body of the sternum and in front of the fibrous pericardium. Contains the thymus, which also extends superiorly.

Posterior mediastinum The area in front of the vertebral bodies and behind the fibrous pericardium. Contains the spinal nerve roots, the descending aorta and oesophagus, the azygos and hemiazygos veins, the thoracic duct, and vagus and splanchnic nerves.

Superior mediastinum The area located between the thoracic inlet superiorly, the manubrium of the sternum anteriorly, by the superior four thoracic vertebrae posteriorly, and inferiorly where a horizontal plane would cross through the sternal angle. It contains the aortic arch and its large branches and the upper half of SVC. It also contains the trachea, the oesophagus, the thoracic duct, and the phrenic, vagus, cardiac, and left recurrent laryngeal nerves.

Middle mediastinum The area containing the heart and pericardium, the ascending aorta, the lower half of the SVC, part of the azygos vein, the pulmonary arteries and veins, the tracheal bifurcation, phrenic nerves, and the IVC.

These areas are easily seen on a lateral CXR (represented in Fig. 33.1).

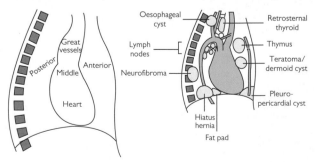

Fig. 33.1 Anterior, posterior, superior, and middle mediastinum.

Likely nature of mediastinal mass according to anatomical site

Anterior mediastinal mass
- Thymoma (superior)
- Thyroid (superior)
- Germ cell tumour
- Lymphoma
- Ascending aortic aneurysm
- Pleuropericardial cyst
- Pericardial fat pad
- Morgagni anterior diaphragmatic hernia (see ➜ p. 342).

Superior mediastinal mass
- Bronchogenic cyst.

Posterior mediastinal mass
- Neural tumour
- Foregut duplication or cyst
- Lipoma
- Descending aortic aneurysm
- Bochdalek posterior diaphragmatic hernia (see ➜ p. 342).

Approach to the patient with a mediastinal mass
- Full history
- Examination, including skin, lymphadenopathy (neck, axillae, groins), and testes
- Look for fatigability: ptosis, ophthalmoplegia, inability to maintain upward gaze
- Look for signs of SVCO or stridor
- Blood tests, including AFP, βHCG, anti-acetylcholine receptor (AChR) antibody
- CXR and lateral CXR (if not already done)
- Arrange CT scan of chest
- Try and locate old CXRs.

Mediastinal abnormalities 1

Neural tumours Mostly occur in the posterior mediastinum. 75% are benign in adults. MRI often helpful in assessment.

- *Schwannomas and neurofibromas* are benign peripheral nerve sheath tumours. They may be multiple. Usually asymptomatic, although can cause segmental pain. Slowly enlarge and rarely can cause cord compression, with dumb-bell-shaped tumours straddling the intervertebral foramen. Can be surgically excised
- *Malignant peripheral nerve sheath tumours or neurosarcomas* include new malignant growths and benign neurofibromas that have undergone malignant change. They may cause systemic features of malignancy and can invade locally and metastasize
- *Autonomic nervous system tumours*, including neuroblastomas and ganglioneuromas, range from benign to malignant. Surgical removal is the treatment of choice, with radiotherapy and chemotherapy if the tumour is malignant.

Thymoma Tumour of epithelial origin arising in the thymus. May contain functioning thymic tissue. ♂=♀. Rare below age 20. Myasthenia gravis is present in 30–40% of patients with a thymoma; this is often unimproved after thymectomy and may even develop after the thymoma is removed. 20% of patients presenting with myasthenia gravis are found to have a thymoma, particularly if patients are over 50 and ♂. This group is likely to have positive AChR autoantibodies, which bind to AChRs at the post-synaptic motor endplate, decreasing available acetylcholine binding sites, causing nerve fatigability.

Patients with thymomas are usually symptomatic with pain, dyspnoea, dysphagia, or myasthenia gravis symptoms. Thymomas contained within the thymic capsule tend to be benign, although they do have malignant potential; those that have extended outside the capsule are malignant and may involve local structures or metastasize. Diagnose with CT, and treat with surgical excision of the thymus, avoiding prior FNA or biopsy, as this may cause tumour seeding outside the capsule. Consider post-operative radiotherapy and chemotherapy for invasive tumours, especially those not completely excised. Thymectomy is indicated in patients with myasthenia gravis, even without thymoma, as it may lead to symptomatic improvement. This gives best results in those with detectable AChR antibody levels and younger patients early in the disease course, particularly those with severe disease.

Thymic cyst may be congenital or acquired 2° to inflammation. Asymptomatic unless large and causing symptoms of compression. Benign but usually treated with surgical excision, as diagnostic certainty may be difficult.

Thymic carcinoid Not associated with myasthenia gravis and behaves aggressively, with local recurrence and metastasis. May be associated with Cushing's syndrome. Treatment with surgery, chemotherapy, or octreotide.

Also: thymic carcinoma, thymic lipoma, and thymic hyperplasia.

Germ cell tumours Arise from immature germ cells, which fail to migrate during development. Tend to be in an anterior and midline location.

- *Mature cystic teratomas* represent 80% of germ cell tumours. These are benign and occur in young adults. ♂=♀. Often asymptomatic but can erode surrounding structures and cause symptoms. CXR shows well-defined mass, which may contain flecks of calcification. Treatment is by surgical excision

- *Seminoma* occurs in men age 20–40y. Mediastinal seminomas are malignant and almost always arise within the thymus and are histologically indistinguishable from those occurring in the testes. Can be 1° mediastinal tumour or metastasis from testicular tumour; therefore, always examine testes and perform USS. Patients frequently present with chest pain. CXR shows non-calcified lobulated anterior mediastinal mass, confirmed with CT. Serum AFP is normal, and this aids diagnosis. Diagnose with surgical biopsy. Surgical excision is not recommended as is usually incomplete. Treatment is with cisplatin-based chemotherapy initially, which can cause infertility, and, therefore, patients may wish to consider sperm banking before treatment. Tumours are radiosensitive, so radiotherapy used if they are bulky. Long-term survival expected in 80%. Better prognosis than non-seminomatous germ cell tumours

- *Non-seminomatous germ cell tumours* (including choriocarcinoma, teratocarcinoma, and yolk sac tumours) are all malignant and occur in men in their 30s. They are symptomatic due to local invasion, and they metastasize. CXR shows mediastinal mass, and diagnosis is with surgical biopsy. βHCG and AFP are raised. Treatment is with cisplatin-based chemotherapy. βHCG and AFP are markers of disease and fall with tumour response.

Thyroid Retrosternal goitre occurs, especially in older women. Usually asymptomatic unless large and compressing the trachea, causing dyspnoea and stridor. May be seen on plain CXR. CT and radioactive iodine isotope scans are helpful in diagnosis. Flow–volume loops are abnormal if there is tracheal compression. Surgery is recommended if there is airway compromise but can lead to tracheomalacia afterwards.

Also: parathyroid adenoma.

Mediastinal abnormalities 2

Lymphoma The mediastinum is frequently involved in patients with Hodgkin's lymphoma. CT scan is necessary to assess the extent of this and to assess response to treatment. To establish the histological diagnosis of lymphoma, an adequate tissue sample is required; this should be from a biopsy, rather than a fine-needle aspirate. This may be best achieved surgically via mediastinoscopy. Examine patient for peripheral lymph nodes, as these may be easier to biopsy. Treatment is with chemotherapy initially.

Enlarged lymph nodes

- *Metastases* from breast, lung, and oesophageal cancer
- *Castleman's disease* Giant lymph node hyperplasia. Rare. Two forms:
  - *Angio-follicular hyperplasia* causing mediastinal or hilar lymph node mass. Often asymptomatic or may cause cough or wheeze due to localized compression. Non-progressive. May have fever and raised ESR. Nodal biopsy shows follicles of pericapillary lymphocytes and proliferation of the plump and eosinophilic capillary endothelial cells. Removal of node(s) may improve symptoms and be curative. Can also occur on pleura
  - *Multicentric Castleman's disease* is a more aggressive disease that usually occurs in association with HIV infection. Lymphoproliferative disorder with prominent systemic symptoms (night sweats, fatigue, weight loss) as well as generalized lymph node enlargement, hepatosplenomegaly, paraproteinaemia, and skin rash. Biopsy shows prominent plasma cell infiltration. Related to IL6 overproduction and human herpesvirus-8 infection. Treatment is with rituximab first line, which induces remission in a high percentage of patients. For patients with aggressive disease or poor performance status, rituximab ± steroids ± chemotherapy (etoposide and vincristine) may be preferred first line, but prognosis is poor. Can progress to non-Hodgkin's lymphoma. Rapidly fatal without treatment
  - *Also*: lymphangioma.

Cysts

- *Foregut duplications or bronchogenic cysts* can be related to the oesophagus or the airways, especially near the carina. Lined by respiratory epithelium. Often diagnosed in childhood, as they cause dyspnoea, stridor, or cough due to limited space to expand. Seen on CXR and CT and treated with surgical excision
- *Pleuropericardial cysts* mostly occur at the cardiophrenic angles and can measure up to 25cm diameter. ♂=♀. Usually asymptomatic but may cause chest pain. CXR shows smooth, round shadow abutting the heart. Excision can be carried out at thoracoscopy, but conservative management is favoured. Also known as springwater cysts.

Inflammation

- *Mediastinitis* occurs after oesophageal perforation or rupture, due to malignancy, instrumentation, or vomiting (Boerhaave's syndrome). Patients are ill, with pain and fever. CXR may show widened mediastinum or air in the mediastinum. Pneumothorax or pleural effusion may also be seen. Treatment includes repairing the defect, parenteral feeding, and antibiotics. High morbidity and mortality

- *Mediastinal fibrosis* Rare idiopathic condition that occurs in middle age. Symptoms depend on which aspects of the mediastinum are involved but may include dyspnoea, wheeze, haemoptysis, hoarse voice, dysphagia, PHT, SVCO. CXR shows a widened mediastinum. Diagnosis made on biopsy, particularly to exclude malignancy. Treatment is supportive; steroids and surgical debulking ineffective. Prognosis variable, depending on sites involved. May be associated with retroperitoneal fibrosis, radiotherapy, methysergide, autoimmune disease, or infection with TB, histoplasmosis, *Aspergillus*, or *Nocardia*.

Mediastinal emphysema or pneumomediastinum. Can be caused by sneezing, straining, Valsalva manoeuvres, vomiting, substance abuse, parturition, positive pressure ventilation, instrumentation, or TBB. Usually symptomless but occasional pain. Hamman's sign may be present (click with each heartbeat on auscultation over lung). Treat with high-flow O_2. Resolves spontaneously.

Vascular Aortic aneurysms are usually asymptomatic, but symptoms relate to compression of adjacent structures. May diagnose on CXR as a widened mediastinum. This is best imaged via CT or MRI. Surgery should be considered to prevent death from rupture.

Further information

Duwe BV et al. Tumors of the mediastinum. Chest 2005;**128**:2893–909.

Chapter 34

Paediatric lung disorders pertinent to adult patients

Chronic lung disease of prematurity

Chronic lung disease of prematurity (CLD), formerly (and still in the USA) known as bronchopulmonary dysplasia (BPD). Advances in neonatal medicine have led to improved survival of premature babies with immature lungs and respiratory disease. Babies born at lower gestational ages are surviving into adulthood, due to therapy with antenatal steroids to prevent respiratory distress syndrome and the use of artificial surfactant to decrease the surface tension of the neonatal alveolar membrane. There have also been improvements in ventilatory techniques, and CLD usually occurs in babies who have been mechanically ventilated. Most long-term studies have been on patients before these improvements in management.

Usually caused by barotrauma from prolonged ventilation, high-pressure ventilation, and/or ventilation with high O_2 concentrations.

Typical presentation Premature baby remaining O_2-dependent after 36 weeks post-conceptional age. Infrequent in those born at 30+ weeks and weighing >1,200g. Mortality 25–30% with severe CLD. May require prolonged home O_2 therapy, up to 1y or beyond. 50% of infants will need hospital re-admission during their first year with respiratory infection. Some have significant pulmonary sequelae during childhood and adolescence: airways hyperreactivity, persistent wheeze, chronic hypoxia, and PHT. Duration of O_2 dependence predicts long-term sequelae. Majority of children with CLD do not have significant ongoing respiratory symptoms. Children may have disabilities associated with prematurity such as cerebral palsy or learning difficulties.

Pathology Cytokine-mediated scarring and repair. *Early inflammatory phase*: bronchial necrosis, alveolar destruction, capillary permeability, and associated obliterative bronchiolitis. *Subacute fibroproliferative phase*: type II pneumocyte hyperplasia, bronchial and bronchial smooth muscle hypertrophy, and interstitial and perialveolar fibrosis. *Chronic fibroproliferative phase*: airway remodelling for up to 1y and bronchial wall thickening. Prior to surfactant use, these changes were more severe.

PFTs Functional respiratory abnormalities persist with increased airway resistance and airway hyperresponsiveness. RV and RV/TLC are raised, indicative of air trapping. Air trapping improves over 3–4y as lung growth occurs; however, small airway abnormalities persist, at least until the age of 10. Expired NO levels are usually not raised, indicating a non-eosinophilic-driven process.

Chest radiology Persisting mild to moderate abnormalities, multifocal areas of reduced lung attenuation and perfusion, bronchial wall thickening, and decreased bronchus/pulmonary artery diameter ratios on CT. Radiological abnormalities correlate with physiological evidence of air trapping.

PAH occurs commonly when persistent lung disease; complex pathophysiological factors. Tends to improve with age.

Adulthood Few longitudinal studies beyond adolescence. Significance of CLD of prematurity to development of later adult lung disease unclear.

Viral wheeze and asthma

A controversial area. Wheezing is common in infants and toddlers and is often due to viral respiratory tract infections, causing a viral-induced wheeze. This has been found to be associated with passive cigarette smoke exposure, contact with other children, and not being breastfed. This transient early wheezing is distinct from childhood asthma and is presumably non-eosinophilic in origin. The children are not atopic and have no family history of such. The wheeze has resolved usually by the age of 3, although they may persist in having airway hyperactivity for many years. Children with asthma tend to have a family history of eczema with concomitant atopic dermatitis and develop their symptoms at any age, but usually slightly later (by the age of 5). Half of them have mild symptoms, which regress by puberty. Those with more severe disease, requiring regular inhaled steroids, often have disease that persists into adult life. Treatment for young children is based on persistent symptoms and atopy. Drugs which may be effective include inhaled corticosteroids and leukotriene receptor antagonists.

Further information

Gough A et al. General and respiratory health outcomes in adult survivors of bronchopulmonary dysplasia: a systematic review. Chest 2012;141:1554–67.

Sigurs N et al. Asthma and allergy patterns over 18 years after severe RSV bronchiolitis in the first years of life. Thorax 2010;65:1045–52.

Congenital abnormalities

Tracheomalacia Floppy trachea, usually associated with oesophageal atresia (but can occur with CLD). Rarely will require intubation or tracheostomy.

Congenital lobar emphysema Overinflation of a lobe due to localized bronchomalacia or bronchial obstruction. May cause wheeze or produce chest deformity. Often resolves spontaneously.

Diaphragmatic hernia A diaphragmatic defect, causing bowel to be present in the chest. This may cause respiratory distress soon after birth and may have been detected during the antenatal period by USS, or it may be completely asymptomatic and found incidentally on CXR, with bowel seen in the chest. There are two types. *Bochdalek hernia* is the congenital absence of posterolateral part of diaphragm, with associated hypoplastic lung due to bowel limiting growth. Treatment is with surgical repair of the diaphragmatic defect, but survival rate is only 50% due to underlying lung problems. *Morgagni hernia* is anteromedial herniation through the foramen of Morgagni, which is more commonly found in adulthood. It may be asymptomatic or cause symptoms of fullness, tightness, or pain in the anterior chest; it does not cause intestinal obstruction. CXR shows a cardiophrenic angle density. Surgical repair is difficult and is usually not necessary.

Cystic adenomatoid lung Excessive overgrowth of bronchioles with multiple cysts occurring in a section of lung. Commonly affects left lower lobe. Can be diagnosed antenatally. Can present in the same way as congenital lobar emphysema. May be mistaken for diaphragmatic hernia. Treatment is by resection of the affected lobe, but there may be space-occupying effects of the abnormal lobe that can cause morbidity and mortality, e.g. due to vena caval obstruction.

Pulmonary sequestration/sequestrated segment Segment of lung parenchyma, with no bronchial connection, that is unventilated. May be supplied by aberrant artery from the aorta and have anomalous pulmonary drainage to the right atrium. Can be intralobar, sharing pleura with the rest of the lung, or extralobar, which is separated from the lung by a lining of pleural tissue. Mostly left-sided; 75% are situated between the diaphragm and left lower lobe. Often associated with other congenital abnormalities. Can be a chance finding on CXR at any age, when cystic change may be seen in this area. Contrast CT or MRI may aid diagnosis. Surgical resection may be necessary if there is repeated infection in this segment.

MacLeod's (or Swyer–James or Brett's) syndrome Hyperlucency of lung or lobe, due to parenchymal and vascular underdevelopment (obliterative bronchiolitis), following childhood bronchitis or bronchiolitis. Usually asymptomatic and is diagnosed on CXR, which shows a hypertranslucent lung with reduced vascular markings and a small pulmonary artery.

Chapter 35

Pleural effusion

Clinical features and imaging

A pleural effusion results from the accumulation of abnormal volumes (>10–20mL) of fluid in the pleural space. Pleural effusions are common and are associated with many different diseases; see Chapter 8 for a step-by-step approach to the diagnosis of a patient with a pleural effusion, differential diagnosis of effusions, and details of pleural fluid analysis.

Clinical features

- May be asymptomatic or associated with breathlessness, dry cough, pleuritic chest pain (suggesting pleural inflammation), chest 'heaviness', and sometimes pain referred to the shoulder or abdomen
- Signs on examination include reduced chest expansion, reduced tactile vocal fremitus, a stony dull percussion note, quiet breath sounds, and sometimes a patch of bronchial breathing above the fluid level. A friction rub may be heard with pleural inflammation.

Imaging

CXR

- Sequential blunting of posterior, lateral, and then anterior costophrenic angles are seen on radiographs as effusions increase in size
- PA CXR will usually detect effusion volumes of 200mL or more; lateral CXR is more sensitive and may detect as little as 50mL pleural fluid
- Classical CXR appearance is of basal opacity obscuring hemidiaphragm, with concave upper border. Massive effusion may result in a 'white-out' of the hemithorax, with mediastinal displacement away from the effusion; lack of mediastinal shift in such cases raises the possibility of associated volume loss due to bronchial obstruction from a lung cancer
- Other CXR appearances include rounded or lentiform shadowing in loculated interlobar effusions and diffuse shadowing throughout the hemithorax on supine films
- CXR appearance may suggest the underlying diagnosis, e.g. bilateral effusions with cardiomegaly in cardiac failure; massive effusions are most commonly seen due to malignancy.

US (see p. 801) has a much higher sensitivity than CXR at detecting and localizing pleural fluid and is useful for distinguishing pleural fluid from pleural masses or thickening. Sonographic appearances can be useful in predicting exudates (echogenic or septated fluid) and for predicting malignancy. Its use for pleural procedures increases success at fluid aspiration and reduces risk of complications.

CT chest with pleural contrast is useful in distinguishing benign and malignant pleural disease: nodular, mediastinal, or circumferential pleural thickening and parietal pleural thickening >1cm are all highly specific for malignant disease. Scans are best performed prior to complete drainage of fluid. CT may also reveal evidence of extrapleural disease, e.g. lymphadenopathy or parenchymal change, which may suggest, e.g. cancer or TB.

Role of MRI is unclear; it may have increasing role in distinguishing benign from malignant pleural disease.

Malignant pleural effusion: causes and investigations

Epidemiology Commonest cause of exudative pleural effusion in patients older than 60y. About 40,000 cases of malignant effusion each year in the UK.

Causes Most malignant effusions are metastatic, with lung and breast the most common 1° sites (see Table 35.1).

Table 35.1 1° sites and frequency

1° site	Approximate frequency (%)
Lung	38
Breast	17
Lymphoma	12
Mesothelioma	10
Genitourinary tract	9
GI tract	7
Unknown 1°	11

Other rarer tumours include sarcoma, melanoma, leukaemia, and myeloma; almost any malignant tumour may spread to the pleural cavity. *Mesothelioma* is an important cause of malignant effusions and is discussed on ➔ pp. 118–9.

Clinical features Breathlessness is the main symptom; chest pain, cough, weight loss, and anorexia may also be present. A small proportion of patients are asymptomatic. Effusions may be unilateral or bilateral and are frequently large volume.

Differential diagnosis Consider other potential causes of pleural effusion in patients known to have cancer, e.g. due to pneumonia, PE, radiotherapy, pericardial disease, or drugs.

Investigations A strategy for investigating the patient with an undiagnosed pleural effusion is detailed on ➔ p. 52. Key investigations in patients suspected to have a malignant effusion are:

Pleural fluid cytology Sensitivity for malignancy is about 60%. Immunostaining of malignant cells may provide clues as to the likely primary site. Visualization of monoclonal cells in fluid on flow cytometry may support a diagnosis of lymphoma.

CT chest with pleural contrast Nodular, mediastinal, or circumferential pleural thickening and parietal pleural thickening >1cm on CT are highly specific for malignant disease. May also demonstrate extrapleural disease, e.g. lymphadenopathy.

Pleural biopsy histology See ➔ p. 777. Required in cytology-negative cases. Options:

- *CT-guided* cutting needle biopsy has been demonstrated to be a more effective diagnostic test for malignant pleural disease than Abrams' pleural biopsy (sensitivity 87% in CT-guided biopsy group vs 47% in Abrams' group)
- *US-guided* needle biopsies are also effective and relatively straightforward to perform
- *Thoracoscopy* (see ➔ p. 813) is an extremely useful investigation allowing direct visualization of the pleural space, with a high sensitivity (>92%) for biopsies. Therapeutic talc poudrage (talc is 'puffed' directly on to the pleural surfaces) may be performed at same time, with a pleurodesis success rate >80%. Usually performed using conscious sedation and local anaesthesia. Complications (such as empyema) are rare.

Serum/pleural fluid tumour markers (e.g. CEA, CA19-9, CA15-3, CA125, PSA) should not be routinely used for investigation of pleural effusions, having a poor combined sensitivity for malignant disease. Mesothelin has a low sensitivity of 48–84% and specificity 70–100% for mesothelioma and is therefore not routinely recommended.

Prognosis Median survival 3–12 months from diagnosis; shortest in lung cancer, longest in mesothelioma and ovarian cancer. Lower pleural fluid pH may be associated with shorter survival, but this is contentious.

Further information

Roberts ME *et al*. Management of a malignant pleural effusion: British Thoracic Society pleural disease guideline 2010. *Thorax* 2010;**65**(Suppl. 2):ii32–40.
Maskell NA *et al*. Standard pleural biopsy vs CT-guided cutting-needle biopsy for diagnosis of malignant disease in pleural effusions: a randomised controlled trial. *Lancet* 2003;**361**:1326–31.

Malignant pleural effusion: management

Key points influencing the management of malignant effusions are:

- Symptoms, performance status, and wishes of the patient
- Sensitivity of the 1° tumour to chemotherapy, e.g. small cell lung carcinoma, lymphoma, ovarian and breast carcinoma may respond to chemotherapy, although, in some cases, pleural effusions remain problematic and require additional treatment
- Extent of lung re-expansion following effusion drainage.

Treatment options

Observation and follow-up if asymptomatic.

Therapeutic pleural aspiration of 1–1.5L pleural fluid to improve breathlessness (see ➲ p. 800). Can be performed at the bedside as a day-case procedure, avoiding hospital admission. Useful in the palliation of breathlessness in patients with a poor prognosis and in rare cases where effusion reaccumulates very slowly. Most effusions recur within 1 month of aspiration, and these patients should be considered for pleurodesis or insertion of an IPC; repeated aspiration may be inconvenient and uncomfortable for the patient and carries a risk of complications such as empyema, pneumothorax, and tumour seeding (in mesothelioma).

If the breathlessness does not improve following fluid aspiration, then there is little to be gained by repeated aspiration, and other causes of breathlessness should be considered, e.g. lymphangitis carcinomatosis, PE.

Intercostal chest drainage and pleurodesis The aim of pleurodesis is to seal the visceral pleura to the parietal pleura with adhesions to prevent pleural fluid accumulating. The success of pleurodesis depends on the degree of apposition of the visceral and parietal pleura, which depends on the degree of lung re-expansion following drainage of the effusion. 'Trapped lung' occurs when tumour encases the visceral pleura and prevents lung expansion. Lung expansion may also be inhibited by a proximal airway obstruction or by a persistent air leak (e.g. after tearing of a friable tumour-infiltrated lung on re-expansion). Trapped lung may also be caused by non-malignant, fibrotic processes, e.g. rheumatoid pleuritis, haemothorax, TB.

The patient should be admitted and the effusion drained with a small-bore (10–14F) intercostal tube. If lung fully re-expands on CXR, proceed to pleurodesis (see ➲ p. 783). If lung fails to re-expand fully (trapped lung; CXR shows a pneumothorax or hydropneumothorax), consider chest drain suction, which may encourage lung expansion and allow pleurodesis.

Treatment options for trapped lung or failed pleurodesis

- *Pleurodesis* may be successful, despite only partial lung re-expansion, and should still be considered if there is >50% apposition of lung against chest wall on CXR. It may be repeated if unsuccessful initially

- *Insertion of a long-term IPC* is likely to be the preferred treatment for patients with significantly trapped lung and avoids the need for recurrent pleural aspiration (see ➔ p. 767). The most frequent complications are symptomatic loculations, catheter blockage, and soft tissue/pleural infection. Can be inserted as a day-case procedure. Needs additional outpatient support (e.g. trained district nurse or respiratory specialist nurse), although most patients perform the drainage themselves after education
- *Repeated therapeutic pleural aspiration* should be avoided, unless prognosis is particularly limited (<1 month)
- *Intrapleural fibrinolytics* (e.g. streptokinase 250,000IU) may be of benefit in the management of multiloculated effusions resistant to drainage and pleurodesis, encouraging free fluid drainage and, in some cases, enabling successful pleurodesis. Haemorrhage is a theoretical complication, although it appears to be uncommon
- *Thoracoscopy* enables the disruption of pleural adhesions and may have a role in facilitating pleurodesis in select patients with trapped lung
- *Pleuroperitoneal shunts* are effective in patients with trapped lung or failed pleurodesis, in the absence of multiple loculations. Shunting of fluid may occur spontaneously, at high pressures, or may require manipulation of a percutaneous pump chamber, inserted at thoracoscopy or mini-thoracotomy. Main problem is shunt occlusion, which occurs in at least 10% of cases, and necessitates shunt removal. Malignant spread may also occur
- *Surgical parietal pleurectomy* may be performed as VATS. The procedure is effective in the management of refractory malignant effusions. May be useful in a minority of patients with good performance status and prognosis. Not suitable for patients with heavily diseased visceral pleura and trapped lung; consider in patients who have failed pleurodesis
- *Palliative care team* involvement should also be considered.

Parapneumonic effusion and empyema: definition and clinical features

Definition and pathophysiology Pleural effusions occur in up to 57% of patients with pneumonia. An initial sterile exudate (simple parapneumonic effusion) may, in some cases, progress to a complicated parapneumonic effusion and eventually empyema (see Fig. 35.1).

Simple parapneumonic effusion	Exudative stage
	Clear sterile fluid with normal pH, glucose, LDH
	Frequently resolves with antibiotics alone
	Drainage not usually required
Complicated parapneumonic effusion	Fibrinopurulent stage
	Fibrin deposited and septations occur
	Fluid infected but not yet purulent; appears clear or cloudy/turbid
	pH <7.2, glucose <2.2mmol/L, and LDH >1,000IU/L
	Gram stain/culture may be positive
	Drainage required
Empyema	Pus in pleural space
	May be free-flowing or multiloculated
	Gram stain/culture may be positive
	Drainage required
	Eventually, fibroblast growth may result in development of thick pleural peel (organizing stage). Treatment at this stage is difficult and decortication may be required

Fig. 35.1 Parapneumonic effusion and empyema: definition and clinical features.

Pleural infection may also occur in the absence of a preceding pneumonic illness ('1° empyema').

Clinical features

Common
- Consider the diagnosis particularly in cases of 'slow-to-respond' pneumonia (e.g. failure of CRP to fall ≥50% in first 3 days), pleural effusion with fever, or high-risk groups with non-specific symptoms such as weight loss
- Similar to clinical presentation of pneumonia: fever, sputum production, chest pain, breathlessness
- Anaerobic empyema may present less acutely, often with weight loss and without fever.

Rare

- Infected pleural fluid may spontaneously drain through the chest wall (*empyema necessitatis*) or into the lung, leading to a bronchopleural fistula and severe pneumonia
- History of atypical chest pain, vomiting, or oesophageal instrumentation suggests possible underlying oesophageal rupture (measure pleural fluid amylase)
- History of a recent sore throat may suggest Lemierre's syndrome (acute oropharyngeal infection with *Fusobacterium* species leads to septic thrombophlebitis of the internal jugular vein and subsequent metastatic infection and abscess formation, commonly in the lungs and pleura; consider US of internal jugular vein if suspected); see ➡ p. 444.

Risk factors for developing empyema include diabetes, alcohol abuse, gastro-oesophageal reflux, and IV drug abuse. Anaerobic infection is associated particularly with aspiration or poor dental hygiene. Empyema may rarely occur following bronchial obstruction from a tumour or foreign body. Many patients, however, have no apparent risk factors. One study identified clinical variables associated with development of pleural infection in those with pneumonia: albumin <30g/L, CRP >100mg/L, platelets >400 × 10^9/L, sodium <130mmol/L, IVDU, and chronic alcohol use.

Differential diagnosis includes malignancy, TB (when the pleural fluid is usually lymphocytic), and rheumatoid pleuritis.

Further information

Davies HE *et al.* Management of pleural infection in adults: British Thoracic Society pleural disease guideline 2010. *Thorax* 2010;**65**(Suppl. 2):ii41–ii53.

Maskell NA *et al.* UK controlled trial of intrapleural streptokinase for pleural infection. *N Engl J Med* 2005;**352**:865–74.

Rahman NM *et al.* Intrapleural use of tissue plasminogen activator and DNase in pleural infection. *N Engl J Med* 2011;**365**:518–26.

Parapneumonic effusion and empyema: bacteriology and investigations

Bacteriology

- *Community-acquired infection* (% of cases):
  - *Streptococcus 'milleri'* group (~30%)
  - Anaerobes (~15–30%)
  - *Streptococcus pneumoniae* (~15%)
  - *Staphylococcus aureus* (~10%)
  - Other less common organisms include other streptococci, enterobacteriaceae, *H. influenzae, Pseudomonas*, TB, and *Nocardia*
- *Hospital-acquired infection* (% of cases):
  - MRSA (~25–30%)
  - *Staphylococcus aureus* (~10–20%)
  - Enterobacteriaceae (~20%)
  - Enterococci (~10%)
  - Others include streptococci, *Pseudomonas*, and anaerobes.

Pleural infection is frequently polymicrobial.

Investigations

- *Diagnostic pleural tap using US* is essential if pleural infection is possible and fluid depth is >10mm (smaller effusions can usually be monitored). Frankly purulent or turbid/cloudy pleural fluid, organisms on pleural fluid Gram stain or culture, or pleural fluid pH <7.2 are all indications for chest tube drainage. 40% of pleural infections are culture-negative. Identification of anaerobes is improved following inoculation of blood culture bottles with pleural fluid. Ultrasound typically shows an echogenic effusion that may be septated, but absence of these features does not rule out pleural infection
- *Contrast-enhanced pleural-phase CT* may be useful both in supporting the diagnosis and visualizing the distribution of fluid, although CT is poor at demonstrating septations. Empyema is associated with pleural enhancement and increased attenuation of extrapleural subcostal fat. The displacement of adjacent lung by empyema may help to distinguish from a parenchymal lung abscess. Empyemas frequently appear lenticular and may exhibit the 'split pleura' sign of enhancing separated visceral and parietal pleura. Absence of pleural thickening on CT is unusual in empyema. CT may also sometimes identify a proximal endobronchial obstructing lesion
- *Blood cultures* positive in only 14% of cases, but, in these cases, they are often the only positive microbiology
- *Bronchoscopy* is only indicated if a bronchial obstructing lesion is suspected.

Parapneumonic effusion and empyema: management and outcome

Management

Antibiotics All patients with pleural infection should be treated with antibiotics; refer to local hospital prescribing guidelines. Typical choices:

- *Community-acquired* empyema—β-lactam/β-lactamase inhibitor (e.g. co-amoxiclav) or second-generation cephalosporin (e.g. cefuroxime), combined with metronidazole for anaerobic cover. Ciprofloxacin and clindamycin together may be appropriate
- *Hospital-acquired* empyema—cover Gram-positive and Gram-negative organisms and anaerobes. MRSA infection is common. Consult with microbiology team. One option is meropenem and vancomycin.

Rationalize with culture and sensitivity results (although note that anaerobes are frequently difficult to culture and may coexist with other organisms). Avoid aminoglycosides, which penetrate the pleural space poorly.

Switch to oral antibiotics when apyrexial and improving clinically. Co-amoxiclav is a useful single agent with anaerobic cover (not if penicillin-allergic). Optimal duration of antibiotic treatment unclear, although likely to be at least 3 weeks.

Chest tube drainage

Indications for chest tube drainage

- Purulent pleural fluid
- Organisms on pleural fluid Gram stain or culture
- Pleural fluid pH <7.2.*

* This is not an absolute cut-off, as pH values vary between pockets of a multiseptated effusion and drainage may be still indicated for higher pH values. Also note that *Proteus* spp. infection gives pH >7.6.

Drain insertion should be carried out under US or CT guidance. Ideal chest tube size remains subject to debate. Small (10–14F), flexible tubes are more comfortable and have been demonstrated to be as effective as large drains in the management of empyema. Usually apply suction (–20cmH$_2$O), and flush regularly (e.g. 20mL normal saline every 6h) to prevent occlusion. Consider drain removal when clinical improvement occurs. If there is no indication for drainage, give antibiotics and monitor closely. If slow to improve or deteriorate, re-sample the effusion and consider chest drain.

Intrapleural fibrinolytics A 2011 RCT (MIST2) showed that the combination of intrapleural alteplase (tPA) and dornase alfa (DNase) significantly improved CXR appearances for patients with pleural infection (1° outcome) and reduced surgical referral and hospital stay with a similar adverse event profile (2° outcomes). Lone tPA or DNase did not confer such benefits (and there was an increased rate of surgical referral for DNase alone). The effects of tPA/DNase combination treatment need further investigation to determine the appropriate circumstances for its use. The 2005 MIST1 RCT showed that intrapleural streptokinase had no effect on mortality and need for surgery or hospital stay, and is therefore not recommended.

Nutritional support Dietician review; consider supplementary NG feeding.

Thromboprophylaxis Given a high risk for developing VTE, all patients should receive LMWH unless contraindicated.

Surgery Consult with thoracic surgeon if there are ongoing features of sepsis and residual pleural collection after 5–7 days despite tube drainage and treatment with antibiotics. Surgical techniques include:

- *VATS* allows the breakdown of adhesions and drainage of residual collection, but it is frequently unsuccessful in chronic empyema with very thickened visceral pleura
- *Thoracotomy and decortication* Removal of fibrinous and infected tissue from the pleural space—a major surgical procedure
- *Open thoracic drainage* Resection of segments of several ribs adjacent to the empyema and insertion of large-bore drains into the cavity: a more minor procedure that can be performed under local anaesthesia but results in open chest wound for long period (typically around 5 months).

Difficulties in management

Chest drainage ceases despite residual pleural collection
- Attempt to flush drain with normal saline
- Ensure that drain is not kinked at skin insertion site or lying subcutaneously
- Consider CT to assess extent of residual collection and drain position
- Remove drain if persistently blocked
- Consider further image-guided chest drain(s), surgery
- If there has been significant clinical improvement, with falling CRP and WCC, further drains may not be warranted despite residual fluid.

Failure to clinically improve despite antibiotics and chest drain
- Review microbiology results, and ensure appropriate antibiotics
- CT to assess extent of residual collection and drain position
- Surgical referral (at days 5–7)
- Options if unfit for surgery:
  - Further image-guided small-bore drains into loculated effusions
  - Large-bore drain
  - Surgical rib resection and open drainage under local anaesthesia.

Outcome About 15% of patients require surgery. Empyema 1y mortality is about 15%. Increased age, renal impairment, low serum albumin, hypotension, and hospital-acquired infection are associated with a poor outcome. CXR may remain abnormal despite successful treatment of empyema, with evidence of calcification or pleural scarring or thickening.

Tuberculous pleural effusion

Definition and epidemiology Tuberculous pleural effusion usually develops from a delayed hypersensitivity reaction to mycobacteria released into the pleural space. It is a common manifestation of 1° TB in regions with a high prevalence, affecting children and young adults; it may also be associated with reactivation of TB in older individuals. May occur more commonly in the setting of HIV co-infection.

Rarely, TB may present as pseudochylothorax or tuberculous empyema.

Clinical features

- Clinical features are similar to those of pulmonary TB, i.e. fever, sweats, weight loss, and dyspnoea, although it may present acutely with pleuritic chest pain and fever, mimicking pneumonia
- Effusions are typically small to moderate in volume although can be massive.

Investigations

- Associated parenchymal infiltrate on *CXR* in less than one-third of cases
- *Tuberculin skin tests* positive in two-thirds of cases
- *Interferon γ release assays* (IGRAs) reported to have high sensitivity (~90%) but fail to distinguish between latent and active TB
- *Pleural fluid* Lymphocytosis, exudative effusion, pH and glucose moderately depressed, mesothelial cells rare. Pleural fluid AFB smears are positive in around 5–10% of cases; pleural fluid cultures are positive in 25% of cases and take 2–6 weeks
- Blind *Abrams' pleural biopsy* alone has a sensitivity of 79%
- *Thoracoscopic biopsies* have a sensitivity of nearly 100%
- Measurement of *adenosine deaminase* (an enzyme released by macrophages after phagocytosis of mycobacteria) in pleural fluid may be of benefit in regions where TB is highly prevalent; a raised value is very sensitive for pleural TB but is non-specific and may also occur in empyema and malignancy. May have a role as a 'rule-out' test
- *PCR* for mycobacterial DNA in the pleural fluid may be useful diagnostically but is not widely available
- *Induced sputum* for AFB may have a diagnostic role in high-risk patients with lymphocytic effusions, even in the absence of parenchymal disease on CXR.

Treatment and outcome

- Tuberculous pleural effusions resolve spontaneously in the majority of cases, but two-thirds of untreated patients go on to develop pulmonary TB within 5y, and so treatment is recommended
- Treatment is the same as for pulmonary TB (see ➔ pp. 492–3)
- Pleural fluid volumes may increase during effective treatment, and therapeutic thoracentesis may be required
- Steroids may reduce fluid volume but do not affect long-term outcome
- Pleural thickening and calcification are common long-term consequences of tuberculous pleural effusion.

Other causes of pleural effusion

Pleural effusion due to PE

- Fourth commonest cause of pleural effusion in the USA
- Consider in all patients with undiagnosed pleural effusion, particularly if there is a history of pleuritic chest pain or of breathlessness/hypoxia out of proportion to the size of the effusion
- Frequently complicates other disease processes, e.g. occurs in 1/5 of patients with cardiac failure and pleural effusions
- Effusions are usually small (<1/3 of hemithorax) and unilateral although may be bilateral
- Pleural fluid analysis is non-diagnostic; appearance varies from clear to bloody; 80% are exudates and 20% transudates. Bloodstained pleural fluid is not a contraindication to anticoagulation
- Imaging investigations, such as CTPA, are required to make the diagnosis; these should be performed prior to thoracentesis if PE is strongly suspected.

RA-associated pleural effusion

- Pulmonary changes may be the first manifestation of RA
- Rheumatoid pleurisy is more common in men (70% are in men)
- Pleural fluid may be yellow-green, serous, turbid, or bloody
- Unilateral or bilateral
- Pleural fluid glucose level frequently low (<1.6mmol/L) and progressively falls in chronic effusions
- Pleural fluid pH commonly reduced (<7.3)
- Low pleural fluid complement levels (C4 <0.04g/L) may also favour the diagnosis
- Pleural fluid RhF titre is not more diagnostically helpful than serum RhF
- Typically persist for months to years, although duration may be several weeks
- Some cases may respond to treatment with steroids.

Haemothorax

- Haemothorax is defined as a pleural effusion with a haematocrit >50% of peripheral blood haematocrit
- Causes include trauma, iatrogenic, malignancy, pulmonary infarction, pneumothorax, thoracic endometriosis, and aortic rupture
- Massive haemothorax defined as >1,500cm³ of blood in hemithorax and is most commonly due to trauma. Traumatic haemothorax requires a chest drain and sometimes thoracotomy; all cases should be discussed immediately with the cardiothoracic surgical team
- Large volumes of residual blood in the pleural space will clot and may lead to pleural thickening, empyema, or trapped lung. Tube drainage may be ineffective, and thoracoscopy or thoracotomy with decortication is often needed.

Pleural effusion after CABG

- Small, typically left-sided pleural effusions occur in the majority of patients post-CABG, and most resolve spontaneously
- Larger (>25% of hemithorax) effusions can be subdivided:
  - Pleural effusions occurring *within 30 days* of surgery. Classically bloody and eosinophilic exudate, with high LDH; probably related to post-operative bleeding into pleural space
  - Pleural effusions *>30 days* after surgery. Typically clear and lymphocytic exudate; cause unknown, perhaps immunological or a form of post-cardiac injury syndrome
- Main symptom in each case is breathlessness; chest pain and fever are unusual
- Management consists of repeated therapeutic thoracentesis to alleviate breathlessness. Recurrent effusions after 1y are rare and may be difficult to treat; NSAIDs, prednisolone, or thoracoscopy and pleurodesis may be considered
- Differential diagnosis of pleural effusion post-CABG includes PE, cardiac failure, pleural infection, post-cardiac injury syndrome, chylothorax.

Pleural effusion following asbestos exposure

The main differential diagnosis is between benign asbestos pleural effusion (see ➋ p. 114) and mesothelioma (see ➋ pp. 118–9).

Pleural thickening

- Pleural fibrosis and thickening may follow previous episodes of pleural inflammation. Causes include previous empyema, tuberculous pleuritis, rheumatoid pleuritis, haemothorax, thoracotomy, and asbestos exposure (diffuse pleural thickening; see ➋ p. 115)
- May be asymptomatic or cause breathlessness
- CXR features include blunting of the costophrenic angle or apices, sometimes with associated calcification
- Ultrasound or CT may be required to distinguish from a pleural effusion
- Treatment is difficult and usually unnecessary; decortication may be considered.

Further information

Light RW. Pleural effusions after coronary artery bypass graft surgery. *Curr Opin Pulm Med* 2002;8:308–11.

Chapter 36

Pneumoconioses

Overview and causative mineral dusts

- Pneumoconioses are non-neoplastic pulmonary diseases caused by the reaction of the lung to the inhalation of mainly mineral, but also organic, dusts (see Table 36.1)
- Inhaled particles of dust size <5 micron reach the terminal airways and alveoli and settle on the epithelial lining. From here, they are slowly cleared by macrophages or alveolar cells. They may pass into the lymphatic system, be cleared via the airway, or remain in the alveolus
- The dust particles can lead to an inflammatory reaction within the lung, depending on their physical and chemical properties
- The inflammation causes characteristic alterations in pulmonary structure and radiological abnormalities
- Of the diseases caused by inhalation of mineral dusts, many are becoming less common in the UK, due to improved protection of workers from dusts and decreasing levels of mining. Newer industrial nations may see increasing numbers of cases of pneumoconiosis
- Organic dusts causing HP and extrinsic asthma are discussed on ⊃ pp. 253–8 and ⊃ pp. 148–9. Asbestos-related diseases are discussed separately on ⊃ p. 111.

Table 36.1 Causative mineral dusts

Mineral dust	Disease	Examples of exposure
Coal dust	Simple pneumoconiosis Progressive massive fibrosis Caplan's syndrome	Coal mining, especially hard coal
Silica	Silicosis Caplan's syndrome	Foundry work, sandblasting, stone cutting, hard rock mining, ceramics
Asbestos	Asbestosis Benign asbestos-related pleural disease Mesothelioma Lung cancer	Mining, milling, and fabrication Installation and removal of insulation
Beryllium	Acute berylliosis Beryllium granulomatosis	Mining, fabrication of electrical and electronic equipment, workers in nuclear and aerospace industry
Iron oxide	Siderosis	Welding
Barium sulphate	Baritosis	Mining
Tin oxide	Stannosis	Mining
Aluminium	Like silicosis (bauxite worker's lung, Shaver's disease)	Mining, firework, painting, and armament manufacture

Types of mineral dust exposure

Non-fibrous mineral dusts
- Silica
- Coal dust
- Mixed mineral dusts containing quartz: slate, kaolin, talc, non-fibrous clays.

Fibrous mineral dusts
- Asbestos
- Other mineral fibres.

Metal dusts and fumes
- Iron, aluminium, beryllium, cobalt

Chest disease in coal miners It was recognized many years ago that coal miners had higher levels of respiratory disease than the general population. Coal miners can get any, or all, of:
- Chronic bronchitis
- COPD
- Pneumoconiosis.

They may be eligible for compensation for all of these. It can be difficult to establish the independent effects of coal dust due to high smoking rates amongst miners. However, it is now thought that coal dust contributes to the COPD and bronchitis caused by smoking, because:
- Miners have an increased prevalence of cough, sputum, and decreased FEV_1 when compared with non-miners. The risk of cough increases with increasing dust exposure
- FEV_1 declines in proportion to the amount of dust exposure
- In smokers, the response to dust is probably different to that of non-smokers, with worse disease at a given level of exposure.

In the past, TB has also been a major problem amongst miners and their families, relating to their socio-economic conditions.

SWORD is the Surveillance of Work-related and Occupational Respiratory Disease scheme run in the UK to monitor the numbers of patients with occupational lung diseases. Patients with a clinical diagnosis of an occupational lung disease are confidentially reported by respiratory or occupational health physicians.

Further information
℘ http://www.dti.gov.uk/coalhealth.

Coal-worker's pneumoconiosis

This is the condition caused by the deposition of coal dust within the lung and its associated inflammatory reaction.

There are two types:
- Simple pneumoconiosis, which can progress to
- Complicated pneumoconiosis, also known as progressive massive fibrosis (PMF).

These diseases are common amongst coal miners who work in poorly ventilated conditions. The risk of pneumoconiosis varies with different compositions of coal from different geographical areas, but the larger the amount of dust to which the miner is exposed, the greater the risk of developing pneumoconiosis. It is now rare for miners under the age of 50 to be diagnosed with pneumoconiosis in the UK.

Pathology

Simple pneumoconiosis Coal dust is inhaled into the alveolus and is engulfed by macrophages, forming a black stellate lesion, the coal macule. This causes cytokine release and subsequent inflammatory cell recruitment, leading to fibroblast activation. These coal macules are found throughout the lung, especially in the upper zones of the upper and lower lobes and often associated with surrounding bronchiolar dilatation. They are not palpable. Regional lymph nodes also become blackened. In time, larger nodules develop, containing reticulin and collagen between the macrophages, and associated bronchiolar dilatation leading to focal emphysema is seen.

PMF occurs on this background but with aggregation of the fibrotic nodules to form larger lesions 2–10cm diameter. Macroscopically, these look like large black scars, extending from the lung parenchyma to the chest wall. The central area of these nodules may be necrotic, and the outer rim is firm and collagenous. It is not understood what causes the progression of small nodules to PMF, although continued exposure to coal dust in the presence of simple pneumoconiosis makes this development more likely.

Clinical features

Simple pneumoconiosis is usually asymptomatic, with no associated clinical signs. This is a relatively benign disease.

PMF is usually associated with cough, productive of mucoid or blackened sputum, and breathlessness, particularly on exertion, and may, in time, lead to the development of cor pulmonale. Examination is unremarkable, with no clubbing and no crepitations audible (the presence of crepitations suggests a different diagnosis).

Investigations

- *CXR* In *simple pneumoconiosis*, there is nodular shadowing, with nodules of varying size, up to 10mm, particularly in the upper and middle zones. Pneumoconiosis can be graded according to the number of different sized nodules: p = <1.5mm, q = 1.5–3mm, and r = 3–10mm. Nodule numbers increase with increasing dust inhalation and usually stop forming when the miner has left the work environment. *PMF* is diagnosed when one or more opacities of >1cm diameter are present, on the background of simple pneumoconiosis. These lesions are often located in the upper lobes and enlarge, becoming increasingly radiodense and clearly demarcated with time. They may distort the adjacent lung and cause emphysema. The lesions continue to progress out of the work environment

- *HRCT* of *simple pneumoconiosis* shows parenchymal nodules 1–10mm in size, with upper zone predominance. In *PMF*, nodules of >1cm are seen, with irregular borders and associated parenchymal distortion and emphysema. Larger lesions may have cavitation and necrosis. They may also have areas of calcification

- *PFTs Simple pneumoconiosis*: FEV_1 and FVC are normal, although TLCO may be slightly decreased. *PMF*: signs of airway obstruction due to emphysema, and restriction due to loss of lung volumes. TLCO is reduced.

Management Minimization of dust exposure with improved mine ventilation, respirator provision, and monitoring of dust levels. Miners have CXR every 4y and are moved to less dusty work, if they show signs of pneumoconiosis, to prevent the development of PMF. Miners with signs of coal-worker's pneumoconiosis are entitled to industrial injury benefits from British Coal (see ➔ p. 669). No increased risk of lung cancer with pneumoconiosis or PMF.

Caplan's syndrome Miners with seropositive RA or positive serum RhF can develop large well-defined nodules. These occur on a background of simple pneumoconiosis and in those with a relatively low coal dust exposure. They may be multiple and may cavitate. They cause no significant functional impairment and have no malignant potential.

Silicosis

This is a chronic nodular, densely fibrosing pneumoconiosis, caused by the prolonged inhalation of silica particles.

- Long lag time of decades between exposure and clinical disease
- Insidious onset, progressive
- Larger radiological opacities than those seen in coal-worker's pneumoconiosis and more rapid progression
- The pattern of disease depends on the level and duration of the silicone dust exposure.

Silica is present mostly as crystalline quartz, which is mined and quarried, and used in industries such as ceramics, brick making, and stone masonry. It is becoming less prevalent in Western societies, due to changes in silica working conditions.

Pathology Quartz and cristobalite forms of crystalline silica cause silicosis. When they accumulate within the airways, lymphocytes and alveolar macrophages engulf the particles and are removed into the lymphatic system. Any remaining silica dust causes focal aggregations of macrophages, which are, in time, converted into fibrosing nodules, the silicotic nodule. Silica dust can cause surfactant secretion from the alveolus due to local irritation. This leads to further macrophage recruitment. Large nodules are formed by the aggregation of smaller nodules.

Different types of silicosis There are four types, and the distinction is often not clear.

- *Acute silicosis* is caused by intense exposure to fine dusts such as those produced by sandblasting. It may become apparent in workers within a few months to a year of starting work. Rapid deterioration over 1–2y, with treatment being ineffective. Rare now, due to regulation of silica levels in the workplace
  - *Clinically* Dry cough, SOB, and a feeling of tightness on breathing deeply. Rapid deterioration over a few weeks. Fine crepitations are heard over the lower zones bilaterally. Respiratory failure
  - *CXR* Patchy bilateral lower airspace consolidation, which may look like pulmonary oedema
  - *Pathology* Irregular fibrosis adjacent to alveolar spaces filled with a lipoproteinaceous exudate, similar to that found in alveolar proteinosis
- *Subacute silicosis* This is the classic picture of silicosis, which is now quite rare. Dry cough, gradual onset of SOB
  - *CXR* Upper and mid-zone nodules are present, measuring between 3 and 5mm diameter. Initially indistinct but become clearer with time. Nodules coalesce and calcify and can progress to PMF where the centre may cavitate. Associated calcified hilar lymphadenopathy (eggshell calcification) and possible pleural thickening. Nodules continue to develop with continued exposure but, due to long lag time, will also develop when patient stops being exposed. In some cases with heavy exposure to silica, patients may develop progressive upper zone fibrosis with sparse nodularity

- *PFTs* Slow decline, including in TLCO, with mild restrictive pattern, unless the silicosis has caused emphysema when obstructive or mixed picture is seen
- *Pathology* Dust particles within the alveoli are phagocytosed by macrophages. They are removed to the lymphatics where they lodge and cause diffuse inflammatory change. Layers of collagen are deposited around the dust particle. Nodules are found within the 2° pulmonary lobule where they cause fibrosis
- *Chronic silicosis* occurs with lower dust concentrations than those seen in active silicosis; appears 10–30y after first exposure
  - *CXR* A few upper and mid-zone nodules occur, which become calcified after 10y or so. There is no associated parenchymal distortion. There may be associated hilar lymphadenopathy.

If there is further silica exposure, this disease may progress, with coalescence of nodules.

- *Silicotuberculosis* Increased likelihood of active TB infection in people with silicosis, most likely due to the reactivation of quiescent lesions. Silica within the lung is thought to affect the efficacy of the macrophage at clearing *Mycobacterium tuberculosis*. TB can be difficult to diagnose, due to multiple pre-existing CXR nodules. Cavitation may occur. Haemoptysis, fever, worsening respiratory function, and new soft CXR opacities should prompt sputum examination and BAL. Confirmed TB should be treated with the usual three- or four-drug regime. NTM infection is also more common.

Management Prevention of silicosis by monitoring and minimizing dust levels with adequate ventilation. Masks can be useful for short-term use if the high levels of dust are transiently unavoidable. Silicosis diagnosed with: history of silica exposure (with amount of exposure and latency taken into account), compatible imaging, and lack of another diagnosis which would fit history and imaging better. Lung biopsy is usually not necessary if these three conditions are met, only if alternative diagnosis being considered. Prescribe bronchodilators if airflow limitation, O_2 if respiratory failure; consider lung transplant if severe. Disability benefits available from the Department for Work and Pensions (see ➋ p. 669). Small increased risk of lung cancer with silicosis and associated PMF.

Berylliosis

Beryllium is a light, strong industrial metal. It is mined and often used as an alloy in the manufacture of fluorescent tubes for lighting and televisions, radiological equipment, in atomic reactors, and in heat-resistant ceramics. Cases of berylliosis are now rare, as beryllium levels have been tightly regulated to avoid sensitization. However, due to the long latent period between exposure and granuloma formation, as well as accidental beryllium exposure, cases are still occurring. There are two types of disease.

- *Acute beryllium disease* is an acute alveolitis due to the direct effects of high-dose inhaled beryllium fumes. There is subsequent widespread airway oedema and pulmonary oedema, which causes dyspnoea, cyanosis, and widespread inspiratory crepitations. CXR shows pulmonary oedema. It may be self-limiting if mild but, if severe, is usually fatal. Corticosteroids may prevent progression, but the patient is often left with residual pulmonary impairment
- *Subacute and chronic berylliosis* is a delayed hypersensitivity-type reaction due to beryllium, occurring a long time after beryllium exposure in a minority of individuals. It can be clinically indistinguishable from sarcoidosis. It has also been seen in the wives of beryllium workers and those who live near beryllium refineries. Inhalation of beryllium or the exposure of beryllium to a skin abrasion causes initial sensitization in 2–19% of exposed individuals. Only low levels of exposure are required for this. There is a T-cell-mediated immune response, with the production of numerous inflammatory cytokines, which cause granulomatous inflammation. Following a long latent period, which may be months to 10y plus after exposure, non-caseating granulomatous tissue reactions occur in the lungs or on the skin. There is a genetic predisposition to the response to beryllium exposure, and it is HLA-mediated (HLA-DPB1(Glu69)). HLA status could be used to identify workers at high risk of berylliosis (but is not routinely used at present).

Clinical features of chronic berylliosis
- *Symptoms* Dry cough, dyspnoea, fever, malaise, night sweats. Macular skin lesions, which do not spontaneously resolve
- *Signs* No clubbing or crepitations in early disease, but both occur with established fibrosis. Hepato/splenomegaly and macular skin lesions. Do not get uveitis or erythema nodosum.

Investigations
- *CXR* Fine reticulonodular appearance throughout both lungs. Finer nodules than those seen in sarcoidosis. Progression to interstitial fibrosis, with irregular linear opacities diffusely or favouring upper lobes. Hilar lymphadenopathy can occur, but always in association with ILD
- *HRCT* Subpleural micronodular change, thickened interlobular septae, traction bronchiectasis, and honeycombing. There may be ground-glass shadowing
- *BAL* High levels of T-lymphocytes
- *PFTs* Restrictive defect, with decreased kCO

- *Pathology* Non-caseating granulomata. Endobronchial and transbronchial biopsies may be adequate, taken from area of abnormal lung on CT. May be indistinguishable from sarcoidosis. May develop irregular fibrosis with bulla and cyst formation
- *Beryllium lymphocyte proliferation test (BeLPT)* assesses whether patient is sensitized to beryllium. This blood test has become the standard industry test to see which beryllium workers are sensitized and therefore part of the diagnostic work-up. Can also be performed on BAL fluid to increase diagnostic accuracy. False negative rate, so borderline and negative tests generally repeated.

It can be difficult to distinguish berylliosis from sarcoidosis.

Management Corticosteroids are given to try and prevent disease progression. Continue indefinitely on the lowest dose which maintains symptom control, as few patients gain complete resolution of symptoms, CXR, or PFTs. Other immunosuppressants have been tried, but evidence limited. Annual screening of beryllium-exposed workers with CXR. If they develop breathlessness or skin rashes, this may be an indication to start oral steroids to delay progression to interstitial fibrosis. Avoid further beryllium exposure once evidence of berylliosis occurs and possibly when evidence of sensitization.

Prognosis Progressive disease, although those with very low exposure who develop CXR changes may find they resolve. Associated delayed skin sensitivity (anergy) to tuberculin. Granulomata do not spontaneously resolve although can be excised if causing problems such as troublesome lesions on the skin. Interstitial fibrosis occurs in the lungs, which is progressive and leads to cyanosis and death. Other complications include pneumothorax, hypercalcaemia, hypercalciuria, and nephrocalcinosis.

Differential diagnosis
- Sarcoidosis
- TB.

In clinic
- Ask patients with suspected sarcoidosis about possible exposure to beryllium
- Monitor PFTs and CXR to assess disease response or progression.

Pneumothorax

Clinical features and investigations

Definition A pneumothorax is air in the pleural space. May occur with apparently normal lungs (1° pneumothorax) or in the presence of underlying lung disease (2° pneumothorax). May occur spontaneously or following trauma.

Epidemiology

- Annual incidence of 1° pneumothorax is around 9 per 100,000
- 1° pneumothoraces occur most commonly in tall thin men aged between 20 and 40. They are less common in women (♂:♀ ≈ 5:1)—consider the possibility of underlying lung disease (e.g. LAM, catamenial pneumothorax)
- Cigarette or cannabis smoking is a major risk factor for pneumothorax, increasing the risk by a factor of 22 in men and 9 in women. The mechanism is unclear; a smoking-induced influx of inflammatory cells may both break down elastic lung fibres (causing bulla formation) and cause small airways obstruction (increasing alveolar pressure and the likelihood of interstitial air leak)
- More common in patients with Marfan's syndrome and homocystinuria
- May rarely be familial (Birt–Hogg–Dubé syndrome; autosomal dominant mutation in folliculin gene (Chr 17); causes renal and skin tumours and pulmonary cysts).

Causes and pathophysiology

1°

Pathogenesis is poorly understood; pneumothoraces are presumed to occur following an air leak from apical subpleural blebs and bullae, although small airway inflammation is often also present and may contribute by increasing airways resistance, causing 'emphysema-like changes' (ELC).

2°

- Underlying diseases include: COPD (60% of cases), asthma, ILD, necrotizing pneumonia, TB, PCP, CF, LCH, LAM, Marfan's syndrome, oesophageal rupture, lung cancer, catamenial pneumothorax, and pulmonary infarction
- Pneumothorax may be the first presentation of the underlying disease.

Clinical features

- Classically presents with acute onset of pleuritic chest pain and/or breathlessness. Breathlessness is often minimal in young patients and is more severe in 2° pneumothorax
- Signs of pneumothorax include tachycardia, hyperinflation, reduced expansion, hyperresonant percussion note, and quiet breath sounds on the pneumothorax side. These are frequently absent in small pneumothoraces. Hamman's sign refers to a 'click' on auscultation in time with the heart sounds, due to movement of pleural surfaces with a left-sided pneumothorax

- May feel 'bubbles' and 'crackles' under the skin of the torso and neck if there is subcutaneous emphysema
- Presents in ventilated patients with acute clinical deterioration and hypoxia or increasing inflation pressures.

Investigations

- *CXR* is the diagnostic test in most cases, revealing a visible lung edge and absent lung markings peripherally. Blunting of the ipsilateral costophrenic angle due to low-volume bleeding into the pleural space is seen. Pneumothoraces are difficult to visualize on supine films: look for a sharply delineated heart border, hemidiaphragm and costophrenic angle depression ('deep sulcus sign'), and increased lucency on the affected side
  - Width of the rim of air surrounding the lung on CXR may be used to classify pneumothoraces into small (rim of air measured at level of hilum ≤2cm) and large (>2cm). A 2cm rim of air approximately equates to a 50% pneumothorax in volume
  - Tiny pneumothoraces that are not apparent on PA CXR may be visible on lateral chest or lateral decubitus radiographs
  - CXR appearance may also show features of underlying lung disease, although this can be difficult to assess in the presence of a large pneumothorax
- *CT chest* may be required to differentiate pneumothorax from bullous disease and is useful in diagnosing unsuspected pneumothorax following trauma and in looking for evidence of underlying lung disease
- *ABGs* frequently show hypoxia and sometimes hypercapnia in 2° pneumothorax.

Prognosis

- Untreated, pneumothoraces without an ongoing air leak resolve at rate of ~2% of volume of hemithorax every 24h
- Average of 30% (range 16–54% in studies) of 1° pneumothoraces recur, most within 2y. Continued smoking increases the risk of recurrence. Risk of recurrence increases with each subsequent pneumothorax; risk of recurrence is around 30% after a first pneumothorax, about 40% after a second, and >50% after a third
- Mortality of 2° pneumothorax is 10%
- Recurrence of 2° pneumothorax occurs in 39–47% and is associated with age, pulmonary fibrosis, and emphysema. Recurrence rates may be as high as 80% in patients with LCH or LAM.

Further information

Sahn SA, Heffner JE. Spontaneous pneumothorax. *N Engl J Med* 2000;**342**:868–74.

Initial management

There is considerable variation amongst clinicians regarding optimal pneumothorax management. The treatment algorithm presented on ➲ p. 378 (see Fig. 37.1) is taken from the BTS guidelines.

General management points

- Determine whether the pneumothorax is 1° or 2° (known lung disease/ evidence of lung disease clinically or age >50 with significant smoking history)
- Management is determined by degree of breathlessness and hypoxia, evidence of haemodynamic compromise, presence and severity of any underlying lung disease, and, to a lesser extent, CXR pneumothorax size
- Severe breathlessness out of proportion to pneumothorax size on a prior CXR may be a feature of impending tension pneumothorax
- 2° pneumothorax has a significant mortality (10%) and should be managed more aggressively. Treat also the underlying disease.

Aspiration

- Procedure described on ➲ pp. 786–7
- Halt the procedure if painful or if the patient coughs excessively; do not aspirate >1.5L of air, as this suggests a large air leak and aspiration is likely to fail
- Aspiration is successful if the lung is fully or nearly re-expanded on CXR and patient feels symptomatically better with improved physiology
- If initial aspiration of a 1° pneumothorax fails, a chest drain is likely to be required if benefits outweigh risks.

Chest drainage

- Procedure described on ➲ pp. 764–5
- Associated with significant morbidity and even mortality, and not required in the majority of patients with 1° spontaneous pneumothorax
- Small (10–14F) drains are sufficient in most cases; consider large-bore (24–28F) drain in 2° pneumothorax with large air leak, severe subcutaneous emphysema, or in mechanically ventilated patients
- Never clamp a bubbling chest drain (risk of tension pneumothorax)
- When air leak appears to have ceased, clamping of the drain for several hours followed by repeat CXR may detect very slow or intermittent air leaks, thereby avoiding inappropriate drain removal; this is controversial, however, and should only be considered on a specialist ward with experienced nursing staff. Addition of washing-up liquid to water in underwater seal bottle aids visualization of bubbling in very slow air leaks
- If water level in drain does not swing with respiration, the drain is either kinked (check underneath dressing as tube enters skin), blocked, clamped, or incorrectly positioned (drainage holes not in pleural space; check CXR)

- Heimlich flutter valves (or thoracic vents) are an alternative to underwater bottle drainage and are being used increasingly in some centres. They allow greater patient mobilization and sometimes outpatient management of pneumothorax.

O_2

All hospitalized patients should receive high-flow (10L/min) inspired O_2 (unless CO_2 retention is a problem). This reduces the partial pressure of nitrogen in blood, encouraging removal of air from the pleural space and speeding up resolution of the pneumothorax.

Persistent air leak

- Arbitrarily defined as continued bubbling of chest drain 48h after insertion
- Consider drain suction (–10 to –20cmH$_2$O), insertion of large-bore drain, and/or thoracic surgical referral
- Check that persistent bubbling is not the result of 'outside' air being sucked down the drain, e.g. following drain displacement such that a hole lies outside the pleural cavity, or if enlargement of the drain track occurs, allowing outside air to enter and then be aspirated down the drain.

Discharge

Prior to discharge, discuss flying and diving (see pp. 241 and 244 respectively), and advise to return to hospital immediately if breathlessness worsens. Document this in medical notes.

Further management

Outpatient follow-up

- Repeat CXR to ensure resolution of pneumothorax and normal appearance of underlying lungs
- Discuss risk of recurrence, and emphasize smoking cessation, if appropriate
- Ascent to altitude with a pneumothorax is potentially hazardous. Guidelines recommend that patients should not fly for at least 1 week from the resolution of spontaneous pneumothorax on CXR. This time interval is arbitrary, however, and patients should understand that there is a high initial risk of recurrence that falls with time, and they may wish to avoid flying for a longer period, e.g. 1y
- Advise never to dive in the future, unless patient has undergone a definitive surgical procedure.

Surgical management

Indications for cardiothoracic surgical referral
- Second ipsilateral pneumothorax
- First contralateral pneumothorax
- Bilateral spontaneous pneumothorax
- Persistent air leak or failure of lung to re-expand (3–5 days of drainage)
- Spontaneous haemothorax
- Professions at risk (e.g. pilots, divers) after first pneumothorax.

Note that these are guidelines only, and patient choice will of course also influence the decision for surgical intervention.

Surgical treatments aim to repair the apical hole or bleb and close the pleural space. Options:
- *VATS* Recurrence rates are higher than for open thoracotomy (4% vs 1.5%) although less invasive procedure and shorter hospital stay. Apical blebs/bullae are stapled, and mechanical pleural abrasion and/or parietal pleurectomy (rather than talc poudrage) is usually favoured for closure of the pleural space. Often the procedure of choice in young patients with 1° pneumothorax
- *Open thoracotomy* Same range of operative interventions undertaken as for VATS but associated with longer recovery (albeit with marginally lower recurrence rates)
- *Transaxillary mini-thoracotomy* uses a relatively small axillary incision and may be a less invasive alternative to open thoracotomy.

Chemical pleurodesis

- Talc or tetracycline most commonly used (although difficulties obtaining tetracycline); procedure described on ➋ pp. 786–7
- Can be performed via intercostal drain or at VATS
- Failure rates around 10–20% and some concern about the long-term safety of intrapleural talc; therefore not recommended in younger patients

- Consider pleurodesis via intercostal drain only as a last resort in older patients with recurrent pneumothorax in whom surgery would be high risk (e.g. patients with severe COPD)
- Likelihood of successful pleurodesis in the setting of an incompletely re-expanded lung with a persistent air leak remains uncertain, although it may be attempted if surgery is not an option.

Algorithm for treatment of spontaneous pneumothorax

Fig. 37.1 is an adapted version of the BTS guidance for treatment of a spontaneous pneumothorax.

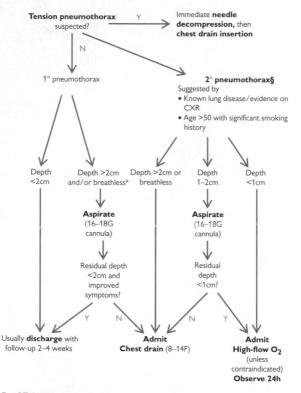

Fig. 37.1 BTS treatment algorithm for spontaneous pneumothorax.

* Disagreement exists regarding this point; in the setting of a relatively asymptomatic patient with a large 1° pneumothorax and no adverse physiology, there may be no justification for intervention. Indeed, the risk of intervention may well outweigh the risk of the pneumothorax, and conservative management is preferable.

§ In our opinion, breathlessness and the degree of physiological compromise are much more important in guiding management than absolute pneumothorax size on CXR. For example, it may be appropriate to insert a CT-guided chest drain in a patient with a <1cm 2° pneumothorax who is particularly compromised while, conversely, an asymptomatic patient with >2cm 2° pneumothorax may be best managed conservatively.

Further information

MacDuff A *et al.* Management of spontaneous pneumothorax: British Thoracic Society pleural disease guideline 2010. *Thorax* 2010;**65**(Suppl. 2):ii18–31.

Specific situations

Tension pneumothorax

- Pneumothorax acts as a one-way valve, with air entering the pleural space on each inspiration and unable to escape on expiration. The progressive increase in pleural pressure compresses both lungs and mediastinum and inhibits venous return to the heart, leading to hypotension and potentially cardiac arrest
- Occurrence is not related to pneumothorax size, and tension can occur with very small pneumothoraces in the context of air trapping in the lung from obstructive lung disease
- Typically presents with acute respiratory distress, agitation, hypotension, raised JVP, and tracheal deviation away from the pneumothorax side. Reduced air entry on affected side
- May present with cardiac arrest (pulseless electrical activity) or with acute deterioration in ventilated patients.

See Box 37.1.

> ▶▶ **Box 37.1 Management of a tension pneumothorax**
> - If strong clinical suspicion, give high-flow O_2 and insert large-bore cannula into second intercostal space in mid-clavicular line on side of pneumothorax
> - Do not wait for a CXR if patient seriously compromised or cardiac arrest has occurred
> - Do not wait for a CXR if the diagnosis is clinically certain
> - Hiss of escaping air confirms diagnosis
> - Aspirate air until the patient is less distressed, and then insert chest drain in safe triangle (see ➲ p. 764), leaving cannula in place until finished and the underwater seal is bubbling satisfactorily.

Iatrogenic pneumothorax

- Causes include TBB, transthoracic needle lung biopsy, subclavian line insertion, mechanical ventilation, pleural aspiration, pleural biopsy, external cardiac massage, and percutaneous liver biopsy
- Presentation may be delayed, even several days after procedure
- Most cases do not require intervention and improve with observation, although aspiration is sometimes required
- Drainage is seldom needed although is more commonly required in patients with COPD. The exception is mechanically ventilated patients, who will require an intercostal drain in the majority of cases.

Traumatic pneumothorax

- Up to half may not be clinically apparent or visible on CXR; chest CT is required for diagnosis
- Majority of patients require intercostal drain. Ensure adequate analgesia; intercostal nerve block may be required
- Consider VATS early if persistent air leak.

Subcutaneous (or 'surgical') emphysema
- Occurs as air tracks below skin under pressure from the pleural space
- May result from large air leaks, particularly in the presence of underlying lung disease such as COPD. Also may occur if chest drain is blocked or displaced so that holes lie subcutaneously
- Harmless in majority of cases although rarely may result in significant respiratory compromise from upper airway compression
- Treat with high-flow (10L/min) inspired O_2 (unless CO_2 retention a problem). Check that the drain is patent (swinging, bubbling)
- Management if unwell: O_2, large-bore chest drain on suction. If the airway is compromised, consider anaesthetizing and incising areas of affected skin, and 'milking' out subcutaneous air; subcutaneous drains are sometimes used, and, in rare cases, tracheostomy is required.

Pneumothorax in pregnancy
- Increased risk of pneumothorax recurrence during pregnancy
- Standard 1° pneumothorax treatment is usually effective, but close liaison with obstetricians and thoracic surgeons
- Elective assisted delivery (forceps/ventouse) near term with epidural anaesthesia is advocated
- Consider VATS after pregnancy.

Pneumothorax in HIV
- Most commonly occurs as a result of PCP. Empirical treatment of PCP is advised (see ➜ pp. 474–5)
- Use of nebulized pentamidine may increase the risk of pneumothorax
- Consider early intercostal drainage and surgical referral.

Pneumothorax in CF
- See ➜ p. 224.

Catamenial pneumothorax
- Pneumothorax occurring at the same time as menstruation
- Usually recurrent
- Pathogenesis is unknown; possibilities include pleural endometriosis or transfer of air into pleural spaces through a diaphragmatic defect from the peritoneal cavity at menstruation
- Treatment options: VATS, pleurodesis, ovulation-suppressing drugs.

Re-expansion pulmonary oedema
- Occurs in up to 14% of cases following treatment and causes breathlessness and cough, with evidence of oedema in the re-expanded lung (and sometimes both lungs) on CXR
- More common in young patients with large 1° pneumothoraces and may be associated with late presentations to hospital
- May be precipitated by early use of suction (<48h)
- Self-resolving in most cases although may rarely be fatal.

Further information
MacDuff A *et al.* Management of spontaneous pneumothorax: British Thoracic Society pleural disease guideline 2010. *Thorax* 2010;**65**(Suppl. 2):ii18–31.

Chapter 38

Pulmonary hypertension

Pulmonary hypertension

Definition PHT is a haemodynamic and pathophysiological state that can be found in multiple clinical conditions (see Box 38.1). It is defined as a mean PAP ≥25mmHg at rest, as assessed by RHC. In clinical groups 1, 3, 4, and 5, the pulmonary capillary wedge pressure is normal at ≤15mmHg. In group 2, this is raised. Resting PHT is significant, as >70% of the vascular bed must be lost for the PAP to rise. Normal resting PAP is around 14mmHg.

Pathophysiology Each group has differing characteristic pathological features, but vasoconstriction, remodelling of the pulmonary vessel wall, medial hypertrophy of distal pulmonary arteries ± fibrotic change and thrombosis lead to raised pulmonary vascular resistance and ultimately right heart failure. An imbalance between NO and prostacyclin (a potent vasodilator and platelet inhibitor) and thromboxane A2 (a potent vasoconstrictor and platelet agonist) has been identified in PAH. Unfavourable imbalances between other regulators of vascular tone and smooth muscle cell growth, including endothelin-1, NO, and serotonin, have also been implicated.

Presenting features The symptoms of PHT are primarily due to RV dysfunction. The symptoms are non-specific, often leading to a delay in diagnosis from first symptoms.
- Exertional breathlessness, due to the inability to increase cardiac output with exercise. WHO functional assessment classification used to quantify; see Box 38.2.
- Chest pain (right heart angina)
- Fatigue and weakness
- Syncope or pre-syncope, due to a fall in systemic BP on exercise
- Palpitations
- Peripheral oedema and other signs of right-sided fluid overload.

Examination Signs of right heart fluid overload and RVH are associated with advanced disease and include:
- RV heave, RV third sound
- Wide splitting of S2 with loud P2
- Pansystolic murmur of TR, diastolic murmur of pulmonary insufficiency
- Raised JVP, with giant V waves
- Hepatomegaly, ascites, peripheral oedema
- Cyanosis
- Possible telangiectasia, digital ulceration, and sclerodactyly in PHT associated with scleroderma
- Stigmata of chronic liver disease with portal hypertension
- Clubbing suggests ILD or congenital heart disease
- Lungs normally clear, unless underlying ILD in association with connective tissue disease or if pulmonary oedema associated with pulmonary veno-occlusive disease.

Box 38.1 Updated clinical classification of PH (Dana Point 2008)

1. PAH

1.1 Idiopathic
1.2 Heritable
    1.2.1 BMPR2 (bone morphogenetic protein receptor, type 2)
    1.2.2 ALK1 (activin receptor-like kinase 1 gene), endoglin (with or without HHT)
    1.2.3 Unknown
1.3 Drug- and toxin-induced
1.4 Associated with (APAH)
    1.4.1 Connective tissue diseases
    1.4.2 HIV infection
    1.4.3 Portal hypertension
    1.4.4 Congenital heart disease
    1.4.5 Schistosomiasis
    1.4.6 Chronic haemolytic anaemia
1.5 Persistent PH of the newborn

1'. Pulmonary veno-occlusive disease and/or pulmonary capillary haemangiomatosis

2. PH due to left heart disease

2.1 Systolic dysfunction
2.2 Diastolic dysfunction
2.3 Valvular disease

3. PH due to lung diseases and/or hypoxia

3.1 COPD
3.2 ILD
3.3 Other pulmonary diseases with mixed restrictive and obstructive pattern
3.4 Sleep-disordered breathing
3.5 Alveolar hypoventilation disorders
3.6 Chronic exposure to high altitude
3.7 Developmental abnormalities

4. Chronic thromboembolic PH (CTEPH)

5. PH with unclear and/or multifactorial mechanisms

5.1 Haematological disorders: myeloproliferative disorders, splenectomy.
5.2 Systemic disorders: sarcoidosis, pulmonary LCH, LAM, neurofibromatosis, vasculitis
5.3 Metabolic disorders: glycogen storage disease, Gaucher's disease, thyroid disorders
5.4 Others: tumoural obstruction, fibrosing mediastinitis, chronic renal failure on dialysis

Updated clinical classification of pulmonary hypertension. *J Am Coll Cardiol* 2009;54:S43–S54.

PHT: investigations

The investigations aim to make a diagnosis of PHT and investigate any possible underlying cause (see Box 38.1). In 85% of patients presenting with symptoms caused by established PHT, a CXR and ECG will be abnormal.

- *CXR* may show enlarged pulmonary arteries and an enlarged cardiac silhouette, with pruning (loss) of peripheral vessels
- *ECG* Right atrial dilatation, RAD, RVH and strain
- *ABG* Slight hypoxia and hypocapnia (correlating with disease severity), with a fall in O_2 saturation on exercise
- *PFTs* The lung volumes may be normal or show a mild restrictive or obstructive defect with a reduced TLCO (late in the disease course). Abnormal if PHT due to underlying lung disease
- *HRCT chest* to exclude underlying lung disease
- *V/Q scanning/CTPA* to exclude chronic thromboembolic disease as a cause. V/Q is more sensitive than CTPA. Normal or low probability V/Q scan effectively excludes CTEPH
- *Echo* The most useful screening tool in PHT. Typically shows enlargement of right-sided cardiac chambers, with paradoxical interventricular septum movement and TR. The systolic PAP can be estimated from the peak velocity of the tricuspid regurgitant jet, using Doppler techniques, and the estimated right atrial pressure from the IVC (assumed to be 5–10mmHg). Pericardial effusions may be present and represent worse prognosis. Bubble echo can help to exclude an intracardiac shunt and also increases the Doppler signal, allowing easier measurement of peak TR velocity
- *Cardiac MRI* to evaluate RV size, morphology, and function
- *Abdominal USS* if liver cirrhosis/portal hypertension suspected
- *RHC* The 'gold standard' test to confirm the diagnosis, assess the PAP, pulmonary capillary wedge pressure, and cardiac output (with a Swann–Ganz catheter, by thermodilution or Fick). Also can exclude a left-to-right intracardiac shunt. *Vasodilator responsiveness* is measured with incremental doses of a short-acting vasodilator such as inhaled NO or IV epoprostenol or adenosine. A positive vasodilator response is defined as a drop in mean PAP by >10mmHg to <40mmHg, with an unchanged or increased cardiac output. Only about 5–10% of patients are responders
- *6MWT* for objective assessment of exercise capacity. Walking distances of <300m and O_2 desaturation of >10% indicate worse prognosis in PAH. Increase in 6MWT distance following treatment often used in assessment and in trials but may not be best outcome measure for PHT subgroups
- *CPET* (see ➔ p. 880) O_2 uptake at the anaerobic threshold and peak exercise are reduced in relation to disease severity
- *Selective pulmonary angiography* is rarely required, as CTPA and V/Q can detect nearly all cases of thromboembolic disease
- *Blood tests* Routine tests, including HIV test, TSH, ACE, autoantibodies (anti-centromere antibody, anti Scl-70, and RNP) if connective tissue disease suspected; thrombophilia screen in CTEPH
- *BNP/NT-proBNP plasma levels* If elevated, associated with worse prognosis in PAH.

A **National Pulmonary Hypertension Service** was established in the UK in 2001 to coordinate diagnosis and treatment in five regional centres, recognizing the need to provide best care (with complex interventions) and optimize funding for expensive treatments. The five UK centres are:
- London—Hammersmith Hospital (general)
  - Royal Brompton Hospital (adult congenital heart disease)
  - Royal Free Hospital (connective tissue disease)
  - Great Ormond Street Hospital for Children (children)
- Cambridge—Papworth Hospital
- Sheffield—Royal Hallamshire Hospital
- Newcastle—Freeman Hospital
- Glasgow—Western Infirmary, Scottish Pulmonary Vascular Unit, Golden Jubilee National Hospital.

Recent guidelines suggest referral to a specialist centre after CXR, ECG, simple spirometry, and echo (but not cardiac catheterization, as this should be done in parallel with a vasodilator study in a specialist centre).

PH centre will: confirm/refine diagnosis, assess severity and prognosis, plan treatment, review progress 3–6-monthly, with appropriate investigations repeated, and gather data for national database to facilitate audit and research.

Recommendations on the management of pulmonary hypertension in clinical practice. *Heart* 2001;**86**:S1.

Box 38.2 WHO functional assessment classification in PAH (modified from NYHA heart failure classification)

Class I Patients with PH but without resulting limitation of physical activity.

Class II Patients with PH resulting in slight limitation of physical activity. They are comfortable at rest. Ordinary physical activity does not cause undue dyspnoea or fatigue, chest pain, or near syncope.

Class III Patients with PH resulting in marked limitation of physical activity. They are comfortable at rest. Less than ordinary physical activity causes undue dyspnoea or fatigue, chest pain, or near syncope.

Class IV Patients with PH with inability to carry out any physical activity without symptoms. These patients manifest signs of right heart failure. Dyspnoea and/or fatigue may even be present at rest. Discomfort is increased by any physical activity.

Reproduced from Galiè N et al. Guidelines for the diagnosis and treatment of pulmonary hypertension. *Eur Heart J* 2009;**30**:2493–537, with permission from OUP.

PHT: features of clinical groups 1

1. PAH

Pathological lesions affect the distal pulmonary arteries, with medial hypertrophy, intimal proliferative and fibrotic changes, adventitial thickening with moderate perivascular inflammatory infiltrates, and thrombotic lesions. Pulmonary veins are unaffected.

1.1 Idiopathic The incidence of IPAH in Europe and the USA is 1–2 cases per million population per year. The mean age at diagnosis is 36, with a ♀ preponderance of about 2:1. Although rare, it is important to diagnose, as it affects a young age group and has an extremely poor outcome without treatment

1.2 Heritable A familial predisposition is seen in 6–10% of IPAH cases where the disease is transmitted in an autosomal dominant fashion. Incomplete penetrance and anticipation are seen, with presentation at a younger age in successive generations. The responsible gene has been localized to Chr 2 (locus 2q 31–32). Abnormal cardiovascular responses to exercise have been demonstrated in asymptomatic carriers of BMPR2.

1.2.1 Bone morphogenetic protein receptor type II (BMPR2) is a receptor in the transforming growth factor beta (TGF-β) receptor superfamily and is an important regulator of apoptosis and proliferation. The identification of a mutation in BMPR2, present in 70% of familial PAH, has improved understanding. It is hypothesized that defective signalling in this pathway may result in abnormal endothelial proliferation and cell growth in response to various insults, with an inability to terminate the proliferative response to injury. Due to incomplete disease penetrance in the presence of a mutation in BMPR2 (15–20%), it is thought that the genetic abnormality may have to be accompanied by some additional environmental factor, e.g. hypoxia, to cause PAH.

1.2.2 ALK1, endoglin (with or without HHT) PAH occurs in around 15% of patients with HHT, an autosomal dominant vascular dysplasia. Mutations in the ALK1 receptor (also in the TGF-β receptor superfamily) are implicated.

1.2.3 Unknown

1.3 Drug- and toxin-induced Damage to the pulmonary artery endothelium can be caused by drugs, e.g. Aminorex, fenfluramine, dexfenfluramine, toxic rapeseed oil, benfluorex, amphetamines, methamphetamines, L-tryptophan, cocaine, phenylpropanolamine, St John's Wort, chemotherapeutic agents, selective serotonin reuptake inhibitors, pergolide. A careful history must be taken. PHT can develop within 4 weeks of starting the drug, with increasing incidence with longer use.

1.4 Associated with (APAH) Conditions which have a similar clinical presentation to IPAH, with identical histological findings. This group accounts for about half the patients looked after in specialist centres.

1.4.1 Connective tissue diseases PAH develops in about 15% of patients with systemic sclerosis and is most frequently seen as an isolated phenomenon in patients with limited cutaneous disease. Also occurs 2° to ILD, with a very poor prognosis. Life expectancy is <1y in patients with systemic sclerosis, isolated PHT, and a gas transfer of <25% of normal. Patients with systemic sclerosis should be screened annually with echo for PHT, even if no symptoms are present. Obliteration of the alveolar capillaries and arteriolar narrowing are induced by both the 1° vascular disease and any interstitial fibrosis. Other connective tissue diseases, including RA, SLE, Sjögren's syndrome, dermatomyositis, can also lead to 2° PHT. There is a strong association with Raynaud's phenomenon, and a ♀ predominance is seen. Immunosuppressive therapy can improve PAH associated with SLE or mixed connective tissue disease.

1.4.2 HIV infection PAH is found in up to 1 in 200 HIV-positive people, more common in men and IVDUs. The incidence is about 0.1%, 6–12 times higher than the general population. The development of PAH is independent of CD4 cell count but is associated with duration of infection. The mechanism is unclear. It is hypothesized that HIV-infected macrophages release vasoactive cytokines that lead to endothelial damage and proliferation.

1.4.3 Portal hypertension PAH is seen in up to 5% of patients with portal hypertension of whatever cause, increasing with duration of liver disease. Porto-pulmonary hypertension is probably due to the failure of the liver to remove vasoactive substances from the portal circulation, with their resultant accumulation and presentation to the pulmonary arterial endothelium (see ❷ p. 250).

1.4.4 Congenital heart disease Pressure overload caused by systemic to pulmonary shunts. Includes large defects (Eisenmenger's syndrome), moderate to large defects, small defects (small ventricular and atrial septal defects). Detailed subclassifications available, based on clinical and anatomical-pathophysiological features, allow individual patients to be better defined.

1.4.5 Schistosomiasis Portal hypertension along with local vascular inflammation caused by *Schistosoma* eggs.

1.4.6 Chronic haemolytic anaemia, such as sickle cell disease, thalassaemia, hereditary spherocytosis, stomatocytosis, and microangiopathic haemolytic anaemia, may result in PAH. The mechanism is related to a high rate of NO consumption, leading to a state of resistance to NO bioactivity

1.5 Persistent PHT of the newborn

1' Pulmonary veno-occlusive disease and/or pulmonary capillary haemangiomatosis Difficult disorders to classify; share some characteristics with IPAH, but also a number of differences. HRCT helpful in diagnosis; characteristic interstitial oedema with diffuse central ground-glass opacification and thickening of interlobular septa. Possible lymphadenopathy and pleural effusion also. Pulmonary capillary haemangiomatosis suggested by diffuse bilateral thickening of interlobular septa and the presence of small, centrilobular, poorly circumscribed nodular opacities. Biopsy is the gold standard for diagnosis but may not be necessary.

PHT: features of clinical groups 2–5

2. PHT due to left heart disease

3. PHT due to lung diseases and/or hypoxia

The majority of patients with PHT seen by a respiratory specialist will have PHT due to chronic hypoxic lung disease such as COPD. Chronic hypoxia causes pulmonary vasoconstriction and, in the longer term, vascular remodelling. Inflammation, mechanical stress of hyperinflated lungs, loss of capillaries, and toxic effects of cigarette smoke all contribute to the pathophysiological mechanisms. Patients with 'out of proportion' PHT due to underlying lung disease should be referred to a specialist centre—that is dyspnoea insufficiently explained by mechanical disturbances, mean PAP ≥40–45mmHg at rest.

3.1 COPD In this case, the PHT is often an incidental finding in a patient with a chronic respiratory disease.
* A significant proportion of COPD patients will develop PHT, possibly up to 25%. The level of PAP in these patients is much lower than that seen in patients with PAH
* COPD with PHT has a much poorer prognosis than COPD without PHT. In patients with a PAP <25mmHg, the 5y survival is >90%. In those with a PAP >45mmHg, the 5y survival is <10%. Whether this is due to the PHT itself or whether the PHT is a marker of worse hypoxia and disease severity is unclear.

PHT in COPD was thought to be due to hypoxia and emphysematous destruction of the vascular bed, but neither of these factors correlates well with PAP. Cigarette smoke may have a direct effect on the intrapulmonary vessels, with the upregulation of mediators leading to aberrant vascular structural remodelling and physiological changes in vascular function

3.2 ILD

3.3 Other pulmonary diseases with mixed restrictive and obstructive pattern

3.4 Sleep-disordered breathing with the obesity hypoventilation syndrome, not just OSA (see ➔ p. 576).

3.5 Alveolar hypoventilation disorders, e.g. due to neuromuscular disease. Both alveolar hypoxia and hypercapnia produce pulmonary vasoconstriction, thereby increasing PAPs.

3.6 Chronic exposure to high altitude

3.7 Developmental abnormalities

4. CTEPH is a frequent cause of PHT, with both proximal and distal clot. Recent data suggest that CTEPH occurs in up to 4% of cases of acute non-fatal PE, higher than previously thought. Pathogenesis is unclear, but abnormalities in the clotting cascade, endothelial cells, or platelets may all contribute. Natural history of pulmonary thromboemboli is resolution or near-total resolution of clot, with restoration of normal pulmonary haemodynamics within 30 days in 90% of patients. Right-sided pressures

return to normal in most patients by 2 weeks. In CTEPH, thromboemboli do not resolve, forming endothelialized fibrotic obstructions of the pulmonary vascular bed. *In situ* thrombosis and vascular remodelling of small distal pulmonary arteries also contribute. Peripheral PAH-like arteriopathic changes are also seen in the distal pulmonary arteries in non-obstructed areas. Collateral vessels from bronchial, intercostal, diaphragmatic, and coronary arteries can develop to partially reperfuse areas distal to complete obstruction. The clinical deterioration parallels the loss of RV functional capacity. Risk factors for CTEPH include increasing age, idiopathic PE, and a larger perfusion defect. Splenectomy is associated possibly by inducing a pro-thrombotic state due to loss of filtering function of the spleen. Antiphospholipid antibodies are present in 10–20% of patients. The diagnosis is not usually made until advanced PHT is present. Progressive PHT seems to result from changes in the small peripheral resistance vessels in the vascular bed, as opposed to being due to progressive pulmonary events. 2° hypertensive changes, probably induced by high PAPs, lead to incremental increases in RV afterload, with increasing PHT, ultimately leading to RV failure. Patients with CTEPH have a 5y survival of <10% if the PAP >50mmHg. CTPA helps determine whether there is any surgically accessible CTEPH.

5. PHT with unclear and/or multifactorial mechanisms
Heterogeneous conditions with different pathological pictures; aetiology unclear or multifactorial.

5.1 Haematological disorders: myeloproliferative disorders, splenectomy

5.2 Systemic disorders: sarcoidosis, pulmonary LCH, LAM, neurofibromatosis, vasculitis

5.3 Metabolic disorders: glycogen storage disease, Gaucher's disease, thyroid disorders

5.4 Others: tumoural obstruction, fibrosing mediastinitis, chronic renal failure on dialysis

PHT management 1: disease-targeted drug therapy

Calcium channel blockers (CCBs)

- Vasoresponders at RHC should be considered for therapy with CCBs. They should not be used in those with a negative vasodilator challenge, as they may increase mortality
- Only a small number of patients with IPAH and vasodilator response at RHC do well with CCBs. High-dose nifedipine (120–240mg daily) and diltiazem (240–720mg daily) are recommended in patients with IPAH with a positive vasodilator response. They should then be followed closely to determine if they are long-term CCB responders, with repeat RHC after 3–4 months of treatment. If their response is inadequate, further PAH therapy should be started
- Vasodilator responsiveness does not predict a favourable long-term response to CCB therapy in patients with APAH and connective tissue disease; high-dose CCBs are often not well tolerated in these patients
- Amlodipine has more selective vasodilating properties and, at doses of up to 20mg daily, may be useful in those intolerant of the other agents or if RV function is impaired
- Calcium antagonists should be started in hospital and titrated with careful monitoring
- Verapamil is not used, because of its negative inotropic effects
- Side effects include hypotension and oedema, which may limit use.

Phosphodiesterase type-5 inhibitors (PDE-5), e.g. sildenafil and tadalafil. Augment the vasodilatory effects of NO, causing pulmonary vasodilatation, and improve exercise capacity and haemodynamics in PAH in patients in functional classes II and III. Common side effects: headache, flushing, epistaxis, nasal congestion

- *Sildenafil* is taken orally tds and has proven benefits in IPAH, APAH with connective tissue disease, congenital heart disease, and CTEPH
- *Tadalafil* oral, once a day.

Prostanoids Prostacylin is produced predominantly by endothelial cells and is a potent vasodilator. It inhibits platelet aggregation and has antiproliferative and cytoprotective properties. Side effects include headache, jaw pain, diarrhoea, flushing, nausea, and arthralgia and are usually dose-related. Prostaglandin treatment doubles the time on the lung transplantation waiting list and improves transplantation outcomes. Improved haemodynamics may lead to some patients coming off transplant waiting lists. Tolerance develops to IV prostaglandin therapy, with increasing dose requirements over time. The mechanism for this is unclear.

- *Epoprostenol* A synthetic prostacyclin analogue potent vasodilator, acting via increasing intracellular cAMP. It is the only drug shown to improve survival in IPAH in RCTs. It probably has its effects as a selective pulmonary vasodilator and potentially through vascular remodelling and platelet adhesion. It also improves symptoms, exercise capacity, and haemodynamics in IPAH and PAH associated with scleroderma. It is inactive in the circulation after 5min and given therefore by continuous IV infusion via a portable pump and tunnelled central venous catheter. Pump failure can be life-threatening

- *Treprostinil* is a prostacyclin analogue that can be given as a continuous subcutaneous or IV infusion, as it has greater *in vivo* stability than epoprostenol. It improves symptoms, exercise capacity, and pulmonary haemodynamics. Pain at the subcutaneous infusion site is the major side effect. Due to its current pricing structure, treprostinil is not routinely prescribed for new patients
- *Iloprost* is a prostacyclin analogue and is more potent than epoprostenol. It has a half-life of 25min and can be given by continuous IV infusion or nebulizer (6–9 times a day). Side effects: headache, cough, mild diarrhoea, and nausea.

Endothelin receptor antagonists (ERA) Endothelin is a powerful vasoconstrictor and pro-inflammatory mediator and causes smooth muscle cell proliferation. Plasma levels raised in some forms of PHT.

- *Bosentan* is an oral endothelin receptor A and B antagonist that has been shown to improve exercise capacity, haemodynamics, functional class, and time to clinical worsening in patients with IPAH, APAH with connective tissue disease, and Eisenmenger's syndrome. It was the first oral therapy approved for the treatment of PHT. 3y survival for a cohort of mainly WHO functional class III patients starting on bosentan was >85%. The major side effect is reversible liver transaminitis, causing discontinuation in ~3%. LFTs should be monitored monthly during treatment. Other side effects include headache and peripheral oedema
- *Ambrisentan* is a selective type A blocker, with a better liver safety profile. Improvements in symptoms, exercise capacity, haemodynamics, and time to clinical worsening in patients with IPAH and APAH with HIV and connective tissue disease.

Current practice There are very clear nationally agreed guidelines on starting treatment for PHT. Disease-targeted drug therapies should only be commenced by a designated specialist PHT centre. Non-specialist clinicians should not routinely prescribe these therapies. Use CCBs in vasodilator responders, but only continue if there is a sustained response. Otherwise— *first-line therapy:* start monotherapy with PDE inhibitor. If this is not clinically appropriate, an endothelin receptor antagonist may be substituted. *Second-line therapy:* patients who have failed to respond to a trial of therapy of adequate dose and duration (typically 8–12 weeks) or failed to tolerate one of the oral therapies should be switched to an alternative oral product as monotherapy. Patients who have initially responded to first-line therapy but then deteriorated despite dose escalation may be considered for dual therapy. Patients with a suboptimal response to first-line therapy may be considered for dual therapy. *Dual therapy:* for patients with progressive disease who have failed to respond to first- and second-line monotherapy or who have initially responded to monotherapy but subsequently deteriorated despite dose escalation or who have had a suboptimal response to monotherapy. *Triple therapy:* only for patients who have been accepted as suitable for transplant.

PHT management 2: general and surgical

General management

- *Anticoagulation* All patients with PHT are at risk of VTE and *in situ* pulmonary arterial thrombosis and therefore should be considered for lifelong warfarin. A small thrombus can have catastrophic effects in a patient who is already severely compromised. Studies show an increased survival with warfarin in PHT, which may reflect reversal of an underlying pro-thrombotic state, as well as the prevention of *in situ* thrombus formation. Additional beneficial effects are seen when combined with a vasodilator
- *Long-term O_2* Hypoxaemia is due to reduced cardiac output, V/Q mismatching, and right-to-left shunting through a patent foramen ovale. Added O_2 may reduce any further rise in PAP resulting from additional hypoxic pulmonary vasoconstriction. Supplemental O_2 should achieve a pO_2 of >8kPa during rest, exercise, and sleep
- *Diuretics and digoxin* Diuretics may be useful for the treatment of oedema, but excess pre-load reduction may limit their usefulness. Digoxin has been shown to improve cardiac output acutely in IPAH, though its longer-term effects are not known
- *Treatment of arrhythmias*
- *Immunization* Annual influenza and one-off pneumococcal vaccination
- *Contraception* may be required, as pregnancy is poorly tolerated in IPAH, with a 30–50% mortality.

Surgical treatments

- *Pulmonary thromboendarterectomy* is the treatment of choice in CTEPH for proximal obstructive disease. This is the surgical removal of organized thrombotic material and aims to strip away the pulmonary arterial endothelium, starting proximally and extending out to remove all clot in the subsegmental levels. It is done on cardiopulmonary bypass with circulatory arrest. The PAP usually falls within 48h of surgery. Operative mortality is <10% in experienced hands. Longer-term effects are not known
- *Atrial septostomy* Creation of a right-to-left shunt by balloon atrial septostomy aims to increase systemic blood flow by bypassing the pulmonary circulation, particularly in patients with syncope or severe right heart failure. It is a palliative procedure and can be used for symptom control prior to transplantation, with the defect being closed at the time of transplant. Also used in people receiving prostanoid therapy having syncope. Arterial desaturation occurs following the procedure but is normally offset by the increased cardiac output seen with increased O_2 delivery. It is not indicated in severe left heart failure or in patients with impaired LV function

- *Transplantation* Improves survival and QoL in patients with PHT. In those with preserved LV function, lung transplant is the procedure of choice. Return of normal RV function is found after transplantation. As for all diseases needing transplantation, timing of referral and operation is crucial, as organ availability is limited. The incidence of obliterative bronchiolitis appears to be higher post-transplantation for PHT than in transplantation for other diseases, although the reason for this is uncertain.

Prognosis in PHT is variable, depending on functional class, haemodynamic compromise with cardiac index, right atrial pressure, and prognosis is linked to mean PAP at presentation. The clinical course is one of progressive deterioration with episodes of acute decompensation. The median survival in NYHA functional class III (symptomatic on mild exertion) is 2.8y and 6 months in NYHA class IV (symptomatic at rest) without treatment.

End-of-life care Palliative care by an MDT may be warranted to improve symptoms such as fatigue, breathlessness, abdominal bloating, nausea, and pain (see ➔ pp. 724–5).

Future developments A number of agents are currently being investigated, including inhaled treprostinil, riociguat, a soluble guanylate cyclase stimulator, and drugs with antiproliferative effects such as simvastatin, imatinib, and sirolimus.

Further information

Guidelines for the diagnosis and treatment of pulmonary hypertension. *Eur Heart J* 2009;**30**:2493–537.

Consensus statement on the management of pulmonary hypertension in clinical practice in the UK and Ireland. *Thorax* 2008;**63**(Suppl II):ii1–41.

Recommendations on the management of pulmonary hypertension in clinical practice. *Heart* 2001;**86**(S1):i1–13.

Kiely DG *et al*. Pulmonary hypertension: diagnosis and management. *BMJ* 2013;**346**:f2028.

Diagnosis and management of pulmonary arterial hypertension: ACCP evidence-based clinical practice guidelines. *Chest* 2004;**126**(suppl).

Pulmonary arterial hypertension. *N Engl J Med* 2004;**351**:1655–65.

Treatment of pulmonary arterial hypertension. *N Engl J Med* 2004;**351**:1425–36.

Patient group. ℘ http://www.phassociation.uk.com and ℘ http://www.phassociation.com

Pulmonary thromboembolic disease

Epidemiology and pathophysiology

Definition A pulmonary embolism (PE) is an obstruction of part of, or the entire, pulmonary vascular tree, usually caused by thrombus from a distant site.

Epidemiology

- The overall annual incidence is 60–70/100,000, with a UK annual death rate of 100/million. The estimated overall population incidence of DVT is 0.5 per 1,000 person years
- PE may account for up to 15% of all post-operative deaths. It is the commonest cause of death following elective surgery, and the commonest cause of maternal death
- Post-mortem studies have consistently shown a frequency of 7–9%, and large inpatient studies have shown a frequency of around 1%, with a mortality of 0.2%. The mortality is much higher in patients with serious underlying comorbid disease
- The incidence is likely to be stable, but improved diagnostic methods mean that it is probably reported more frequently.

Pathophysiology

- 75% of thrombi are generated in the deep venous system of the lower limbs and pelvis, probably initiated by platelet aggregation around venous valve sinuses. Activation of the clotting cascade leads to thrombus formation, with Virchow's triad (venous stasis, injury to the vessel wall, and increased blood coagulability) predisposing to thrombus formation. Venous stasis is increased by immobility and dehydration. In addition, coagulation factors may be altered in various disease states, e.g. in the acute phase response, malignancy, and autoimmune disease
- 20% of leg thrombi embolize, with a higher incidence in above than below knee clots. Large clots may lodge at the bifurcation of the main pulmonary arteries, causing haemodynamic compromise. Smaller clots will travel more distally, infarcting the lung and causing pleuritic pain. These are more commonly multiple and bilateral and are found most often in the lower lobes where blood flow is greatest
- Thrombi can also develop in the right heart following MI
- Paradoxical emboli start within the venous system and enter the arterial circulation, usually via a patent foramen ovale (causing right-to-left shunt). They typically present with features of cerebral ischaemia and these should be considered as the cause for a cerebrovascular event in the young
- Septic emboli are found in endocarditis, in association with intraventricular septal defects/AV shunts or central venous access.

Haemodynamic effects of PE depend on the size of the clot and which area of the pulmonary vascular tree it subsequently obstructs, as well as the pre-existing state of the myocardium.

- As the pulmonary vasculature in a healthy lung has a large capacitance, the mean PAP does not rise until at least 50% of the vascular bed has been occluded
- As the PAP rises, RV afterload increases, with a resulting increase in RV end diastolic pressure. The RV will start to fail as the PAP reaches over 40mmHg *acutely*
- This causes a reduction in pulmonary blood flow, leading to reduced LV filling and a reduction in systemic BP
- Adequate blood volume for right-sided heart filling is vital. The 2° effects are much worse if right-sided filling cannot be maintained, e.g. if the patient is dehydrated, hypovolaemic, or erect
- Arterial hypoxia results from several factors: reduced cardiac output, consequently a low mixed venous PaO_2, a higher perfusion to the remaining alveoli, resulting in inadequate oxygenation of this blood
- Hypoxia will be worse if there is a larger premorbid V/Q spread, e.g. in the elderly and in those with pre-existing lung disease. The increased blood flow, with a lower mixed venous PaO_2 passing through low V/Q areas, overwhelms their oxygenating ability. It is therefore possible for a young person with healthy lungs to have a normal PaO_2 and A–a gradient following a significant PE
- Death is due to circulatory collapse from the inability of the right heart to acutely maintain an adequate cardiac output.

Aetiology

Risk factors can be divided into major and minor factors (see Table 39.1). This division is important for an assessment of clinical probability.

Table 39.1 Risk factors for VTE

Major risk factors (relative risk × 5–20)	
Surgery	Major abdominal/pelvic surgery
	Orthopaedic surgery (especially lower limb)
	Post-operative intensive care
Obstetrics	Pregnancy (higher incidence with multiple births)
	Caesarean section
	Pre-eclampsia
Malignancy	Pelvic/abdominal
	Metastatic/advanced
Lower limb problems	Fracture, varicose veins
Reduced mobility	Hospitalization
	Institutional care
	Long haul flight
Previous proven VTE	
Minor risk factors (relative risk × 2–4)	
Cardiovascular	Congenital heart disease
	CCF
	Hypertension
	Central venous access
	Superficial venous thrombosis
Oestrogens	Oral contraceptive pill (OCP) (especially third-generation higher oestrogen-containing)
	Hormone replacement therapy (HRT)
Miscellaneous	Occult malignancy
	Neurological disability
	Thrombotic disorders
	Obesity
	IBD
	Nephrotic syndrome
	Dialysis
	Myeloproliferative disorders
	Behçet's disease

Risk of malignancy Occult cancer will be present in 7–12% of patients presenting with idiopathic VTE. New NICE guidance (2012) recommends considering further investigations for cancer with an abdomino-pelvic CT and a mammogram for women in all those aged >40 with a first episode of unprovoked PE or DVT. No studies so far show that this strategy leads to a reduction in cancer-related mortality.

Inherited thrombophilias

- 25–50% of patients with VTE have an identifiable inherited thrombophilia, e.g. antiphospholipid syndrome, deficiency of antithrombin III, a prothrombin gene defect, protein C or protein S deficiency
- These usually need to interact with an additional acquired risk factor to cause VTE
- Factor V Leiden is present in 5% of the population and 20% of patients presenting with thrombosis
- Current recommendations do not advocate routine screening for inheritable thrombophilias, unless in specific circumstances (see further text on thrombophilia testing), as the number needed to test to prevent an episode of VTE would be very high. In addition, detecting a heritable thrombophilia does not predict a significantly higher rate or earlier occurrence of VTE in the absence of a 2° risk factor.

Consider thrombophilia testing in:
- Patients with recurrent venous thrombosis
- Patients <40 with venous thrombosis with no obvious risk factors
- Thrombosis 2° to pregnancy, OCP, HRT
- Thrombosis at an unusual site—cerebral, mesenteric, portal, or hepatic veins
- Do not offer testing in those continuing lifelong anticoagulation or in those with provoked clot.

All, but factor V Leiden deficiency and the prothrombin gene mutation, need to be tested for when the patient is *off* anticoagulants.

'Economy class syndrome' refers to thromboembolic disease associated with long-distance sedentary travel, with an increasing incidence of disease with increasing distance travelled. A 2001 study of >135 million passengers showed an incidence of PE of 1.5 cases/million for travel over 5,000km, compared with 0.01 cases/million for travel under 5,000km. For travel over 10,000km, the incidence increased to 4.8 cases/million.

Clinical features

Acute PE typically presents in four main ways.
- *Pulmonary infarction and haemoptysis* ± pleuritic pain. ABGs may be normal and ECG changes uncommon. Localizing signs may be present, e.g. pleural rub
- *Isolated dyspnoea* (in 25%) Defined as acute breathlessness in the absence of haemorrhage or circulatory collapse. The thrombus is more likely to be central, with hypoxia on blood gases. The patient may have sudden-onset and unexplained breathlessness, in the presence of risk factors for VTE. There may also be angina from increased right heart work and inadequate O_2 delivery to its muscle
- *Collapse, poor reserve* (in 10%) May be due to a small PE, often in an elderly patient with limited cardiorespiratory reserve. These patients can rapidly decompensate with even a relatively small PE. The clinical findings may be non-specific and reflect more the underlying disease process and thus fail to arouse suspicion of a PE
- *Circulatory collapse in a previously well patient* Hypotension ± loss of consciousness in 1%. Usually due to extensive pulmonary artery occlusion from massive PE, causing marked hypoxia and hypocapnia (due to hyperventilation) and acute right heart failure, with chest pain due to right heart angina, raised JVP, and fainting on sitting up. ECG may be normal, show sinus tachycardia or right heart strain. Echo shows PHT and RV failure. These patients have the highest mortality, up to 30%.

Chronic thromboembolic disease This typically presents with more insidious onset of breathlessness over the course of weeks to months due to increasing load of recurrent small-volume clots (see ➲ pp. 390–1).

Dyspnoea and tachypnoea (RR >20) are the commonest presenting features and are absent in only 10% of patients.

Remember to consider PE in the differential diagnosis of:
- Unexplained SOB
- Collapse
- New-onset AF
- Signs consistent with acute right heart failure
- Pleural effusion.

Examination of a patient with PE
- May be normal
- Tachycardia and tachypnoea are common
- AF
- Reduced chest movement (due to pain)
- Pleural rub
- Classically loud P2 and splitting of the second heart sound, with a gallop rhythm (acute right heart strain)

- Hypoxia (with hypocapnia due to hyperventilation, and an increased A–a gradient), *but* PaO_2 may be in the normal range in young healthy individuals
- Low-grade fever
- Signs of DVT (common, in around 25%)
- Acute right heart failure—low cardiac output and raised JVP, with reduced BP and perfusion pressure
- Deterioration in cardiac output on sitting up, when filling pressure falls.

Diagnosis of acute PE

The diagnosis of a PE can be difficult and involves a clinical assessment of probability. This takes risk factors, clinical presentation, and clinical signs into account. Investigations are then performed, that may add weight to the clinical decision, rather than being stand-alone diagnostic tests. Therefore, the estimation of the pre-test clinical probability of DVT and PE is of vital importance in interpreting the results of the tests performed.

Pre-test clinical probability scoring systems
(See Tables 39.2 and 39.3.)

Table 39.2 Wells' score for DVT

Clinical feature	Score
Active cancer (treatment ongoing, within 6 months, or palliative)	1
Paralysis, paresis, or recent plaster immobilization of the lower extremities	1
Recently bedridden for 3 days or more or major surgery within 12 weeks requiring general or regional anaesthesia	1
Localized tenderness along the distribution of the deep venous system	1
Entire leg swollen	1
Calf swelling at least 3cm larger than asymptomatic side	1
Pitting oedema confined to the symptomatic leg	1
Collateral superficial veins (non-varicose)	1
Previously documented DVT	1
An alternative diagnosis is at least as likely as DVT	−2
Likelihood of DVT	
DVT *likely*	≥2 points
DVT *unlikely*	≤1 point

Local alternative scoring systems may be in place.
  These scoring systems should always be used with the D-dimer result.

D-dimer has an important role in diagnosing and excluding PE and should only be used with a pre-test clinical probability assessment following careful clinical evaluation by an experienced clinician. D-dimers are sensitive for DVT and thromboembolism but not specific. They are rarely in the normal range in cases of acute thromboembolism but are not a valid screening test for PE alone. D-dimers are generated as a result of fibrinolysis, which occurs in many clinical situations, including sepsis, post-surgery, pneumonia, neoplasia, inflammatory disease, pregnancy, and advanced age.
• Only a normal result (which virtually excludes PE) is of clinical value

- An abnormal result (however high) does not necessarily imply a significantly increased probability of PE
- The sensitivity ranges from 87% to 99%, depending on the assay used; these should be known before incorporating into diagnostic algorithms
- D-dimer testing for excluding PE has been validated as an outpatient test but not in inpatient groups.

Assessment and documentation of pre-test clinical probability in PE is paramount. This enables accurate clinical assessment and may obviate the need for imaging.

An alternative explanation for the symptoms should be sought when a PE is excluded.

Table 39.3 Wells' score for PE

Clinical feature	Score
Clinical signs and symptoms of DVT (minimum of leg swelling and pain with palpation of the deep veins)	3
An alternative diagnosis is less likely than PE	3
HR >100bpm	1.5
Immobilization for >3 days or surgery in the previous 4 weeks	1.5
Previous DVT or PE	1.5
Haemoptysis	1
Malignancy (on treatment, treated in the past 6 months, or palliative)	1
Likelihood of PE	
PE *likely*	>4 points
PE *unlikely*	≤4 points

Investigations

- *ECG* Non-specific changes are frequent. Most commonly, sinus tachycardia. AF, RBBB, anterior T-wave inversion (indicating RV strain) are common. The $S_1Q_3T_3$ pattern is uncommon
- *CXR* A good-quality departmental CXR is required. No specific features are characteristic in PE, but it may reveal another pathology. Small effusions are present in 40% (80% are exudates, 20% transudates). Focal infiltrates, segmental collapse, and a raised hemidiaphragm can also occur
- *ABG* may be normal, especially in the young and healthy. Hypoxia and hypocapnia, due to hyperventilation, with an increased A–a gradient are more common
- *D-dimer* (see ➜ pp. 404–5)
- *Brain natriuretic peptide* (BNP) levels in acute PE reflect severity of RV strain and haemodynamic compromise, providing additional prognostic information to that of echo
- Elevated *cardiac troponin* levels are associated with worse short-term prognosis in acute PE. Heart-type fatty acid-binding protein (H-FABP), an early marker of myocardial injury, is reported to be superior to troponin or myoglobin measurements for risk stratification of PE on admission. There are currently no universally accepted criteria for the measurement of myocardial injury in acute PE
- *CTPA* is the gold standard investigation and is recommended as the initial imaging technique in suspected non-massive PE. It has a sensitivity of >95% and may enable an alternative diagnosis to be made if PE is excluded. Advances in imaging mean that a 16-slice multi-detector row scanner can image the entire chest with resolution approaching 1mm, requiring a breath-hold of <10s. Emboli can be detected in sixth-order pulmonary vessels, which are so small that their clinical relevance is uncertain. CTPA should be performed within 1h in suspected massive PE and within 24h of suspected non-massive PE. The sensitivity and specificity of CTPA depends on the location of the emboli, with lower sensitivity for clot confined to the segmental or subsegmental pulmonary vessels, compared with more central clot. CTPA needs specialist reporting.

In those with a high clinical probability, but negative CTPA, the options are:
- PE has been excluded; stop anticoagulation, or
- Perform further imaging (leg US, conventional pulmonary angiogram, venous phase CT to include the legs).

In one large prospective multicentre study, with all patients investigated with CTPA and leg US, those with negative tests and low or intermediate clinical probability were not anticoagulated. Only 0.2% had a definite PE after 3 months of follow-up. Those with negative tests, but high clinical probability, were investigated further, and PE was identified in 5% (Musset D *et al. Lancet* 2002;**360**:1914).

A volume of 100–150mL contrast media is required for CTPA, which poses a substantial risk of nephropathy (in patients with renal insufficiency and diabetes) and sometimes fluid overload (patients with impaired LV function). In these patients, leg US and/or isotope lung scanning might be safer first-line investigations.

- *Isotope lung scanning* (V/Q scan)—mostly now superseded by CTPA. Some units may just perform the Q (perfusion) part of the scan. May be useful as a first-line imaging investigation in patients with a normal CXR and with no concurrent cardiopulmonary disease, in whom a negative scan can reliably exclude a PE. Scans are reported as low, intermediate, or high probability, and the report's meaning must be interpreted in light of the pre-test clinical probability score. Further imaging is necessary for those in whom:
  - The scan is indeterminate
  - There is a discordant scan result and clinical probability.

The clinical significance of the V/Q scan report is:

- Normal = no PE
- Low or intermediate pre-test clinical probability *plus* low probability scan = PE excluded
- High pre-test clinical probability *plus* high probability scan = PE diagnosed
- Any other = need further imaging.

Other imaging techniques

- *Leg US* Around 70% of patients with a proven PE have a proximal DVT; hence, leg imaging can be used as an alternative to lung imaging in those with clinical DVT. A single examination is not adequate to exclude subclinical DVT (venography is more sensitive). It is safe to withhold anticoagulation in patients with suspected DVT and a single negative leg US, but these data cannot yet be extrapolated to those presenting with suspected PE. If a leg US is positive in a patient with clinical features of PE, this excludes the need for further imaging. Up to 50% of patients with a clinically obvious DVT will have a high-probability V/Q scan
- *Conventional pulmonary angiogram* is available in a few specialist centres only where catheter fragmentation of large clots may be of therapeutic benefit. Now mostly superseded by CTPA
- *CT venography* is an emerging area. It can be combined with CTPA to image the pelvic leg veins simultaneously
- *Echo* is diagnostic in submassive and massive PE. The transoesophageal route is more sensitive, enabling visualization of intrapulmonary and intracardiac clot. Gives prognostic information and aids risk stratification
- *Transthoracic US* is used uncommonly. May show peripheral infarcts with peripheral PEs.

Treatment

Risk stratification

The PE severity index (PESI score; see Table 39.4) allows stratification of immediate risk following PE, dividing patients into high risk and non-high risk, and clearly defines a low-risk population suitable for outpatient management.

* *High-risk PE* Shock or hypotension, with positive biomarkers of RV dysfunction, is a life-threatening emergency and has a mortality of >15%
* *Non-high-risk PE* can be stratified with the use of cardiac biomarkers of RV dysfunction or myocardial injury into intermediate- (one or more positive markers but no shock, mortality 3–15%, requires in-hospital management) and low-risk PE (negative markers, mortality <1%).

Echocardiographic features of RV dysfunction occur in up to 25% of all patients with PE and are associated with a 2-fold increased risk of death. There is no agreed definition of the echo features of RV dysfunction.

Table 39.4 PESI score*

Clinical feature	Score
Age—add 1 point per year of age	Age
♂ patient	10
History of cancer	30
History of heart failure	10
History of chronic lung disease	10
HR ≥110	20
Systolic BP <100mmHg	30
RR ≥30/min	20
Temperature <36°C	20
Altered mental status? (disoriented, lethargy, stupor, or coma)	60
SaO₂ on room air <90%	20
≤65 Class 1 Very low risk	
66–85 Class 2 Low risk	
86–105 Class 3 Intermediate risk	
106–125 Class 4 High risk	
>125 Class 5 Very high risk	

* Predicts 30-day outcome of patients with PE (Aujesky D et al. Am J Respir Crit Care Med 2005;**172**:1041).

LMWH is as effective as standard unfractionated IV heparin and should be given to patients with intermediate or a high pre-test clinical probability immediately, prior to imaging.

Unfractionated heparin should be considered in massive PE (faster onset of action); first dose bolus prior to commencement of LMWH. Renal impairment (eGFR <30); use either unfractionated heparin or LMWH with anti-factor Xa monitoring. Use unfractionated heparin if risk of bleeding.

Oral anticoagulation should only be commenced once PE is proven, after initial heparin treatment. Target INR 2.0–3.0 (heparin can be stopped after 5 days or once INR >2). Some centres now advocate outpatient antico-agulation for PE as well as DVT. Recent data suggest that this is as safe as inpatient anticoagulation in a carefully selected population in centres with a well-established outpatient DVT service.

Length of warfarin anticoagulation
- Temporary provoking risk factor: 3 months
- First episode of idiopathic PE—review anticoagulation at 3 months. Discuss with patient, including consideration of risk of bleeding and risk of recurrence. Some advocate 6 months' treatment or lifelong treatment—in which case this decision should be reviewed annually, as the relative risks and benefits of anticoagulation may change
- For patients with active cancer—6 months of LMWH before a decision as to whether to continue with a vitamin K antagonist (VKA) long term
- Recurrent idiopathic PE—no guidelines exist; length of treatment depends on individual circumstances, with risk of bleeding balanced with risk of recurrent event, and often long-term anticoagulation
- Persisting risk factors: lifelong anticoagulation may be recommended
- New direct thrombin inhibitors, e.g. dabigatran, and factor Xa inhibitors, e.g. rivaroxaban (predictable dose response curves and no need for laboratory monitoring), are now licensed for PE treatment.

Side effects
- The risk of bleeding increases with age and concurrent illness
- Higher bleeding rate with concomitant aspirin use and previous GI bleed
- Risk of bleeding relates to duration and intensity of anticoagulation.

Thrombolysis There is emerging evidence to support the use of throm-bolysis in certain subgroups of patients with PE; however, this is a contro-versial area, and the risk/benefit analysis of this treatment must always be carefully considered.

Massive PE causing circulatory collapse (systolic BP <90mmHg or a pressure drop of 40mmHg with no other explanation). Current NICE guidance (2012) recommends unfractionated heparin and subsequent sys-temic thrombolysis. In practice, thrombolysis is usually given to the acutely unwell/peri-arrest patient, when the history and physical findings are suggestive of massive PE, in the absence of another reasonable explana-tion. There is rarely time for imaging or investigations in this situation. See Box 39.1.

▶▶ Box 39.1 Management of acute massive PE

Acute massive PE has a mortality of 20%; involve senior colleagues early, and arrange transfer of the patient to a critical care area.

- O_2—100%, via non-rebreathe mask
- IV access. Send baseline bloods, including clotting. Perform ECG
- Analgesia, if required; consider opiates
- Management of cardiogenic shock—fluids and inotropes may be required in submassive or massive PE to maintain RV filling
- Start IV heparin unless active GI bleeding or intracerebral haemorrhage:
  - Bolus dose 5,000–10,000U or 80IU/kg
  - Maintenance infusion of 1,300IU/h or 18U/kg/h
  - Adjust infusion rate until APTT is 1.5–2.5× control. Check APTT 4–6h after initial bolus and 6–10h after any dose change. When APTT is in the therapeutic range, check it daily
- Investigation to confirm PE depends on the clinical state of patient. Ideally perform urgent echo, and, if this is non-diagnostic, perform a CTPA but not delaying for >1h. It may, however, be unwise to move a sick patient to the radiology department for a CTPA. If there is circulatory collapse and the patient is peri-arrest and PE is the most likely cause, confirmation of the diagnosis should not be sought but treatment prioritized. Remember aortic dissection, cardiac tamponade, and acute MI can mimic PE
- Thrombolysis if collapsed or hypotensive, if no active GI bleeding or intracerebral haemorrhage:
  - Alteplase 100mg over 2h, given peripherally, or
  - Streptokinase 250,000U in 30min, with 100,000U/h for 24h (plus hydrocortisone to prevent further circulatory instability), or
  - Urokinase 4,400IU/kg in 10min and 4,400IU/kg/h for 12h
  - Stop the heparin during thrombolysis, and restart afterwards
  - In cardiac arrest due to suspected massive PE, 50mg IV alteplase immediately may be lifesaving
- Consider liaising with cardiothoracic centre to consider embolectomy, particularly if thrombolysis is contraindicated or has failed.

Non-massive PE is more controversial. Most would only recommend thrombolysis for patients with clinically massive PE. Increasing evidence suggests that individuals with a large clot volume, in the absence of haemodynamic compromise, have better clinical outcomes with thrombolysis. This is due to the prevention of chronic thromboembolic disease, as larger clot volume is a risk factor for this. More data are required.

Contraindications None absolute; rarely a consideration in the life-threatening situation. Risk of major haemorrhage is 3–4 times that of heparin (around 13% in large studies), with a higher incidence of bleeding in the elderly. Active bleeding or recent intracerebral bleed are contraindications.

Embolectomy Rarely done, and only in life-threatening massive PE. Options include surgical embolectomy (few regional centres only) and mechanical clot fragmentation via RHC.

IVC filter placement There is little evidence to show improved survival or reduction in recurrent PE rate with IVC filters, and changing to LMWH may be as effective. They are potentially pro-thrombotic and should be removed as soon as possible once no longer required. IVC filters may be indicated in:

- Acute VTE in patients with an absolute contraindication to anticoagulation
- Patients with recent massive PE who survive (a second PE may be fatal)
- Recurrent VTE despite adequate anticoagulation
- Post-pulmonary thromboendarterectomy in PHT.

Further information

Konstantinides S et al. Heparin plus alteplase compared with heparin alone in patients with submassisve pulmonary embolism. *N Engl J Med* 2002;**347**:1143–50.

Torbicki A et al. European Society of Cardiology acute PE guidelines. *Eur Heart J* 2008;**29**:2276–315. http://eurheartj.oxfordjournals.org/content/29/18/2276.full.pdf+html.

Special circumstances

Pregnancy and thromboembolic disease

- The incidence of DVT ± PE in pregnancy is 1 in 1,000, rising to 2 in 1,000 in the puerperium. The risk of PE in pregnancy is greater with increasing maternal age and with increasing gestational age. More PEs occur during pregnancy than after delivery. There is a 20–30 times increased risk with Caesarean section, compared with normal vaginal delivery. PE is one of the commonest causes of maternal death in pregnancy (1/100,000 pregnancies)
- D-dimers are raised in the normal pregnancy and so are unhelpful in the investigation of thromboembolic disease, unless negative
- The CTPA whole body radiation dose is 2–4mGy, with an absorbed dose to the foetus of 0.01mSv. This equates to a risk of fatal cancer to age 15 of <1 in 1 million. The absorbed dose to the breast is 10mSv (higher in pregnancy). CTPA increases the lifetime breast cancer risk in premenopausal women from 10% to 11.4%, with an even higher risk in pregnancy
- The V/Q scan whole body radiation dose is 1.5–2mGy, with an absorbed dose to the foetus of 0.12mSv. This equates to a risk of fatal cancer to age 15 of 1 in 280,000. The absorbed dose to the breast is 0.28mSv
- The overall radiation risk depends on the gestation of the foetus and the metabolic activity of the pregnant breast tissue. There is considerable debate as to which imaging technique is best in pregnancy, in terms of radiation risk to both the mother (including breast tissue) and the foetus. The lowest overall risk favours a Q scan as the first-line investigation, especially as this young healthy population are likely to have normal lungs. Some experts suggest a leg US first (see ➔ p. 407)
- In those with antenatal thromboembolic disease, LMWH is used. Close to delivery, this is changed to unfractionated heparin, as it is easier to monitor and to reverse its effects. It is unclear whether heparin should be stopped or the dose reduced at the time of delivery. LMWH levels can be monitored with anti-Xa levels
- There are case reports of successful thrombolysis, catheter-directed thrombolysis, and embolectomy in massive PE, but no relevant trials
- Warfarin is teratogenic and is contraindicated in pregnancy, although it is safe in breastfeeding
- Anticoagulation should be continued for 6 weeks after delivery or 3 months following the initial episode, whichever is longer.

Thromboembolic disease and the OCP/HRT

- Oestrogen-containing OCPs, pregnancy, and HRT increase the risk of PE, but the incidence of fatal PE is low—estimated at 1/100,000 OCP users, with a median age of 29
- Risk of fatal PE is twice as high in those taking third-generation pills
- Previous history of DVT or PE is a contraindication to the OCP
- Meta-analyses show a relative risk of VTE of 2.1 in HRT users, which is highest in the first year of use.

Flight prophylaxis for thromboembolic disease

- For patients with high risk of a PE, i.e. previous VTE, within 6 weeks of surgery, or current malignancy, the 1997 BTS guidelines recommend low-dose aspirin, LMWH, or formal anticoagulation (INR 2–3) prior to flying
- For those with moderate or low risk, graduated or compression stockings, with or without pre-flight aspirin, is suggested.

Future developments

Low-intensity warfarin therapy A reduced target INR of 1.5–2.0 may be used. A study of a cohort of patients treated for up to 4.3y, following 6 months of standard warfarin therapy for idiopathic VTE, led to a 48% reduction in recurrent VTE, major haemorrhage, or death, compared with placebo (Ridker PM *et al. N Engl J Med* 2003;**348**:1425).

Further information

NICE Guidance GC144 June 2012. Venous thromboembolic diseases: the management of venous thromboembolic diseases and the role of thrombophilia testing. ℘ http://www.nice.org.uk/nicemedia/live/13767/59711/59711.pdf and summary in *BMJ* 2012;**345**:43–5.

Kaeron *et al. Chest* 2012;**141**(2)Suppl:e419S–e494S.

Goldhaber SZ. Seminar: pulmonary embolism. *Lancet* 2004;**363**:1295–305.

Rare causes

Air embolism Air within the arterial or venous circulation. Small amounts of air can be tolerated, but large amounts can lodge in the pulmonary vasculature and cause mechanical obstruction and death. This is rare.

Causes Neck vein cannulation, intrauterine manipulations (such as criminal abortion where a frothy liquid is passed under pressure into the uterus), bronchial trauma, or barotrauma causing air to enter the pulmonary vein and left heart. Air in the LV causes impairment to venous filling and subsequent poor coronary perfusion as air enters the coronary arteries.

Diagnosis Arterial air emboli may cause dizziness, loss of consciousness, and convulsions. Air may be seen in the retinal arteries or from transected vessels. *Venous* air emboli may cause raised venous pressure, cyanosis, hypotension, tachycardia, syncope, and a 'mill-wheel' murmur over the praecordium.

Treatment Patients should lie on their right side, with head down and feet up, to allow air to collect and stay at the cardiac apex. From here, it can be aspirated via thoracotomy.

Amniotic fluid embolism is estimated to occur in 1 in 25,000–80,000 live births. It is the third commonest cause of maternal death, and the most common cause of death in the immediate post-partum period. Usually catastrophic, 80% of women die, 20–50% of these in the first hour. An anaphylactic-type response to amniotic fluid entering the circulation is seen. Amniotic fluid enters the circulation because of torn foetal membranes, which can occur in Caesarean section, uterine or cervical trauma, or uterine rupture. It has a thromboplastic effect, causing DIC and thrombi to form in pulmonary vessels. Not all women react in this way to amniotic fluid. It is more common in older multiparous mothers, who have had short tumultuous labour, often involving uterine stimulants.

Clinically presents with sudden-onset respiratory distress, hypoxia, bronchospasm, cyanosis, cardiovascular collapse, pulmonary oedema, convulsions, coma, and cardiac arrest. Coagulopathy with intractable uterine bleeding and uterine atony is seen.

Diagnosis is clinical. Foetal debris/cells can be identified in blood sampled from the maternal pulmonary artery, but this is not pathognomonic.

Treatment is supportive, whilst the thrombi clear from the maternal lungs. Maintain the circulation with fluids and inotropes. Respiratory support with O_2 and ventilation may be needed. Correct coagulopathy with fresh frozen plasma and packed cells. Control placental bleeding.

Fat embolism Common pathological finding following long bone fractures. Occurs especially with lower limb fractures—pelvis and femur. Commoner in fractures that have not been immobilized. Can also occur after prosthetic joint replacement, cardiac massage, liver trauma, burns, bone marrow transplant, rapid high-altitude decompression, and liposuction. Generally occurs in the young and previously healthy. Presents 24–72h post-fracture. Marrow fat enters the circulation and lodges in the lungs, causing mechanical obstruction.

Classically presents with hypoxia, coagulopathy, with a transient petechial rash on the neck, axillae, and skinfolds, and neurological disturbance such as confusion, disorientation, or sometimes coma. Stable patients may deteriorate with low-grade fever, petechial rash, hypoxia, and confusion. Jaundice and renal dysfunction are possible.

Diagnosis is usually made clinically in a patient with a lower limb fracture presenting with tachypnoea and hypoxia. Fat globules can be identified in the urine. CXR shows bilateral alveolar infiltrates. ARDS can develop.

Treatment is with early immobilization of fracture, fluid replacement, O_2, and supportive care.

Septic, hydatid, and tumour emboli are also rare causes. Uterine leiomyosarcoma has vascular tropism and can invade the IVC and obstruct the pulmonary arteries. Teratomas can invade the IVC and pulmonary arteries.

Chapter 40

Respiratory infection—bacterial

Community-acquired pneumonia (CAP)

CAP is a common disease, associated with significant morbidity and mortality.

Definition A syndrome of infection that is usually bacterial, with symptoms and signs of consolidation of part(s) of the lung parenchyma. This is different to bronchitis (see ➔ p. 649).

Epidemiology

- CAP is the commonest infectious cause of death and the 6th leading cause of death in the UK and USA (with age-adjusted death rates of between 1 and 24/100,000)
- Up to 42% of UK adults with CAP require hospital admission. Hospital mortality varies between 5% and 12%
- A BTS multicentre UK study showed that 5–10% of patients with CAP require ICU admission
- Mortality is up to 50% in those admitted to ICU
- CAP managed in the community has a mortality of <1%.

Pathophysiology The lung and tracheobronchial tree are usually sterile below the level of the larynx, so an infecting agent must reach this site via a breach in host defences. This may be by micro-aspiration (which occurs in around 45% of healthy individuals overnight), haematogenous spread, direct spread from an adjacent structure, inhalation, or activation of previously dormant infection.

Aetiology See Box 40.1. Broadly similar pathogens are seen in patients managed in the community and in hospital. A single pathogen is identified in 85% of cases. The proportion of cases with >1 pathogen is unknown.

Risk factors for CAP

- *Aspiration* Typically caused by anaerobes and Gram-negative organisms
- *Alcoholism and diabetes* Typically associated with bacteraemic pneumococcal pneumonia. Anaerobes and mixed infections are more common in alcoholics
- *Oral steroids/immunosuppression* Legionella infection may be more common
- *Cigarette smoking* is the strongest independent risk factor for invasive pneumococcal disease in immunocompetent patients
- *COPD* Haemophilus influenzae and Moraxella catarrhalis are more common, and COPD is more common in those with bacterial pneumonia
- *Nursing home residents* have an increased frequency of CAP, with aspiration, Gram-negative organisms, and anaerobes more common than in age-matched elderly people. Haemophilus influenzae is the most common causative organism. Mycoplasma pneumoniae and Legionella are less common.

Box 40.1 Organisms causing CAP

- *Streptococcus pneumoniae* ('pneumococcus')—the most frequently identified organism, commonest in winter, accounting for two-thirds of all cases of bacteraemic pneumonia. Previous epidemics in the UK have been associated with overcrowding, e.g. in prisons—these are now very rare
- *Legionella pneumophilia*—most common in the autumn. 52% are travel-related. Epidemics occur related to water-containing systems in buildings, typically in the Mediterranean
- *Staphylococcus aureus*—commonest in winter months. Coincident influenza infection in 39% of those requiring hospital admission and 50% of those admitted to ICU
- *Influenza*—annual epidemics in the winter months, complicated by pneumonia in 3% of community cases. 10% of those admitted to hospital have coincident *Staphylococcus aureus* infection
- *Mycoplasma pneumoniae*—epidemics occur every 4y in the UK
- *Chlamydophila pneumoniae*—epidemics in the community; whether it has a direct pathogenic role or is an associated infectious agent is not clear
- *Chlamydophila psittaci*—infection acquired from birds and animals, with 20% of cases having a history of bird contact. Human-to-human spread may occur. Uncommon
- *Coxiella burnetii (Q fever)*—epidemics in relation to animal sources (usually sheep), but occupational exposure only present in 8%. Uncommon.

See ➲ p. 459 for zoonotic causes of CAP.

CAP: clinical features

- Fever
- Cough
- Sputum
- SOB
- Pleuritic chest pain
- Non-specific features in the elderly. May present 'off legs' or with confusion, in the absence of fever.

Examination

- Raised RR (may be the only sign in the elderly)
- Tachycardia
- Localizing signs on chest examination. Reduced chest expansion on the affected side, with signs consistent with consolidation (reduced air entry, with bronchial breathing, reduced percussion note, increased vocal resonance) and crackles. A normal chest examination makes the diagnosis unlikely.

Diagnosis of CAP is made on the basis of:

- Symptoms and signs of an acute lower respiratory tract infection
- New focal chest signs
- New radiographic shadowing, for which there is no other explanation
- At least one systemic feature (e.g. sweating, fevers, aches, and pains)
- No other explanation for the illness.

Most helpful in diagnosis

- Fever, pleuritic pain, dyspnoea, and tachypnoea
- Signs on chest examination.

Specific clinical features of pathogens The aetiological agent cannot be accurately predicted from the clinical features alone, although some features are more statistically likely with one pathogen than another. The exception to this is the presence of chest pain or fever (>39°C) in those admitted to ICU, which predicts a higher likelihood of streptococcal pneumonia.

- *Streptococcus pneumoniae* Increasing age, comorbidity (especially cardiovascular), acute onset, high fever, and pleuritic chest pain
- Bacteraemic *Streptococcus pneumoniae* Alcohol, diabetes, COPD, dry or no cough, ♀
- *Legionella* Younger patients, smokers, absence of comorbidity, more severe infection, neurological symptoms, evidence of multi-system disease (e.g. abnormal liver enzymes and raised CK)
- *Mycoplasma pneumoniae* Younger patients, prior antibiotics, less multi-system involvement but extrapulmonary involvement, including haemolysis, cold agglutinins, hepatitis, skin and joint problems
- *Staphylococcus aureus* Recent influenza-like illness
- *Chlamydophila psittaci* Longer duration of symptoms prior to admission, headache

- *Coxiella burnetii* (Q fever) Dry cough, high fever, headache, ♂, animal exposure, e.g. sheep and goats
- *Klebsiella pneumoniae* Low platelet count and leucopenia, ♂.

Rare causes
- *Acinetobacter* Older patients, history of alcoholism, high mortality
- *Streptococcus 'milleri' group* Dental or abdominal source of infection
- *Streptococcus viridans* Aspiration is a risk factor.

CAP: severity assessment

- CAP has a wide range of severity. An assessment of severity enables the most appropriate care to be delivered in the most appropriate clinical setting
- Early identification of patients at high risk of death allows early decisions about hospital admission and possible need for assisted ventilation to be made
- Assessment of disease severity depends on the experience of the clinician; a number of predictive assessment models have been trialled. These severity models should be regarded as adjuncts to clinical assessment, and regular reassessment of the disease is needed.

Poor prognostic factors Those with two or more adverse prognostic factors are at high risk of death and should be managed as for severe CAP.
- *Age* ≥65
- *Coexisting disease* Including cardiac disease, diabetes, COPD, stroke
- *RR* ≥30/min—this is one of the most reliable predictors of disease severity
- *Confusion* Abbreviated mental test score (AMTS) ≤8
- *BP* Systolic ≤90mmHg and/or diastolic ≤60mmHg
- *Hypoxaemia* Respiratory failure, with PaO_2 <8kPa and the need for assisted ventilation, predicts mortality
- *Urea* ≥7mmol/L
- *Albumin* <35g/L
- *WCC* >20 or <4 × 10^9/L are both predictive
- *Radiology* Bilateral or multilobe involvement. In patients admitted to ICU, progression of CXR changes is a poor prognostic marker
- *Microbiology* Positive blood culture, whatever the pathogen isolated.

A commonly used severity assessment score is *CURB-65*, which aims to predict morbidity and mortality in CAP. A CURB-65 derivative CRB-65 does not rely on laboratory blood tests and may be used in the community to help assess which patients require hospital admission. The Pneumonia Severity Index (PSI) is an alternative, which may be more sensitive, but is much more complicated and includes information on comorbid disease and laboratory tests before stratifying patients into five risk classes.

CURB-65 score core factors
- *Confusion* New mental confusion defined as AMTS ≤8 (see Box 40.2)
- *Urea* >7mmol/L
- *RR* Raised ≥30/min
- *BP* Systolic BP <90 and/or diastolic BP ≤60
- *65* Age ≥65.

The presence of the CURB-65 factors correlates with mortality:
- 3–5 factors present gives a mortality of 15–40%, 2 factors 9%, 1 factor 2.1%, and 1.2% in the presence of no factors
- Low risk of death: age <50, no coexisting disease, CURB-65 score 0–1 patients may be suitable for home treatment
- CRB-65 may be used by GPs in the community to help assess patients: a score of 0 suggests patients with a low risk of death who may be appropriately treated in the community; scores of ≥1 should be considered for hospital admission
- Pneumonia severity scores aim to contribute to, rather than supersede, a clinical judgement; they include a potential over-emphasis on age.

Box 40.2 Abbrieviated mental test score (AMTS)
(1 point per question, max = 10)
- Age
- Date of birth
- Time (to nearest hour)
- Year
- Hospital name
- Recognition of two people (e.g. nurse, doctor)
- Recall address
- Date of First World War
- Name of monarch
- Count backwards 20 to 1.

CAP: investigations

General investigations are aimed at confirming the diagnosis, assessing disease severity, guiding appropriate treatment, assessing the presence of underlying disease, enabling identification of complications, and monitoring progress.

- *Oxygenation assessment* Those with an O_2 saturation of <92% on admission or with features of severe pneumonia should have ABGs measured. The inspired O_2 concentration must be documented
- *CXR*
  - Consolidation, most commonly in the lower lobes. Also interstitial infiltrates and cavitation
  - Multilobe involvement, more common in bacteraemic pneumococcal infection
  - Pleural effusion, more common in bacteraemic pneumococcal infection
  - Lymphadenopathy, uncommon, but most likely with *Mycoplasma* infection
  - Multilobe involvement, cavitation, or spontaneous pneumothorax suggest *Staphylococcus aureus* infection
  - Upper lobe preponderance suggests *Klebsiella*
- *CT chest* Unlikely to add additional information. May be useful if the diagnosis is in doubt or the patient is severely ill and failing to respond to treatment in order to exclude abscess formation, empyema, underlying malignancy, or other interstitial disease process
- *Blood tests*
  - FBC—a WCC >15 × 10^9 suggests bacterial (particularly pneumococcal) infection. Counts of >20 or <4 indicate severe infection
  - Deranged renal and liver function tests can be indicative of severe infection or point to the presence of underlying disease. LFTs may be abnormal, particularly with right lower lobe pneumonia. A raised urea is a marker of more severe pneumonia
  - Metabolic acidosis is associated with severe illness
  - CRP may be useful in management, with high levels being a more sensitive marker of infection than the WCC or temperature. Serial measures may be useful in assessing response to treatment.

Microbiological investigations The microbiological cause for CAP is not found in 25–60% of patients and therefore often does not contribute to patient management. Microbiological investigations can help to aid selection of optimal antibiotics, hence limiting antibiotic resistance and the possible problems of *Clostridium difficile*-associated diarrhoea. They also inform public health or infection control teams, aiding in the monitoring of pathogen trends causing CAP over time.

- *Blood cultures* Recommended for all patients with CAP, ideally before antibiotics are started. About 10% of patients with CAP will have positive blood cultures. The early availability of blood culture results (within 24h of admission) improves outcome

- *Sputum culture and sensitivity* Useful for those patients who have failed to improve with empirical antibiotic treatment and in those with non-severe pneumonia admitted to hospital who are expectorating purulent samples and have not received prior antibiotics. Also useful in severe pneumonia. Not routinely recommended for those treated in the community. Sputum examination is recommended for possible TB in those with weight loss, a persistent cough, night sweats, and risk factors for TB, e.g. ethnic origin, social deprivation
- *Pleural fluid* (if present) for M, C, & S and pH to exclude empyema (see ➔ p. 352)
- *Viral and 'atypical' pathogens* In severe CAP only
- *Serological testing* Paired samples (from within 7 days of the onset of the illness, repeated 10–14 days later) should be tested together, in those with severe CAP and in those unresponsive to β-lactam antibiotics. They are unlikely to guide initial treatment though.

Tests for specific pathogens

- *Pneumococcal pneumonia*
  - Urinary antigen has a sensitivity of 100% and specificity of 60–90% for invasive pneumococcal disease, and testing is recommended in all patients with severe CAP
- *Legionnaires' disease* A number of immunological tests exist to aid in the prompt and accurate diagnosis of *Legionella pneumophilia*:
  - Urinary antigen detection is about 80% sensitive and >95% specific for serogroup A, and rapid results can be obtained early. A positive urinary antigen test correlates with subsequent ITU admission
  - Direct immunofluorescence tests (DIFs)—*Legionella pneumophilia* can be detected on bronchial aspirates
  - Culture is 100% specific (sputum, endotracheal aspirate, BAL, pleural fluid, lung)
  - Serology—antibody levels and PCR are also available
- *Mycoplasma pneumoniae*
  - PCR is the method of choice for diagnosis. The complement fixation test (CFT) is the commonest serological assay. Culture of *Mycoplasma pneumoniae* is not generally available
- *Chlamydophila*
  - *Chlamydophila* can be detected using PCR or antigen detection using DIF on respiratory samples or by CFT
- *Others*
  - Influenza A and B, adenovirus, RSV—PCR or serological testing. *Coxiella burnetii* indirect immunofluorescence antibody test.

CAP: management

General management

- *O2* Hypoxia is due to V/Q mismatching, as blood flows through unventilated lung. Aim for O_2 saturation ≥94% (PaO_2 ≥8kPa). If there is severe concomitant COPD, controlled O_2 therapy and close monitoring of blood gases are mandatory. A rising CO_2 in a patient without prior respiratory disease may indicate they are tiring and need respiratory support—discuss with ITU early
- *Non-invasive ventilatory support* A number of studies demonstrate beneficial effects of NIV in severe CAP. However, following initial improvement in physiological parameters, >50% of patients subsequently deteriorate, requiring intubation. A higher initial RR (>30) is associated with failure of NIV support (CPAP or bi-level ventilation). NIV may have a place in the management of severe CAP but should only be used in a high dependency setting, with very close observation
- *Fluids* Assessment of volume status by JVP (with or without central venous access) and BP is paramount. Encourage oral fluids. IV fluids may be needed if volume-depleted and severely unwell. Monitor urine output
- *Analgesia* Paracetamol or NSAIDs initially, if required. Paracetamol also has an antipyretic role
- *Nutrition* Nutritional status is important to the outcome, and nutritional supplements may be of benefit in prolonged illness. Poor nutritional status may increase the risk of acquiring pneumonia
- *Physiotherapy* Airway clearance techniques may be considered in patients having difficulty expectorating sputum
- *VTE prophylaxis.*

Additional treatments

Bronchoscopy May be helpful, especially after intubation on ITU, to suction retained secretions, particularly if these are causing lobar collapse, to obtain further samples for culture, and to exclude an endobronchial abnormality.

Steroids Not recommended for the standard treatment of severe CAP.

Monitoring Temperature, RR, HR, BP, mental status, O_2 saturation, and inspired O_2 concentration should be monitored twice daily, and more often in the severely ill.

ICU admission Those fulfilling criteria for severe CAP on admission or who fail to respond rapidly to treatment should be considered for transfer for close monitoring, either to a HDU or to ICU. Persisting hypoxia (PaO_2 8kPa), acidosis, hypercapnia, hypotension, or depressed conscious level, despite maximal therapy, are indications for assisted ventilation. CPAP may be of benefit whilst awaiting for the arrival of the anaesthetist (although this may just be a more effective way of delivering 100% O_2).

When to discuss patient with CAP with ITU
- Always sooner, rather than later
- Respiratory failure (PaO_2 <8kPa) despite high-flow O_2
- Tiring patient, with a rising CO_2
- Worsening metabolic acidosis, despite antibiotics and optimum fluid management
- Hypotension despite adequate fluid resuscitation.

CAP: antibiotics

- Most antibiotics are used empirically at diagnosis of CAP in the absence of microbiological information. The clinical scenario also guides antibiotic choice such as the addition of anaerobic cover in an alcoholic who has a high chance of aspiration
- Severity assessment guides antibiotic therapy and the method of antibiotic administration (see Table 40.1). When pathogens are identified, consider narrowing antibiotic coverage (see Table 40.2)
- Local protocols and antibiotic resistance patterns may also guide choice
- Liaise closely with microbiologist.

General points

- Early antibiotic administration is associated with an improved outcome
- Antibiotics given before admission can influence the results of subsequent microbiological investigations, but this should not delay antibiotic administration in the community if the patient is unwell
- It is vital there is no delay in the administration of the first antibiotic dose in patients with confirmed CAP. Confirmation of pneumonia with CXR and antibiotic administration should occur within 4h of admission
- *IV antibiotics* will be needed in 30–50% of patients admitted to hospital. Consider IV antibiotics if:
  - Severe pneumonia
  - Loss of swallow reflex
  - Impaired absorption
  - Impaired conscious level
- *Oral antibiotics* should be used in those with community-managed pneumonia or those with non-severe hospital-managed pneumonia, with no other contraindications
- *Panton-Valentine leukocidin-producing Staphylococcus aureus* (PVL-SA) is a rare cause of rapidly progressive necrotizing pneumonia. If strongly suspected, discuss with microbiology and add linezolid, clindamycin, and rifampicin (all IV)
- *Add anaerobic antibiotic cover*, e.g. metronidazole if possible aspiration pneumonia or if suspicion of lung abscess on CXR/CT
- Switch IV to oral antibiotics as soon as possible, usually when a patient has shown clear response to treatment, being apyrexial for 24h
- A switch to oral co-amoxiclav, and not an oral cephalosporin, is recommended after treatment with IV cephalosporin
- For those treated with benzylpenicillin plus levofloxacin, a switch to oral levofloxacin ± oral amoxicillin is recommended.

Length of treatment

There is no evidence to guide treatment length, but consensus suggests:
- 7 days—non-severe, uncomplicated pneumonia
- 7–10 days—severe microbiologically undefined pneumonia
- 14–21 days—if *Legionella*, staphylococcal disease, or Gram-negative enteric bacteria suspected
- Consult local antibiotic guidelines (also see Tables 40.1 and 40.2); concern regarding increasing rates of *Clostridium difficile* has led to reduced antibiotic course length and alternative empirical antibiotic choice in some centres. There is no evidence that any specific antibiotic (other than clindamycin) is more likely to cause *C. difficile* than any other.

Newer fluoroquinolones Moxifloxacin is licensed in the UK for the treatment of CAP. It is not recommended for first-line treatment for CAP for community use, given the current low level of pneumococcal resistance in the UK. Levofloxacin is available in oral and IV preparations and is licensed for severe CAP. Other fluoroquinolones, e.g. gemifloxacin and gatifloxacin, are likely to extend the choice of oral antibiotics for CAP when they are licensed in the UK. The ketolides (e.g. telithromycin) are novel macrolides, with efficacy against penicillin- and erythromycin-resistant pathogens.

Antibiotic resistance Studies suggest that the UK prevalence of penicillin-resistant *S. pneumoniae* is now about 6–8%. Macrolide-resistant organisms may be as high as 12–15%. Worldwide prevalence of pneumococcal resistance to fluoroquinolones is low, at <2%, though this has increased substantially in some countries (e.g. Hong Kong) in recent years (because of the spread of a fluoroquinolone-resistant clone).

Table 40.1 Suggested empirical antibiotics for CAP treatment

	Preferred treatment	Alternative (if intolerant of, or allergic to, preferred treatment)
Community treatment	Amoxicillin 500mg–1g tds PO	Doxycycline 100mg od (after 200mg loading dose) PO or clarithromycin 500mg bd PO
Hospital treatment: low severity (CURB-65 = 0–1)	Amoxicillin 500mg tds PO (or same dose IV if oral treatment impossible)	Doxycycline 100mg od (after 200mg loading dose) PO or clarithromycin 500mg bd PO
Hospital treatment: moderate severity (CURB-65 = 2)	Amoxicillin 500mg–1g tds PO *and* clarithromycin 500mg bd PO If oral treatment impossible: amoxicillin 500mg tds IV *or* benzylpenicillin 1.2g qds IV *and* clarithromycin 500mg bd IV	Doxycycline 100mg od (after 200mg loading dose) PO *or* levofloxacin 500mg od PO *or* moxifloxacin 400mg od PO
Hospital treatment: high severity (CURB-65 = 3–5)	Co-amoxiclav 1.2g tds IV *and* clarithromycin 500mg bd IV (add levofloxacin if *Legionella* strongly suspected)	Benzylpenicillin 1.2g qds IV *and* either levofloxacin 500mg bd IV or ciprofloxacin 400mg bd IV OR Cefuroxime 1.5g tds IV/ cefotaxime 1g tds IV/ ceftriaxone 2g od IV *and* clarithromycin 500mg bd IV (add levofloxacin if *Legionella* strongly suspected)

CAP: treatment failure

A CRP that does not fall by >50% at 3–4 days suggests either treatment failure or the development of a complication such as a lung abscess or empyema.

Causes of failure to improve

- Slow clinical response, particularly in the elderly patient
- Incorrect initial diagnosis:
  - Pulmonary thromboembolic disease
  - Pulmonary oedema
  - Bronchial carcinoma
  - Bronchiectasis
  - Also consider eosinophilic pneumonia, foreign body aspiration, alveolar haemorrhage, COP, vasculitis or connective tissue disease, drug-induced lung disease
  - Review the history, examination, and radiology
  - Consider repeat imaging, e.g. CT chest
- 2° complication:
  - Pulmonary, e.g. parapneumonic effusion (occurs in 36–57%, simple effusions resolve spontaneously, chest drainage for complicated parapneumonic effusions), empyema, abscess formation, ARDS
  - Extrapulmonary, e.g. septicaemia, metastatic infection (e.g. meningitis, endocarditis, septic arthritis), sequelae of initial insult, e.g. renal failure, MI
- Inappropriate antibiotics or unexpected pathogen:
  - Review dose, compliance, and route of administration. Send further microbiological specimens
  - Review microbiological data; exclude less common pathogens, e.g. *Legionella, Mycoplasma*, staphylococcal disease
  - Pathogen may be resistant to common antibiotics; 10% of CAP will have a mixed infection
  - Consider TB, fungal infection
- Impaired immunity
  - Systemic, e.g. hypogammaglobulinaemia, HIV infection, myeloma
  - Local, e.g. bronchiectasis, aspiration, underlying bronchial carcinoma
  - Overwhelming infection.

Table 40.2 Recommended antibiotic treatment of specific causative organisms

Pathogen	Preferred antibiotic	Alternative antibiotic
Streptococcus pneumoniae	Amoxicillin 500mg–1g tds PO *or* benzylpenicillin 1.2g qds IV	Clarithromycin 500mg bd PO *or* cefuroxime 0.75–1.5g tds IV *or* cefotaxime 1–2g tds IV *or* ceftriaxone 2g od IV
Mycoplasma pneumoniae and *Chlamydophila pneumoniae*	Clarithromycin 500mg bd PO/IV	Doxycycline 100mg od PO (after 200mg loading dose) *or* fluoroquinolone PO/IV
Chlamydophila psittaci and *Coxiella burnetii*	Doxycycline 100mg od PO (after 200mg loading dose)	Clarithromycin 500mg bd PO/IV
Legionella spp.	Fluoroquinolone PO/IV	Clarithromycin 500mg bd PO/IV (azithromycin may be an option)
Haemophilus influenzae	*Non-lactamase-producing* amoxicillin 500mg tds PO/IV *Lactamase-producing* co-amoxiclav 625mg tds PO *or* 1.2g tds IV	Cefuroxime 750mg–1.5g tds IV *or* cefotaxime 1–2g tds IV *or* ceftriaxone 2g od IV *or* fluoroquinolone PO/IV
Gram-negative enteric bacilli	Cefuroxime 1.5g tds *or* cefotaxime 1–2g tds IV *or* ceftriaxone 1–2g bd IV	Fluoroquinolone IV *or* imipenem 500mg qds IV *or* meropenem 0.5–1.0g tds IV
Pseudomonas aeruginosa	Ceftazidime 2g tds IV and gentamicin *or* tobramycin (dose monitoring)	Ciprofloxacin 400mg bd IV *or* piperacillin 4g tds IV and gentamicin *or* tobramycin (dose monitoring)
Staphylococcus aureus	*Non-MRSA* flucloxacillin 1–2g qds IV ± rifampicin 600mg od/bd PO/IV	*MRSA* vancomycin 1g bd (dose monitoring) *or* linezolid 600mg bd IV *or* teicoplanin 400mg bd IV ± rifampicin 600mg od/bd PO/IV
Aspiration pneumonia	Co-amoxiclav 1.2g tds IV	

CAP: follow-up

CXR resolution Radiographic improvement lags behind clinical improvement. There is no need to repeat a CXR before hospital discharge in those who have made a satisfactory clinical recovery.

- In one study of CAP, complete radiographic resolution occurred after 6 weeks in 73% of patients, but only in 51% at 2 weeks
- Radiographic resolution is slower in the elderly, those with multi-lobe involvement at presentation, smokers, and hospital inpatients
- *Legionella* and pneumococcal pneumonia are slower to resolve (may take 12 weeks or more).

CXR follow-up is recommended around 6 weeks after CAP:

- In all patients with persisting symptoms or clinical signs
- In all patients at higher risk of underlying lung malignancy, i.e. smokers and those over the age of 50.

This is to exclude an underlying condition that may have led to CAP such as lung cancer. Further investigations, such as bronchoscopy, should be considered at this time in patients with persisting symptoms and/or a persistently abnormal CXR.

- One study showed lung cancer is diagnosed on follow-up in 17% of smokers aged over 60 treated for CAP in the community
- Other studies have shown a prevalence of lung cancer of 11% in current and ex-smokers aged over 50, who are inpatients with CAP and who undergo bronchoscopy prior to discharge.

Vaccination

Influenza vaccination This reduces hospital deaths from pneumonia and influenza by about 65% and respiratory deaths by 45%. It also leads to fewer hospital admissions.

Recommended for 'high-risk' individuals

- Chronic lung disease
- Cardiac, renal, and liver disease
- Diabetes
- Immunosuppression due to disease or treatment
- Those aged over 65
- Long-stay residential care
- Health care workers
- Contraindicated in people with hen egg hypersensitivity (the virus is cultured in chick embryos).

The vaccination contains both A and B subtype viruses and provides partial protection against influenza illnesses. It is modified annually, based on recent viral strains. The protection rate from influenza by vaccination is over 75% for influenza A and 51–97% for influenza B. Antibody levels appear to reduce about 6y after vaccination.

Pneumococcal vaccination

Recommended for:

- Those aged over 65
- Asplenic individuals (including coeliac disease and sickle cell disease)
- Chronic renal, cardiac, and liver disease
- Diabetes
- Immunodeficiency or immunosuppression (due to disease, including HIV infection, or drugs).

It should not be given during acute infection or in pregnancy. Re-immunization is contraindicated within 3y.

Further information

Lim WS *et al*. British Thoracic Society guidelines for the management of community acquired pneumonia in adults: update 2009 *Thorax* 2009;**64**(Suppl III):iii1–55.

Thomas MF. Community acquired pneumonia. *Lancet* 2003;**362**:1991–2001.

Hospital-acquired pneumonia: clinical features

Definition New radiographic infiltrate in the presence of evidence of infection (fever, purulent sputum, leucocytosis), with onset at least 48h after hospital admission. It represents around 15% of hospital-acquired infections. Most occur outside the ICU, but those at highest risk are mechanically ventilated patients. Hospital-acquired pneumonia is expensive and prolongs the hospital stay. It requires different antibiotic treatment to CAP and is the leading cause of death from hospital-acquired infection. It is also known as nosocomial pneumonia.

Pathophysiology Hospital-acquired pneumonia occurs from aspiration of infected upper airway secretions, from the inhalation of bacteria from contaminated equipment, or haematogenous spread of organisms.

Aspiration is thought to be the most important cause. Around 45% of normal people aspirate during sleep, and this is increased in hospital inpatients (who may be more frail) and in those with chronic disease. These patients' upper airways become colonized with Gram-negative bacteria (in up to 75% within 48h of admission), and this proportion is even higher in those who have received broad-spectrum antibiotics. In addition, the severely ill may have impaired host defences, making them more susceptible to hospital-acquired pneumonia. Alteration in the gastric pH with illness and various drugs means that the GI tract is no longer sterile, thereby providing a potential source of bacterial infection. A cerebrovascular event and reduced conscious level are the major risk factors for aspiration.

Risk factors for nosocomial pneumonia
- Age >70
- Chronic lung disease and/or other comorbidity (especially diabetes)
- Reduced conscious level/cerebrovascular accident
- Chest/abdominal surgery
- Mechanical ventilation
- NG feeding
- Previous antibiotic exposure
- Poor dental hygiene
- Steroids and cytotoxic drugs.

Risk factors for specific organisms

- *Streptococcus pneumoniae and Haemophilus influenzae* Increased risk in trauma
- *Staphylococcus aureus* Increased risk in ventilated neurosurgical patients (especially closed head injury), blunt trauma, and coma
- *Pseudomonas aeruginosa* Increased risk with intubation >8 days, COPD, prolonged antibiotics
- *Acinetobacter spp.* Increased risk with prolonged ventilation and previous broad-spectrum antibiotics
- *Anaerobic bacteria* Increased with recent abdominal surgery, aspiration.

Clinical features It presents typically with:
- Fever
- Productive cough
- Raised inflammatory parameters
- New CXR infiltrate
- Deterioration in gas exchange.

Diagnosis is often a clinical one, and identification of the infecting agent can be difficult, especially if the patient has already received broad-spectrum antibiotics.

Investigations

- *CXR* usually shows a non-specific infiltrate
- *Blood, sputum, and pleural fluid* should be cultured
- *ABG* to determine severity
- *Renal and liver function tests* to assess other organ dysfunction
- *Serological tests* are of little use in nosocomial pneumonia.

Hospital-acquired pneumonia: management

Severity assessment The CURB-65 pneumonia severity score (see ➲ pp. 422–3) for CAP has not been validated in hospital-acquired pneumonia but may be useful in guiding the treatment needed.

Microbiology

- About 50% are mixed infections
- 30% are due to aerobic bacteria alone (most commonly, Gram-negative enteric bacilli and *Pseudomonas*)
- Anaerobes alone are found in about 25%
- *Pseudomonas aeruginosa* and *Staphylococcus aureus* are common causes
- *Peptostreptococcus, Fusobacterium*, and *Bacteroides* spp. are commonly isolated, as well as *Enterobacter* spp., *Escherichia coli, Serratia marcescens, Klebsiella*, and *Proteus* spp.
- *Acinetobacter* is a new emerging pathogen
- MRSA is increasing in prevalence
- Viruses are recognized as causes.

Management

- Patients developing pneumonia within 48h of arrival in hospital can be treated with standard CAP antibiotics (see ➲ p. 429), as the pneumonia is likely to be due to bacteria acquired in the community
- Patients developing pneumonia >48h after hospital admission need antibiotics to cover different organisms
- Prolonged IV treatment is usually needed, with cover for Gram-negative bacteria. Empirical antibiotics are chosen, based on knowledge of local microbial resistance patterns, but typical choices include co-amoxiclav, ceftriaxone, piperacillin-tazobactam, or a carbapenem. A stat (or ongoing) dose of gentamicin (e.g. 5–7mg/kg, guided by renal function) may be appropriate for severe sepsis. Addition of an antibiotic with MRSA coverage should be considered, particularly if the patient is known to be recently colonized with MRSA
- Supportive treatment is also required, with O_2, fluids, and ventilation, if necessary
- In penicillin-allergic patients, clindamycin or ciprofloxacin can be used (as long as *Streptococcus pneumoniae* is not thought to be the infecting agent). Levofloxacin has better pneumococcal cover
- Complications of nosocomial pneumonia are the same as for CAP, including lung abscess and empyema. Drug fever, sepsis with multi-organ failure, and PE with 2° infection are all more common in nosocomial pneumonia
- In this situation, chest US (to look for empyema) or CT scanning may demonstrate abscess, underlying tumour, or infection at extrathoracic sites.

Prognosis Associated with a high mortality, ranging between 20 and 50%.

Prevention Meticulous hygiene and hand washing by medical staff, in addition to careful infection control measures, have been shown to reduce hospital-acquired pneumonia.

Post-operatively, early mobilization, careful cleaning and maintenance of respiratory equipment, and preoperative smoking cessation reduce infection rates. Some ICUs use antibiotics to selectively decontaminate the GI tract of Gram-negative bacilli. This has been shown to reduce infection rates, but there is no proven effect on mortality or length of ICU admission.

Ventilator-associated pneumonia (VAP)

Definition Pneumonia in a mechanically ventilated patient, developing 48h after intubation. It has a prevalence of up to 65% in some units. It is an independent predictor of mortality and is the commonest nosocomial infection >ITU. Up to two-thirds of patients requiring mechanical ventilation for >48h will develop VAP. It has a mortality of 15–50%, increasing the length of ITU stay by an average of 6.1 days.

The major cause is bacterial contamination of the lower respiratory tract from the aspiration of oropharyngeal secretions, which is not prevented by cuffed endotracheal tube or tracheostomy.

Diagnosis is suggested by:
- New or progressive CXR infiltrate
- Association with fever, high WCC, purulent secretions, and worsening ventilatory parameters (increasing RR, decreasing tidal volumes, and increasing O_2 requirements)
- There are many non-infectious causes of fever and CXR infiltrate in ITU patients, so the diagnosis is not always straightforward. Other sources of fever are also common in ventilated patients, including infected lines, sinusitis, UTI, and pseudomembranous colitis, and may warrant further investigation.

Differential diagnosis of fever and CXR infiltrate in ITU
- Chemical aspiration without infection
- Atelectasis
- ARDS
- LVF
- PE with lung infarction
- Pulmonary haemorrhage
- COP
- Drug reaction
- Tumour
- Lung contusion.

Investigations
- *CXR* often shows a non-specific infiltrate, with air bronchograms being the best predictor of the disease
- *Airway sampling for microbiology:*
  - *Bronchoscopic sampling* Protected specimen brush (PSB) samples (with the tip of the bronchoscope placed opposite the orifice of an involved segmental bronchus, and PSB advanced through its protective sheath into the airway) or BAL samples (from a subsegmental bronchus, with the end of the bronchoscope wedged into the airway, ideally >150mL saline wash) are the best methods to obtain lower airway samples with minimal contamination. VAP is diagnosed when an arbitrary threshold of organisms are grown on a BAL or PSB sample. The usual cut-offs are 1,000 colony-forming units/mL (cfu/mL) for PSB samples and 10,000 cfu/mL for BAL samples. Thresholds vary between units, as do thresholds for starting treatment. Meta-analysis of three RCTs

showed no significant mortality differences between quantitative and qualitative culture assessments. Airway neutrophil counts may also aid in making the diagnosis

- *Non-bronchoscopic airway sampling*, e.g. blind bronchial sampling of lower respiratory tract secretions (so-called 'mini-BAL') is cheaper and does not need an expert operator. A catheter is advanced through the endotracheal tube until there is resistance, and saline (~20mL) is infused and then aspirated. A meta-analysis of five RCTs showed no significant differences in mortality with non-invasive vs. invasive (bronchoscopic) airway sampling; further, there were no significant differences in number of days of mechanical ventilation, length of ICU stay, or antibiotic changes (Berton DC *et al. Cochrane Database Syst Rev* 2012;**1**:CD006482)
- *Serial sampling* is favoured in some units. Regular non-invasive serial airway sampling may aid early diagnosis of VAP. It needs careful interpretation, as the microbiology of the respiratory tract changes over time in critically ill mechanically ventilated patients
- *Tracheal aspiration samples* are easy to obtain but non-specific in diagnosing VAP, as upper airway colonization is very common.

Antibiotic treatment Problems with the emergence of resistant bacteria mean that empirical treatment with antibiotics is used less commonly. Local policies are often in place, and advice should always be sought from microbiology. The most common drug-resistant pathogens are *P. aeruginosa*, MRSA, *Acinetobacter* spp., and *Klebsiella* spp. Delay in commencing antibiotics is associated with a poorer outcome.

> **Risk factors for resistant organisms include:**
> - Hospitalization in the previous 90 days
> - Nursing home residence
> - Current hospital admission >5 days
> - Mechanical ventilation >7 days
> - Prior broad-spectrum antibiotic use (e.g. third-generation cephalosporin)
> - High frequency of local antibiotic resistance.

Antibiotics should be chosen on the basis of:
- Recent antibiotic treatment
- Local policy and known local flora
- Culture data.

Empirical antibiotic choice often includes coverage for anaerobes and **MRSA**, **Legionella** (if long stay), *P. aeruginosa*, and *Acinetobacter*.

Length of treatment depends on the clinical response, with one trial showing that 8-day treatment had similar efficacy to 15-day treatment, although patients with *P. aeruginosa* infection had a greater risk of recurrence following discontinuation of antibiotics at 8 days. Failure to respond should lead to a change of antibiotics and a search for additional infection or another cause for the radiographic infiltrate. Further cultures should be sent.

Aspiration pneumonia

Definition Pneumonia that follows the aspiration of exogenous material or endogenous secretions into the lower respiratory tract.

Epidemiology Aspiration pneumonia is the commonest cause of death in patients with dysphagia due to neurological disorders and is the cause of up to 20% of pneumonias in nursing home residents. It occurs in about 10% of patients admitted to hospital with a drug overdose.

Pathophysiology Micro-aspiration is common in healthy individuals, but, for an aspiration pneumonia to occur, there must be compromise of the normal defences protecting the lower airways (i.e. glottic closure, cough reflex), with inoculation of the lower respiratory tract of a significant amount of material. Most pneumonias are a result of aspiration of micro-organisms from the oral cavity or nasopharynx.

Situations predisposing to aspiration pneumonia
- *Reduced conscious level* (cough reflex and impaired glottic closure)
  - Alcohol
  - Drug overdose
  - Post-seizure
  - Post-anaesthesia
  - Massive cerebrovascular accident (CVA)
- *Dysphagia*
  - Motor neurone disease (MND)
  - Following a neurological event; those with impaired swallow reflex post-CVA are seven times more likely to develop a pneumonia than those in whom the gag reflex is unimpaired
- *Upper GI tract disease*
  - Surgery to the stomach or oesophagus
  - Mechanical impairment of glottic or cardiac sphincter closure, e.g. tracheostomy, nasogastric feeding, bronchoscopy
  - Pharyngeal anaesthesia
- *Increased reflux*
  - Large-volume vomiting
  - Large-volume NG feed
  - Feeding gastrostomy
  - Recumbent position
- *Nursing home residents*
  - The risk of aspiration is lower in those without teeth, who receive aggressive oral hygiene
  - There is a higher incidence of silent aspiration in the otherwise healthy elderly
  - Strong correlation between volume of aspirate and the risk of developing pneumonia.

Aspiration pneumonia: clinical features

Three pulmonary syndromes result from aspiration. The amount and nature of the aspirated material, the site and frequency of the aspiration, and the host's response to it will determine which pulmonary syndrome occurs.

Chemical pneumonitis

This is aspiration of substances toxic to the lower airways, in the absence of bacterial infection.

This causes a chemical burn of the tracheobronchial tree, causing an intense parenchymal inflammatory reaction, with release of inflammatory mediators that may lead to ARDS. Animal studies show that an inoculum with a pH <2.5 of relatively large volume (about 25mL in adults) is needed to initiate an inflammatory reaction. Animal models show rapid pathological changes within 3min, with atelectasis, pulmonary haemorrhage, and pulmonary oedema. (This was first described by Mendelson, referring to the aspiration of sterile gastric contents and its toxic effects. The original case series was in obstetric anaesthesia.)

Clinical features
- Rapid onset of symptoms, with breathlessness (within 1–2h)
- Low-grade fever
- Severe hypoxaemia and diffuse lung infiltrates involving dependent segments
- CXR changes within 2h.

Treatment
- If aspiration is observed—suction and/or bronchoscopy to clear aspirated secretions or food. This may not prevent chemical injury from acid, which is similar to a flash burn
- Support of cardiac and respiratory function—with IV fluids, $O_2 \pm$ ventilation
- Steroids—controversial. No benefit has been shown in human studies
- Antibiotics—usually given, even in the absence of evidence of infection, because 2° bacterial infection is common and may be a contributing or 1° factor in the aspiration. Acid-damaged lung is more susceptible to the effects of 2° bacterial infection; up to 25% will develop 2° bacterial infection. Activity against Gram-negative and anaerobic organisms is needed, e.g. cefuroxime plus metronidazole, or penicillin plus clindamycin.

Bacterial infection Aspiration of bacteria normally resident in the upper airways or stomach. The normal bacterial flora are anaerobes, in a host susceptible to aspiration, and less virulent than the bacteria causing CAP.

Clinical features depend on the infecting organism:
- Cough, fever, purulent sputum, breathlessness
- The process may evolve over weeks and months, rather than hours
- May be more chronic, with weight loss and anaemia
- Absence of fever or rigors
- Foul-smelling sputum

- Periodontal disease
- Involvement of dependent pulmonary lobes
- Anaerobic bacteria are more difficult to culture so may be present, but not identified in microbiological culture
- May present with later manifestations, e.g. empyema, lung abscess.

Major pathogens are *Peptostreptococcus*, *Fusobacterium nucleatum*, *Prevotella*, and *Bacteroides* spp. Mixed infection is common.

Treatment
- Antibiotics to include anaerobic cover, e.g. co-amoxiclav, clindamycin, or a carbapenem
- Swallow assessment/neurological review if no obvious underlying cause found.

Mechanical obstruction Aspiration of matter that is not directly toxic to the lung may lead to damage by causing airway obstruction or reflex airway closure. Causative agents include:
- Saline
- Barium
- Most ingested fluids, including water
- Gastric contents with a pH >2.5
- Mechanical obstruction, such as occurs in drowning, or those who are unable to clear a potential inoculum, e.g. neurological deficit, impaired cough reflex, reduced conscious level
- Inhalation of an object, with the severity of the obstruction depending on the size and site of the aspirated particle. This is commoner in children but does occur in adults, e.g. teeth, peanuts.

Treatment
- Tracheal suction
- Remove obstructing object if necessary
- No further treatment is needed if no CXR infiltrates.

Lung abscess: clinical features

Definition A localized area of lung suppuration leading to necrosis of the pulmonary parenchyma, with or without cavity formation.

Lung abscesses may be single or multiple, acute or chronic (>1 month), 1° or 2°. They may occur spontaneously, but, more commonly, an underlying disease exists. Lung abscess is now rare in the developed world but has a high mortality of 20–30%. They are most common in alcoholic men aged >50.

Pathophysiology Most are the result of aspiration pneumonia. Predisposing factors for abscess are those for aspiration pneumonia (see ⊃ p. 440).
- Dental disease
- Impaired consciousness—alcohol, post-anaesthesia, dysphagia
- Diabetes
- Bronchial carcinoma (with bronchial obstruction)
- 2° to pneumonia (cavitation occurs in about 16% of *Staphylococcus aureus* pneumonia)
- Immunocompromise—abscesses due to *Pneumocystis jirovecii* (PCP), *Cryptococcus neoformans*, *Rhodococcus* spp., and fungi in HIV-positive patients
- Septic embolization (right heart endocarditis due to, e.g. *Staphylococcus aureus* in IV drug abusers).

The bacterial inoculum reaches the lung parenchyma, often in a dependent lung area. Pneumonitis, followed by necrosis, occurs over 7–14 days. Cavitation occurs when parenchymal necrosis leads to communication with the bronchus, with the entry of air and expectoration of necrotic material leading to the formation of an air-fluid level. Bronchial obstruction leads to atelectasis with stasis and subsequent infection, which can predispose to abscess formation.

Presentation
- Often insidious onset
- Productive cough, haemoptysis
- Breathlessness
- Fevers
- Night sweats
- Non-specific feature of chronic infection—anaemia, weight loss, malaise (especially in the elderly)
- Foul sputum or purulent pleural fluid.

Lemierre's syndrome (necrobacillosis) Jugular vein suppurative thrombophlebitis. This is a rare pharyngeal infection in young adults, most commonly due to the anaerobe *Fusobacterium necrophorum*. It presents with a classical history of painful pharyngitis, in the presence of bacteraemia. Infection spreads to the neck and carotid sheath, often leading to thrombosis of the internal jugular vein. This may not be obvious clinically (neck vein USS or Doppler may be needed). Septic embolization to the lung, with subsequent cavitation, leads to abscess formation. Empyema and abscesses in the bone, joints, liver, and kidneys can complicate.

Lung abscess: diagnosis

The diagnosis is usually made from the history, along with the appearance of a cavity with an associated air-fluid level on CXR.

Investigations

- Microbiological culture, ideally before commencing antibiotics. Useful to exclude TB
  - Blood cultures
  - Sputum or bronchoscopic specimen (BAL or brushings rarely needed)
  - Transthoracic percutaneous needle aspiration (CT- or US-guided) may provide samples. Risk of bleeding, pneumothorax, and seeding of infection to pleural space, if abscess not adjacent to the pleura.

In practice, blood cultures and sputum microbiology usually suffice. Samples are usually only obtained by more invasive means if appropriate antibiotics are not leading to an adequate clinical response.

- *Imaging*—exclude aspirated foreign body, underlying neoplasm, or bronchial stenosis and obstruction
  - *CXR* may show consolidation, cavitation, air-fluid level (if the patient is unwell, the CXR is likely to be taken in a semi-recumbent position, so an air-fluid level may not be visible). 50% of abscesses are in the posterior segment of the right upper lobe or the apical basal segments of either lower lobe
  - *CT* is useful if the diagnosis is in doubt and cannot be confirmed from the CXR appearance or if the clinical response to treatment is inadequate. It can also help to define the exact position of the abscess (which may be useful for physiotherapy or if surgery is being considered—rarely needed)

CT also is useful to differentiate an abscess from a pleural collection—a *lung abscess* appears as a rounded intrapulmonary mass, with no compression of adjacent lung, with a thickened irregular wall, making an acute angle at its contact with the chest wall. An *empyema* typically has a 'lenticular' shape and compresses adjacent lung, which creates an obtuse angle as it follows the contour of the chest wall.

CT can determine the presence of obstructing endobronchial disease, due to malignancy or foreign body, and may be useful in defining the extent of disease in a very sick patient who has had significant haemoptysis. Even with CT, differentiating an abscess from a cavitating malignancy can be very difficult (no radiological features differentiate them).

Microbiology Commonly mixed infection, usually anaerobes.
- The most common organisms are those colonizing the oral cavity and gingival crevices—*Peptostreptococcus, Prevotella, Bacteroides,* and *Fusobacterium* spp.
- Aerobes—*Streptococcus 'milleri'* group, *Staphylococcus aureus, Klebsiella* spp., *Streptococcus pyogenes, Haemophilus influenzae, Nocardia*

- Non-bacterial pathogens are also reported—fungi (*Aspergillus,*
  Cryptococcus, Histoplasma, Blastomyces) and mycobacteria
- Opportunistic infections in immunocompromised—*Nocardia*,
  mycobacteria, *Aspergillus*.

Differential diagnosis of a cavitating mass, with or without an air-fluid level

- Cavitating carcinoma—1° or metastatic
- Cavitatory TB
- GPA (Wegener's)
- Infected pulmonary cyst or bulla (can produce a fluid level, usually
  thinner-walled)
- Aspergilloma
- Pulmonary infarct
- Rheumatoid nodule
- Sarcoidosis
- Bronchiectasis.

Lung abscess: management

Antibiotics to cover aerobic and anaerobic infection, including β-lactam/β-lactamase inhibitors, e.g. co-amoxiclav and clindamycin. Long courses are needed. Risk of *Clostridium difficile* diarrhoea.
- Infections are usually mixed, therefore antibiotics to cover these
- Metronidazole to cover anaerobes
- No data to guide length of treatment. Common practice would be 1–2 weeks IV treatment, with a further 2–6 weeks oral antibiotics, often until outpatient clinic review.

Drainage Spontaneous drainage is common, with the production of purulent sputum. This can be increased with postural drainage and physiotherapy.
- No data to support use of bronchoscopic drainage
- Percutaneous drainage with radiologically placed small percutaneous drains for peripheral abscesses may be useful in those failing to respond to antibiotic and supportive treatment. These are usually placed under US guidance (though are rarely indicated).

Surgery is rarely required if appropriate antibiotic treatment is given. It is usually reserved for complicated infections failing to respond to standard treatment after at least 6 weeks of treatment.
May be needed if:
- Very large abscess (>6cm diameter)
- Resistant organisms
- Haemorrhage
- Recurrent disease
- Lobectomy or pneumonectomy is occasionally needed if severe infection with an abscess leaves a large volume of damaged lung that is hard to sterilize.

Complications Haemorrhage (erosion of blood vessels as the abscess extends into the lung parenchyma). This can be massive and life-threatening (see ➲ p. 47) and is an indication for urgent surgery.
If slow to respond, consider:
- Underlying malignancy
- Unusual microbiology, e.g. mycobacterium, fungi
- Immunosuppression
- Large cavity (>6cm) may rarely require drainage
- Non-bacterial cause, e.g. cavitating malignancy, GPA (Wegener's)
- Other cause of persistent fever, e.g. *Clostridium difficile* diarrhoea, antibiotic-associated fever.

Prognosis 85% cure rate in the absence of underlying disease. Mortality is reported as high as 75% in immunocompromised patients. The prognosis is much worse in the presence of underlying lung disease, with increasing age and large abscesses (>6cm) with *Staphylococcus aureus* infection.

Nocardiosis

Definition *Nocardia* are Gram-positive, partially acid-fast, aerobic bacilli that form branching filaments. They are found in soil, decaying organic plant matter, and water and have been isolated from house dust, garden soil, and swimming pools. Infection typically follows inhalation, although percutaneous inoculation also occurs. The *Nocardia asteroides* spp. complex accounts for the majority of clinical infections.

Consider *Nocardia* infection when soft tissue abscesses and/or CNS manifestations occur in the setting of a pulmonary infection. The combination of respiratory, skin, and/or CNS involvement may lead to a misdiagnosis of vasculitis, and the respiratory manifestations may mimic cancer, TB, or fungal disease.

Epidemiology *Nocardia* occurs worldwide, and the frequency of subclinical exposure is unknown. Clinically apparent infection is rare and usually occurs in patients with immunocompromise (haematological malignancy, steroid therapy, organ transplant, diabetes, alcoholism, and HIV infection, especially IVDUs) or pre-existing lung disease (particularly pulmonary alveolar proteinosis, TB). Infection also occurs in apparently healthy people (10–25% of cases). Nosocomial infection and disease outbreaks have been reported.

Clinical features

Pulmonary disease

- The lung is the most common site of involvement
- Patients typically present with productive cough, fever, anorexia, weight loss, and malaise; dyspnoea, pleuritic pain, and haemoptysis may occur but are less common
- Empyema occurs in up to a quarter of cases, and direct intrathoracic spread causing pericarditis, mediastinitis, rib osteomyelitis, or SVCO is also reported

Extrapulmonary disease

- Dissemination from the lungs occurs in 50% of patients
- CNS is the most common site of dissemination, occurring in 25% of pulmonary nocardiosis cases. Single or multiple abscesses occur and may be accompanied by meningitis
- Other sites include the skin and subcutaneous tissues, kidneys, bone, joints and muscle, peritoneum, eyes, pericardium, and heart valves.

Investigations

- Identification by smear and culture is the principal method of diagnosis. *Nocardia* grows on routine media, usually within 2–7 days, although more prolonged culture (2–3 weeks) may be required

- Direct smear of appropriate specimens (e.g. aspirates of abscesses, biopsies) is highly sensitive and typically shows Gram-positive beaded branching filaments, which are usually acid-fast on modified Ziehl–Neelsen (ZN) stain. Examination of BAL fluid may also be diagnostic
- Sensitivity testing of isolates and identification to species level is done by reference laboratories
- Biopsies typically show a mixed cellular infiltrate; granulomata occur rarely and may result in misdiagnosis as TB or histoplasmosis
- CXR and CT may demonstrate parenchymal infiltrates, single or multiple nodules (sometimes with cavitation), or features of pleural infection
- Sputum smear is usually unhelpful. Sputum culture has a greater yield, but *Nocardia* growth may be obscured in mixed cultures. The significance of *Nocardia* growth on sputum culture in asymptomatic patients is unclear; it may represent contamination or colonization in the setting of underlying lung disease
- Blood cultures are almost always negative, although *Nocardia* bacteraemia may occur in the setting of profound immunocompromise
- Consider MRI of the brain to exclude asymptomatic CNS involvement in patients with pulmonary nocardiosis.

Management

- Discuss treatment with an infectious diseases specialist
- Drug treatment choices include sulfonamides/co-trimoxazole, minocycline, imipenem, cefotaxime, ceftriaxone, or amikacin. Sulfa drugs, in particular co-trimoxazole, have traditionally been the mainstay of therapy. Imipenem and amikacin combination therapy has been shown to be active *in vitro* and in animal models and is recommended for pulmonary nocardiosis and for very ill patients. Extended-spectrum cephalosporins, such as ceftriaxone and cefotaxime, have the advantages of good CNS penetration and low toxicity
- Optimal treatment duration is unclear: typically given for 6 months in non-immunocompromised patients, and for 12 months or longer for CNS involvement or immunocompromised patients
- Surgery may be required for abscess drainage.

Prognosis Clinical outcome is dependent on the site and extent of disease and on underlying host factors. Disease remissions and exacerbations are common. Cure rates are ~90% in pleuropulmonary disease and 50% in brain abscess. Mortality of *Nocardia* infection is generally low, although it approaches 50% in cases of bacteraemia.

Further information

Saubolle MA, Sussland D. Nocardiosis: review of clinical and laboratory experience. *J Clin Microbiol* 2003;**41**:4497–501.
Lerner PI. Nocardiosis. *Clin Inf Dis* 1996;**22**:891–905.

Actinomycosis

Definition Actinomycosis is caused by a group of anaerobic Gram-positive bacilli, of which *Actinomyces israelii* is the commonest. These organisms are present in the mouth, GI tract, and vagina. Clinical infection may follow dental procedures or aspiration of infected secretions. Infection is slowly progressive and may disseminate via the bloodstream or invade tissue locally, sometimes resulting in sinus tract formation.

Consider this diagnosis particularly in patients with pulmonary disease accompanied by soft tissue infection of the head and neck. The diagnosis of actinomycosis is often unsuspected, and the clinical and radiological features may mimic cancer, TB, or fungal disease.

Epidemiology Actinomycosis is rare. It can occur at any age and is more common in men. Predisposing factors include corticosteroid use, chemotherapy, organ transplant, and HIV infection.

Clinical features

Thoracic disease Thoracic disease occurs in about 15% of cases. Symptoms of pulmonary involvement are non-specific and include cough, chest pain, haemoptysis, fever, anorexia, and weight loss. Chest wall involvement may occur, with sinus formation or rib infection, and empyema is common. Mediastinal involvement is documented.

Extrathoracic disease Soft tissue infection of the head and neck, particularly the mandible, is the commonest disease presentation (about 50% of cases). Discharging sinuses may form. Other extrathoracic disease sites include the abdomen (particularly the ileocaecal region), pelvis, liver, bone, and CNS (manifest as single or multiple abscesses).

Investigations
- CXR and CT appearances are variable, including masses (sometimes with cavitation), parenchymal infiltrates, consolidation, mediastinal disease, and/or pleural involvement
- Diagnosis is based on the microscopy and anaerobic culture of infected material. Warn the microbiology laboratory if the diagnosis is suspected, as specific stains and culture conditions are required. Examination of infected material may reveal yellow 'sulfur granules' containing aggregated organisms. Sample sputum, pleural fluid, and pus from sinus tracts; inoculate into anaerobic transport media, and rapidly transport to lab. Endobronchial biopsies have a low sensitivity. Most infections are polymicrobial, with accompanying aerobic or anaerobic bacteria.

Management
- Discuss treatment with an infectious diseases specialist
- Drug treatment choices include penicillin, amoxicillin, clindamycin, or erythromycin. Administration should initially be IV. Optimal treatment duration is unclear (typically given for 6–12 months)
- Surgery may be required for abscess drainage
- Monitor response to treatment with serial CT or MRI scans
- Treat any associated periodontal disease.

Prognosis Disease relapse is common if prolonged treatment is not administered.

Further information
Mabeza GF, Mcfarlane J. Pulmonary actinomycosis. *Eur Resp J* 2003;**21**:545–51.

Anthrax

Definition and epidemiology
- *Bacillus anthracis* is an aerobic Gram-positive spore-forming bacterium that causes human disease, principally following either inhalation or cutaneous contact. Spores can survive in soil for many years. Person-to-person transmission does not occur
- Considerable recent interest has focused on the use of anthrax in bioterrorism; five envelopes containing anthrax spores were sent through the USA postal service in 2001, and there were 11 confirmed cases of inhalational anthrax (including five deaths) and seven confirmed cases of cutaneous anthrax. A previous outbreak occurred in Sverdlovsk in the former Soviet Union in 1979, following the release of spores from a biological weapons plant, and resulted in 68 deaths
- Anthrax infection also occurs very rarely in association with occupational exposure to *Bacillus anthracis* in animal wool or hides. The majority of occupational cases result in cutaneous disease, and a diagnosis of inhalational anthrax strongly suggests a bioterrorist attack.

Clinical features
Inhalational anthrax
- Incubation period is variable, although, in the USA, in 2001, it typically ranged 4–6 days following exposure from opening mail
- Patients typically experience a prodrome of flu-like symptoms such as fever and cough. GI symptoms (vomiting, diarrhoea, abdominal pain), drenching sweats, and altered mental status are often prominent symptoms. Breathlessness, fever, and septic shock develop several days later. Haemorrhagic meningitis is a common complication
- Large haemorrhagic pleural effusions are a characteristic feature.

Cutaneous anthrax
- Initial symptoms include itch and development of a papule at the infection site. A necrotic ulcer with a black centre, and often surrounding oedema, subsequently develops. Systemic symptoms, such as fever and sweats, may be present.

Investigations
- *Bacillus anthracis* grows on conventional media and is readily cultured if sampling precedes antibiotic treatment; a definitive diagnosis requires specialized laboratory tests (e.g. PCR, immunohistochemistry of biopsy samples, or serological studies)
- Blood tests typically reveal leucocytosis
- Blood cultures are positive in nearly all cases of inhalational anthrax when taken prior to antibiotic treatment. Staining and culture of pleural fluid may be diagnostic
- CXR in inhalational anthrax classically shows a widened mediastinum (due to necrosis of mediastinal lymph nodes and haemorrhagic mediastinitis); pleural effusions and pulmonary infiltrates may be present. CT may also demonstrate mediastinal and hilar lymphadenopathy
- Gram stain and culture of the ulcer is usually diagnostic in cutaneous anthrax, although biopsy is sometimes required.

Management

- Discuss with infectious diseases and public health specialists if the diagnosis is suspected
- Antibiotic treatment should be administered immediately after taking blood cultures. Recommendations are for initial treatment with either ciprofloxacin or doxycycline IV, in combination with 1–2 additional antibiotics (choices include clindamycin, vancomycin, meropenem, or penicillin). Subsequent treatment should be with either ciprofloxacin or doxycycline orally for 60 days. Oral treatment alone may be sufficient in cases of mild cutaneous disease
- Corticosteroid treatment should be considered in patients with meningitis or severe neck or mediastinal oedema
- Supportive care, including ventilatory support, treatment of shock with IV fluids and/or inotropes, and chest tube drainage of large pleural effusions may be needed.

Prognosis Inhalational anthrax is associated with a high mortality; five of the recent 11 cases in the USA died. The mortality of previously documented cases has been even higher, perhaps reflecting a delay or lack of antibiotic treatment.

Prophylaxis USA recommendations advise prophylaxis with oral ciprofloxacin or doxycycline for individuals considered to have been exposed to anthrax spores in contaminated areas. A vaccine is available, although its value in post-exposure prophylaxis is unknown.

Tularaemia

Definition and epidemiology Tularaemia is a rare zoonosis caused by infection with the Gram-negative bacteria *Francisella tularensis*. Two major subspecies are described: subspp. *tularensis* (type A) is highly virulent and found in North America; subspp. *holarctica* (type B) is less virulent and found in North America, Europe, and Asia. Small mammals (particularly rabbits and hares) acquire infection from arthropod bites and act as reservoirs; human infection follows inhalation, direct contact with infected rodents, ingestion of contaminated food, or arthropod bites. Tularaemia is most frequently encountered in rural areas, following activities, such as farming and hunting, although laboratory workers are also at risk. There has been considerable interest in the development of *F. tularensis* as a biological weapon, and more recently concerns have arisen as to its possible use in bioterrorism.

Clinical features Typically abrupt onset of fever, headache, dry cough, and malaise. Development of a tender ulcer and regional lymphadenopathy ('ulceroglandular tularaemia') around an infected arthropod bite is common. Tularaemia pneumonia, following infection with type A, is characterized by cough (productive or dry), breathlessness, and sweating, with often minimal signs on examination; may progress rapidly to respiratory failure and death. Symptoms of pneumonia are milder after infection with type B.

Investigations

- Serology is the principal method of diagnosis, although PCR-based techniques are increasingly used
- *F. tularensis* may be identified in culture of wound specimens, although the laboratory should be warned—type A is sufficiently virulent for some laboratories not to perform culture. Sputum cultures may be diagnostic
- CXR may demonstrate parenchymal infiltrates, often progressing to lobar consolidation. Pleural effusions, hilar lymphadenopathy, and lung abscess may occur.

Management

- Discuss treatment with an infectious diseases specialist
- Drug treatment choices include streptomycin or gentamicin for 10 days. Doxycycline or chloramphenicol are alternatives, although treatment failure rates are higher and a course of 14 days is recommended
- In the setting of a large-scale outbreak (e.g. following use in bioterrorism), doxycycline or ciprofloxacin may be used for treatment or following exposure.

Prognosis Mortality is 1–2% from type A; type B is benign in humans.

Further information

Tarnvik A, Berglund L. Tularaemia. *Eur Resp J* 2003;21:361–73.

Melioidosis

Definition and epidemiology Melioidosis is caused by *Burkholderia pseudomallei*, a Gram-negative bacillus that is found in soil and water in South-East Asia, northern Australia, China, and India; clinical disease is particularly common in Thailand where it may account for up to a third of all pneumonia deaths. Infection is thought to follow entry via skin abrasions or inhalation, and pneumonia is the most common clinical presentation. Most cases represent recent infection; reactivation of infection is rare but can occur many years after exposure. Risk factors for melioidosis include diabetes, alcohol excess, renal disease, and chronic lung disease (including CF).

> Consider melioidosis in returning travellers from Asia or Australia with CAP or a subacute/chronic 'TB-like' respiratory illness.

Clinical features include:
- *Acute septicaemic melioidosis* Patients present acutely unwell, with a severe pneumonia and widespread nodular consolidation on CXR, may progress rapidly to death
- *Localized subacute melioidosis* Subacute cavitating lobar (often upper) pneumonia, mimicking TB
- *Chronic suppurative melioidosis* Chronic lung abscess ± empyema; suppurative infection may involve other organs, including skin, brain, joints, bones, liver, spleen, kidney, adrenal, prostate, lymph nodes.

Diagnosis
Identification by culture is the principal method of diagnosis. Blood cultures may be diagnostic; alert the laboratory to the possibility of this infection. ELISAs are relatively insensitive.

Management
- *B. pseudomallei* is resistant to multiple antibiotics. Treat with high-dose IV ceftazidime, meropenem, or imipenem for at least 10–14 days (longer if severe pulmonary disease or organ abscesses), then oral antibiotic (e.g. co-trimoxazole, alone or in combination with doxycycline) for at least 12 weeks to ensure eradication
- Supportive care, with ITU admission for septic shock or severe pneumonia.

Prognosis Documented mortality rates range 19–46%.

Further information
Currie BJ. Melioidosis: an important cause of pneumonia in residents of and travelers returned from endemic regions. *Eur Resp J* 2003;**22**:542–50.

Leptospirosis

Definition and epidemiology Leptospirosis is a zoonosis transmitted from water or soil contaminated with urine of infected animals (e.g. rats, dogs, cats, pigs, cattle, hamsters, bats) through skin abrasions or mucosa. Present worldwide, more common in tropical countries, but well described in UK. Individuals most at risk in the UK include farmers, vets, sewage workers, returning travellers from the topics, military personnel, and canoeists. Incidence peaks in spring/summer. In the tropics, epidemics may occur following storms or floods.

Consider leptospirosis in all patients with diffuse alveolar haemorrhage and in at-risk individuals with pneumonia or ARDS.

Clinical features Disease manifestations are highly variable, ranging from asymptomatic infection to multi-organ failure, pulmonary haemorrhage, and death. Patients may present solely with pulmonary haemorrhage, without other features of Weil's disease. Manifestations include:
- *Acute (anicteric) leptospirosis* Self-limiting flu-like illness; myalgia, rash, and aseptic meningitis may occur
- *Weil's disease (icterohaemorrhagic fever)* Classic form of leptospirosis. Features include fever, myalgia, conjunctival haemorrhage, rash, jaundice/hepatic failure, renal failure, coagulopathy, and thrombocytopenia, shock, myocarditis/cardiac arrhythmias
- *Pulmonary disease* Occurs in at least a third of hospitalized patients with acute leptospirosis or Weil's disease. Manifestations include mild symptoms/signs (cough, wheeze, and crackles), pneumonia, pulmonary oedema 2° to myocarditis, and ARDS or fulminant alveolar haemorrhage syndrome.

Investigations
- May be isolated in blood cultures
- Serology confirms the diagnosis and is performed in a single Leptospira Reference Unit in the UK. Both ELISA and microscopic agglutination tests may be performed
- CXR and CT typically demonstrate patchy consolidation and ground-glass shadowing, commonly bilateral with lower lobe predominance.

Management
- Discuss treatment with infectious diseases and renal specialists. Antibiotic choices include penicillin, ceftriaxone, or doxycycline
- Ventilatory support required for alveolar haemorrhage and ARDS
- Ensure adequate hydration; blood products may be required
- High-dose glucocorticoids are occasionally used, although there is no convincing evidence of benefit. Plasma exchange and desmopressin infusions have been tried.

Prognosis Acute leptospirosis typically resolves spontaneously after about 14 days. Severe pulmonary disease can progress very rapidly (over hours), with reported mortality rates approaching 50%.

Differential diagnosis of zoonotic microbial causes of CAP (with exposures)
- Avian influenza virus (birds, animals)
- *Bacillus anthracis* (anthrax; animals)
- Brucellosis (animals)
- *Chlamydophila psittaci* (psittacosis; poultry, birds)
- *Coxiella burnetii* (Q fever; parturient cats, cattle, sheep, goats, rabbits)
- *Cryptococcus neoformans* (birds)
- *Francisella tularensis* (tularaemia; rabbits, cats, rodents)
- Hantavirus (rodents, the Americas)
- *Histoplasma capsulatum* (histoplasmosis; birds or bats, the Americas)
- Leptospirosis (water contaminated with infected animal urine)
- *Pasteurella multocida* (pasteurellosis; animals, birds)
- *Ricketsia rickettsii* (Rocky mountain spotted fever; tick bite or exposure to tick-infested habitats, USA)
- *Yersinia pestis* (pneumonic plague; rodents, cats).

Chapter 41

Respiratory
infection—fungal

Aspergillus lung disease: classification

Types of disease *Aspergillus fumigatus* and other *Aspergillus* moulds are ubiquitous fungi that can be isolated from the air in most houses, and this increases with increasing indoor humidity. Inhalation of spores (conidia) can produce a range of diseases, some of which are related to each other and some of which are not. The finding of fungal hyphae (rather than just spores) in the sputum should provoke an assessment.

Classification

IgE-mediated allergic asthma from inhaled *Aspergillus* spores. One of many common antigens provoking airway inflammation and bronchospasm.

Exuberant IgE and IgG reaction to *Aspergillus* in the airways of (usually) asthmatics, provoking mucous plugging with distal consolidation that may flit from area to area. This is one of the causes of pulmonary eosinophilia.

Allergic bronchopulmonary aspergillosis (APBA) A probable evolution and progression of exuberant IgE and IgG reaction to *Aspergillus* in (usually) asthmatics, with inflammatory damage to the airways and resultant bronchiectasis (but no actual invasion of *Aspergillus* into the airway walls).

Invasive Aspergillus pneumonia due to invasion of Aspergillus into lung tissue 2° to immunosuppression. This can be a multi-system disorder with *Aspergillus* invading almost any part of the body.

Semi-invasive aspergillosis, a much lower-grade process than invasive *Aspergillus* pneumonia, usually seen in older individuals with no apparent immunosuppression, but usually some underlying chronic lung disease.

Aspergilloma where *Aspergillus* lives and grows as a separate ball of fungus in a pre-existing lung cavity. There is usually an inflammatory response to limited hyphae invasion into the tissue walls of the cavity.

Hypersensitivity pneumonitis (or extrinsic allergic alveolitis) due to an immune inflammatory reaction to inhalation of large numbers of spores (see ➲ pp. 254–5).

The presentation and clinical setting of these various *Aspergillus*-related disorders are clearly different and thus are detailed separately.

Atopic allergy to fungal spores

Approximately 10% of asthmatics are skin prick-positive to *Aspergillus* species, compared with about 70% to house dust mite. It is assumed that this allergy contributes to allergic inflammation in the airways, but, in the few relevant studies, symptoms have not always correlated with exposure. However, in some studies, asthma admissions to hospital correlated better with fungal spore counts than with pollen counts. Fungal spore release may explain an association between thunderstorms and asthma attacks. Particularly high exposure results from working with mouldy vegetable matter, e.g. in compost heaps, during late summer/early autumn.

Asthma and positive IgG precipitins to *Aspergillus*

Definition Asthmatics with IgE responses to *Aspergillus* can also develop IgG antibodies (precipitins). Why this happens is not clear. *Aspergillus* hyphae can sometimes be isolated from the sputum, and it has been suggested that *Aspergillus* spores are able to germinate and grow in the mucus within the airways. This may explain the mucous plugging and flitting areas of pulmonary consolidation.

Clinical features and investigations

Associated features may include:

- Serum IgE >1,000ng/mL
- Blood eosinophilia >0.5 × 10⁹/L
- Skin prick +ve to *Aspergillus*
- IgG precipitins to *Aspergillus* (many different allergenic proteins)
- Long history of asthma, perhaps recently deteriorated.

Therefore, suspect this development in:

A patient with long-term asthma whose control deteriorates, with CXR changes, IgE and IgG to *Aspergillus*, eosinophilia, and perhaps hyphae in the sputum.

Management may only require an increase in inhaled steroids. However, there is a suggestion that courses of oral steroids are particularly effective and may prevent progression to bronchiectasis (see next section). Steroids limit the host's immunological response but do not seem to lead to *Aspergillus* invasion of the tissues. Poorly documented evidence of improvement with antifungal agents such as itraconazole.

Allergic bronchopulmonary aspergillosis

Definition This condition is probably an extension of exuberant IgE and IgG reaction to *Aspergillus* where the inflammatory response to the *Aspergillus* in the airways provokes a more exuberant response, with damage to the bronchial walls and bronchiectasis. Some authors reserve the use of the term ABPA for when bronchiectasis is present; others may include exuberant IgE and IgG reaction to *Aspergillus* and subdivide into ABPA-S (seropositive only) and ABPA-CB (central bronchiectasis).

The prevalence of ABPA in asthmatic populations has varied considerably between studies and clearly will depend on whether the definition includes bronchiectasis or not. It probably occurs in about 1–2% of asthmatics. A related condition occurs in patients with CF where it appears about 7% have evidence of colonization and potential ongoing damage.

Pathophysiology The factors promoting the evolution from atopic asthmatic to ABPA are not known. A particular HLA association has been shown, with the suggestion that a CD4/Th2 response to a particular *Aspergillus* antigen (Asp f 1 antigen), with release of IL4 and IL5, may be critical. Proteolytic enzymes are released by *Aspergillus* as part of its exophytic feeding strategy, and these enzymes may damage airway mucosa. However, most believe that the damage results from host defence mechanisms. Septated hyphae (rather than just spores) may be visible in the mucus and grown from sputum, but there does not appear to be actual invasion of the bronchial mucosa. This immune inflammatory activity produces mucoid impaction in the airways, eosinophilic pneumonitis, and bronchocentric granuloma formation.

Main criteria for diagnosis (the first four are the most important)
- Long history of asthma
- Skin prick/IgE +ve to *Aspergillus fumigatus*
- IgG precipitins to *Aspergillus fumigatus*
- Central (proximal) bronchiectasis
- Blood/sputum eosinophilia
- Total serum IgE >1,000ng/mL
- Lung infiltrates—flitting.

Other clinical features
- Long-standing asthma, recent deterioration
- Recurrent episodes of mucous plugging
- Fever/malaise
- Expectoration of dark mucous plugs, sometimes as casts of the airways
- Eosinophilia (sputum and blood)
- Occasional haemoptysis.

The major complication is poorly controlled asthma that requires repeated courses of oral steroids.

Investigations

- *Spirometry* Degree of airways obstruction
- *Skin prick sensitivity* to Aspergillus (IgE)
- *Sputum* Aspergillus hyphae and eosinophils
- *Blood*
  - IgG precipitins
  - IgE RAST to Aspergillus
  - Total serum IgE
  - Eosinophil count (suppressed if on steroids)
- *CXR*
  - Flitting infiltrates
  - Bronchiectasis, mucous impaction (gloved finger shadows)
- *CT* Central (proximal) bronchiectasis with upper lobe predominance.

Management The management is essentially that of severe chronic asthma, but with generous use of courses of oral steroids. Several RCTs have shown courses of itraconazole (200mg bd for 4 months) are well tolerated, reduce steroid requirements, and improve exercise tolerance. There appears to be a sustained effect after the itraconazole is stopped, suggesting at least temporary eradication of the Aspergillus. Response and relapse can be monitored with IgG precipitins to Aspergillus. Itraconazole can cause liver dysfunction, so LFTs need monitoring.

Differential diagnosis This list revolves mainly around the pulmonary infiltrates and eosinophilia.
- Acute/chronic eosinophilic pneumonia
- Churg–Strauss/EGPA syndrome
- Various parasites (e.g. filariasis, ascaris; Löffler's syndrome)
- Drug-induced eosinophilic pneumonia.

Further information

Denning DW et al. The link between fungi and severe asthma: a summary of the evidence. *Eur Resp J* 2006;**27**:615–26.

Wark PA et al. Azoles for allergic bronchopulmonary aspergillosis associated with asthma. *Cochrane Database Syst Rev* 2004;**3**:CD001108.

Invasive aspergillosis

Definition The term 'invasive aspergillosis' is reserved for the situation where *Aspergillus* hyphae actually invade tissue (hyalohyphomycosis). This usually occurs with severe immune suppression, particularly neutropenia and steroid use. The port of entry is probably the lungs, but spread can be to almost any area of the body. The species most commonly seen are *Aspergillus fumigatus, flavus, terreus,* and *niger*. Mortality is very high. The source of *Aspergillus* is unclear but has been found in hospital water supplies.

Pathogenesis Alveolar macrophages probably normally destroy *Aspergillus* spores. Macrophage failure may allow more spores to germinate, and any subsequent invasion with hyphae seems to be prevented by neutrophils. Inadequate neutrophil function allows invasion across tissue planes and into vessels, with infarction and further spread throughout the body. There is some evidence that CMV may inactivate macrophages, allowing spores to germinate. The fungal digestive proteases do the damage, rather than the host's limited immunological responses.

Clinical features

Typical setting
Fever, chest pain, cough, haemoptysis, dyspnoea, and pulmonary infiltrate in a neutropenic patient failing to respond to broad-spectrum antibiotics.

Risk factors
- Following chemotherapy, particularly provoking severe neutropenia (<100 cells/microlitre)
- Bone marrow suppression for allogeneic stem cell transplants
- Advanced HIV infection and AIDS
- Immune suppression following transplant
- Infliximab (or other anti-TNF-α) therapy.

Spread can occur anywhere, with the following well recognized:
- Sinuses (paranasal) and spread into the brain
- Endocarditis
- Eyes
- Skin (papular, ranging to ulcerative, lesions).

Careful examination and particular investigations may be needed to detect spread to these areas.

Investigations
- *Isolate Aspergillus branching septate hyphae* from respiratory tract by:
  - Sputum
  - Expressed sputum (3% saline via nebulizer)
  - BAL
  - TBB.

(Hyphae may be present when not the 1° cause of the infiltrate.)

- *Biopsies* from other sites (most convincing when acute-angle branching, septated non-pigmented hyphae are seen)
- Circulating levels of *galactomannan*, an exoantigen of *Aspergillus* (commercial EIA kit available; sensitivity for invasive aspergillosis 71%, specificity 89%; false positives due to some antibiotics, e.g. co-amoxiclav and piperacillin-tazobactam). Serial sampling is recommended. May also have a role in examining BAL fluid
- Presence of β-*glucan* in serum represents fungal invasion but is not *Aspergillus*-specific; false positives due to blood processing and some antibiotics may affect results
- *CXR/CT* CXR changes are usually non-specific. CT may show a halo of low attenuation surrounding a nodular lesion early on. An 'air crescent' sign may develop on CXR, with air appearing at the edge of an area of consolidation. Usually occurs when neutrophil count rising and probably represents gradual containment of the infection into a cavity, not unlike an aspergilloma. Radiological findings may also be seen with other angioinvasive filamentous fungi, *Nocardia* spp., and *Pseudomonas aeruginosa*.

Ultimately, it is the clinical picture that dominates the diagnosis.

Management Reduction of immunosuppression when possible; consider colony-stimulating factors. Prompt use of antifungals is essential, for a minimum of 6–12 weeks

- IV voriconazole is the treatment of choice (may cause visual disturbances, deranged LFTs, skin rash)
- Liposomal amphotericin B is an alternative first-line treatment
- Patients who are intolerant of voriconazole/liposomal amphotericin or who have refractory disease can be treated with lipid-based amphotericin posaconazole, itraconazole, caspofungin, or micafungin

Some centres use oral posaconazole as prophylaxis when commencing substantial immune suppression.

Surgical resection of the infected focus should be considered in some (e.g. lung lesions contiguous with the heart or great vessels, chest wall invasion, osteomyelitis, pericardial infection, and endocarditis).

Differential diagnosis

The differential will be the large number of other opportunistic infections seen in immunosuppressed patients. Another invasive mycosis *Candida albicans* is now less common due to its susceptibility to fluconazole.

Further information

Walsh TJ et al. Treatment of aspergillosis: Clinical Practice Guidelines of the Infectious Diseases Society of America. *Clin Infect Dis* 2008;**46**:327–60.

Upton A et al. Invasive aspergillosis following hematopoietic cell transplantation. *Clin Infect Dis* 2007;**44**:531–40.

Patterson TF. Advances and challenges in the management of invasive mycoses. *Lancet* 2005;**366**:1013–25.

Semi-invasive aspergillosis

(also known as chronic necrotizing aspergillosis, chronic pulmonary aspergillosis, or subacute invasive pulmonary aspergillosis)

Definition This entity is poorly defined, but it is clear that a low-grade chronic invasion of *Aspergillus* into airway walls and surrounding lung can occur. In the original descriptions, some cause of mild immuno-incompetence was present such as diabetes, steroid therapy, chronic lung disease, poor nutrition, etc. Previous asthma is not usually present, unlike ABPA.

Pathogenesis It is assumed that this form of aspergillosis results from lowered immunity in those with a tendency to make Th2 eosinophilic responses to antigens. There is infiltration of hyphae into lung tissue, ranging from minor patchy consolidation to multiple cavities. There is little, if any, angioinvasion. It is assumed that the fungal digestive proteases gradually do the damage, rather than the host's immunological response.

Clinical features

Suspect semi-invasive aspergillosis when:
• Middle-aged
• Reason for mild immunosuppression, e.g. diabetes, alcoholism, and steroid usage
• A pre-existing chronic lung disease
• Fever
• Productive cough
• Patchy indolent CXR changes.

Investigations
• Sputum samples may allow isolation of hyphae
• CT will show an airway-centred type of picture with 'tree-in-bud' appearance. With increasing severity, this gives way to denser areas and small cavities that occasionally may contain a fungus ball
• Likely to have IgG precipitins to *Aspergillus*, but not always.

Management On the assumption that mild immune suppression is the dominant cause, steroids are not usually recommended for fear of further immune suppression. This is in contrast to ABPA where the damage is due to the host's immune defence mechanisms. Oral treatment with voriconazole is usually appropriate, but IV therapy is required for severely ill patients. Alternative treatment options are as for invasive aspergillosis.

Respiratory infection—fungal

Aspergillum mycetoma

Definition

Pathogenesis

Clinical features

Investigations

Management

Aspergilloma/mycetoma

(known as chronic cavitary pulmonary aspergillosis when there are multiple cavities)

Definition The term aspergilloma is used to describe a ball of fungal hyphae within a cavity in the lung. It is assumed that this is colonization of a prior cavity ('saphrophytic infection'), rather than arrested invasion. Aspergillomas can occur in other organs, including the pleural space.

Chronic cavitary pulmonary aspergillosis (CCPA) demonstrates multiple cavities, often with aspergillomas, in association with pulmonary and systemic symptoms and raised inflammatory markers. Usually associated with prolonged symptoms and defects in innate immunity.

Pathogenesis Cavities can occur in the lung following a variety of insults such as TB, sarcoid, ordinary pneumonia/lung abscess, treated tumours, and CF. Fungal spores entering the cavity germinate and survive in a relatively protected environment. The ball consists of hyphae, inflammatory cells, fibrin, and debris. Around the cavity is an intense inflammatory response, often with considerable extra vascularization from bronchial arteries and occasional fungal hyphae.

Clinical features Aspergillomas are often asymptomatic. Up to 75% will present with haemoptysis, assumed to come from damaged vessels on the inner surface of the cavity wall, via a communication with a bronchus. Sometimes, there are systemic symptoms, malaise, and fever, as well as chest pain. Superadded infection may provoke exacerbations.

Investigations
- *CXR* Apical cavity with ball within that changes position if CXR is performed decubitus
- *CT* Obvious cavity with fungus ball and possible invasion into surrounding lung (uncommon)
- *Sputum culture*
- *Aspergillus IgG precipitins* Often higher levels than seen in other *Aspergillus* diseases.

Management
- Single aspergilloma:
  - May not require treatment
  - Consideration of surgical resection
  - Systemic symptoms of fever and malaise may be hard to ascribe to a mycetoma and require a therapeutic trial of voriconazole/itraconazole
  - The most significant complication is life-threatening haemoptysis. The emergency management of haemoptysis is described on ➜ p. 47
  - Itraconazole or voriconazole will not eradicate the fungus but seem to reduce cavity size and lessen the tendency to haemoptysis. It is assumed that they kill any fungus in the walls and inhibit growth in the cavity

- CCPA:
  - Treat with itraconazole or voriconazole
  - Avoid surgery (associated with high morbidity and mortality, with complications, including haemorrhage, bronchopleural fistulae, and soiling of the pleural space).

Haemoptysis

- Bronchial arteriograms should reveal a leash of vessels supplying part of the cavity wall that can be embolized, even if not actively bleeding. Short-term success rate is good; long term, less good
- Surgery can be difficult, as mycetomas may be stuck to the chest wall. Problems of seeding the pleural space are seen less often than in the past, probably due to better antifungal agents
- A few case reports exist of successful reduction of haemoptysis with radiotherapy
- Older approaches involving intracavity injections of amphotericin are rarely used now, although a recent case series of 40 patients seemed promising.

Overview of *Aspergillus* lung disease

The essential differences between the *Aspergillus* lung diseases depends on whether the damage to the lung is mediated by host defence mechanisms (atopic asthma, flitting consolidation, ABPA, possibly aspergilloma) or by the fungus' own digestive proteolytic enzymes (invasive aspergillosis, semi-invasive, aspergilloma). These two disease states are clearly different, but there probably exists a continuum between each of the subdivisions within each group, and the dominant mechanism in aspergilloma is not entirely clear. Therefore, it is likely that patients with mixed and transitional features will be encountered.

Future developments

- Evaluation of combination antifungal therapies
- Antifungal action of older drugs—flucytosine, rifampicin
- Place of early surgery
- Place of prophylaxis
- Further evaluation of the role of galactomannan and β-glucan levels in blood and BAL fluid for diagnosis.

Further information

Aspergillus/Fungal Research Trust website. ℘ http://www.aspergillus.org.uk.
Soubani A et al. The clinical spectrum of pulmonary aspergillosis. *Chest* 2002;**121**:1988–99.

General approach to chronic haemoptysis

- Tranexamic acid (must be taken during clot formation, as binds to fibrin to prevent action of endogenous fibrinolytics)
- Treat associated bacterial infections.

Specific to aspergilloma

- Itraconazole/voriconazole
- Arterial embolization (usually bronchial circulation)
- Surgical resection.

Pneumocystis pneumonia (PCP): diagnosis

Definition PCP is the clinical syndrome of pneumonia resulting from infection with the fungus *Pneumocystis jirovecii* (previously termed *Pneumocystis carinii*). *Pneumocystis jirovecii* is widespread in the environment, and most people are infected by the age of 2y; PCP is thought, however, to follow new infection, rather than reactivation of latent infection. Most cases of infection are likely to be person-to-person airborne transmission, rather than environmental.

Causes Risk factors for PCP include HIV infection (particularly with CD4 count <200 × 10⁶/L), treatment with chemotherapy (especially fludarabine), corticosteroids or other immunosuppressive agents, and malnutrition in children. Neutropenia does not appear to be a particular risk factor. PCP occurring in the setting of AIDS is associated with both a greater number of organisms and fewer inflammatory cells in the lungs when compared with infection associated with other causes of immunocompromise. PCP is much less common following the routine use of co-trimoxazole prophylaxis in HIV and post-transplantation, although cases still occur, e.g. in patients presenting with advanced HIV or in those non-compliant with prophylaxis. The threshold steroid dose for predisposition to PCP is unclear, although a dose equivalent to 16mg prednisolone or greater for 8 weeks appears to significantly increase risk; the risk is likely also to reflect the underlying condition, e.g. PCP may develop in patients with haematological malignancy taking as little as 5mg prednisolone daily. PCP often appears to present as immunosuppressant drug doses are tapered or increased.

Clinical features Gradual onset of dry cough and exertional breathlessness, sometimes with retrosternal tightness. Fever and tachypnoea may occur; chest examination is typically normal. May present with pneumothorax. Extrapulmonary disease is very rare.

Investigations

- *CXR* Pattern is classically of bilateral perihilar infiltrates that progress to alveolar shadowing. Less common patterns include small nodular infiltrates or focal consolidation. CXR is normal in about 10%. Pleural effusions are very rare. CT is not routinely required, except in cases of a normal CXR when it may demonstrate a bilateral ground-glass pattern or cystic lesions
- *Hypoxia* is common. Desaturation on exercise may suggest the diagnosis in at-risk individuals with normal saturations at rest
- *White blood count* is usually normal. Serum LDH is typically raised (sensitive but non-specific)
- *Induced sputum* (see ⮞ p. 776) has a diagnostic yield of about 60% in HIV infection but is much less sensitive when performed in the setting of non-HIV immunocompromise where the organism burden is lower. It should not be performed on the open ward or outpatient department

- *Bronchoscopy with BAL* is the diagnostic investigation of choice in non-HIV-infected patients and in patients with HIV in whom induced sputum analysis is non-diagnostic. BAL with silver or immunofluorescent staining has a specificity of nearly 100% and sensitivity of 80–90%. This sensitivity is lower in non-HIV-infected immunocompromised patients, reflecting their lower pathogen loads
- *Transbronchial lung biopsy* has a slightly higher sensitivity (around 95%) but is associated with an increased risk of complications so is reserved for cases where BAL is non-diagnostic. Surgical lung biopsy may be required for diagnosis in a minority of HIV-negative patients.

PCP: treatment

Antimicrobial

- Liaise with infectious diseases or HIV specialist
- High-dose co-trimoxazole (trimethoprim and sulfamethoxazole) remains the drug of choice. Administer 120mg/kg daily in four divided doses PO or IV (dilute 480mg ampoules in at least 75mL 5% glucose; infuse over 60min). Use IV route initially and then PO during clinical improvement; PO may be used initially in mild cases. Side effects (e.g. rash, nausea, vomiting, blood disorders) are common, particularly in HIV-infected patients. Consider routine use of antiemetics
- Second-line choices, if intolerant or unresponsive to co-trimoxazole, include IV pentamidine, clindamycin and primaquine, dapsone and trimethoprim, atovaquone
- All treatments should be for 2–3 weeks
- If PCP is strongly suspected and the patient is unwell, treatment can be started immediately, as BAL pneumocystis stains remain positive for up to 2 weeks. Empirical treatment is also required in the occasional situation where the diagnosis is suspected but bronchoscopy is non-diagnostic or not tolerated
- In cases of HIV presenting with PCP, early introduction of highly active antiretroviral therapy (HAART) has been contentious, with theoretical risks of drug interactions, increasing toxicities, and the potential for IRIS. However, a randomized trial and a retrospective analysis both demonstrated a 50% reduction in mortality when HAART was started within 2 weeks of PCP treatment. Suspected IRIS should be treated with corticosteroids ± reintroduction of PCP therapy.

Steroids

- High-dose steroids (prednisolone 40mg bd PO or IV hydrocortisone) are recommended for all patients in respiratory failure. Treat at high dose for 5 days; taper dose over 1–3 weeks (e.g. prednisolone 40mg daily for days 6–11, then 20mg daily for days 12–21).

Supportive therapy

- Hypoxia is common; administer supplementary high-flow O_2, and consider use of CPAP. Mechanical ventilation, if considered appropriate, may be required; make this decision prior to initiating CPAP.

Outcome

- Mortality 10–20% in the setting of AIDS, but 35–50% in patients with other forms of immunocompromise, probably reflecting the adverse consequences of the greater pulmonary inflammatory response to pneumocystis which is observed in non-HIV immunocompromise. Mortality from PCP requiring mechanical ventilation in HIV-infected patients is about 60% although may be significantly higher in patients with low CD4 counts.

- Relapse rate in AIDS is high (60% in 1y), so 2° prophylaxis with co-trimoxazole is recommended. 1° prophylaxis is offered to HIV-positive patients with CD4 count <200 × 10⁶/L. The indications for prophylaxis in non-HIV patients are less well defined; consider prophylaxis for patients who are likely to receive high doses of prednisolone for prolonged periods.

Future developments

- The effect of co-infection with CMV on the outcome of PCP in HIV-infected patients is unclear. In patients with severe PCP treated with steroids, the presence of CMV in BAL fluid is associated with a worse outcome; the role of anti-CMV therapy, such as ganciclovir, in such cases is unknown
- The use of PCR to detect pneumocystis may further increase diagnostic sensitivity, although, in a proportion of cases, detection using PCR is not accompanied by evidence of clinical infection and appears to represent colonization. It is unclear if asymptomatic carriage precedes infection in such patients, and the consequences of carriage in immunocompetent individuals are also unknown
- Pneumocystis is one of only a handful of cells known to be unable to synthesize the metabolic intermediate molecule S-adenosylmethionine (AdoMet) and, as a result, must scavenge this molecule from its host. In a small study, lower plasma levels of AdoMet were demonstrated in PCP when compared with healthy controls and individuals with other pulmonary infections, suggesting a possible role for AdoMet in diagnosis. This finding has not yet been replicated in a larger study, however.

Further information

Kovacs JA et al. New insights into transmission, diagnosis, and drug treatment of *Pneumocystis carinii* pneumonia. *JAMA* 2001;**286**:2450–60.

Thomas CF, Limper AH. Pneumocystis pneumonia. *N Engl J Med* 2004;**350**:2487–98.

Cryptococcosis

Epidemiology

- *Cryptococcus neoformans* is found worldwide in bird droppings. Following inhalation, yeasts propagate within the alveoli, without usually causing symptoms. Migration to the CNS may then occur, and meningoencephalitis is the most common clinical manifestation of infection
- Patients with impaired cell-mediated immunity (e.g. AIDS, steroid use, lymphoma) are particularly vulnerable to cryptococcal infection.

Clinical features

- Clinically evident cryptococcal lung disease is rare, but well described, even in HIV-negative patients. Symptoms are non-specific, including fever and cough, and presentations may be acute or chronic. The CXR may show non-calcified nodules, lymphadenopathy, lobar infiltrates, or pleural involvement
- Pulmonary involvement is associated with meningoencephalitis in those with underlying immunosuppression, and clinical signs of meningism are characteristically absent. CT head (to exclude a space-occupying lesion), followed by lumbar puncture, should therefore be considered in all patients with pulmonary cryptococcal disease who have any condition predisposing to dissemination or neurological signs.

Diagnosis Diagnostic techniques include:

- India ink stain on CSF, or latex agglutination test for capsular antigen in BAL or pleural fluid, blood, or CSF. Serum cryptococcal antigen test is extremely sensitive and specific for the diagnosis
- Stains and culture of sputum, blood, urine, or BAL fluid. Positive culture from sputum may indicate colonization, rather than active disease, and should be interpreted in the clinical context.

Treatment of cryptococcal infection in the immunocompromised is with amphotericin B IV and flucytosine IV for 2–3 weeks, followed by fluconazole. The natural history of disease in immunocompetent patients is poorly understood, and observation alone is often recommended; disseminated disease may occur, however, and some experts advise treatment with fluconazole.

Candidal pneumonia

- *Candida* occurs as part of the normal human flora and is found in the GI tract and on the skin. Invasive disease may occur in the immunocompromised, particularly in neutropenic patients. Prophylaxis with fluconazole is used following bone marrow transplantation
- *Candida* is often isolated from respiratory secretions but very rarely causes respiratory disease. Haematogenous seeding to the lungs causing infiltrates or enlarging nodules may occur with disseminated candidal infection
- Risk factors for candidaemia include immunocompromise, central venous lines, parenteral nutrition, and GI surgery. In lung transplant recipients, a positive donor tracheal culture for *Candida* is a marker for post-transplant candidal infection
- The clinical and radiological features of pulmonary involvement are non-specific. Extrapulmonary manifestations of infection are common, e.g. skin, eye, hepatic, or CNS involvement. Candidaemia is typically associated with a high fever
- Definitive diagnosis of pulmonary disease requires identification of tissue invasion by *Candida* on TBB or surgical lung biopsy
- Treat with an echinocandin (e.g. caspofungin, micafungin), amphotericin B, or fluconazole, and remove any central lines
- Candidaemia carries a mortality of 30–40%.

Further information

Pappas PG *et al.* Clinical practice guidelines for the management of candidiasis: 2009 update by the Infectious Diseases Society of America. *Clin Infect Dis* 2009;**48**:503–35.

Endemic mycoses: introduction

Several types of dimorphic fungi are known to commonly cause pulmonary disease in endemic regions, particularly in North America: *histoplasmosis*, *blastomycosis*, *coccidioidomycosis*, and *paracoccidioidomycosis*. Endemic fungi can rarely present in non-endemic areas, and diagnosis is often delayed because of their non-specific and varied clinical features and the failure to obtain a detailed travel history. Fungal infection may mimic other diseases, such as TB and lung cancer, often leading to inappropriate investigations and treatment. Fungal infections can also cause granulomata on lung biopsy, which sometimes results in diagnostic confusion (e.g. with sarcoidosis).

Infection in immunocompetent individuals is usually either asymptomatic or mild and self-limiting, although severe infection may rarely occur in apparently immunocompetent individuals. Outbreaks of disease may occur, as well as sporadic cases. Unlike invasive candidiasis and aspergillosis, where neutrophils are the key host defence mechanism, T-cell-mediated immunity is essential for defence against the endemic mycoses. Patients with impaired T-cell-mediated immunity (e.g. AIDS, lymphoma, steroid use) are therefore at particular risk of developing severe or disseminated infection.

Endemic mycoses: histoplasmosis

Epidemiology *Histoplasma capsulatum* is found in bird and bat dropping-contaminated soil in the Midwest and south-east USA, particularly the Ohio and Mississippi valleys, as well as in Mexico and parts of South America. The mycelial form is inhaled and subsequently develops into the yeast form ('dimorphism') within the lung before spread via the lymphatics and the activation of T-cell-mediated immunity with granuloma development.

Clinical features Manifestations of infection are highly variable.

- *Asymptomatic* infection occurs in the majority of cases. CXR may be normal or demonstrate single or multiple nodules, which may calcify in a characteristic 'target lesion' pattern. Lymphadenopathy may occur with eggshell calcification
- *Acute* symptoms may follow heavy or recurrent exposure (e.g. pigeon fanciers, cavers). Range from a self-limiting flu-like illness of fever, cough, and malaise to fulminant disease with respiratory failure. CXR may be normal or show consolidation, bilateral alveolar shadowing, multiple small nodules, and sometimes lymphadenopathy
- *Chronic* progressive lung disease occurs particularly in patients with underlying COPD; lung cavitation is common, sometimes leading to an incorrect diagnosis of TB or cancer
- *Disseminated* disease may affect the immunocompromised (particularly AIDS) and the elderly. Presentation may be acute or chronic, and manifestations include fever, weight loss, and diffuse lung involvement, although almost any organ system may be affected; other features may include hepatosplenomegaly, GI symptoms, headache and meningism, cytopenias, endocarditis, and adrenal failure
- Other unusual manifestations include broncholithiasis, mediastinal fibrosis (with compression of large airways, oesophagus, or SVC), or isolated extrapulmonary disease (e.g. arthritis, pericarditis, erythema nodosum, erythema multiforme).

Diagnosis

- Smears or culture of infected material, e.g. sputum or BAL fluid (for chronic pulmonary disease, insensitive for acute disease), blood, urine, or bone marrow (for disseminated disease). May take several weeks
- Serology in acute disease—typically negative at presentation and becomes positive after several weeks. A variety of serological tests are in use, including:
  - Complement fixation, designed to detect antibodies to *Histoplasma* mycelial antigen or *Histoplasma* yeast antigen. A positive result (serum titre ≥1:16 for mycelial antigen, ≥1:32 for yeast antigen) for either antigen, in a compatible clinical setting, is considered diagnostic of active disease
  - Immunodiffusion may distinguish active disease from previous exposure but is less sensitive than complement fixation, and a negative result does not exclude the diagnosis

- Serum, urine, or BAL fluid *Histoplasma* polysaccharide antigen test—useful for diagnosis of disseminated disease and also pulmonary disease. Positive in 85–95% cases in AIDS patients. Antigenuria is seen in 90%, and antigenaemia in <50% of non-AIDS patients.

Treatment

- Infection in immunocompetent individuals is typically self-limiting, and symptoms usually resolve within 2–4 weeks without treatment
- Indications for antifungal treatment are:
  - Persistent symptoms (usually lasting >1 month)
  - Progressive disseminated disease
  - Heavy exposure leading to ARDS
  - Infection in the setting of immunocompromise
- Oral itraconazole is appropriate for persistent symptoms in mild to moderate disease and for disseminated disease, including patients with AIDS who have mild disease. Treat for 6–12 weeks in acute histoplasmosis, and for 1–2y in chronic disease. In the setting of AIDS, treatment should be lifelong or until CD4 count >200 for at least 6 months after starting HAART. Check itraconazole drug interactions, and monitor liver function (ideally monthly) if taking for >1 month. Hypokalaemia may be associated with long-term use
- IV lipid formulations of amphotericin B should be used to treat severe infection in the setting of ARDS or immunocompromise.

Endemic mycoses: blastomycosis

Epidemiology Infection with *Blastomyces dermatitidis* follows the inhalation of spores from contaminated soil, and clinical infection may follow outdoor activities. Blastomycosis is endemic in a distribution similar to that of histoplasmosis in the USA, although extending further north; it is endemic in the south-east USA and the Mississippi, Ohio, and St Lawrence river valleys. Blastomycosis also occurs in Africa, India, and the Middle East. It is significantly less common than histoplasmosis.

Clinical features Clinical presentation is variable and may mimic other diseases such as bacterial pneumonia, TB, and lung cancer. Clinical manifestations include:

- *Asymptomatic* in at least 50% of those infected
- *Acute* presentation is typically with fever, cough, productive of mucopurulent sputum, and sometimes pleuritic chest pain; misdiagnosis as bacterial pneumonia is common. Acute presentation of fulminant respiratory disease with ARDS may occur. Other acute presentations include a flu-like illness with fever, myalgia, arthralgia, and erythema nodosum
- *Chronic* presentation with fever, productive cough, and weight loss
- *Disseminated* disease occurs in a minority of patients (especially in the immunocompromised) and most commonly involves the lungs, skin, bone, joints, and CNS.

CXR Airspace infiltrates are the most common finding, but a very wide range of appearances are seen, including nodular pattern, lobar consolidation, diffuse infiltrates, or large peripheral masses (often with air bronchograms). Lymphadenopathy and pleural effusions may rarely occur.

Diagnosis

- Diagnosis is by the staining or culture of infected material. A pyogenic inflammatory response to the fungus is common (unlike in histoplasmosis) and facilitates diagnosis
- Culture of sputum has a high yield and is diagnostic in most cases of acute pulmonary disease. Multiple specimens may be required, however. A drawback of sputum culture is that several weeks may be required before the fungus is identified. Cytological examination of sputum may provide a rapid diagnosis if the examiner is trained appropriately and alerted to the possible diagnosis
- Bronchoscopy has a similar diagnostic yield to sputum culture (92% in one study) and is recommended for patients with negative sputum results; note that lidocaine may inhibit the fungal growth, and minimal concentrations should be used
- More invasive procedures, such as surgical lung biopsy or thoracoscopy, are only rarely needed. Histological specimens require particular stains (e.g. silver stain) to facilitate identification of the fungus
- Currently available serological tests lack sensitivity and are rarely helpful.

Treatment is usually with itraconazole for at least 6 months. Observation without treatment is not generally recommended, although this is controversial, and symptoms are usually self-limiting in immunocompetent individuals. Lipid formulations of amphotericin B should be used to treat very ill patients.

Endemic mycoses: coccidioidomycosis

Coccidioidomycosis is endemic in parts of south-west USA (Arizona, California, Texas, New Mexico, Utah, Nevada), northern Mexico, and Central and South America. Infection follows inhalation of *Coccidioides immitis* or *C. posadasii* spores from soil. Manifestations of infection are variable, including:

- *Asymptomatic* infection, which appears to be common in endemic regions
- *Acute* pulmonary disease. Presents in a similar manner to bacterial pneumonia, with fever, cough, pleuritic chest pain, and often skin rash (e.g. erythema nodosum or erythema multiforme). Eosinophilia may be present. CXR appearance is variable and may show areas of consolidation, lymphadenopathy, and pleural effusion, or be normal. The disease is self-limiting in most cases (Valley Fever); a minority progress to ARDS or chronic disease
- *Chronic* pulmonary disease. Uncommon, may be asymptomatic. CXR typically shows single or multiple nodules that may cavitate; upper lobe infiltrates, similar to those seen in TB, may develop
- *Disseminated* disease. Rare, occurs particularly in the immunocompromised. Presentation may be acute or chronic. Pulmonary disease occurs in association with involvement of the skin, bones, joints, genitourinary system, or CNS.

Diagnosis is with stains or culture of infected tissues. Sputum cultures are often positive in cavitating disease. BAL fluid culture and lung biopsies may also be diagnostic. Serological tests are also available.

Treatment is not required in the majority of patients who have mild self-limiting disease. Fluconazole is the antifungal of choice, when required.

Endemic mycoses: paracoccidioidomycosis

- Paracoccidioidomycosis is endemic in parts of Central and South America and Mexico
- Caused by the dimorphic fungus *Paracoccidioides brasiliensis*
- Typically presents as chronic pulmonary disease, although acute disseminated disease may occur in the immunocompromised
- Diagnosis is made on culture of sputum or BAL fluid, or following staining of lung biopsy samples
- Treatment is with itraconazole, and long courses of up to 6 months may be needed. Severe disease is treated with amphotericin B.

Chapter 42

Respiratory infection—mycobacterial

Tuberculosis: epidemiology and pathophysiology

Tuberculosis (TB) is the second leading infectious cause of death world-wide (after AIDS), despite being a potentially curable disease. It kills around 1.4 million people per year, of whom 0.43 million are HIV +ve and 64,000 are children. Rising rates of HIV and immigration mean TB remains a large proportion of the workload for respiratory physicians in some parts of the UK. The disease is a great 'mimicker' and should often be considered as part of the differential diagnosis in patients with respiratory disease.

Epidemiology Globally, the WHO estimates there are 125 cases of TB per 100,000 population (2011). The highest incidence is in sub-Saharan Africa (262 cases per 100,000 population). High population density countries in Asia (India, China, Pakistan, and Indonesia) account for half the global burden. The countries comprising the former Soviet Union have rapidly increasing rates because of economic decline and failing health services, with around 25% multidrug resistance in this area. Globally, a significant proportion of people are co-infected with HIV; this number is particularly high in sub-Saharan Africa.

In the UK, there were 8,800 cases of TB in 2011, 14 per 100,000. This number has been relatively stable for the past 5–10y. UK death rates from TB are decreasing. The majority of cases in the UK are in people born abroad, but a significant amount of TB is in UK-born Caucasians. Around 8% of cases are co-infected with HIV. TB is concentrated in the major cities, with 40% of cases in London.

Pathophysiology The disease is spread by airborne droplets containing *Mycobacterium tuberculosis* (MTB). Droplets remain airborne for hours after expectoration because of their small size. Infectious droplets are inhaled and become lodged in the distal airways. MTB is taken up by alveolar macrophages, triggering the innate immune system, and spreads via the lymphatics to hilar lymph nodes. Later, a cell-mediated immune process leads to granuloma formation by activated T-lymphocytes and macrophages, which limits further bacterial replication and disease spread. Most (over 90%) immunocompetent individuals successfully contain the infection (either eliminated or contained in a latent state); 10% progress to active 1° disease (1° progressive TB).

Many factors influence whether or not infection leads to active disease, including age, host immunity, and time since infection (risk highest in first few years after infection). The estimated lifetime risk of clinical disease in a child newly infected with MTB is about 10%.

Active disease occurs when the host's immune response is unable to contain MTB replication, with absent or poorly formed granulomas. Active disease occurs most often in the lung parenchyma (due to high O_2 content, in which the bacillus grows well) and hilar lymph nodes. It can occur in any organ from haematogenous spread. This is most common in young children and immunosuppressed adults. Most disease in adults is due to reactivation of childhood disease, so-called 'post-primary disease', from activation of latent TB (the Ghon focus) lying dormant in the lung.

The term *smear-positive TB* refers to the identification of AFB on sputum smear (ZN stain). Infectious. Patient will require isolation if admitted to hospital.

Culture-positive TB refers to AFB not seen on smear (smear-negative). TB grown on culture (may take up to 9 weeks). Much less infectious than smear-positive disease, although transmission can still occur.

Main risk factors for active TB in the UK

- Place and date of birth:
  - Caucasian population; increasing prevalence with age ($\circlearrowleft > \circleorarrow$)
  - Afro-Caribbean immigrants; highest prevalence in the young ($\circlearrowleft = \circleorarrow$)
  - Indian subcontinent; highest prevalence in middle age ($\circlearrowleft = \circleorarrow$)
- HIV/AIDS
- Poverty, undernutrition, and overcrowding
- Heavy alcohol consumption and smoking
- Medical factors—diabetes, end-stage renal failure, malignant disease, systemic chemotherapy, steroids and TNF-α antagonists, e.g. infliximab, vitamin D deficiency (vitamin D has pleiotropic effects on the immune system, including macrophage activation).

TB: pulmonary disease

Symptoms
Most cases present with pulmonary disease, classically:
- Productive cough
- Haemoptysis
- Breathlessness
- Systemic symptoms—weight loss, night sweats, and malaise
- Chest pain.

Haemoptysis is more common with cavitatory disease, and up to two-thirds will be smear-positive. Most haemoptysis is small volume. Massive haemoptysis is rare and is most common as a consequence of destruction of a lobe, with consequent bronchiectasis formation (possibly with 2° *Aspergillus* infection or mycetoma in a healed TB cavity). This is seen in those untreated in the pre-chemotherapy era. Most haemoptysis will resolve with antituberculous chemotherapy.

Signs are often non-specific.
- Examination may be normal
- Lymphadenopathy (particularly cervical)
- Crackles
- Signs of a pleural effusion
- Signs of consolidation (with extensive disease)
- Signs of weight loss/underlying immunocompromise
- Look for evidence of extrapulmonary disease, e.g. skin, joints, CNS, retina, and spinal disease.

Complications Long-term sequelae of inadequately treated infection include:
- *Bronchiectasis*, bronchial obstruction, and airway stenosis (uncommon) may result from endobronchial disease, though this is much less common in the post-chemotherapy era. It is more common in the presence of extensive parenchymal disease and is associated with lymph node enlargement, with compromise of airway size
- *Pleural disease* (see → p. 356) is due to either 1° progressive disease or reactivation of latent infection. It probably represents an increased immune response—a delayed-type hypersensitivity reaction to mycobacterial antigens, rather than a diminished one, which is the case in other forms of TB infection. Culture is more likely from pleural tissue than fluid (where the organism burden is lower)
- *Pneumothorax* is rare (<1% in the developed world) and results from the rupture of a peripheral cavity. Can lead to the formation of a bronchopleural fistula
- Draining *abscess*
- *Right middle lobe syndrome*—compression of the right middle lobe bronchus by hilar lymph nodes leads to lobar collapse
- The previous treatment with *thoracoplasty* can lead to respiratory failure in later life due to compromised VC.

TB: extrapulmonary disease

Extrapulmonary disease is seen in about 20% of patients with TB. This proportion is higher in HIV-positive patients.

The tuberculin skin test (see ➔ pp. 490–1) is more frequently positive in extrapulmonary disease, as this most commonly represents reactivated disease and less commonly 1° disease. Anergy is more likely in those with poor nutritional status, underlying disease (including HIV), and the elderly.

CNS disease is the most serious manifestation and includes meningeal involvement and space-occupying lesions (tuberculoma) that may lead to cranial nerve lesions. The clinical manifestations are due to the presence of MTB and the host's inflammatory immune response.

TB meningitis presents with headache, fever, altered conscious level, and focal neurological signs, including cranial nerve palsies. Fits are common.

CSF contains lymphocytes, high protein, and low glucose. PCR of CSF may be useful but is not 100% sensitive.

Pericardial TB The yield is low from pericardial fluid and biopsy. 85% have a positive tuberculin test. A large effusion may lead to cardiac tamponade and may need to be drained.

Spinal disease can affect any bone or joint; spine involvement (Pott's disease) is most common in the thoracic spine. Surgery may be needed if there is evidence of cord compression or instability.

Genitourinary disease from seeding during haematogenous spread. Involvement of the renal and genital tracts is uncommon.

In men—may cause prostatitis and epididymitis.

In women—genitourinary TB is a cause of infertility. Sterile pyuria (white and red blood cells in the urine, in the absence of bacterial infection) may indicate TB infection.

Peripheral cold abscess can occur at almost any body site.

Disseminated disease is more common in immunosuppressed individuals. Pulmonary disease is typically a miliary (millet seed) pattern, but pulmonary disease is not universal in disseminated disease. This has a higher mortality than localized disease.

TB: investigations

The diagnosis is usually made in one of three ways: *smear or culture* of sputum (or other sample, e.g. pus, CSF, urine, biopsy tissue), or *histology* with the identification of caseating granulomas on biopsy.

- *CXR* classically shows upper lobe infiltrates with cavitation
  - May be associated with hilar or paratracheal lymphadenopathy
  - May show changes consistent with prior TB infection, with fibrous scar tissue and calcification
  - HIV-infected patients typically have less florid CXR changes and are less likely to have cavitary disease. Miliary pattern is more common in later stages of AIDS
  - All patients with non-pulmonary TB should have a CXR to exclude or confirm pulmonary disease
- *Sputum ZN stain and culture* is required for definitive diagnosis and is vital for drug resistance testing. ZN is only 50–80% sensitive
  - New sputum processing techniques, along with fluorescence microscopy, have improved smear sensitivity and efficient reading of slides
  - Smear-negative disease accounts for about 20% of disease transmission; smear-positive cases are more infectious
  - Induced sputum is as effective as BAL, especially if the CXR shows changes consistent with active disease (but should not be used for potential MDR-TB, due to the danger to health workers)
  - Conventional culture takes 6 weeks or longer, although use of the mycobacterial growth indicator tube (MGIT) culture system can lead to positive cultures within days
  - Nucleic acid amplification techniques are increasingly used to confirm mycobacteria serotype and drug susceptibility. The Xpert MTB/RIF assay can simultaneously detect MTB and identify rifampicin resistance (which is strongly associated with MDR-TB) within 2h and has been recommended by the WHO for use in regions with high rates of HIV/TB co-infection or MDR-TB
- *Tuberculin skin test (Mantoux)* are only useful if strongly positive (suggesting active disease) or if negative (see Box 42.1). The skin test must be interpreted with the clinical picture and with knowledge of the patient's ethnic origin, exposure, and BCG vaccination history
- *IGRAs* (see ➔ p. 508) High sensitivity, but low specificity, of IGRAs mean a negative/low result rules out active or latent TB, but a positive result cannot differentiate between the two
- *Bronchoscopy/EBUS* may be needed to obtain BAL or lymph node samples if there is a high index of clinical suspicion but a non-productive cough or unhelpful sputum culture. In extensive disease, macroscopic bronchoscopic abnormality may be present, with erythematous or ulcerated airways. Granulation tissue or enlarged lymph nodes may be visible. Nodes can perforate or protrude into the bronchial lumen, extruding caseous material into the airway

- *Biopsy from extrapulmonary sites*, e.g. neck lymph nodes, or mediastinoscopy may be warranted. Lymph node biopsy samples, pleural biopsies, and pus aspirated from lymph nodes should be transported to the laboratory in a dry pot (not formalin). Bone marrow or liver biopsy may aid diagnosis in miliary TB. The bone marrow culture yield is higher in pancytopenia
- *Gastric washings* reflect TB swallowed overnight. Rarely performed if bronchoscopy is readily available. Used more commonly in children
- *Urine* Early morning urine (EMU) only if renal disease suspected
- *Blood tests* Baseline FBC, renal and liver function tests. Useful to document normal baseline levels before starting antituberculous chemotherapy
- *HIV test* should be offered to all patients
- *CT scan* is more sensitive than CXR, especially for smaller areas of disease. It may show cavitatory disease and signs of airway disease—the 'tree-in-bud' appearance, useful for differentiating between active disease and non-active old disease and guiding area for BAL. May also be needed to assess mediastinal or hilar lympadenopathy.

A tuberculoma is an encapsulated focus of reactivated TB. These lesions rarely cavitate, and the differential diagnosis is wide, including malignancy (pulmonary nodule, see ➲ p. 312) and vasculitis. Diagnosis may only be possible by percutaneous biopsy, as, in the absence of a main airway component, cultures may be negative.

Box 42.1 Mantoux skin test
- Read at 48h
- Intradermal. Use 0.1mL of 1 in 1,000 (= 0.1mL of 100TU/mL = 10TU)
- Graded:
  - <5mm, negative
  - 5–14mm, positive
  - >15mm, strongly positive.

TB: management 1

Treatment aims to cure disease without relapse, prevent transmission, and prevent emergence of drug resistance. Long-term treatment with a number of drugs is required, as TB can remain dormant for long periods prior to treatment, making the emergence of naturally resistant mutants possible.

- Send material for bacteriological diagnosis prior to initiating treatment, if possible, to allow for subsequent drug susceptibility testing
- In practice, if there is a high clinical suspicion of TB, treatment should be started before culture and full sensitivities are available.
- Never treat with a single drug
- Never add a single drug to a failing regime
- The majority of patients can be treated as outpatients
- Every TB patient should have an easily contactable key worker
- Smear-positive HIV-negative patients should become smear-negative within 2 weeks of starting treatment (this does not apply to MDR-TB). These patients should be isolated either in hospital (if they are admitted) or at home for this time period
- All patients should be discussed and managed within a TB MDT
- From 2007, there are no prescription costs for TB drugs in the UK
- All new cases must be *notified* (including those diagnosed after death), as this initiates contact tracing. In some districts, notification triggers specialist nursing input. The doctor making the diagnosis has a legal responsibility to notify. It also provides epidemiological and surveillance data, enabling treatment and screening services to be planned. A patient can be denotified if the mycobacterium cultured turns out to be an NTM.

Drug treatment is usually in two phases:

- *Phase 1—initial intensive phase* Designed to kill actively growing bacteria
  - This phase lasts 2 months and shortens the duration of infectivity
  - At least three drugs are needed, e.g. isoniazid, rifampicin, and pyrazinamide, and guidelines recommend four drugs, with ethambutol added because of risks of drug resistance
- *Phase 2—continuation phase* is usually with two drugs, typically isoniazid and rifampicin for 4 months
  - Fewer bacteria are present in this phase, and there is therefore a lower chance that drug-resistant mutants will emerge, so drug resistance is less of a problem.

Compliance is of major importance, and all patients should have a risk assessment for treatment adherence. If the clinical response is not satisfactory, check sputum 2 months before the end of the planned treatment period. Compliance can be monitored with urine colour testing (turns red with rifampicin) and tablet counts. If concerns about compliance, consider directly observed treatment (DOT).

DOT aims to increase compliance by nurse-supervised and observed daily or weekly tablet swallowing. This has been shown to increase treatment completion, reduce relapses, and reduce development of drug resistance, as the ingestion of each dose is witnessed. This is recommended for patients unlikely to comply, including alcoholics, drug abusers, the homeless, those with serious mental illness (the so-called 'hard to reach'), and those with MDR-TB. Some areas consider other incentives to improve adherence such as providing food and transport costs.

Compulsory detention under Sections 37 and 38 of the Public Health Act (England) is allowed for infectious pulmonary TB, but compulsory treatment is not allowed. This is only used in extreme circumstances to protect public health.

TB: management 2

Standard treatment regimes for drug-sensitive TB
(see ➔ p. 496)

- The standard first-line regime is for 6 months—four drugs in the initial 2-month phase (rifampicin (R), isoniazid (H), pyrazinamide (Z), and ethambutol (E) (or streptomycin)) and two drugs in the last 4 months (rifampicin and isoniazid) in patients with fully sensitive organisms
- Rifampicin should always be given throughout the 6-month course in first-line therapy
- If drug sensitivity is unavailable at 2 months, continue the four-drug regime until it is available
- The fourth drug (usually ethambutol) can be omitted in those at low risk of isoniazid resistance (not previously treated, HIV-negative, UK-born Caucasians, with no drug-resistant contacts). There is a higher risk of isoniazid resistance in ethnic minority groups, immigrants, refugees, those who have had previous treatment, and those who are HIV-positive. This depends on local policy and the ethnic make-up of the local area. If in doubt, treat with four drugs
- Other treatment regimes are also effective (e.g. daily for 2 months, then two or three times weekly for 4 months with DOT, or three times weekly for the whole 6 months with DOT), though are used less commonly
- Check baseline renal and liver function in all patients. If normal and not at high risk of adverse drug reaction, they do not need to be re-checked. Treatment in the setting of liver and renal disease is described on ➔ p. 504 and p. 505
- Dosages are weight-dependent and may need to be changed for weight loss or gain during the treatment course
- A 6-month treatment course is effective for all other forms of non-CNS extrapulmonary TB (including lymph node and spinal disease), with the same drugs as for respiratory disease. Surgery may be needed, in addition, for spinal disease
- CNS disease needs a 12-month treatment course
- Steroids may be indicated for large pleural effusions, pericardial effusions (60mg/day for constrictive pericarditis), and CNS disease, especially if associated with neurological impairment (see further text). Steroids may also be indicated in ureteric disease and to suppress hypersensitivity reactions to the antituberculous drugs
- Peripheral lymph nodes may enlarge and abscesses may form during treatment; this does not imply failure of treatment but should prompt a compliance check
- Pyridoxine is not required, unless subjects are at higher risk of pyrazinamide-related peripheral neuropathy—in diabetes, renal failure, HIV, and alcoholics.

Meningitis A 12-month course of rifampicin and isoniazid, with pyrazinamide and a fourth drug (e.g. ethambutol) for at least the first 2 months, is effective. If pyrazinamide not used, extend treatment period to 18 months. Steroids may be needed for severe disease, equivalent to prednisolone

20–40mg od if on rifampicin, otherwise 10–20mg od. Steroids can usually be tapered after the initial 2–3 weeks of treatment. Ethambutol should be used with caution in unconscious patients, as visual acuity cannot be tested and there is a small risk of ocular toxicity.

Cerebral tuberculoma without meningitis 12-month regime.

Disseminated TB/miliary TB 6-month regime unless CNS involvement. Exclude CNS disease in miliary TB with CSF examination, whether or not symptoms are present. Start treatment, even if LFTs are abnormal (this may be due to intrahepatic granulomas). Seek advice if LFTs deteriorate significantly on treatment (see ➔ p. 551. See Box 42.2).

Bone and spinal TB 6-month standard regime. A CT or MRI should be performed in patients with active spinal disease who have neurological symptoms and signs. If there is direct spinal cord involvement (e.g. a spinal cord tuberculoma), treatment should be as for meningeal TB. There is no place for routine spinal surgery (e.g. anterior spinal fusion) in the absence of spinal instability.

Pericardial TB Standard 6-month regime. Steroids, e.g. prednisolone 60mg od if on rifampicin, tapered after 2–3 weeks of treatment, may be required. Repeat echo may be needed.

Peripheral lymph node TB Standard 6-month regime, which should be used, even if the infected node has been surgically removed. Stop treatment at the end of the 6-month course, regardless of the appearance of new nodes, residual nodes, or draining sinuses.

Patient advice to document on starting TB chemotherapy

- Possibility of nausea and abdominal pain
- Persistent vomiting and/or jaundice—stop drugs *immediately*, and contact doctor
- Red urine with rifampicin
- Red contact lenses with rifampicin
- Contraception advice, if on the OCP as efficacy reduced
- Visual acuity (Snellen chart) (ethambutol)
- Visual disturbance (ethambutol)—stop drugs *immediately*, and contact doctor
- Potential drug interactions (see Table 42.2).

First-line anti-TB drugs

- *Isoniazid (H)* Bactericidal. Single daily dose, well tolerated. Major side effect is age-dependent hepatitis. Increased toxicity with alcohol. Peripheral neuropathy is uncommon, although increased risk with diabetes and pregnancy; reduce incidence with 10mg pyridoxine daily
- *Rifampicin (R)* Bactericidal. Single daily dose, well tolerated. Increases hepatic microsomal enzymes; therefore, increases clearance of hepatic metabolized drugs, including prednisolone and the OCP, thus the risks of pregnancy must be highlighted. Red discoloration of urine and contact lenses occurs, and GI upset
- *Pyrazinamide (Z)* Bactericidal. Single daily dose. GI upset common. Major side effect is hepatic toxicity. Renal excretion leads to hyperuricaemia
- *Ethambutol (E)* has some bactericidal effect, mostly bacteriostatic at usual doses. Single daily dose, well tolerated. Side effect—optic neuritis, uncommon. Document visual acuity (Snellen chart) before starting, and warn patient to stop drugs immediately and contact doctor if any visual disturbance
- *Streptomycin* Bactericidal. Given parenterally. Increased risk of ototoxicity in the foetus and the elderly.

Combined preparations

- *Rifinah® 150* (contains rifampicin 150mg and isoniazid 100mg), *Rifinah® 300* (contains rifampicin 300mg and isoniazid 150mg)
- *Rifater®* (contains 120mg rifampicin, 50mg isoniazid, and 300mg pyrazinamide).

Table 42.1 shows the recommended doses of the main four drugs.

Table 42.1 Recommended doses of standard anti-TB drugs

Drug		Daily dose	Intermittent dose
Isoniazid (H)		300mg	15mg/kg three times weekly
Rifampicin (R)	<50kg	450mg	600–900mg three times weekly
	≥50kg	600mg	
Pyrazinamide (Z)	<50kg	1.5g	<50kg—2.0g
	≥50kg	2.0g	≥50kg—2.5g three times weekly or 3.5g twice weekly
Ethambutol (E)		15mg/kg	30mg/kg three times weekly or 45mg/kg twice weekly

For example, a 75kg adult commencing quadruple therapy would be given:
- Isoniazid 300mg od
- Rifampicin 600mg od
- Pyrazinamide 2.0g od
- Ethambutol 1.2g od ± pyridoxine 10mg od.

If using a combined preparation, e.g. Rifater®, with ethambutol:
- 45kg adult: Rifater® four tablets and ethambutol 700mg od
- 60kg adult: Rifater® five tablets and ethambutol 900mg od
- 80kg adult: Rifater® six tablets and ethambutol 1.2 g od.

Drug regimes are often abbreviated to the number of months each phase of treatment lasts, followed by the letters for the drugs being administered during that treatment phase, e.g. 2HRZE/4HR is the standard 6-month recommended regime; 2HRE/7HR is 2 months of isoniazid, rifampicin, and ethambutol, followed by 7 months of isoniazid and rifampicin.

Potential TB drug interactions are listed in Table 42.2.

Table 42.2 Interactions of TB drugs

Drug	Increases level of	Decreases level of
rifampicin	(Level decreased by ketoconazole and PAS)	warfarin
		OCP
		phenytoin
		glucocorticoids
		theophyllines
		digoxin
		Methadone
		sulfonylureas
		ciclosporin
isoniazid	phenytoin	azoles, e.g. ketoconazole
	carbamazepine	
	warfarin	
	diazepam	
pyrazinamide	probenecid	

TB: adverse drug reactions

These occur in around 10% of patients, often requiring a change of therapy. Reactions are more common in those on non-standard therapy and in HIV-positive individuals.

Isoniazid peripheral neuropathy can be prevented by pyridoxine 10mg daily (recommended in those at highest risk—diabetes, renal failure, alcoholics, HIV-positive).

Rifampicin may cause shock, acute renal failure, thrombocytopenia. Withdraw, and do not reintroduce the drug. Double maintenance steroid doses at the start of treatment (because of enzyme induction).

Ethambutol causes rare optic toxicity; recommend baseline visual acuity assessment with a Snellen chart. Use only in those with adequate visual acuity and those able to report changes in visual acuity or new visual symptoms. Document that the patient has been told to cease the drug immediately at the onset of new visual symptoms. Check baseline renal function before starting ethambutol, and avoid in renal failure.

HIV-positive patients Rifampicin and isoniazid lead to reduced serum concentrations of antifungals. Ketoconazole can inhibit rifampicin absorption. Rifampicin may reduce drug levels of protease inhibitors (as they are metabolized via the cytochrome P450 pathway, which is induced by rifampicin). Rifabutin can cause a severe iritis. Liaise closely with HIV specialist.

Drug resistance occurs in <2% of Caucasian cases in the UK, with higher levels in ethnic minority groups.

- Isoniazid resistance is seen in up to 6% in patients of African and Indian subcontinent origin
- Increased drug resistance is seen in HIV-positive patients (fourfold increased risk)
- Second-line drugs are generally more toxic and less effective than first-line drugs, and the treatment of drug resistance can therefore often be complex and difficult—seek specialist advice
- The regime must include at least three drugs to which the organism is known to be susceptible. An injectable drug is often added, as this has shown improved outcomes
- The initial regime will depend on the incidence of drug resistance in the community and should be altered, depending on local drug susceptibility patterns
- In general, always add at least two drugs to which the MTB is susceptible
- Parenteral treatment is usually recommended when there is resistance to two or more drugs.

See Table 42.3.

Table 42.3 Recommended drug regimes for non-MDR drug-resistant TB

Drug resistance	Initial phase	Continuation phase
S	2RHZE	4RH
H known before treatment	2RZSE	7RE
H known after treatment	2RZE	10RE
Z	2RHE	7HR
E	2RHZ	4RH
R (only if confirmed as isolated resistance)	2HZE	16HE
S and H	2RZE	10RE

Isoniazid (H), rifampicin (R), pyrazinamide (Z), ethambutol (E)

Rifampicin monoresistance is uncommon but does require regime modification. In most cases, rifampicin resistance is a marker of MDR-TB (see ➔ pp. 506–7) and should be treated as such, until full sensitivities are known.

TB: inpatient admission

- This is rarely needed, but, if necessary, patients with suspected pulmonary TB should initially be admitted to a side room vented to the outside air (until proven non-infectious)
- Patients with smear-positive non-MDR-TB should be managed as infectious (in a side room, with face mask). This especially applies if they are on a ward with immunosuppressed patients (who may be at higher risk)
- A risk assessment (including an assessment of the immune status of other ward patients) can be made once the infectiousness and likelihood of drug resistance of the patient are known
- Patients with non-pulmonary TB can be nursed on a general ward (but aerosol-generating procedures, e.g. abscess irrigation, may need patient isolation)
- Staff should wear face masks if the patient is potentially infectious
- Inpatients with smear-positive pulmonary TB should be asked to wear a face mask whenever they leave their room, unless they have received 2 weeks' drug treatment
- Barrier nursing is unnecessary for smear-negative non-MDR-TB
- Liaise closely with infection control/microbiology/public health specialists
- If a patient on an open ward is found to have infectious TB, the risk to the other patients is small. Patients whose exposure is considered comparable to that of a household contact should be screened. Only those in the same bay as a coughing infectious case, for at least 8h, are considered at risk. Exposure should be documented and the patient and the GP contacted
- Non-MDR-TB HIV-negative patients usually become non-infectious after 2 weeks' chemotherapy. Any bacilli seen in smears after that time are likely to be dead
- Patients with HIV and those with TB should not be nursed in close proximity
- All patients with known or suspected MDR-TB should be admitted to negative pressure ventilated side room. Staff should wear protective face masks (FFP3)
- At discharge, a clear plan must be in place for the administration and supervision of all chemotherapy; this is particularly important for patients with MDR-TB where close liaison with the infection control team and consultant in communicable disease control is paramount.

Treatment failure/disease relapse

- This is usually due to poor compliance
- Drug resistance may have developed
- Never add a single drug to a failing regime. Add only two or three, ideally those to which the patient has not been previously exposed
- Assume drug resistance to all, or some, of the drugs in the failed regime
- Repeat cultures and sensitivity testing in this situation. Consider specific molecular tests for rifampicin/isoniazid resistance. If found, then treat as for MDR-TB (see ➲ pp. 506–7)

- UK TB death rates have decreased since 2001, but death is still the most common cause for not completing treatment course. Higher proportions of deaths were found in older patients of white ethnicity who were born in the UK. A higher proportion of deaths were in patients with pulmonary TB than with extrapulmonary. One-quarter of patients who died were diagnosed with TB post-mortem where it was thought to cause or contribute to death in 33%.

TB: treatment follow-up

- CXR is advised at the end of therapy for pulmonary disease
- Relapse is uncommon in those compliant with standard treatment regimes in the UK (0–3%); therefore, long-term follow-up is not recommended
- Follow-up at 12 months after treatment completion is recommended for patients treated for drug-resistant TB
- Relapse after good compliance is usually due to fully sensitive organism; therefore, treatment can be with the same regime again
- Relapse due to poor compliance needs a fully supervised regime.

MDR-TB follow-up

Prolonged follow-up is recommended; lifelong for HIV-positive patients.

TB in pregnancy

There is no increased risk of developing clinical disease in pregnancy. Presentation is the same as in non-pregnant individuals, but the diagnosis may be delayed by the non-specific nature of the symptoms in the early stages of disease, with malaise and fatigue being common in the early stages of pregnancy. A CXR is more likely to be delayed.

The tuberculin skin test result is not affected by pregnancy; this applies to HIV-positive and negative subjects. A negative skin test should not lead to BCG vaccination, as live vaccines are contraindicated in pregnancy. In this situation, the skin test should be repeated after delivery and BCG given then after a second negative test.

TB outcome in pregnancy

- If diagnosed in the first trimester, the disease has the same outcome as for non-pregnant women
- If diagnosed in the second or third trimester, studies give more variable outcomes (some studies show a good foetal outcome; some show higher rates of small-for-date babies, pre-eclampsia, and spontaneous abortion), but these effects tend to be related to late diagnosis and incomplete drug treatment. Some studies also show a poorer foetal outcome in extrapulmonary disease
- Late diagnosis of pulmonary TB can lead to a 4-fold increased obstetric mortality and 9-fold increased pre-term labour in some developing countries.

Treatment in pregnancy

- Isoniazid, rifampicin, and ethambutol are not teratogenic and can be used safely in pregnancy. The 'standard' short-course therapy is recommended (i.e. 6-month treatment)
- Limited pyrazinamide data on the risk of teratogenicity
- Streptomycin may be ototoxic to the foetus
- Active TB must be treated in pregnancy because of the risk of untreated disease to the mother and foetus
- Reserve drugs may be toxic, and the risk/benefit ratio of each case must be assessed individually if second-line drugs are needed
- Babies of sputum-positive mothers, who have had <2 weeks' treatment by delivery, should be treated with isoniazid and have a skin test at 6 weeks. If the skin test is negative, the chemoprophylaxis should be stopped and BCG given 1 week later (as BCG is sensitive to isoniazid)
- Congenital infection is very rare (<300 reported cases). The child can be infected at delivery (this is rare).

Breastfeeding

- Most anti-TB drugs are safe. Isoniazid—monitor infant for possible toxicity, as there is a theoretical risk of convulsions and neuropathy. Give prophylactic pyridoxine to the mother and infant
- Concentrations of drugs reaching breast milk are too low to prevent or treat infection in the infant.

TB chemotherapy with comorbid disease

Liver disease

- Drug-induced hepatitis can be fatal. A raised ALT (see Box 42.2) is more common in those who regularly consume alcohol, have viral hepatitis or other chronic liver disease, take concomitant hepatotoxic drugs, are pregnant, or are within 3 months post-partum
- About 20% of those treated with isoniazid alone will have an asymptomatic transient rise in ALT. In the majority, this represents hepatic adaptation. Acetylator status (fast or slow) may influence this
- Isoniazid-induced hepatitis can be symptomatic or asymptomatic and usually occurs within weeks or months of treatment and is age-related
- Isoniazid inhibits several cytochrome P450 enzymes, potentially increasing the plasma concentrations of other hepatotoxic drugs
- Rifampicin can cause subclinical hyperbilirubinaemia without hepatocellular damage. It can also cause direct hepatocellular damage and potentiate the hepatotoxicity of other TB drugs
- Decompensated liver disease—use a drug regime without rifampicin
- Avoid pyrazinamide in patients with known chronic liver disease
- Baseline and regular monitoring of liver function is necessary (weekly LFTs for the first 2 weeks, then at 2-weekly intervals) in patients with chronic liver disease.

Box 42.2 TB drugs and abnormal LFTs

- New drug-induced hepatitis
  - Virological tests to exclude concomitant viral hepatitis
  - AST/ALT rise 2× normal—monitor LFTs weekly for 2 weeks, then 2-weekly until normal
  - AST/ALT rise under 2× normal—repeat LFT at 2 weeks
  - AST/ALT rise 5× normal or bilirubin rise—cease rifampicin, isoniazid, and pyrazinamide, unless the patient is unwell. If the patient is unwell or sputum still positive, consider admission for parenteral therapy, e.g. streptomycin and ethambutol, with appropriate monitoring
- Drug re-challenge once LFTs are normal—reintroduce sequentially, in order:
  - Isoniazid: at 50mg/day, sequential increase to 300mg/day after 2–3 days if no reaction
  - Rifampicin: at 75mg/day, increase to 300mg/day after 2–3 days if no reaction, then to maximum dose/kg
  - Pyrazinamide: start at 250mg/day, increase to 1g/day after 2–3 days, and to maximum dose/kg if no reaction
  - Daily monitoring of LFTs and clinical condition
  - If no further reaction, continue chemotherapy
  - If there is a further reaction, exclude the offending drug, and change to an alternative regime
- If intolerant of pyrazinamide, use rifampicin and isoniazid for 9 months, with ethambutol for 2 months.

Renal failure

- Isoniazid and rifampicin have biliary excretion so can be given in normal doses in renal disease
- Pyrazinamide metabolites are renally cleared; the dose may need to be less frequent in those with renal insufficiency
- Give pyridoxine, in addition to isoniazid, in those with severe renal disease to prevent isoniazid-induced peripheral neuropathy
- Ethambutol can accumulate, causing optic neuropathy; use only with caution and at a lower dose
- Dialysis patients should receive drugs after dialysis
- Post-renal transplant immunosuppressive drug doses also need alteration.

HIV infection

- Regimes are the same for HIV-positive as HIV-negative patients: standard four-drug regime. Liaise closely with HIV specialists
- Identification of HIV allows additional package of care to be added, including co-trimoxazole prophylaxis and early antiretroviral therapy (ART), which improves mortality—hence the importance of HIV testing in all patients with TB
- In newly diagnosed HIV-positive individuals, the usual practice is to start TB chemotherapy before HIV chemotherapy. ART should be started within the first 8 weeks of TB treatment, and patients with CD4 counts $<50 \times 10^6$/L should start ART within the first 2 weeks; an exception is treatment of tuberculous meningitis when early ART should be avoided
- Protease inhibitors should not be used with rifampicin (they interfere with each other's metabolism)
- Paradoxical worsening of disease (worsening fever, CXR infiltrates, increased lymphadenopathy, or new manifestations of the disease) at the initiation of HIV treatment is common (in ~15%)—so-called TB IRIS. This reflects the restoration of pathogen-specific immune responses. Steroids reduce the morbidity associated with IRIS
- Death during TB chemotherapy is more common in HIV-infected patients, who also have higher relapse rates than non-HIV-infected subjects
- Atypical presentations of TB are common in patients with CD4 counts $<200 \times 10^6$/L and disseminated TB with multi-organ involvement and mycobacteraemia, but sparing the lung may occur with CD4 counts $<75 \times 10^6$/L. Active TB may be asymptomatic in the setting of HIV
- Patients co-infected with TB and HIV should be considered potentially infectious to others at each admission, until proved otherwise, and should be segregated. Review the immune status of other patients and their likely drug resistances and their potential infectivity.

Diabetes

- Increased risk of TB and the disease may be more extensive. Note that rifampicin reduces the efficacy of sulfonylureas.

Multidrug-resistant TB (MDR-TB)

Defined as MTB resistant to two or more first-line agents, usually isoniazid and rifampicin.

- Treatment is complex and time-consuming
- MDR-TB is not more infectious than other forms of TB, but the consequences of acquiring it are more serious
- 3.6% of new TB cases in the world have MDR-TB. The frequency varies between countries. Of 450,000 new MDR-TB cases in 2012, half were in China, India and the Russian Federation
- Specialist advice essential; patients should be managed by experts with experience of managing resistant cases, in a hospital with isolation facilities. The MDRTBservice@lhch.nhs.uk email address, based in Liverpool, can be used to seek advice from a panel of experts in the management of MDR disease. An MDR-TB UK database is run from the Cardiothoracic Centre in Liverpool
- Rapid molecular tests for rifampicin resistance should be carried out in all patients suspected of having MDR-TB. Liaise closely with the reference laboratory
- Close monitoring (because of increased drug toxicity) is needed
- Compliance is paramount, and all patients should receive DOT (see ❍ p. 493)
- Start treatment with at least four drugs with certain or almost certain effectiveness. Often >4 drugs are started if the susceptibility pattern is unknown (see Table 42.4). Smears and cultures should be performed monthly, even after they become negative. Treatment should be given for a minimum of 18 months after culture conversion, but 24 months may be indicated in chronic disease with extensive pulmonary damage
- If the drug choice is limited by drug resistance and intolerance, consider desensitization and reintroduction of the offending drug. Desensitization must be carried out with concurrent treatment with two other drugs (to minimize emergence of resistant strains)
- Surgery may be indicated
- Successful outcomes reported in 48% of patients worldwide.

Contacts of MDR-TB Chemoprophylaxis for contacts should include at least two drugs. Base the drug choice on the sensitivities of the index case for a minimum of 6 months (although there are no data to support this treatment period). If there is extensive resistance, no regime may be suitable, and regular follow-up needed instead.

Risk factors for resistant disease

- Previous anti-TB treatment, prior treatment failure
- Lack of response to intensive phase of standard short-course therapy/treatment failure
- HIV infection
- Contact with patients with drug-resistant disease
- History of poor adherence, aggravated by social deprivation or substance abuse
- Residence in regions with high prevalence of drug-resistant disease.

Extensively drug-resistant TB' (XDR-TB) is MDR-TB with added resistance to all fluoroquinolones and one of three injectable anti-TB drugs (capreomycin, kanamycin, and amikacin) represents 10% of MDR-TB cases. In September 2013, 92 countries had reported at least one case to WHO. Genotyping data suggest the emergence of XDR-TB is due to the transmission of XDR strains between individuals and is not a consequence of previous unsuccessful treatment. 85% of South African XDR isolates are from the KZN family of TB strains, which were mostly fully susceptible when first described in 1996. Outcomes are variable, but association with advanced HIV infection in a localized outbreak in South Africa was universally fatal. Some TB strains have also been reported which are resistant to all anti-TB drugs.

Table 42.4 second-line TB chemotherapy

Drug	Dose	Potential side effects
Amikacin	15mg/kg	Tinnitus, ataxia, renal impairment, vertigo
Azithromycin	500mg od	GI upset
Capreomycin	15mg/kg	As for amikacin
Ciprofloxacin	750mg bd	Abdominal upset, headache, drug interactions
Clarithromycin	500mg bd	GI upset
Ethionamide (or protionamide)	<50kg: 375mg bd ≥50kg: 500mg bd	GI upset, hepatitis. Avoid in pregnancy
Kanamycin	15mg/kg	As for amikacin
Ofloxacin	400mg bd	Abdominal upset, headache
PAS	10g od or 5g bd	GI upset, fever, rash, hepatitis
Rifabutin	300–450mg od	As for rifampicin. Uveitis (particulary with HIV infection) with drug interactions, e.g. with macrolides
Streptomycin	15mg/kg (max dose 1g od)	As for amikacin
Thiocetazone	150mg	GI upset, rash, conjunctivitis, vertigo. Avoid if HIV-positive (risk of Stevens–Johnson syndrome)

Latent TB infection

Defined as a positive skin test or IGRA, showing MTB infection but with a normal CXR and no symptoms. This represents the presence of a small total number of mycobacteria, with the host immune system retaining control over mycobacterial replication. It should be distinguished from active disease, which is usually accompanied by symptoms and an abnormal CXR and for which the mainstay of diagnosis is sputum microscopy and culture; IGRA and skin tests have no role in the diagnosis of active disease.

An estimated 2 billion people worldwide have latent TB. Treatment of latent TB with chemoprophylaxis (see further text) reduces the risk of subsequent development of active disease by about 90%, but a proportion of people will be treated who would never have developed active disease.

Tuberculin skin test A positive skin test (Mantoux) results from the development of cell-mediated immunity against TB. Potential problems with skin testing are:
• Low sensitivity in the immunocompromised and cross-reactivity with BCG
• The patient has to return to have the test read after 48–72h
• Criteria for a positive test depend on the population in which it is being used.

IGRA Two blood tests (T-SPOT.TB, Oxford Immunotec Ltd., and QuantiFERON-TB Gold, QIAGEN) are available and are based on the detection of IFN-γ released by T-cells in response to MTB-specific antigens. The T-SPOT.TB test is an ELISpot test, counting individual T-cells producing IFN-γ; the QuantiFERON test is based on a whole blood ELISA and measures the IFN-γ level in the supernatant of the stimulated whole blood sample. Both assays use two proteins (ESAT-6 and CFP10) encoded by a unique genomic sequence of MTB, which is absent from *M. bovis* BCG and the majority of opportunistic mycobacteria. These proteins are the main targets for IFN-γ-secreting T-lymphocytes in individuals infected with MTB. These tests have several advantages over the tuberculin skin test: no return visit for test reading is required, the result is available the next day, and repeated testing does not cause boosting. With both tests, blood must be collected in a heparinized tube and processed within 6–8h of venepuncture. The blood should be transferred to the laboratory at room temperature. Both tests are more sensitive for the diagnosis of latent TB than the tuberculin skin test, particularly in children and HIV-positive individuals, and, on current available evidence, there is little difference between the two, although the T-SPOT.TB test may be more sensitive in HIV-positive individuals.

HIV infection The tuberculin skin test may be falsely negative, and radiological changes may be atypical. Current WHO guidelines recommend isoniazid chemoprophylaxis for HIV-infected patients in low-income, high-burden countries, with positive or unknown skin tests in the absence of active disease. Uptake of this recommendation is slow, partly because of the difficulties in distinguishing active from latent disease in the setting of HIV co-infection and concern regarding emergence of resistant strains. Exposure to smear-positive disease should lead to chemoprophylaxis in the absence of active disease. Recommended follow-up is at 3 and 12 months for those not receiving chemoprophylaxis (but who were eligible for it). HIV-positive patients should receive long-term follow-up as part of their ongoing HIV management.

Chemoprophylaxis is given to contacts or screened immigrants with a strongly positive skin test or positive IGRA, who have no radiological or clinical evidence of active disease. The risk of developing disease after exposure depends on a number of factors, including BCG and HIV/immune status, and whether infection was recent. Younger patients must have had relatively recent infection and have a longer life expectancy from which to gain the benefits of chemoprophylaxis.

Chemoprophylaxis is recommended for:
- Those aged <35 (because of the increased risk of drug hepatotoxicity with age)
- Those with recent documented tuberculin conversion
- HIV-infected contacts of smear-positive cases (any age)
- Any age health care worker
- Children aged <16 with a strongly positive Mantoux (>15mm if prior BCG)
- Individuals with HIV, injecting drugs, with haematological malignancy, chronic renal failure or on dialysis, with silicosis, gastrectomy, solid organ transplant, or receiving anti-TNF-α therapy have a higher risk of developing active TB.

Drug regimes
- Rifampicin and isoniazid daily for 3 months (3RH). Improved compliance but slightly higher side effect profile
- Isoniazid daily for 6 months (6H). Lowest toxicity regime. Has a 60–90% effectiveness in reducing progression of latent infection to clinical disease
- 6H is recommended for people with HIV
- 6R is recommended for contacts of patients with isoniazid-resistant disease
- Individuals who decline chemoprophylaxis should be given 'inform and advise' information, regarding TB risks and symptoms and have a CXR at 3 and 12 months.

TB and anti-TNF-α treatment

Humanized monoclonal anti-TNF-α antibody is approved for the treatment of rheumatoid arthritis, Crohn's disease, psoriatic arthropathy, and juvenile idiopathic arthritis. Etanercept is a fusion protein that binds free TNF-α, using a soluble portion of the TNF-α receptor, and is licensed for use in RA. Adalimumab is a recombinant humanized monoclonal antibody against TNF-α, also licensed for use in RA. Infliximab is a human chimera monoclonal antibody, licensed for the treatment of RA, Crohn's disease, and ankylosing spondylitis.

These drugs cause profound immunosuppression, and patients treated with them have an increased risk of developing TB. Most TB cases have been seen with infliximab (242 at time of publication), with most occurring within three treatment cycles (within a mean of 12 weeks of starting treatment). TB is the most frequently described opportunistic infection in this context. 50% of the reported cases are extrapulmonary disease. The initial high incidence of cases has now plateaued, presumably due to improved assessment and awareness and the use of isoniazid chemoprophylaxis. The calculated TB prevalence in etanercept/infliximab-treated RA patients in America is 41 per 100,000, 9 per 100,000 for Crohn's disease. Overall, there is an average 5-fold increased risk of developing TB with anti-TNF-α therapy. *All patients due to start anti-TNF-α antibody treatment should be screened for active and latent TB.*

- All patients should have a clinical examination, with history of previous TB treatment and exposure carefully documented. All should have a CXR and tuberculin test or IGRA. The IGRA is less sensitive in those taking concomitant prednisolone and/or disease-modifying drugs, e.g. azathioprine
- Both those with an abnormal CXR consistent with previous TB, or those who have a history of extrapulmonary TB, who have received adequate treatment (as assessed by an expert), can start anti-TNF-α therapy but need monitoring every 3 months with a CXR and symptom assessment. The onset of any new respiratory symptoms, especially within 3 months of starting anti-TNF-α therapy, should be investigated promptly
- Both those with an abnormal CXR consistent with previous TB, or those who have a prior history of extrapulmonary TB, who have NOT had adequate treatment, need to have active TB excluded by appropriate investigations. They should receive chemoprophylaxis before anti-TNF-α therapy commences (assuming active disease is not identified). If there is clinical concern because of the delay in starting anti-TNF-α treatment, a shorter course of chemoprophylaxis can be given, but this may be more toxic
- Any TB diagnosed (pulmonary or extrapulmonary) should be treated with standard chemotherapy
- If active TB is present, patients should receive a minimum of 2 months' anti-TB chemotherapy before starting anti-TNF-α therapy
- If the CXR is normal, the tuberculin test or IGRA may be helpful if the patient is not on immunosuppressants. The skin test must be interpreted knowing the BCG history. A tuberculin skin test is unhelpful

if the patient is on immunosuppressants. In this situation, an individual assessment should be made (see Table 42.5); if the risk of drug-induced hepatitis is less than the annual risk of developing TB, chemoprophylaxis should be given. However, if the risk of hepatitis is greater, the patient should be monitored regularly and any suggestive symptoms investigated promptly

- No chemoprophylaxis regime is 100% effective; the protective efficacy of 6H is reported at 60 and 50% for 3HR
- In those without previous BCG, Mantoux 1 in 10,000, 0–5mm is negative, and Mantoux 1 in 10,000, >6mm is positive and should lead to a risk assessment
- In those with prior BCG, Mantoux 1 in 10,000, 0–14mm is negative, and Mantoux 1 in 10,000, >15mm may represent either latent infection or BCG effect and therefore needs further investigation
- In general, all black African patients aged >15 and all South Asians born outside the UK should be considered for chemoprophylaxis with 6 months' isoniazid
- If a patient develops TB whilst on anti-TNF-α therapy, treat with the full standard course of anti-TB chemotherapy. The anti-TNF-α can be continued, if indicated
- Close liaison between the prescriber of the TNF-α antibody treatment and TB specialists is needed.

Table 42.5 Sample calculations for aiding TB risk assessment for patients starting anti-TNF-α treatment

Case type	Annual risk of TB disease/ 100,000	TB risk adjusted × 5 for anti-TNF-α effect	Risk of hepatitis following 6H chemoprophy- laxis/100,000	Risk/benefit conclusion
White, UK born, age 55–74	7	35	278	Observation
ISC, in UK >3y, age >35	593	2965	278	Prophylaxis
Black African age 35–54	168	840	278	Prophylaxis
Other ethnic group, in UK >5y, age >35	39	195	278	Observation

ISC = Indian subcontinent. The risk of hepatitis with 3RH chemoprophylaxis is 1,766/100,000.

Further information

BTS recommendations for assessing risk and for managing *Mycobacterium tuberculosis* infection and disease in patients due to start anti-TNF-α treatment. *Thorax* 2005;**60**:800–5.

TB: screening and contact tracing

Immigrant screening Immigrants are screened, as ethnic minority groups in the UK constitute 50% of TB cases. New entrants are screened at port of arrival. The incidence of TB is highest in the first few years after arrival to the UK. Return visits to countries with a high background prevalence are a risk factor for acquiring disease. Immigrants with symptoms suggestive of TB and those who are asymptomatic with a grade 3 or 4 tuberculin skin test should be referred to the local chest clinic for CXR and assessment. BCG vaccination is recommended for tuberculin-negative immigrants (but not in those who are HIV-positive because of the risk of generalized BCG infection).

Contact tracing identifies those with TB and those who are infected but without evidence of disease. It also identifies those suitable for BCG vaccination.

Close contacts are usually those within the same household, sharing kitchen facilities, and frequent household visitors.

Casual contacts usually include most occupational contacts. Examination is usually only needed if the index case was smear-positive or if the contacts are at high risk. This also applies if >10% of the close contacts have been infected, i.e. the index case is considered highly infectious.

- 10% of TB is diagnosed by contact tracing, with disease occurring in about 1% of contacts
- Smear-negative patients are much less infectious, but contact tracing is still recommended in these patients
- Contacts should be traced for the period the index case has been infectious or for 3 months prior to the first positive sputum or culture, if the time period is uncertain
- Most disease in contacts is found at the first screening visit
- Subjects should be advised to report suspicious symptoms
- Follow-up is recommended at 3 and 12 months for those not receiving chemoprophylaxis
- School index cases—if a pupil is diagnosed with smear-positive TB, the rest of the class and year group who share classes should be assessed as part of routine contact tracing. If a school teacher is diagnosed with smear-positive TB, the pupils in their class during the previous 3 months should be assessed as part of routine contact tracing. The extension of contact tracing to include non-teaching staff will depend on the infectivity and proximity of the index case and whether the contacts are likely to be especially susceptible to infection.

Airplane transmission rates are low, even on long-haul flights. Contact tracing of passengers and crew is only necessary if the index case was smear-positive and coughing during a flight of at least 8h. In this situation, screening is only recommended in those at high risk—immunocompromised travellers and children or if the index case was unusually infectious or had MDR-TB.

Extrapulmonary disease Contact screening is not recommended.

Contact examination This usually involves symptom enquiry, BCG vaccination status, Mantoux test and/or IGRA, and CXR.

HIV-infected contacts CXR is indicated, as a negative Mantoux test may be due to anergy and may therefore be a false negative. Mantoux testing is not contraindicated in HIV (PPD is dead). BCG is contraindicated (it is a live vaccine). IGRA usually useful.

BCG vaccination remains the only licensed vaccine for TB. The UK national schools' vaccination programme ceased in 2005 and now aims to target vaccination to selected 'at-risk' groups. Vaccination is offered to:
- All infants whose parents or grandparents originate from a country with a TB incidence of 40/100,000 or higher or those living in areas with a TB incidence of 40/100,000 or higher
- All Mantoux-negative contacts of patients with respiratory TB if they are previously unvaccinated and aged <35y. Laboratory and health care workers who are contacts meeting the same criteria should be vaccinated if they are aged >36
- Previously unvaccinated entrants from high incidence areas aged <16. If originating from sub-Saharan Africa or a country with a TB incidence of 500 per 100,000, those aged 16–35 should also be offered vaccination
- All Mantoux-negative health care workers, irrespective of age, who are previously unvaccinated and who will be exposed to patients and clinical materials
- Mantoux-negative, previously unvaccinated individuals aged <35, if potentially at risk of TB exposure because of their occupation, including veterinary and abattoir workers, prison staff, staff in care homes for the elderly, staff of accommodation for refugees and the homeless, and those going to work in a high-incidence country for >1 month
- BCG has an efficacy of around 70% against TB in children, but difficulties with vaccine supply and regional policies have meant that not all children in the UK have been vaccinated in the past. It is less effective in adults and is not used in America
- Adverse events include pain and suppuration at the injection site and localized lymphadenitis. A course of rifampicin and/or isoniazid for 3–6 months, depending on response, may be needed.

M. bovis Cattle TB is due to *M. bovis*. Humans are at low risk, as the majority of milk consumed is pasteurized. *M. bovis* is distinguishable from MTB in the laboratory, although initial diagnosis can be difficult (only distinguishable on culture). Around 40 cases are isolated per year. BCG is live attenuated *M. bovis*.

Disseminated BCG infection (BCGosis)

Live attenuated BCG immunotherapy is the most effective intravesical agent for the treatment and prophylaxis of superficial bladder cancer. BCG leads to a T-cell-mediated immune response, which has anti-tumour activity. After intravesical instillation, live mycobacteria attach to the urothelial lining. BCG organisms are internalized by bladder epithelial cells, leaving bacterial cell surface glycoproteins attached to the epithelial cell membrane. These antigens are thought to mediate the immune response.

- The standard treatment regime is 6-weekly instillations of 100 million to 1 billion cfu of BCG. Some advocate a further 3-week course, 6 weeks after cessation of the first cycle. The dose-response curve is bell-shaped, with excess BCG probably promoting increased tumour activity
- Local side effects are common, with cystitis reported in around 90% of patients; low-grade fever and malaise are frequent. Cystitis persisting >48h after treatment should be treated with a fluoroquinolone or isoniazid 300mg od; rifampicin 600mg od should be added if the symptoms persist at 1 week
- Breaks in the uroepithelium are a risk factor for systemic infection, and, therefore, patients with persistent cystitis or haematuria should have their treatment delayed
- Significant reactions are reported in around 5%, with high fever commonest. A high fever post-treatment (>39°C) may represent the onset of systemic BCG infection or hypersensitivity, and hospital admission is recommended
- BCG sepsis is reported in around 0.4–0.7%, with ten deaths attributed to intravesical BCG to date. The major differential diagnosis is Gram-negative sepsis; thus, patients should be treated with broad-spectrum antibiotics
- Later-onset symptoms (at up to 8–12 weeks, though may occur much earlier), including fever, malaise, arthralgia, and breathlessness, may represent systemic BCG infection, though there is debate as to whether these sorts of systemic symptoms are due to systemic BCG infection or hypersensitivity to BCG. Non-caseating granulomas can be identified on lung and liver biopsy. Culture of organisms is rarely reported, but tissue *M. bovis* can be identified by PCR
- Disseminated infection—treat with rifampicin 600mg od and isoniazid 300mg od for 6 months. Some advocate the addition of ethambutol. Prednisolone 40mg od may be added, and response to corticosteroids is said to support the diagnosis of hypersensitivity. There are no trial data to support these treatment regimes or length of treatment, but *M. bovis* is susceptible to most anti-TB drugs, except pyrazinamide and cycloserine. There is no evidence that isoniazid reduces the anti-tumour effects of BCG

- BCG HP is suggested by pulmonary infiltrates; micronodular and miliary appearances are reported with or without eosinophilia
- Granulomatous hepatitis is reported. Standard TB treatment (6 months) is suggested, with prednisolone if symptoms of hypersensitivity predominate
- Systemic BCG infection is reported in HIV-positive infants and infants with severe immune deficiency, undiagnosed at the time of BCG vaccination. Systemic BCG infection is reported after BCG injection into melanoma.

Future developments in TB

- Molecular techniques are increasingly employed in TB diagnostics and for the detection of drug resistance, and recently the use of whole genome sequencing for rapid MTB antibiotic susceptibility testing was reported. Whole genome sequencing of mycobacteria also allows delineation of TB outbreaks
- Current clinical trials are investigating the use of fluoroquinolones and higher doses of rifamycins as part of shorter treatment regimens. A number of antibiotics are under investigation for the treatment of drug-resistant disease, including bedaquiline, the nitroimidazoles delamanid and PA-824, and linezolid
- 12 vaccines are currently in clinical trials. Most recently, a large placebo-controlled trial showed a lack of efficacy of the vaccine MVA85A against TB in infants
- The role of vitamin D supplementation in the treatment and prevention of TB needs further assessment
- Additional treatments aimed at immunomodulation may facilitate bacillary clearance and increase cure rates, particularly in MDR disease. Small studies suggest that IL2 and nebulized interferon gamma-1b may have some benefit in this setting and in patients with HIV co-infection. A larger study in HIV-negative patients with pulmonary TB has not shown improved bacillary clearance. In MDR-TB, however, there may be greater benefits of treatment
- A change is planned to roll out the UK CXR-based pre-entry screening programme to 82 countries, as entry screening at UK airports has not been found to be cost-effective. For those people who apply for a ≥6 month UK visa from countries with TB incidence of 40/100,000 or above, they will only be eligible for a visa if they have proven clearance of active TB disease.

Further information

NICE Guideline CG117: Clinical diagnosis and management of tuberculosis, and measures for its prevention and control 2011. ℜ http://www.nice.org.uk/CG117.

Zumla A et al. Tuberculosis. N Engl J Med 2013;**368**:745–55.

Chemotherapy and management of tuberculosis in the UK: recommendations 1998. Thorax 1998;**53**:536–48.

Control and prevention of tuberculosis in the UK: Code of practice 2000. Thorax 2000;**55**:887–901.

UK's national tuberculosis charity. ℜ http://www.tbalert.org and ℜ http://www.thetruthabouttb. org.

TB National Knowledge Service. ℜ http://www.hpa.org.uk/tbknowledge.

Non-tuberculous mycobacteria (NTM)

NTM (also called atypical mycobacteria, opportunistic mycobacteria, environmental mycobacteria) are found in the environment, including in soil and water, and may cause disease in susceptible individuals. They are divided into rapid and slowly growing species (for clinically relevant examples, see ⊃ pp. 520–1). NTM are less virulent than MTB and—unlike MTB—are unable to adhere to intact, undamaged airway mucosa.

Risk factors for NTM disease

- Chronic lung disease such as CF, bronchiectasis, COPD, cavitary lung disease 2° to prior TB
- Immunodeficiency, e.g. HIV, organ transplantation, anti-TNF-α therapy, rare genetic mutations in IL12/IL23/IFN-γ signalling, autoantibodies against IFN-γ
- GORD, pectus excavatum, and kyphoscoliosis may be risk factors
- NTM disease is well described in otherwise healthy, thin, tall, middle-aged women; the pathogenesis is obscure, although one hypothesis is habitual voluntary cough suppression, leading to failure to clear airway secretions (so-called 'Lady Windermere syndrome')
- Monotherapy with macrolides (e.g. in the setting of CF) may increase the risk of NTM infection through inhibition of autophagy, a key process in anti-mycobacterial host defence; stop macrolide if NTM is suspected.

Clinical features

- Symptoms are non-specific: typically chronic productive cough, fatigue, sometimes with weight loss, dyspnoea, fever
- Often complicates known underlying lung disease, such as COPD, leading to atypical disease progression
- Colonization of abnormal lung may not cause symptoms but can progress to cause disease later
- Disseminated infection may occur, especially in immunocompromised
- HP 2° to NTM may occur following use of hot tubs, indoor swimming pools, or contaminated metalworking fluids; breathlessness tends to be a prominent symptom.

Investigations

- *CXR* can be indistinguishable from that of MTB, with upper zone infiltrate with cavitation. Airway nodularity and associated bronchiectasis are recognized. CXR may be difficult to interpret in the presence of pre-existing lung disease
- *Sputum samples* Microbiology for AFB stain, culture, and further identification. If there is growth of an atypical AFB, send at least two further sputum samples at intervals of 7 days for AFB smear and culture
- *Bronchoscopy* with lavage may be required
- *HRCT* chest typically shows thin-walled upper lobe cavities, with marked pleural involvement, or small nodules with tree-in-bud pattern and cylindrical bronchiectasis; bilateral diffuse ground-glass infiltrates, nodules, or mosaic pattern may be seen with NTM-associated HP.

Diagnosis Distinguishing contamination or colonization with NTM from clinical disease may be challenging. A single positive NTM sputum culture is unlikely to be of significance, although such patients should be followed up with periodic sputum cultures. Treat patients who are deteriorating clinically and who have repeatedly positive cultures or smears for NTM. At least two separate positive sputum cultures or a single positive bronchial wash/lavage or biopsy culture are usually considered sufficient to justify treatment in the appropriate clinical context. Compatible histopathology (granulomatous inflammation), when available, further supports a decision to commence treatment. HRCT may be useful in facilitating treatment decisions, as an abnormal baseline HRCT consistent with NTM infection appears to be predictive of disease progression.

Management

- The decision to treat is complex and is based on the likelihood of clinical disease, weighed against the side effects and potential toxicity of treatment
- No need to notify or contact-trace, as there is low risk of cross-infection
- Typical drug regimens for specific NTM species are described on ➔ pp. 520–1. Prolonged courses of treatment are required, and drug side effects frequently limit therapy
- Avoid macrolide monotherapy, which encourages macrolide resistance
- Be alert to the possibility of drug interactions. In the setting of HIV, there are potential drug interactions between rifampicin, macrolides, and protease inhibitors and non-nucleoside reverse transcriptase inhibitors (NNRTIs). Rifampicin induces liver enzymes, and, therefore, the elimination of other drugs (e.g. oral contraceptives, warfarin, phenytoin, prednisolone, ciclosporin, etc.) may be increased. Macrolides may cause QT interval prolongation, particularly when taken alongside other QT-prolonging drugs
- Curative therapy is not always possible, reflecting antibiotic resistance in the NTM species, drug intolerance due to side effects, and/or significant comorbid disease
- Although rarely employed in the UK, surgical resection of focal disease, in combination with drug therapy, may be curative in patients who are able to tolerate resection—consider in patients with highly resistant isolates who have failed to respond to standard therapy.

Further information

Griffith DE et al. ATS/IDSA Statement: diagnosis, treatment and prevention of NTM. Am J Respir Crit Care Med 2007;**175**:367–416.

NTM species and lung disease

Slowly growing species

Mycobacterium avium complex (MAC)

- MAC includes the different *M. avium* subspecies as well as *M. intracellulare*; it is also referred to as *M. avium intracellulare* (MAI)
- Classical presentations include upper lobe fibrocavitary disease in elderly ♂ smokers and nodular/bronchiectatic disease in non-smoking ♀
- Initial treatment should be triple therapy with a macrolide (clarithromycin or azithromycin), rifampicin, and ethambutol. A three times weekly regimen may be used in less severe disease. Consider adding nebulized/IV amikacin or IV streptomycin in severe (usually cavitary) disease
- Antibiotic susceptibility testing is not predictive of clinical response in MAC, with the exception of macrolide susceptibility, and so routine susceptibility testing of MAC isolates is performed for clarithromycin only. Macrolide resistance is associated with a poor prognosis, and its management is complex—seek microbiology advice. The major risk factor for macrolide resistance is macrolide monotherapy, and macrolides should *never* be used as monotherapy for treatment of MAC
- Antibiotic treatment should be continued for 12–18 months of negative sputum cultures whilst on therapy
- MAC is the leading cause of NTM infection in the setting of HIV and may occur late in the disease when CD4 count <50 or during the first 2 months of ART. Disease is rarely confined to the lungs in this setting, and lymphadenitis and disseminated infection are common.

Mycobacterium kansasii

- *M. kansasii* classically presents with progressive upper lobe fibrocavitary disease similar to TB, and isolation of *M. kansasii* is usually associated with disease (rather than reflecting contamination)
- Treatment is usually with rifampicin, ethambutol, and isoniazid for a minimum of 12 months of negative sputum cultures. Clarithromycin and moxifloxacin may be useful agents, e.g. for rifampicin-resistant isolates. Usually good response to treatment: >90% 5y cure and <10% relapse with full compliance.

Mycobacterium malmoense

- *M. malmoense* typically causes cavitary disease, often in patients with underlying COPD, and isolation of *M. malmoense* is usually associated with disease (rather than contamination)
- Treatment is usually with 2–4 drugs, including ethambutol and rifampicin, and often a macrolide, for 12–24 months.

Mycobacterium xenopi

- *M. xenopi* typically causes upper lobe cavitary disease resembling TB
- Treatment regimens include ethambutol, isoniazid, and rifampicin for at least 24 months; macrolides may be useful. Disease may progress, despite treatment, and mortality appears to be relatively high.

Mycobacterium gordonae
- *M. gordonae* is frequently isolated from sputum but is usually a contaminant and only rarely causes progressive lung disease.

Rapidly growing species

Mycobacterium abscessus
- *M. abscessus* comprises three species *M. abscessus* (*sensu stricto*), *M. massiliense*, and *M. boletii*, which may differ in treatment response (with a better prognosis in *M. massiliense*, compared to *M. abscessus*)
- *M. abscessus* has emerged as a major pathogen in CF where it is the leading mycobacterial cause of progressive lung disease. Recent reports suggest the existence of person-to-person spread of *M. abscessus* between CF patients, and segregation in CF centres is increasingly recommended
- *M. abscessus* also causes nodular/bronchiectatic disease in patients without CF, classically non-smoking ♀
- *M. abscessus* is uniformly resistant to standard antituberculous agents, and there is currently no proven curative antibiotic regimen for *M. abscessus* lung disease. Regimens based on *in vitro* drug susceptibilities are recommended; a typical treatment protocol in CF might comprise induction therapy for at least 3–4 weeks with IV amikacin, IV cefoxitin or imipenem, and PO azithromycin, followed by long-term maintenance therapy with nebulized amikacin, PO azithromycin, and another PO agent to which the isolate is sensitive (e.g. a quinolone). Azithromycin appears to induce less macrolide resistance and is probably more effective than clarithromycin against *M. abscessus*. Tigecycline may be a useful second-line agent for induction, although nausea often limits its use
- Although guidelines recommend continuing antibiotic treatment for 12–18 months once cultures are negative, in practice, achieving this level of suppression of *M. abscessus* is often unrealistic. This is a chronic incurable infection for many CF patients, and intermittent courses of IV agents (e.g. amikacin, cefoxitin, or imipenem) are typically required to treat exacerbations and control symptoms/minimize progression of lung disease.

Mycobacterium chelonae
- Rarely causes lung disease. Treat with at least two drugs to which the isolate displays *in vitro* susceptibility; often susceptible to macrolides, tobramycin, amikacin, imipenem; resistant to cefoxitin.

Mycobacterium fortuitum
- Often does not cause progressive lung disease in the absence of treatment; when therapy is needed, usually susceptible to macrolides, quinolones, imipenem, cefoxitin.

Chapter 43

Respiratory infection—parasitic

Introduction to parasitic respiratory infections

A wide variety of parasitic organisms may infect the lungs, although clinical disease is rare in the UK. In general, parasites may cause lung disease by two different mechanisms:

- Hypersensitivity reactions, e.g. Löffler's syndrome and eosinophilic lung disease, most commonly from helminths such as *ascaris, toxocara*, and liver flukes
- Direct infection and invasion, e.g. amoebic disease, pulmonary hydatid disease.

Some of the more important examples are noted in this chapter.

Pulmonary hydatid disease

- Hydatidosis is the commonest parasitic lung disease worldwide
- Human infection follows ingestion of parasite eggs, with the adult worm found in dogs, sheep, goats, horses, camels, and moose; infection is common in sheep-raising regions, particularly Central Europe and the Mediterranean, as well as Alaska and Arctic Canada
- Caused by a cestode (tapeworm). Two main forms:
  - *Echinococcus granulosus*, which causes cystic hydatid disease as the larvae grow in the lungs. Common. Symptoms include cough (sometimes productive of cyst contents, 'hydatidoptysis'), haemoptysis, and chest pain. CXR shows rounded cysts, sometimes with calcified walls, most commonly in lower lobes; CT may show 'daughter cysts'. Cyst rupture may occur, with wheeze, eosinophilia, and bronchial or pleural spread
  - *Echinococcus multilocularis*, which leads to alveolar hydatid disease following tissue invasion. Rare. Lung masses are less clearly delineated on CT than in cystic disease
- Diagnose from serology or sputum analysis. Serology is insensitive for the diagnosis of pulmonary disease (around 50%). Demonstration of liver cysts supports the diagnosis. Avoid needle aspiration of cysts, which may result in hypersensitivity or dissemination.
- Treatment is with surgical excision in most cases. Medical treatment with albendazole if the patient is unfit for surgery or following cyst rupture and dissemination.

Amoebic pulmonary disease

- Caused by the protozoa *Entamoeba histolytica*
- Intestinal and liver infection are common, with lung involvement in a minority
- Lung disease can develop either directly via transdiaphragmatic spread from the liver or via the bloodstream or lymphatics
- Pulmonary manifestations include right lower lobe consolidation, empyema, lung abscess, or hepatobronchial fistulae (resulting in large volumes of brown or 'anchovy' sputum). May be associated pericardial disease
- Diagnose using serology (sensitivity >90%) or following identification of trophozoites in stool, sputum, or pleural fluid
- Treatment is with metronidazole plus diloxanide.

Pulmonary ascariasis

- An intestinal nematode (roundworm) distributed worldwide
- Following oral ingestion of *Ascaris lumbricoides* eggs, larvae haematogenously migrate to lungs where they mature over 1–2 weeks
- Clinically presents as a hypersensitivity reaction, with cough, wheeze, fever, retrosternal discomfort, CXR infiltrates, and peripheral eosinophilia (Löffler's syndrome)
- Examination of gastric aspirates or respiratory secretions for larvae is required to definitively diagnose. Stool for eggs may confirm the diagnosis although often not detectable for ~2 months
- Usually resolves spontaneously after 1–2 weeks. Consider treatment with albendazole/mebendazole for GI infection once larvae have reached maturity.

Strongyloidiasis

- Caused by the nematode (roundworm) *Strongyloides stercoralis*, found in Central and South America and Africa. Filariform larvae (in faecally contaminated soil) migrate through skin and travel to lungs haematogenously
- Pulmonary involvement may lead to a Löffler-type syndrome, with wheeze, skin rash, eosinophilia, and CXR infiltrate. In the setting of immunocompromise, disseminated autoinfection may occur, leading to the 'hyperinfection syndrome'. ARDS may develop, and 2° bacterial sepsis is common
- Diagnose using serology (sensitivity ~85%; false negatives in immunosuppression) or following microbiological analysis of stool (relatively low sensitivity) or duodenal fluid. In disseminated strongyloidiasis, larvae may be found in sputum, BAL fluid, and pleural fluid
- Treatment is with ivermectin or albendazole.

Toxocariasis

- Caused by roundworm *Toxocara canis*, distributed worldwide in dogs (*T. cati* from cats also causes disease)
- Ingestion of eggs from contaminated soil/food may result in visceral larva migrans. Migration of larvae through the lungs results in an immune response, with wheeze, cough, and eosinophilia. Heavy ingestion causes fever, anorexia, hepatomegaly, and urticarial rashes
- Diagnosis may be made from serology (sensitivity ~80%)
- Treatment often not required; moderate/severe cases are given albendazole; steroids may be beneficial in severe cases.

Dirofilariasis

- Nematode (roundworm) found in USA, Japan, South America
- Infection is caused by *Dirofilaria immitis* following mosquito transfer from animals, especially dogs. Worms lodge in the pulmonary arteries and elicit an inflammatory response, leading to a necrotic nodule
- Presentation is classically asymptomatic, with a single peripheral nodule on CXR mimicking cancer. Patients may present with cough, chest pain, and haemoptysis, presumably due to pulmonary infarction
- Definitive diagnosis requires lung biopsy. Serology lacks sensitivity and specificity
- Treatment is not usually required.

Schistosomiasis

- Found in the Middle East, South America, South-East Asia, Africa, and the Caribbean
- *Schistosoma* species are trematodes (flukes) carried by snails, and infection follows skin penetration, often during swimming
- Pulmonary involvement may reflect acute tissue migration, causing cough, wheeze, and CXR infiltrates. Chronic infection can lead to interstitial infiltrates or AV fistulae. In some, portal hypertension opens up portosystemic collaterals, and eggs then embolize into the pulmonary circulation. A granulomatous pulmonary endarteritis develops, causing PHT and cor pulmonale
- Diagnosis from observation of ova in sputum, BAL, urine, or stool, or from lung biopsy. Serology testing is possible, but such tests are not standardized
- Treatment is with praziquantel.

Paragonimiasis

- Caused by *Paragonimus* spp., particularly *P. westermani* (oriental lung fluke), a trematode (fluke) distributed in West Africa, the Far East, India, and Central and South America
- Following ingestion of undercooked seafood, flukes migrate to the lung or pleura and become encapsulated, developing into adults in ~6 weeks
- Clinical features may be acute or chronic and include chest pain, pneumothorax, pleural effusion, Löffler's syndrome, and recurrent haemoptysis. Serum eosinophilia is common
- Diagnose with serology (sensitivity ~90%) or observation of eggs (late phase of infection) in sputum, TBB, BAL, pleural fluid, or stool
- Treatment is with praziquantel.

Tropical (filarial) pulmonary eosinophilia

- Follows infection with *Wuchereria bancrofti*, *Brugia malayi*, or *Brugia timori* in the tropics
- These roundworms reside in the lymphatics and bloodstream
- Pulmonary involvement is common and represents a hypersensitivity reaction to the organism trapped in the lung, with cough, wheeze, CXR infiltrates, peripheral eosinophilia, and raised serum IgE. See pp. 234–5
- Diagnosis is serological (modest sensitivity)
- Treatment is with diethylcarbamazine.

Chapter 44

Respiratory infection—viral

Overview of viral pneumonia

- Viral URTIs are common, but typically self-limiting, and are usually managed in the community. Viral pneumonia is less common but is more serious and usually requires hospitalization. Viral pneumonia in the immunocompetent is rare and typically affects children or the elderly; influenza strains are the commonest cause in adults. Studies suggest that viruses are detectable in 15–30% of patients hospitalized with pneumonia
- Viruses may cause serious respiratory infection in the immunocompromised (particularly patients with depressed T-cell function, e.g. following organ transplantation). CMV is the commonest serious viral pathogen that affects immunocompromised patients. Influenza, parainfluenza, RSV, measles, and adenovirus may also cause pneumonia in the immunocompromised, although diagnosis of these viruses is difficult and infection is commonly undetected
- The clinical and radiological features of viral pneumonia are non-specific. Worsening cough and breathlessness following an URTI suggest the development of pneumonia; wheeze may accompany bronchiolitis. CXR typically shows non-specific diffuse interstitial infiltrates, and hypoxia may occur. 2° bacterial infection may complicate viral pneumonia
- A variety of diagnostic techniques are available, including PCR, viral culture, antigen testing (e.g. EIA and direct fluorescent antibody (DFA) testing), and serology
- Treatment consists of supportive care and, in some cases, antivirals. Infection with certain viruses may require isolation. Treat 2° bacterial infection with antibiotics
- Specific features of the common and/or important viruses are noted in the remainder of the chapter.

Influenza: background

- Single-stranded enveloped RNA viruses
- Commonest cause of viral pneumonia in immunocompetent adults. It is transmitted via respiratory secretions and is extremely contagious
- Three pathogenic serotypes: A, B, and C. Type A causes more severe disease and occurs in annual epidemics and intermittent pandemics. Types B and C cause epidemics
- The surface antigens haemagglutinin and neuraminidase determine influenza serotype. Genetic mutations may result in antigenic shifts (major genetic rearrangements between strains, associated with pandemics of influenza A—1918 (H1N1), 1957 (H2N2), 1968 (H3N2), and 2009 (H1N1) pandemics) and antigenic drifts (more minor genetic variations associated with epidemics)
- Genetic rearrangement of virus occurs in animal and bird reservoirs, and the virus may then be transferred to humans, e.g. 2009 H1N1 was caused by reassortment of two swine, one human, and one avian strains
- Seasonal influenza is very well recognized in the UK, particularly during the winter months. Seasonal influenza may affect previously well individuals, although it occurs more commonly in the elderly, particularly in the setting of chronic heart or lung disease or immunocompromise
- Pandemic 2009 influenza A/H1N1 was first detected in Mexico and lasted until August 2010, affecting >214 countries and territories and an estimated 201,000 respiratory deaths associated with influenza (18,500 of these were laboratory-confirmed cases). The majority of infection and deaths occurred in those aged 18–64 years old, with lower rates in elderly patients probably due to exposure to similar strains earlier in life. High death rates particularly seen in pregnant patients
- Outbreaks of highly pathogenic H5N1 avian influenza have occurred in many countries, raising fears of the development of sustained human-to-human transmission and a new global pandemic. >600 cases have been reported worldwide since 2003, associated with a 60% mortality
- Novel avian influenza A/H7N9 was first reported in March 2013 in eastern China, with likely transmission via secretions/excretions of infected poultry, with no evidence (as yet) of sustained human-to-human transmission. Serological studies have found no evidence of human infection with novel H7N9 prior to November 2012 in Chinese poultry workers. The virus seems to have been created by reassortment of at least four avian influenza viruses (probably obtaining its haemagglutinin gene from H7N3 in domestic ducks, its neuraminidase gene from H7N9 in wild birds, and six remaining genes from multiple related H9N2 viruses in domestic poultry). Early reports suggest that the median patient age is ~60 years old (contrasted with median H5N1 patient age of ~25 years old) and is associated with a 27% mortality.

Regularly updated information on seasonal, avian, and pandemic influenza is available from the Health Protection Agency, the World Health Organization, and the US Centers for Disease Control and Prevention websites:

- ℠ http://www.hpa.org.uk/Topics/InfectiousDiseases/InfectionsAZ/Influenza/
- ℠ http://www.who.int/csr/don/en/index.html
- ℠ http://www.cdc.gov/flu/weekly.

Additional guidelines are available for the management of suspected influenza in the setting of a pandemic with UK Pandemic Alert Levels 2–4 (cases of pandemic influenza identified in UK):

- ℠ http://www.brit-thoracic.org.uk/Guidelines/Pandemic-Flu-Guideline.aspx.

Influenza: diagnosis

Clinical and laboratory features Incubation period typically 1–4 days; adults contagious for 7 days and children for 21 days from illness onset. The clinical picture following infection is variable and may be influenced, in part, by the influenza subtype. Features include:

- *Asymptomatic* infection
- *'Flu'* (acute onset of fever, cough, headache, coryzal symptoms, myalgia, sore throat)
- Complications include:
  - Bronchitis/bronchiolitis
  - *1° influenza viral pneumonia* (onset typically within 48h of initial fever; cough dry or productive, haemoptysis may occur, bilateral crackles, and/or wheeze; may progress very rapidly to respiratory failure and death; described in many patients infected with avian influenza H5N1 and H7N9 and more likely among pandemic H1N1 than for seasonal influenza; often associated with lymphopenia, thrombocytopenia, abnormal liver function, and multi-organ failure)
  - *2° bacterial pneumonia* (significantly more common than viral pneumonia; onset typically 4–5 days after initial fever, during early convalescence, although may occur earlier; pathogens include S. pneumoniae, S. aureus—particularly associated with lung abscess— and H. influenzae; mixed bacterial/viral pneumonia may occur)
  - GI symptoms (e.g. watery diarrhoea; more frequently described during influenza A H1N1 and avian H5N1 than seasonal infection)
  - Otitis media (particularly in children), conjunctivitis; rarely parotitis
  - Myositis (CK may be elevated; rarely myoglobinuria with renal failure)
  - Neurological (encephalitis, acute necrotizing encephalopathy, transverse myelitis, Guillain–Barré syndrome—all rare; Reye's syndrome with encephalopathy and fatty liver following aspirin use is well described in children and adolescents)
  - Cardiovascular (ECG abnormalities common, myocarditis or pericarditis rare).

Imaging

- *CXR* typically shows bilateral mid-zone interstitial infiltrates in 1° viral pneumonia, although focal consolidation is also well described. Lobar consolidation occurs in 2° bacterial pneumonia.

Differential diagnosis of 'flu-like' illness includes adenovirus, RSV, rhinovirus, parainfluenza, *Chlamydophila pneumoniae*, *Legionella*, *Mycoplasma*, and *S. pneumoniae*. A very high fever is said to favour a diagnosis of influenza. Consider Middle East respiratory syndrome (MERS) (see → p. 548) in patients with an appropriate travel history.

Diagnosis is often suggested by knowledge of a local outbreak. Diagnostic investigations include:
- *Virology* (not routinely required if pandemic established with widespread infection across the UK—Alert Level 4—when diagnosis will be clinical—'influenza-like illness')
  - Presentation <7 days after illness onset: nose and throat swabs in virus transport medium (for direct immunofluorescence, ELISA, virus culture, and/or reverse transcriptase PCR (RT-PCR))
  - Presentation >7 days after illness onset: 'acute' serum and subsequently 'convalescent' serum after 10–14 days (for influenza serological testing)
- *Bacteriology* (in patients with influenza-related pneumonia)
  - Blood culture
  - Pneumococcal and *Legionella* urinary antigen
  - Sputum M, C, & S (if purulent sputum and either no prior antibiotics or failure to respond to empirical antibiotics)
  - 'Acute' serum and subsequently 'convalescent' serum after 10–14 days for influenza/other agents serological testing.

Influenza: management

Severity assessment

- Patients with uncomplicated influenza do not require admission
- For influenza-related pneumonia, a CURB-65 score (see ➋ pp. 422–3) of ≥3 indicates severe pneumonia and a high risk of death; patients with a score of 0 or 1 may be considered for home treatment
- Bilateral CXR infiltrates consistent with 1° viral pneumonia should be considered as severe pneumonia, irrespective of CURB-65 score.

Infection control

- Outside the setting of a UK pandemic, most suspected cases of influenza are likely to be seasonal
- H5N1 avian influenza should be seriously considered in patients with:
  - Fever (≥38°C) and lower respiratory tract symptoms or CXR showing consolidation/ARDS or a severe illness suggestive of an infectious process, *and*
  - Close contact (<1m) within 7 days with *either* live or dead domestic poultry or wild birds in countries affected by H5N1 (or known infected animals, e.g. cats or pigs) *or* close contact with human cases of severe unexplained respiratory illness or unexplained illness resulting in death in patients from countries with H5N1
- H7N9 avian influenza should be suspected in patients with:
  - Fever (≥38°C) and clinical or CXR findings of consolidation/ARDS or a severe illness suggestive of an infectious process, *and*
  - Travel to China within 10 days before symptom onset

In such cases of suspected avian influenza, the patient should be assessed either at their home or in a hospital side room, with both patient and staff wearing surgical masks and staff wearing surgical gown and gloves. Immediately inform local Health Protection Unit as well as hospital infection control and occupational health. If hospitalization is required, patients should be in strict respiratory isolation, preferably in a negative pressure room (although patients should not be transferred for this reason alone), and staff should wear high-filtration mask (FFP3), gown, gloves, and eye protection (consider also cap and plastic apron, depending on situation). Mark all laboratory samples as 'high risk', and inform local laboratory of the sample status.

Treatment

- *Supportive care* O_2, IV fluids, nutritional support. Consider ITU/HDU admission for patients with one or more of more of: 1° viral pneumonia; CURB-65 score of 4 or 5; PaO_2 <8kPa despite high-flow O_2; progressive hypercapnia; pH <7.26; septic shock. NIV may be used for patients with COPD and decompensated type II respiratory failure, although infection control measures should be in place and protective equipment worn by staff to minimize any spread of infection from respiratory droplets
- *Antiviral* treatment with neuraminidase inhibitors is indicated for patients with an influenza-like illness and fever >38°C within 48h of symptom onset; consider also treating immunocompromised

or very elderly patients in the absence of fever, and severely ill or immunocompromised patients if >48h from disease onset. Also treat patients with suspected H5N1 or H7N9, regardless of duration of symptoms. Treat with: oseltamivir 75mg bd for 5 days (75mg od if creatinine clearance <30mL/min); anti-emetics may be needed for nausea. Inhaled zanamivir 10mg bd via inhaler for 5 days (up to 10 days if resistance to oseltamivir) is another option for non-severe disease. Antivirals appear to reduce illness duration (by 1 day), hospitalization, and subsequent antibiotic requirements; possible effects on mortality have not been adequately studied. The neuraminidase inhibitor zanamivir may be given intravenously (e.g. for ventilated patients), but its effectiveness in this situation is unproven. Antiviral prophylaxis may be considered for health care workers caring for patients with suspected avian influenza, as well as the patient's household contacts

- Treat influenza-related pneumonia with *antibiotics*, according to severity, e.g. oral co-amoxiclav, a tetracycline (e.g. doxycycline), or a macrolide if non-severe; IV co-amoxiclav or cefuroxime or cefotaxime, together with a macrolide, if severe.

Outcome Uncomplicated influenza typically resolves within 7 days, although cough and malaise may persist for several weeks. The reported mortality from 1° influenza viral pneumonia is >40% and up to 24% from 2° bacterial pneumonia. Risks of viral pneumonia are increased in older patients with cardiorespiratory disease or diabetes. Pandemics are associated with a shift in the age distribution—the 2009 pandemic saw high rates of mortality and morbidity among children and young adults.

Vaccination

- The influenza inactivated vaccine is modified annually, based on recent viral strains (and now includes antigen from the 2009 pandemic H1N1), and provides partial protection against influenza illness, hospitalization, and death. Vaccination if age >65, chronic comorbidity, nursing home residents, or health workers. Vaccination will not protect against H5N1 avian influenza but may make simultaneous co-infection with human and avian influenza less likely and so reduce the likelihood of viral genetic reassortment
- Administration of oseltamivir 75mg od to high-risk individuals throughout periods of exposure may also prevent infection
- Live attenuated influenza vaccines are currently under investigation.

Further information

Gao et al. Clinical findings in 111 cases of influenza A (H7N9) virus infection. N Engl J Med 2013;368:2277–85.

Gao et al. Human infection with a novel avian-origin influenza A (H7N9) virus. N Engl J Med 2013;368:1888–97.

Cytomegalovirus pneumonia

Epidemiology

- Enveloped dsDNA virus
- CMV is the commonest serious viral pathogen in the immunocompromised and is a particular problem following transplantation where prophylaxis is now widely used
- Individuals are described as 'seropositive' for CMV if they have evidence of IgG antibodies, indicating latent infection following previous exposure; seropositivity increases with age. Infection in transplant recipients results from either transmission from a CMV positive donor to a CMV antibody negative recipient (via the organ or a blood transfusion) or reactivation of latent CMV in a seropositive recipient as a result of immunosuppression
- Infection occurs most frequently during the first 4 months following organ or bone marrow transplantation, corresponding to the period of maximal T-cell suppression. GVHD increases the risk of CMV infection.

Clinical and laboratory features

- 'Flu-like' symptoms in immunocompetent patients
- Symptoms of CMV pneumonia in the immunocompromised are non-specific: fever, dry cough, dyspnoea, and malaise
- Extrapulmonary manifestations of CMV infection (e.g. gastro-oesophagitis; hepatitis) may suggest the diagnosis
- Hypoxia may occur. Leucopenia, thrombocytopenia, and abnormal LFTs are characteristic.

Imaging

- *CXR* Typically bilateral diffuse interstitial infiltrate, although lobar consolidation and localized haziness also described; can be normal. A nodular infiltrate may suggest co-infection with *Aspergillus*
- *CT* Features include localized or diffuse ground-glass and nodular shadowing that may progress to airspace consolidation.

Diagnosis Antibody tests are used to estimate risk following transplantation, but diagnosis of active disease requires evidence of either viraemia (by antigen or PCR testing of blood) or tissue invasion (by biopsy). A wide range of diagnostic tests are available, and the choice of tests varies between centres—discuss with your local virologist. The nature of the transplant and immunosuppression also influence the interpretation of test results. Methods include:

- Early antigen fluorescence test on BAL fluid (high sensitivity, low specificity)
- Qualitative PCR on blood or BAL fluid (highly sensitive but unable to differentiate between latent and replicating CMV; negative result practically excludes the diagnosis, positive result is unhelpful)
- CMV antigenaemia on blood (rapid, differentiates between latent and replicating virus)
- Quantitative PCR on blood or BAL fluid (rapid, differentiates between latent and replicating virus)

- Indirect immunofluorescence with monoclonal antibodies to CMV in BAL fluid (rapid, highly sensitive, and specific)
- Histology of lung tissue from transbronchial or surgical biopsies (demonstrate CMV inclusion bodies—the 'owl's eye' appearance— within infected cells; considered gold standard investigation).

In some cases, a definitive diagnosis is not possible and treatment is empirical.

Treatment Reduce immunosuppression where possible. Ganciclovir 5mg/kg IV bd for 2–4 weeks (side effects include neutropenia, anaemia). Consider additional treatment with anti-CMV hyperimmune globulin or prolonged oral valganciclovir in cases of severe or relapsed disease. Foscarnet 60mg/kg tds for 2–3 weeks is an alternative to ganciclovir for resistant cases, but toxicity (nephrotoxicity, metabolic disturbance) can limit treatment.

Complications

- Opportunistic infection (e.g. PCP, aspergillosis) due to further suppression of T-cell function by the CMV infection itself
- Increased risk of organ rejection, as allografts are more susceptible to CMV infection than native organs.

Outcome The reported mortality from CMV pneumonia varies although may be as high as 85%. Relapse occurs in up to one-third of patients.

Adenovirus

- Non-enveloped dsDNA viruses
- Worldwide distribution, occur throughout the year
- >50 serotypes, the relative frequency of which is unclear. Some studies suggest serotypes 1–3 are most common, but studies in the armed services found high frequencies of serotypes 4, 7, and 14 (all of these are associated with upper and lower respiratory tract infections)
- Most common symptoms are those of self-limiting upper airways infection, which frequently mimics group A streptococcal infection, particularly in childhood
- Can cause pneumonia and ARDS in adults
- Occasional complications—myocarditis, hepatitis, nephritis, meningoencephalitis, and DIC
- Disseminated disease may occur in the immunocompromised (sometimes due to virus reactivation)
- Diagnosis is by nasopharyngeal fluid, sputum, or BAL fluid viral culture, antigen testing or PCR, or quantitative PCR on blood (particularly in the immunocompromised). Serology and histology (showing intranuclear inclusions) may also be helpful
- Treatment is usually supportive, but the seriously unwell (particularly the immunocompromised) may be treated with cidofovir (unlicensed; nephrotoxicity; poor evidence) ± IV immunoglobulin. Ganciclovir has limited activity against adenoviruses.

Measles

- Enveloped single-stranded RNA virus
- Very rare in adults. Symptomatic respiratory involvement (e.g. croup, bronchiolitis, and pneumonia) occur most commonly in the very young and those >20 years old and is a common cause of mortality
- Symptoms of fever and URTI are followed by a diffuse maculopapular rash. Leucopenia is common
- CXR may show reticulonodular infiltrates, hilar lymphadenopathy, and pleural effusions
- 2° bacterial infection is common
- Diagnosis is serological; viral culture is possible but rarely performed
- Treatment is supportive. Treat 2° bacterial infection with antibiotics.

Human metapneumovirus

- Single-stranded enveloped RNA virus
- First isolated in 2001, ubiquitous worldwide
- Seasonal variation—peaks in late winter and early spring
- Most children are infected by 5 years old
- Usually causes mild self-limiting upper airways infection ~5 days after infection but may progress to wheezing and pneumonia or ARDS in some adults (especially the immunocompromised or elderly patients with comorbidities)
- Ongoing airways hyperreactivity may last for several weeks
- PCR/serological evidence of metapneumovirus in ~4% of adults admitted with acute lower respiratory tract infection
- Diagnosis is usually using in full reverse transcriptase PCR (RT-PCR), serology, or viral culture of nasopharyngeal or BAL specimens
- Treatment is supportive. Ribavirin may have activity *in vivo*, but this is still under investigation.

Parainfluenza

- Single-stranded enveloped RNA viruses; serotypes 1–4
- >90% of adults have antibodies to parainfluenza, but these are only partially protective
- Types 1–3 usually cause self-limiting upper respiratory infection but can cause pneumonia, particularly among the elderly or immunocompromised. Type 4 usually causes URTI
- Associated with asthma and COPD exacerbations
- Rarely causes myocarditis, meningitis, and Guillain–Barré syndrome
- Diagnosed using PCR, antigen detection, or viral culture on nasopharyngeal secretions or BAL fluid
- Treatment is supportive, with reduction of immunosuppression (particularly glucocorticoids) when possible.

Respiratory syncytial virus

- Single-stranded enveloped RNA virus; subtypes A and B. Subtype A is associated with more severe disease
- Very common cause of bronchiolitis and pneumonia in children, causing winter outbreaks. Role in adult respiratory disease is more significant than previously appreciated, and infection often goes unrecognized, with ~5% of adults developing RSV each year
- Clinical features in adults are usually of URTI or tracheobronchitis, but this may progress to pneumonia, particularly in the setting of underlying cardiac or respiratory disease, malignancy, or immunosuppression; outbreaks affecting adults in hospitals and nursing homes also occur. RSV may be a relatively common viral cause of pneumonia in patients who have recently undergone bone marrow transplantation
- Nasopharyngeal secretions and BAL fluid are often diagnostic; detection of RSV antigen in BAL fluid has a sensitivity of nearly 90%. PCR-based diagnostic techniques and serological testing may have a role
- Bacterial superinfection may be a frequent complication
- Treatment is principally supportive. Role of aerosolized ribavirin and steroids in the treatment of severe disease in adults is unclear. Reports of successful outcomes in bone marrow transplant recipients following treatment with ribavirin and immunoglobulin.

Varicella pneumonia

- Caused by varicella-zoster virus (an enveloped dsDNA virus)
- Pneumonia occurs in a small proportion of adults with chickenpox or shingles but accounts for the majority of mortality associated with adult disease. Risk factors for its development include smoking, increased number of skin spots (>100), pregnancy (third trimester), steroid treatment, and immunocompromise
- There is typically a history of recent exposure to a contact infected with chickenpox or shingles. Chest symptoms tend to occur several days after the onset of rash (erythematous macules progressing to papules and then vesicles), although rarely may precede the rash. Cough and breathlessness are common, and pleuritic pain and haemoptysis may occur
- CXR typically shows a diffuse small nodular infiltrate; hilar lymphadenopathy and pleural effusions may uncommonly occur. Nodules may subsequently calcify and persist
- Multi-organ involvement may occur
- Diagnosis is usually suspected on the basis of the history of exposure, presence of rash, and CXR features. Cytological examination of smears from skin lesions, serology, or viral culture or PCR on BAL fluid may confirm the diagnosis
- Treatment of varicella pneumonia is with early administration of aciclovir 10–12.5mg/kg IV tds for 7–10 days. Aciclovir is not licensed for use in pregnancy but does not appear to be associated with increased foetal abnormalities, and the benefits of treatment almost certainly outweigh any risk. Varicella is very infectious until lesions enter the 'crusting' stage; inpatients should be isolated. Extracorporeal membrane oxygenation/life support has been used successfully in individuals with fulminant respiratory failure. Consider early administration of varicella-zoster immune globulin for immunocompromised and pregnant patients exposed to varicella
- Most cases resolve spontaneously, but a minority progresses to respiratory failure and death (10–30%). Mortality may be significantly higher in pregnancy.

Hantavirus pulmonary syndrome

- Also known as hantavirus cardiopulmonary syndrome
- Caused by single-stranded enveloped RNA hantaviruses
- First described following an outbreak in the south-western USA in 1993. Several different hantaviruses (e.g. Sin Nombre virus) have been associated with this syndrome. Previously described hantavirus-associated diseases occurred more commonly in Scandinavia and north-eastern Asia and tended to cause haemorrhagic fever and renal failure, with relative sparing of the lung
- Very rare, and affected individuals are almost exclusively from America, particularly from the Four Corners Region of USA where Arizona, Colorado, Utah, and New Mexico meet. A 2012 outbreak, affecting ten people who visited Yosemite National Park (California), was thought to be associated with rodent infestation in cabin insulation
- Disease develops following inhalation of aerosolized viruses from rodent faeces, urine, or saliva and typically affects previously well young adults
- Common presenting symptoms are fever, chills, cough, myalgia, and GI symptoms such as vomiting and abdominal pain. Breathlessness occurs later in the disease course and is often quickly followed by respiratory failure and the development of ARDS. Shock may occur and is associated with a poor prognosis
- Laboratory testing classically reveals neutrophilia, thrombocytopenia, elevated LDH, and sometimes renal impairment and mildly abnormal LFTs. Leucocytosis and immunoblasts in peripheral blood are associated with severe disease
- CXR typically shows initially bilateral basal infiltrates that progress to involve all regions of the lung; a minority are normal
- Diagnosis may be confirmed using serology, PCR for the virus, or by detection of viral antigen using immunochemistry
- Treatment is supportive within an ICU, including the use of extracorporeal membrane oxygenation when appropriate. It is unclear if person-to-person transmission occurs, and patients should be in respiratory isolation. IV ribavirin may be administered, although this has not been demonstrated to improve outcome
- Mortality 10–50%, with death usually occurring within several days of presentation.

Severe acute respiratory syndrome (SARS)

Caused by SARS-coronavirus (SARS-CoV; an enveloped RNA virus).

Epidemiology Rapidly progressive acute respiratory illness, first recognized in November 2002 in the Guangdong province of China. By late February 2003, it had spread internationally, with 792 cases reported. First outbreak mainly affected health care workers and contacts. Disease spread to Hong Kong via a Guangdong province physician, who infected individuals in a Hong Kong hotel lift. Spread to Singapore, Thailand, Vietnam, and Canada via travellers. By July 2003, the worldwide epidemic had ended. There were a few cases in 2004, mostly laboratory-related, and no further cases thereafter.

A total of 8,098 cases were reported to the WHO by August 2003, with 774 deaths, giving a case fatality rate of 9.5%. The fatality rate for those aged ≥60 was 43%. Twenty-nine countries on all five continents were affected; 83% of the worldwide cases were in China and Hong Kong. No deaths occurred in the USA or the UK; 41 deaths (of 251 cases) were in Canada.

Case definition WHO defined criteria for those presenting with the disease after July 2004 (⅏ http://www.who.int/csr/sars/en):
- Fever >38°C, *plus*
- One or more symptom of lower respiratory tract illness (cough, difficulty breathing, SOB), *plus*
- Radiographic evidence of lung infiltrate, consistent with pneumonia or ARDS, *or* autopsy findings consistent with the pathology of pneumonia *or* ARDS without identifiable cause, *plus*
- No alternative diagnosis to explain the illness.

Laboratory case definition
- A person with symptoms or signs suggestive of SARS, *plus*
- Positive laboratory findings for SARS-CoV, based on one or more of:
  - PCR positive for SARS-CoV for two separate samples
  - Seroconversion by ELISA or immunofluorescence assay
  - Virus isolation.

Pathophysiology A previously undescribed coronavirus (SARS-CoV) is the causal agent. It is thought that animals, possibly palm civets (similar to cats) or bats, act as the main reservoir.

SARS is mostly spread by large droplets and person-to-person contact. There have been no reports of foodborne or waterborne transmission. However, SARS-CoV is shed in large quantities in stool, and profuse watery diarrhoea is a common symptom.

Lung post-mortem studies show diffuse alveolar damage, 2° bacterial pneumonia, and interstitial giant cell and macrophage infiltration. Pathological findings similar to those of bronchiolitis obliterans are recognized. There are no specific diagnostic features.

Incubation period is 2–10 days prior to the onset of the first symptom, which is typically fever.

Clinical features A two-stage illness, commencing with a prodrome of fever (>38°C), with or without rigors, with non-specific systemic symptoms, e.g. malaise, headache, and myalgia.

The respiratory stage of the illness starts 3–7 days after the prodromal phase, with dry cough and breathlessness. Progression to respiratory failure needing ventilation is well recognized. Up to 70% of patients develop large-volume watery diarrhoea without blood or mucus.

Destruction of lung tissue is thought to result from an excessive immune response to the virus, rather than from the direct effects of virus replication. Peak viral load is at day 12–14 of infection, with virus shed not only in respiratory secretions, but in faeces and other body fluids.

Retrospectively devised, but non-validated, scoring systems show that the presence of cough, myalgia, diarrhoea, and rhinorrhoea or sore throat are 100% sensitive and 76% specific at identifying a patient with SARS.

Children experience a milder form of the disease, with a low death rate.

Investigations

- Blood tests:
  - White blood count is normal or reduced; low lymphocyte count is common. Leucopenia and thrombocytopenia also recognized
  - Raised CK and ALT. Raised LDH is associated with a poorer outcome
- CXR—ranges from normal to diffuse bilateral interstitial infiltrate. Areas of focal consolidation, initially peripherally and lower zone in distribution, are also described. Cavitation, hilar lymphadenopathy, and pleural effusion are uncommon at presentation
- CT—interstitial infiltrate, ground-glass opacities, and interlobular septal thickening in those with a normal CXR. Spontaneous pneumothorax, pneumomediastinum, subpleural fibrosis, and/or cystic changes can occur in later stages
- SARS-CoV can be detected by RT-PCR (sensitivity 70%, dependent on specimen type and duration of illness). Useful specimens include nasopharyngeal aspirate, throat swab, urine, and faeces. An initial positive result on PCR must be confirmed by another clinical sample. Serology is sensitive, but seroconversion takes ~20 days.

Treatment There is no specific treatment for SARS, other than general supportive care. Ribavirin has been used but no clear benefit and toxicities common. Lopinavir-ritonavir may have some activity, but evidence of benefit is lacking.

Hospital admission Nosocomial transmission of SARS-CoV has been a striking feature in most outbreaks. Infected and suspected cases should be managed in negative pressure side rooms. Full protective clothing, including protective eye wear and face masks, is recommended for all visitors and health care workers. Aerosol-generating procedures (endotracheal intubation, nebulization, bronchoscopy) may amplify transmission.

Prognosis Older age is associated with a poorer outcome. Diabetes and other comorbid illness are independent risk factors for death.

Middle East respiratory syndrome (MERS)

- Caused by the novel MERS-coronavirus (MERS-CoV), an enveloped RNA virus first reported in Saudi Arabia in September 2012
- Closely related to bat coronaviruses
- 53 cases reported as of early June 2013, predominantly in Middle East countries (particularly Saudi Arabia) and in travellers returning from the Middle East
- Most patients are severely ill with pneumonia and ARDS, and many have acute kidney injury
- Diarrhoea, DIC, and pericarditis also seen
- Mortality >50%.

Diagnosis

- Using RT-PCR to detect MERS-CoV in respiratory samples (e.g. nasopharygeal fluid, sputum, or BAL fluid)
- Testing recommended by WHO for the following:
  - People with acute respiratory infection requiring admission and any of:
    - Disease occurring as part of a cluster occurring within 10 days, unless another aetiology found
    - Disease occurring in a health care worker working in an environment where patients with severe acute respiratory infections are cared for, unless another aetiology found
    - Disease occurring within 10 days of travel to the Middle East, unless another aetiology found
    - Disease follows an unexpectedly severe course despite appropriate treatment
    - People with acute respiratory illness of any severity who had exposure to a probable case of MERS-CoV within 10 days
    - Patients requiring mechanical ventilation in countries where MERS-CoV has been detected.

Treatment

Supportive. Antiviral agents are not currently recommended. Infection control precautions are essential.

Further information

Zaki AM et al. Isolation of a novel coronavirus from a man with pneumonia in Saudi Arabia. *N Engl J Med* 2012;**367**:1814–20.

WHO website. ℘ http://www.who.int/csr/disease/coronavirus_infections/en/.

Sarcoidosis

Epidemiology, aetiology, and immunopathology

Definition
- A multi-system disorder of unknown cause, likely resulting from the interplay of environmental and genetic factors
- Characterized by non-caseating granulomata and CD4+ Th1-biased T-cell response in affected organs
- Commonly involves the respiratory system but can affect nearly all organs
- 50–60% of people have spontaneous remissions; others may develop chronic, and sometimes progressive, disease.

Epidemiology Incidence varies across population studies, from 5 to 100/100,000, according to geographic distribution. UK incidence is about 5–10/100,000. Commoner in African Americans, West Indians, and the Irish. Commonly presents between ages of 20 and 40. Unusual in children and the elderly. Typically more aggressive disease in black populations than in Caucasians—higher incidence of skin disease, peripheral lymphadenopathy, bone marrow, and liver involvement; higher relapse rates and worse long-term prognosis.

Aetiology Sarcoidosis is the result of an abnormal immunological response to a benign environmental trigger(s) or antigen(s). The environmental trigger is likely to be a poorly degradable antigen but not a specific antigen or infectious agent. This abnormal immunology occurs in a genetically predisposed host.

Genetics Familial and ethnic clustering of cases suggest a genetic predisposition. Best evidence of HLA association comes from large multicentre ACCESS study, showing HLA-DRB1*1101 is associated with susceptibility to disease in blacks and whites; HLA-DRB1*0301 has been associated with acute and remitting disease. Genome-wide association studies have identified polymorphisms in *BTNL2*, *ANXA11*, and *FAM178A* as susceptibility genes in both familial and sporadic cases.

Immunopathology
- Unknown antigen triggers CD4 (helper) T-cell activation and expansion. This response is exaggerated and Th1-biased, with resultant interferon γ and IL2 production from these T-cells
- Activated T-cells proliferate and release mediators, attracting additional inflammatory cells, with concomitant macrophage activation and aggregation
- This leads to immune granuloma formation, which is enhanced by interferon γ
- Granulomata themselves cause increased local fibroblast stimulation and hence eventual fibrosis

- Metabolic activity of macrophages causes raised ACE levels in serum, lung tissue, and bronchoalveolar fluid. Increase in T-cell activity causes B-lymphocyte stimulation, which can cause raised serum immunoglobulins and immune complexes
- In most patients, response resolves over 2–5y.

Delayed-type hypersensitivity reactions are depressed in sarcoidosis. This is thought to be due to the migration of activated lymphocytes to the active compartment (lungs), with resultant peripheral blood lymphopenia. Seen as a decreased response to tuberculin, mumps virus, and *Candida albicans* antigens. This is not thought to be clinically significant.

Sarcoid-like reactions are reported in association with malignancy (mainly lymphoma, cervical, liver, lung, testes, and uterus). Non-caseating pulmonary granulomas are found, but there are no other symptoms or signs of sarcoidosis.

The main differential diagnoses of granuloma on a lung biopsy are shown in Box 45.1.

Box 45.1 Differential diagnosis of granuloma on lung biopsy

- Sarcoidosis
- TB
- HP
- Wegener's granulomatosis
- Drug reactions
- NTM
- Fungal infections:
  - Cryptococcosis
  - Aspergillosis
  - Coccidioidomycosis
  - Blastomycosis
- Aspiration of foreign material
- Primary biliary cirrhosis
- Sarcoid-like reaction to malignancy.

Further information

Iannuzzi MC. Advances in genetics of sarcoidosis. *Proc Am Thorac Soc* 2007;4:457–60.

Schurmann M et al. Familial sarcoidosis is linked to the major histocompatibility complex region. *Am J Respir Crit Care Med* 2000;162:861–4.

Schurmann M et al. HLA-DQB1 and HLA-DPB1 genotypes in familial sarcoidosis. *Respir Med* 1998;92:649–52.

Chest disease: clinical features

More than 90% of patients with sarcoidosis have thoracic involvement, with an abnormal CXR (see Boxes 45.2 and 45.3). Pulmonary sarcoidosis can be an incidental CXR finding in ~30% of patients. There is spontaneous remission in two-thirds, and 10–30% have a chronic course.

Clinical features There are probably at least two distinct clinical courses:

- *Löfgren's syndrome* Acute disease, which is usually self-limiting. Presents with fever, bilateral hilar lymphadenopathy, erythema nodosum, and arthralgia. Occurs particularly in Caucasians. Has a good prognosis and resolves completely and spontaneously in 80% within 1–2y. A minority may develop lung disease
- *Persistent or progressive* infiltrative lung disease.

Hilar/mediastinal lymphadenopathy May be asymptomatic or cause cough or chest pain. Usually bilateral and symmetrical, rarely unilateral and asymmetrical (this would suggest alternative diagnosis more likely). Can be associated with systemic symptoms of malaise and arthralgia, which are helped by NSAIDs. Benign course.

Important to exclude other causes of lymphadenopathy such as TB and lymphoma (see Box 45.3). May need CT and lymph node aspirate or biopsy.

Does not require systemic steroid treatment.

Stage I: 85% resolve spontaneously over 2y; 15% develop lung infiltrates. The average time for bilateral hilar lymphadenopathy resolution is 8 months.

Interstitial lung involvement May be asymptomatic or cause morbidity and mortality, with dyspnoea, cough, chest ache, or frank pain, malaise, fatigue, and impaired QoL. Rarely have crackles or clubbing on examination. Pulmonary infiltrates on CXR. Can return to normal over time or progress to fibrosis and respiratory failure. Lung function tests may be normal or may show a restrictive defect with reduced transfer factor.

Differential diagnosis: other ILD, malignancy, infection.

Box 45.2 Scadding radiological classification of thoracic sarcoidosis

Stage 0	Normal
Stage I	Hilar lymphadenopathy only
Stage II	Hilar lymphadenopathy and parenchymal infiltrate
Stage III	Parenchymal infiltrate
Stage IV	Fibrosis

Seeing a patient with possible sarcoidosis in clinic
- Make diagnosis—clinically, HRCT ± histology
- Assess extent/severity/presence of extrapulmonary involvement—CXR, PFT, ECG, eyes, rash, renal function, serum calcium, liver function, immunoglobulins, and ACE (last two can be raised in active sarcoidosis)
- Stable or progressive?—CXR, PFT (VC ± kCO), oximetry, ACE, urea (if renal involvement)
- Treatment?

Box 45.3 Differential diagnosis of bilateral hilar lymphadenopathy on CXR
- Sarcoidosis
- TB
- Lymphoma
- Lung cancer, especially small cell
- Coccidioidomycosis and histoplasmosis
- Berylliosis
- Mycoplasma
- HP.

Chest disease: diagnosis and monitoring

Diagnosis is based on a characteristic clinical picture, plus:
- Histological evidence of non-caseating granuloma in any tissue
- Characteristic picture on imaging (thoracic HRCT scan or gallium scan)
- Lymphocytosis on BAL.

Other diseases capable of producing similar clinical and histological picture, particularly TB and lymphoma, should be excluded.

Investigations

- *HRCT* Micronodules in a subpleural and bronchovascular distribution. Fissural nodularity and bronchial distortion. Irregular linear opacities, ground-glass shadowing related to bronchovascular bundles, and nodular or ill-defined shadows. Air trapping due to small airway granulomata common. Endobronchial disease in 55%. Minority has UIP pattern, associated with worse prognosis. Hilar and mediastinal lymphadenopathy. CT-guided FNA of subcarinal or mediastinal nodes may be possible and yield a tissue diagnosis
- *Bronchoscopy (TBB, TBNA, bronchial biopsy, EBUS, or BAL)* may not be necessary if no diagnostic doubt. May be important to exclude infectious agents. Positive yield of bronchial biopsy is 41–57%. Higher if visible abnormal mucosa. Positive yield of TBB is 40–90% (yield still high even if lungs appear normal on HRCT). Initial procedure of choice for suspected pulmonary sarcoidosis. TBNA of mediastinal lymph nodes yields a diagnosis in 63–90% of cases. TBB and TBNA have a higher yield together than either alone. However, presence of non-caseating granulomas on TBB or bronchial biopsy more significant than on lymph node sampling, as granuloma can accompany tumour infiltration of lymph nodes. BAL in sarcoidosis shows a CD4:CD8 ratio of >3.5. A lymphocytosis of $>2 \times 10^5$ cells/mL supports the diagnosis but is not diagnostic (also seen in HP and drug-induced alveolitis)
- *Mediastinoscopy* for central or paratracheal nodes or open lung biopsy: 90% positive yield. May be necessary to exclude lymphoma. Surgical biopsy is not usually necessary, but, if other procedures have not yielded a definitive diagnosis, it may be required. Lymph node ± lung (usually via VATS) can be biopsied
- *Biopsy other affected areas*, such as skin, liver, etc., if indicated, as these may be easier to biopsy in order to make a diagnosis
- *Mantoux/Heaf test* is typically grade 0 in sarcoidosis (peripheral cutaneous anergy to tuberculin due to migration of T-cells to active sites of disease). Positive Mantoux or Heaf test make sarcoidosis a less likely diagnosis although does not necessarily make TB more likely. Heaf testing not widely used now
- *Kveim test* No longer performed clinically, due to risks of transmissible diseases. It involved injecting homogenized splenic tissue from a patient with sarcoidosis to see if a granulomatous reaction occurred.

Monitoring disease There is no single measurement to assess all the aspects of patients with sarcoidosis. Clinical examination and serial measurements are key.

- *PFT* Pulmonary sarcoidosis gives a restrictive defect with decreased TLC and VC. TLCO provides the most sensitive measurement of change, although many use a properly performed VC as an alternative. Likely to improve with steroids. Airflow obstruction may also occur
- *CXR* may improve with time or treatment
- *HRCT* can help with determining burden of active disease
- *ACE* levels increased in up to 80% of patients with acute sarcoidosis although can be normal in active disease. It may be a surrogate marker of the total granuloma burden. Levels become normal as disease resolves. Can be useful to monitor the clinical course, if activity is uncertain, but levels should not be used in isolation to determine treatment. Levels suppressed by steroids, and, when steroids are stopped, levels usually increase, unrelated to sarcoidosis activity. This is not a specific test. False positives include TB
- *Calcium* may rise with active sarcoidosis or in the summer months. This may cause renal impairment, so urea or creatinine should also be checked
- *BAL* not performed routinely to assess progress of sarcoidosis, but reduction in lymphocytosis would indicate improvement
- *PET* scan may be positive in areas of disease activity. Not reliable for studying brain or heart. Limited studies of serial data
- *Gallium scan* rarely used now, as non-specific and expensive. Areas of active inflammation are positive, with a classic 'panda pattern'. Positive areas soon become negative with steroid use. Bowel and liver positive anyway, so disease cannot be charted in these areas.

Management

Most patients with pulmonary sarcoidosis do not require treatment. Asymptomatic CXR infiltrates are usually just monitored. The BTS have recently issued guidelines (see Box 45.4).

> **Box 45.4 BTS recommendations for the management of sarcoidosis (2008)**
>
> - Because of the high rate of spontaneous remission, treatment is not indicated for asymptomatic stage I disease
> - Because of high rates of remission, treatment is not indicated in asymptomatic stage II or III disease with mildly abnormal lung function and stable disease
> - Oral corticosteroids are the first line of therapy in patients with progressive disease determined by radiology or on lung function, significant symptoms, or extrapulmonary disease requiring treatment
> - Treatment with prednisolone (or equivalent) 0.5mg/kg/day for 4 weeks, then reduced to a maintenance dose which will control symptoms and disease progression, should be used for a period of 6–24 months
> - Biphosphonates should be used to minimize steroid-induced osteoporosis
> - Inhaled corticosteroids, either as initial treatment or maintenance therapy, are not of significant benefit. They may be considered for symptom control (cough) in a subgroup of patients
> - Other immunosuppressive or anti-inflammatory treatments only have a limited role but should be considered in patients when corticosteroids are not controlling the disease or side effects are intolerable. At present, methotrexate is the treatment of choice
> - Lung transplantation should be considered in end-stage pulmonary sarcoidosis.

Starting drug treatment

- When required, treatment is usually with steroids initially. Good evidence for short- to medium-term improvement in symptoms, respiratory function, and radiology, but long-term benefits less clear
- Give high doses, such as 30mg prednisolone/day, to control active disease. Rarely need >40mg/day. Usually give this high dose for 2–3 weeks, and then reduce if there has been a response
- *Maintenance dose* of around 5–20mg to control symptoms and prevent progression of disease. Leave on this dose for a few months, and then slowly reduce steroid dose further. Maintain on low dose of prednisolone (5–7.5mg/day or alternate days) for prolonged period of up to 12 months to consolidate resolution, before considering complete withdrawal. Remember bone protection
- Some patients, e.g. with progressive pulmonary sarcoidosis, may require longer treatment (years) of low-dose prednisolone to prevent relapse

- *Inhaled steroids* are of limited efficacy in sarcoidosis but may be useful if there is cough or bronchial hyperreactivity
- *Relapses* often occur when treatment is stopped and may require the reintroduction of steroids or the increase of steroid dose. Duration and dose of steroids is dictated by site and response to treatment
- *If steroid treatment fails* or sarcoidosis life-threatening, other immunosuppressive regimens may be indicated (see Box 45.5), e.g. pulsed high-dose IV methylprednisolone, especially for neurosarcoidosis
- In cases where *prolonged immunosuppression* is required, or if steroid side effects cannot be tolerated, other immunosuppressive drugs should be considered. Possibilities include azathioprine and methotrexate. There are limited data for their use in sarcoidosis
- Patients who have troublesome symptoms related to sarcoidosis, such as arthralgia, skin disease, fever, sweats, ocular symptoms, systemic symptoms such as fatigue, may require symptomatic steroid treatment. Lower initial doses, such as 20mg/day, are likely to be sufficient to gain symptomatic control, and doses can then be reduced
- Prescribe gastric and bone protection with steroids when necessary.

Box 45.5 Indications for immunosuppressive treatment
- Increasing symptoms, deteriorating PFTs, and worsening CXR infiltrates
- Cardiac sarcoidosis
- Neurosarcoidosis
- Sight-threatening ocular sarcoidosis
- Hypercalcaemia
- Lupus pernio
- Splenic, hepatic, or renal sarcoidosis.

Other drugs used in sarcoidosis

(See ➲ p. 673 for more information regarding immunosuppressive drugs.)
If there is progressive pulmonary sarcoidosis refractory to steroids, consider:
- *Methotrexate* Given once/week 10–15mg PO for 6-month trial. Use instead of, or in addition to, low-dose prednisolone. Avoid if hepatic or renal failure. Side effects: GI upset, stomatitis, pneumonitis, myelosuppression. Teratogenic. Monitor FBC and MCV, AST, ALT every 2 weeks for 3 months, then monthly. Do not use for >2y without review. Useful for chronic sarcoidosis and cutaneous disease
- *Azathioprine* Used in neurosarcoidosis and stages II/III pulmonary sarcoidosis with partial/no steroid response. 100–150mg/day. Use instead of, or in addition to, low-dose prednisolone. Side effects: myelosuppression, GI upset, stomatitis, idiosyncratic reaction—fever, rash. Low oncogenic potential. No gonadal toxicity. Check FBC every 2 weeks for 3 months, then monthly. Thiopurine methyltransferase (TPMT) testing should be performed prior to commencement (see ➲ pp. 676–7)

- *Anti-malarials* Hydroxychloroquine 200mg od/bd. For skin and particularly hypercalcaemia. Steroid-sparing. Can be given with steroids and other immunosuppressant in severe sarcoidosis. Side effects: rarely ocular toxicity
- *Others* Leflunomide, ciclosporin, thalidomide, TNF-α inhibitors (etanercept, infliximab, adalimumab, golimimumab), to be used in conjunction with specialist centres.

Prognosis There are no prognostic markers in sarcoidosis, apart from:
- *Good prognosis* Löfgren's syndrome has complete resolution in 80% of people. Associated with HLA-DQB1*0201
- *Poorer prognosis with chronic disease* Lupus pernio, nasal mucosa involvement, chronic uveitis, chronic hypercalcaemia, nephrocalcinosis, neural involvement, age >40, and black race
- Prognosis according to CXR appearance:
  - Stage II: 50% cases recover spontaneously in 2y; 30–40% require systemic steroids; 10–15% require long-term steroids
  - Stage III: worse prognosis. Only 30% show significant improvement with steroids
- Gene expression from mRNA profiling has shown early promise in differentiating progressive from non-progressive disease.

Transplant Consider if patient has end-stage lung disease, rapidly progressive disease despite treatment, or if they are O_2-dependent. Sarcoidosis is a rare indication for lung transplant. Granulomata recur in transplanted lung but do not cause higher rates of graft failure.

Extrathoracic disease 1

Varies according to ethnic origin and sex of patient.

Systemic symptoms are common, such as fever, sweats, loss of appetite, weight loss, fatigue, malaise, chest pain, dyspnoea, and cough. Polyarthralgia often affects the knees, ankles, wrists, and elbows and can be improved by NSAIDs.

Hypercalcaemia Granulomata convert vitamin D3 to active 1,25-dihydroxycholecalciferol. This causes enhanced calcium absorption from intestine. Sunlight also increases levels of vitamin D and calcium. High calcium may cause systemic effects and is often associated with renal damage and hypercalciuria. Commoner in Caucasians and in men.

Treatment If mildly raised, limit dietary calcium intake; avoid sun exposure, and drink plenty of fluids. Otherwise, steroids, often low dose once calcium level controlled (should be within 2 weeks—if not, investigate for other cause for hypercalcaemia). Decrease dose when calcium level satisfactory. Some patients may only need steroids during the summer months. Hydroxychloroquine can also be used.

Skin 25% of patients have skin involvement. More common in women.

Erythema nodosum Raised papules, nodules, or plaques, usually on shins. Also tender, indurated, or bruised appearance. Firm and often have shiny appearance. Nodular change involving different tattoo colours recognized and is characteristic of sarcoidosis. Sarcoid tissue may arise in old scars or cause scar hypertrophy.

Lupus pernio is a bluish tinge that occurs on nose, cheeks, and ears. It is associated with chronic disease.

Diagnosis Usually easily biopsied.

Treatment Initially with topical preparations. Lupus pernio should be treated with systemic steroids. Hydroxychloroquine or methotrexate may be necessary. Role of long-term tetracyclines for cutaneous sarcoidosis under investigation.

Eye Common, occurring in 25% plus of cases, especially women and African-Caribbeans

Uveitis (acute or chronic), episcleritis, scleritis, glaucoma, conjunctivitis, and retinal involvement can occur. May be asymptomatic or cause painful red eye, with photophobia, lacrimation, and blurred vision. Pupil irregular or constricted. Untreated, can cause visual impairment.

Lacrimal involvement in sarcoidosis gives keratoconjunctivitis sicca—dry eye with diminished tear secretion. Painful red eyes. Treat with artificial tears.

Diagnosis Assessment by an ophthalmologist with slit lamp examination if any ocular symptoms. Some recommend that all newly diagnosed patients with sarcoidosis have slit lamp examination. Mild asymptomatic eye involvement is common. May need conjunctival biopsy if no evidence of sarcoid elsewhere.

Treatment Local steroids are commonly used if there is no other indication for systemic steroids. However, if it does not respond, systemic steroids should be used.

Heart Cardiac sarcoidosis occurs in 5% of patients with pulmonary disease. Post-mortem studies show cardiac sarcoidosis is present in 25% so is often undiagnosed. Patients may present with chest pain or, more commonly, are found to have conduction defects on the ECG. These may be benign and asymptomatic, like first-degree heart block, but more significant arrhythmias can occur, the first indication of which may be sudden death. Myocardial granulomata can occur in any part of the heart. Commonly, they occur in the interventricular septum where they can affect nodal and conducting tissue. The LV wall can be affected, with fibrosis causing reduced compliance and contractile difficulties, leading to cardiac failure. Aneurysms can form, and pericarditis can occur. Valvular dysfunction due to infiltration of the papillary muscles is rare. The clinical course can be uncertain.

Diagnosis Echo may show signs of cardiomyopathy—usually restrictive. MRI, technetium scan, or gallium scan show non-segmental fixed defects. Biopsy is diagnostic but can be difficult, as sarcoidosis is patchy. Not recommended in general. ECG and 24h tape may be helpful in identifying potentially fatal arrhythmias and conduction defects.

Treatment Must be treated with systemic steroids 20–40mg prednisolone/ day, which improve symptoms and ECG and echo features. These should be slowly reduced, but intractable arrhythmias may need continued high dosage. May need other immunosuppressants. Investigate with 24h tape and electrophysiological studies if uncertain. Amiodarone, a pacemaker, implantable defibrillator, or heart transplant may be necessary.

In clinic Perform a screening ECG on all patients with sarcoidosis, perhaps every 6 months.

Extrathoracic disease 2

Kidney A degree of renal involvement is found in 35% of patients with sarcoidosis. Rarely can present with renal failure (especially following onset of hypercalcaemia), obstructive uropathy, nephrolithiasis, or urinary tract disorder. Nephrocalcinosis is a common cause of chronic renal failure. Often associated hypercalcaemia or other manifestation of sarcoidosis.

Diagnosis Renal biopsy with granulomata found in interstitium, but this is rarely needed in this context. Search for pulmonary sarcoidosis.

Treatment Steroids ± hydroxychloroquine for hypercalcaemia.

CNS Involved in 4–18% of patients. Can affect any part of the peripheral or central nervous system. Can present as a peripheral nerve or cranial nerve lesion. Most common is lower motor neurone facial nerve palsy, with optic nerve involvement being next most common. Mononeuritis multiplex recognized. May be less specific, with psychiatric features. Hypothalamic granulomata may cause diabetes insipidus, appetite disturbance, or hypersomnolence.

Diagnosis Difficult but may be made easier if there is another sign of systemic sarcoidosis, e.g. bilateral hilar lymphadenopathy. Lumbar puncture may show a raised CSF ACE and an increased lymphocyte count. Confirm with biopsy, if possible—cerebral or meningeal tissue if no pulmonary involvement.

Treatment Must be treated with steroids, but often resistant to treatment. May need to try further immunosuppressants, e.g. TNF-α inhibitors.

Musculoskeletal Arthralgia is common in sarcoidosis, but arthritis is unusual. Arthralgia commonly affects the ankles and feet in men, but also hands, wrists, and elbows. A subacute proximal myopathy can occur as well as bone cysts, especially of terminal phalanges. The latter show little response to systemic steroids.

Diagnosis Granuloma seen on muscle biopsy.

Treatment NSAIDs, steroids may be necessary.

GI 60% of liver biopsies on patients with sarcoidosis show granuloma. Frequently asymptomatic. Hepatomegaly unusual but can get portal fibrosis and cirrhosis. LFTs suggestive if 3× normal, especially ALP and γGT.

Diagnosis Biopsy.

Treatment Steroids—may reduce size of liver and improve LFTs.

Haematological Splenomegaly can occur and may be massive, causing abdominal discomfort. A massive spleen may require splenectomy to avoid rupture. Associated anaemia, neutropenia, and thrombocytopenia. Lymphopenia often seen.

ENT Nasal or laryngeal granuloma. Sinus invasion. Parotid and other salivary gland enlargement, dry mouth.

Rarely Breast disease, ovarian or testicular masses.

Further information

Baughman RP et al. A concise review of pulmonary sarcoidosis. *Am J Respir Crit Care Med* 2011;**183**:573–81.

Dempsey OJ et al. Sarcoidosis. *BMJ* 2009;**339**:620–5.

American Thoracic Society/European Respiratory Society/World Association of Sarcoidosis and other Granulomatous Disorders statement on sarcoidosis. *Eur Respir J* 1999;**14**:735–7.

BTS interstitial lung disease guideline 2008. ℘ http://www.brit-thoracic.org.uk/portals/0/guidelines/dpldguidelines/thorax%20sept%2008.pdf.

Judson MA et al. Two year prognosis of sarcoidosis: the ACCESS experience. *Sarcoidosis Vasc Diffuse Lung Dis* 2003;**20**:204–11.

World Association of Sarcoidosis and other Granulomatous Disorders website. ℘ http://www.wasog.org/.

Lockstone HE et al. Gene set analysis of lung samples provides insight into pathogenesis of progressive, fibrotic pulmonary sarcoidosis. *Am J Respir Crit Care Med* 2010;**181**:1367–75.

Chapter 46

Sickle cell disease— pulmonary complications

Overview

Background

Sickle cell disease is an autosomal recessive condition resulting in a substitution of a valine for glycine in the β-globin subunit of Hb, forming HbS. HbS is less soluble under reduced O_2 tensions and leads to deformation of red blood cells (sickling) when deoxygenated (e.g. in atelectatic lung), resulting in chronic haemolysis and vascular occlusion with tissue infarction in individuals homozygous for the β-globin gene mutation (sickle cell anaemia/disease). Hb electrophoresis or high-performance liquid chromatography (HPLC) in sickle cell disease demonstrates HbS ~80–99% and no normal Hb HbA; anaemia Hb 6–9g/dL is usual. Heterozygote carriers of the β-globin gene mutation are referred to as having 'sickle cell trait' and are largely asymptomatic, although sickle crises may occur during extreme hypoxia (e.g. during anaesthesia); HPLC analysis demonstrates HbS ~35–40%, and HbA (normal Hb) ~50%. Sickle Hb solubility testing does not distinguish between trait and homozygous disease.

Pulmonary complications

- *Pneumonia* is more common, particularly from *Chlamydia pneumoniae*, *S. pneumoniae*, *H. influenzae*, *Mycoplasma*, *Legionella*, and respiratory viruses; may precipitate acute chest syndrome. Invasive pneumococcal disease is significantly more common. Patients should take lifelong prophylactic penicillin, as functionally asplenic
- *Asthma* appears to be a common comorbidity and may be associated with increased vaso-occlusive crises and episodes of acute chest syndrome
- *Nocturnal oxyhaemoglobin desaturation* is common, pathogenesis unclear—tonsillar hypertrophy is common, and OSA may be a contributing factor
- *Pulmonary thromboembolism* appears to be more common and may precipitate acute chest syndrome
- *Acute chest syndrome* (see ➲ pp. 567–8)
- *Sickle cell chronic lung disease* is a poorly described entity, characterized by progressive breathlessness and abnormal pulmonary function, sometimes with PHT. Thought to follow recurrent episodes of lung infarction/infection, although there may not be a history of previous acute chest syndrome. Radiologically, characterized by multifocal interstitial infiltrate. PFTs typically restrictive, although airways obstruction also described
- *PHT* is a relatively common complication of sickle cell disease and other forms of haemolytic anaemia. Management is largely as for IPAH in a specialist centre (see ➲ p. 392). Hydroxyurea and transfusions reduce episodes of vaso-occlusive crisis and acute chest syndrome and may be of benefit. Inhaled NO may have a role; studies are ongoing. A minority of these patients have CTEPH.

Acute chest syndrome

Definition and clinical features Defined as a new pulmonary infiltrate on CXR, consistent with consolidation but not atelectasis, typically associated with symptoms such as fever, cough, chest pain, and breathlessness. A form of acute lung injury, which may progress to ARDS. One of the leading causes of death in sickle cell disease, although mortality has fallen due to use of maintenance hydroxyurea therapy and earlier treatment with transfusion. Risk factors include young age, high steady state leucocyte counts and Hb levels, smoking, and past history of acute chest syndrome. May follow surgery and anaesthesia.

Causes may not be apparent and include one or more of infection (including viruses, atypical bacteria, encapsulated bacteria, MRSA), pulmonary fat embolism (preceded by bony pain), *in situ* thrombosis or PE, atelectasis following hypoventilation (from acute painful crisis of chest wall or excessive opiates), and possibly pulmonary oedema due to excessive hydration. Each leads to hypoxia with increased sickling and vascular occlusion, and initially mild disease can escalate rapidly to ARDS and death. All patients with a painful vaso-occlusive crisis should be monitored closely for the development of the acute chest syndrome; routine use of incentive spirometry may help prevent its development in these patients.

Investigations

- *Blood tests* Raised WCC, anaemia; check HbS %
- *Hypoxia* is common and may be underestimated using pulse oximetry; A–a gradient predicts clinical severity; consider ICU transfer if worsens
- *Culture* blood and sputum
- *CXR* shows multifocal pulmonary infiltrates, sometimes with pleural effusion
- *BAL* may be considered in patients not responding to treatment
- *Echo* reveals evidence of PHT and right heart strain in a significant minority of patients, associated with a higher mortality; such patients may also develop excessive haemolysis and thrombocytopenia and may benefit from a more aggressive exchange transfusion policy.

▶▶ Management of sickle cell acute chest syndrome

Supportive care on ICU may be required. Liaise with haematology team. Treatment comprises:

- O_2 to correct hypoxia; monitor ABGs
- Empirical broad-spectrum *antibiotics* (including a macrolide)
- *Rehydration* (IV fluids may be needed; care to avoid overhydration)
- *Bronchodilators* are often used; airflow obstruction is common, may contribute to high airway pressures during mechanical ventilation
- Ensure adequate *analgesia* for bony pain (consider NSAIDs; IM or SC opiates often required)
- *Incentive spirometry* and chest physiotherapy to prevent atelectasis. Pain may limit their use, and CPAP may be better tolerated
- *Simple* and *exchange blood transfusion* both reduce the HbS concentration and improve oxygenation in acute chest syndrome, and early transfusion therapy is recommended. Simple transfusion is indicated if anaemic with Hb <10g/dL, although Hb should not be raised above 11g/dL, as the increase in blood viscosity exacerbates sickling. Exchange transfusion should be used in patients with a relatively high Hb, aiming for HbS <20%, and is also recommended in severe or rapidly progressive disease
- Other treatments Successful use of inhaled *NO* for the treatment of a handful of refractory cases has been reported, but a clinical trial has failed to demonstrate a reduction in the development of acute chest syndrome following treatment of vaso-occlusive crises with NO. *Corticosteroids* may be of benefit in reducing length of hospital admission, but rebound painful crises are more common, and routine use of corticosteroids is not usually recommended. *Hydroxycarbamide* increases foetal Hb and reduces sickling and significantly reduces the incidence of acute chest syndrome; it is recommended for patients with recurrent episodes.

Prognosis ~13% of patients with acute chest syndrome require mechanical ventilation; overall mortality 4–9%.

Further information

Miller AC, Gladwin MT. Pulmonary complications of sickle cell disease. *Am J Respir Crit Care Med* 2012;**185**:1154–65.

Chapter 47

Sleep apnoea and hypoventilation

Obstructive sleep apnoea (OSA)

Definition and epidemiology OSA, or obstructive sleep apnoea/hypopnoea (OSAH) are currently the preferred terms for the problem of dynamic upper airway obstruction during sleep.

- OSA is part of a spectrum, with trivial snoring at one end and repetitive complete obstruction throughout the night (such that the patient cannot sleep and breathe at the same time) at the other
- Along this spectrum is a point at which the degree of obstruction/recovery and the attendant arousal fragments sleep sufficiently to cause daytime symptoms
- Distinction should be made between just the findings on sleep study of OSA episodes (OSA) and an abnormal sleep study *plus* the presence of symptoms (i.e. *obstructive sleep apnoea syndrome*, OSAS). Asymptomatic OSA is commoner than symptomatic (OSAS).

Thresholds defining 'abnormality' are arbitrary (e.g. 10s to define an apnoea). Numerical definitions of OSA, based on counting individual events during a sleep study, are not very helpful. The current definition of the clinical syndrome should be:

Upper airway narrowing, provoked by sleep, causing sufficient sleep fragmentation to result in significant daytime symptoms, usually excessive sleepiness.

- Prevalence depends on the chosen thresholds for defining both an abnormality on the sleep study and significant symptoms
- 0.5–1% of adult men in the UK (and about a fifth as many women) have OSAS, sufficient to be candidates for treatment with nasal CPAP
- Prevalence figures depend on levels of obesity and will be higher in the USA and probably rise inexorably in the UK in the future
- The prevalence in women is thought to be lower due to their different fat distribution. Upper body obesity (and thus neck obesity) is more a ♂ pattern
- OSA is the third most common serious respiratory condition, after asthma and COPD. In some respiratory units, it has now become the commonest reason for specialist referral.

Pathophysiology and associated conditions Control of the upper airway musculature is complex; upper airway patency depends on dilator muscle activity. All postural muscles relax during sleep (including pharyngeal dilators); some narrowing of the upper airway is normal. Excessive narrowing with the onset of sleep is due to the following factors.

Causes of a small pharyngeal size when awake (such that normal muscle relaxation with sleep is enough to provoke critical narrowing)

- Fatty infiltration of pharyngeal tissues and external pressure from increased neck fat and/or muscle bulk
- Large tonsils
- Subtle 'abnormalities' of craniofacial shape, e.g. minor micrognathia or retrognathia
- Extra submucosal tissue, e.g. myxoedema, mucopolysaccharidoses.

Causes of excessive narrowing of the airway occurring with muscle relaxation at sleep onset

- Mass loading from an obese or muscular neck may simply 'overwhelm' residual dilator action as well as reduce the starting size
- Neuromuscular diseases with pharyngeal involvement may lead to greater loss of dilator muscle tone, e.g. stroke, myotonic dystrophy, Duchenne dystrophy, MND
- Muscle relaxants such as sedatives and alcohol
- Increasing age.

Other theories

In a small number of examples of OSA, a heightened tendency to arouse, before the breathing and the upper airway stabilize, may be important in maintaining ventilatory instability. There may also be years of damage to the mucosa from snoring, which reduce the protective reflex dilation of the pharynx in response to narrowing activated by surface receptors.

Predisposing conditions OSA is found more commonly in certain conditions, such as acromegaly and hypothyroidism, but the reasons are not well understood. It is unclear whether there need to be any other non-anatomical factors to provoke OSA. Most associated abnormalities that have been described are likely to be 2° to long periods of snoring and OSA, rather than 1° causal factors.

Short-term consequences of OSA In severe OSA, repetitive collapse of the upper airway, with the arousal required to reactivate the pharyngeal dilators, occurs approximately every minute throughout the sleeping period (60 events/h or over 400/night); they are usually attended by hypoxia (see Fig. 47.2) and hypercapnia that are corrected during the inter-apnoeic hyperventilatory period. Obstructive events, short of complete obstruction, also provoke arousal, as it is usually the compensatory reflex increase in inspiratory effort, rather than the blood gas deterioration directly, that wakens the brain. In this situation, the drops in O_2 saturation may be very much less and, in younger thinner individuals, almost imperceptible on oximetry tracings (see Fig. 47.6). This is because the compensation afforded by the increased inspiratory effort may be adequate, and the bigger O_2 stores in the lungs of the less obese will buffer any brief hypoventilation.

- Recurrent arousals lead to highly fragmented and unrefreshing sleep
- Excessive daytime sleepiness results
- The correlation between the sleep fragmentation and the resultant degree of sleepiness is not tight, with some patients being sleepy with low levels of fragmentation, and vice versa
- This is thought to result partly from inter-individual differences in sensitivity to the effects of sleep fragmentation
- With every arousal, there is a rise in BP, often over 50mmHg. It is unclear if these BP rises do any damage to the cardiovascular system. There is also a carry-over of hypertension (average of 3mmHg) into the waking hours, which falls after treatment at 1 month
- There is true nocturia, mechanism unclear; there may be raised atrial natriuretic peptide (ANP) levels from increased central blood volume, from the subatmospheric intrathoracic pressures during the obstructed breathing; or it may be simply a reflection of highly fragmented sleep, preventing the normal reduction in urine flow associated with sleep.

OSA: clinical features

Chapter 14 covers many of the essential features in the history and discusses the differential diagnosis of excessive daytime sleepiness.

Most patients present with:

- Excessive sleepiness, measured crudely using the ESS; >9 is considered abnormally sleepy (see ➲ pp. 90–1)
- Loud snoring and apnoeic episodes recognized by the bed partner
- The patient recognizes that he wakes up choking from time to time
- Poor concentration
- Unrefreshing sleep and waking unrefreshed
- Nocturia (true nocturia with reversal of the usual day/night ratio).

Less often there will be:

- Nocturnal sweating
- Reduced libido
- Oesophageal reflux
- Increasingly common are patients arriving with spouses worried by the apnoeic pauses they have observed.

Sleepiness

- Sometimes difficult to assess; failure by the patient to recognize the problem or denial due to concerns over driving and licensing
- The Epworth scale (see ➲ p. 93) assesses *tendency to fall asleep*, rather than *perceived sleepiness per se*, as some patients may regard their situation as normal
- It is important to separate the symptom of tiredness from sleepiness (see ➲ pp. 90–1), the latter being much more typical of OSA, although sometimes complained of (rather than sleepiness) more by women with OSA.

Examination and investigations

The examination (often unrewarding) and the investigations are detailed in Chapter 14 (see ➲ pp. 92–3). Look for the presence of additional lower airways obstruction, with associated CO_2 retention, so-called 'overlap syndrome'. CO_2 retention in pure OSA is very uncommon (except in the very, very obese). It appears that the additive effect of some lower airways obstruction (often not enough in its own right to precipitate CO_2 retention) is required, which perhaps limits the inter-apnoeic hyperventilation and thus gradually encourages tolerance to raised levels of CO_2.

The majority of patients with significant OSA are ♂, tend to have a combination of upper body obesity (neck circumference >17in) and a relatively undersized or set-back mandible. Airway size can be assessed and documented with scoring systems, e.g. see ➲ p. 595.

Sleep study

The sleep study assesses if there is anything likely to be the cause of the patient's symptoms. The considerable grey area between normality and abnormality means that sometimes it is unclear whether the symptoms can be blamed on the sleep study findings. There is also considerable night-to-night variation in sleep study indices that further blurs the distinction between normality and abnormality. In this situation, it may be necessary to undertake a therapeutic trial of CPAP and let the patient decide if the benefits of treatment outweigh the disadvantages.

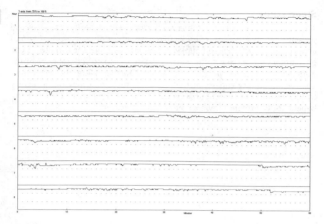

Fig. 47.1 Normal overnight oximetry. Normal baseline and a few dips. Vertical axis, 70–100% SaO$_2$ for each panel; horizontal axis, 60min each panel, 8h total.

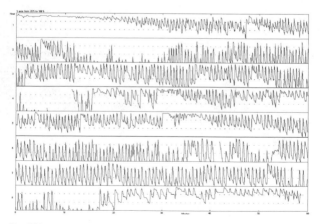

Fig. 47.2 Severe OSA. Large numbers of regular dips, sawtooth-shaped (faster rise in SaO$_2$ than fall).

OSA: types of sleep study

- Overnight oximetry alone, including HR (see Figs. 47.1 to 47.8)
- More than just oximetry, with other channels such as sound, body movement, oronasal airflow, chest and abdominal movements, leg movements: so-called 'limited' sleep studies or 'respiratory polysomnography (PSG)'
- Full PSG, with electroencephalogram (EEG), electro-oculogram (EOG), and EMG, to stage sleep electrophysiologically, in addition to the channels listed.

There is no evidence that OSA diagnosis needs full PSG (PSG with EEG); it is very rarely indicated, and its routine use is a waste of resources. Oximetry (SaO_2 and pulse rate) identifies most moderate to severe cases, allowing referral for CPAP. Abnormal oximetry, sometimes mimicking OSA, occurs with Cheyne–Stokes breathing (heart failure, post-stroke), in the very obese, and when there is a low baseline SaO_2 (e.g. COPD); this allows the SaO_2 to oscillate more with small changes in PaO_2, due to the increasing steepness of the Hb dissociation curve at lower SaO_2. False negatives, discussed earlier, can occur with younger and thinner patients.

With appropriate expertise, a good history, and recognition of its limitations, domiciliary oximetry alone is a valuable tool in the diagnosis and management of OSA. The addition of sound and/or oronasal flow channels reduces the number of equivocal results needing a further study.

Limited sleep studies (respiratory PSG) are the usual routine investigation. Different units have expertise in interpreting different sorts of sleep studies. Experience is more important than the particular sleep study equipment used. Any system should assess the degree of sleep fragmentation and the degree of upper airway narrowing; this can be done using many different direct and indirect techniques.

Management

Not all patients need treatment. The evidence for significant treatment benefits rests on *symptoms*, which drive treatment, rather than the degree of OSA on a sleep study. Treatment decisions require a close dialogue between physician and patient. Recent evidence suggests that many patients underestimate their symptoms so that, when in doubt, erring on the side of a CPAP trial is sensible.

Key features in making a treatment choice
- How sleepy is the patient? Does it affect QoL? Is it critical to the patient's livelihood (e.g. HGV driving)? Is there motivation for treatment?
- Has the patient underestimated the impact of their sleepiness or misled the doctor because of concerns over driving issues?

- Is there any evidence of the 'overlap' syndrome where additional lower airways obstruction has contributed to type II ventilatory failure? If so, is this a stable state or part of an acute decline with a respiratory acidosis?
- Is obesity the dominant risk factor, or is there a surgically remediable component (e.g. tonsillar hypertrophy)?

There is no RCT evidence that cardiovascular disease, nocturnal angina, or poorly controlled hypertension should influence the decision to treat. Many, however, would lower the treatment threshold under these circumstances. OSA is a risk factor for recurrent AF; some evidence exists that treating OSA, when there is left heart failure, improves ejection fraction and possibly survival.

Simple approaches
- Weight loss. This is difficult; slimming clubs have the best record for non-surgical approaches
- Reduce evening alcohol consumption
- Sleep decubitus, rather than supine, and with the bedhead elevated.

For snorers and mild OSA
- Mandibular advancement devices, assuming adequate dentition
- Pharyngeal surgery as a last resort (poor RCT data and what there is suggests poor outcomes, not recommended).

For significant OSA
- CPAP therapy
- Bariatric surgery (e.g. gastric band or gastric bypass operations)
- Tracheostomy (rarely indicated)
- Mandibular/maxillary advancement surgery in highly selected cases.

Severe OSA with CO_2 retention
- May require a period of non-invasive positive pressure ventilation (NIPPV) prior to CPAP, particularly if acidotic
- Compensated CO_2 retention may reverse with CPAP alone.

If there are large tonsils, then their removal may be appropriate although much more successful in children than adults. Pharyngeal surgery is a poor option for either snoring or OSA; the minimal evidence suggests that the outcomes are little better than placebo. There is no real place for alerting agents (such as modafinil) in the routine management of sleepiness in OSA. It is unclear if these drugs do help; they may possibly reduce the perception of sleepiness more than the sleepiness itself and have only been studied properly in the residual sleepiness sometimes found in patients even when treated successfully with CPAP.

Mandibular advancement devices
- Worn in the mouth at night, holding the lower jaw forward: similar to 'jaw thrust' in an unconscious patient. Generally used to control snoring and OSA at the milder end of the spectrum
- Many different designs, but essentially one half clips to the upper teeth and the other half to the lower, and connected together with the lower jaw held forward by 5–10mm
- Some give adjustable forward displacement; some are fixed

- The more sophisticated need to be customized to match the patient's dentition, which usually requires the services of a dentist
- DIY devices exist that are heated and moulded to the teeth directly
- One-size-fits-all devices exist that can work for snoring, but only if they advance the lower jaw
- Side effects include excessive salivation, tooth pain, and jaw ache, which often lessen with time
- Long-term use may be associated with movement of the teeth and alterations to the bite
- The initial cost (usually over £400 for customized versions) is more than that of a CPAP machine (£300), and they usually only last about a year.

OSA: CPAP

CPAP consists of a blower/pressure generator that sits by the patient's bed and is connected to a mask by a length of large-bore tubing. The masks are usually just nasal, but nose and mouth masks are also used. The blower raises the pressure at which the patient is breathing (to about $10cmH_2O$) and splints open the pharynx, preventing its collapse, sleep fragmentation, and the consequent daytime sleepiness. *CPAP is a highly effective therapy, with resolution of the sleepiness and large gains in QoL.* It is a sufficiently curious and initially uncomfortable therapy to require a *careful induction programme.* Without this, the take-up and compliance rates are poor. Most centres have found that a dedicated CPAP nurse or technician is required. Many centres use special patient education aids, such as video presentations, and provide helplines. The best method of establishing a patient on CPAP and deriving the required mask pressure is not known, and many different approaches appear to work. Recent innovations include CPAP machines that automatically hunt for the required pressure and do not require an attended overnight titration. New mask designs appear at regular intervals, with a slow improvement in their comfort and fit (important to prevent air leaks). Patients require access to long-term support to maintain their CPAP equipment and attend to problems. There are now significant problems supporting the very large numbers of patients on CPAP that accumulate, the longer a service has been in operation.

The commonest problems encountered include:

- Mouth leaks lead to increased air through the nose and out of the mouth, with excessive drying of the mucosa, nasal congestion, rhinitis, and sneezing. Usually solved with the addition of a heated humidifier
- Pain and ulceration of the skin on the nasal bridge. Try different masks or patient 'interfaces' not resting on the nasal bridge
- Claustrophobia. This usually settles but may require a different interface
- Temporary nasal congestion, usually during a cold. Try nasal decongestants for these short periods only such as xylometazoline.

Alternative diagnoses

Most patients who snore are sleepy and have an abnormal sleep study, will have ordinary OSA, and respond to CPAP. Sometimes, differentiating OSA from central apnoeas (see ➲ pp. 586–7) can be difficult, because some patients with Cheyne–Stokes breathing may have a few obstructed breaths at the end of each apnoeic cycle, even though the problem is primarily central. Poor response to CPAP should at least prompt a reappraisal of the diagnosis. Not all OSA is due to pharyngeal collapse; a very small number of patients have laryngeal closure. This can occur with:

- Shy–Drager syndrome (multi-system atrophy). This causes laryngeal abductor weakness with laryngeal closure during sleep, with stridulous obstruction, rather than the usual noise of snoring
- RA can damage the larynx, with resultant OSA

- Arnold–Chiari malformation can compress the brainstem and interfere with the control of the larynx and pharynx, as well as the control of ventilation, with mixed findings on the sleep study
- These forms of obstruction also respond to CPAP therapy, as the larynx is also 'blown open' by raising airway pressure.

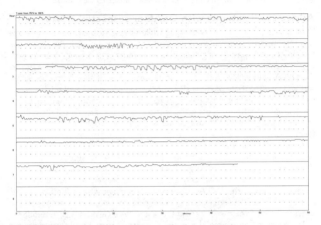

Fig. 47.3 Sleep-onset periodic ventilation. Short bursts of dipping, otherwise normal.

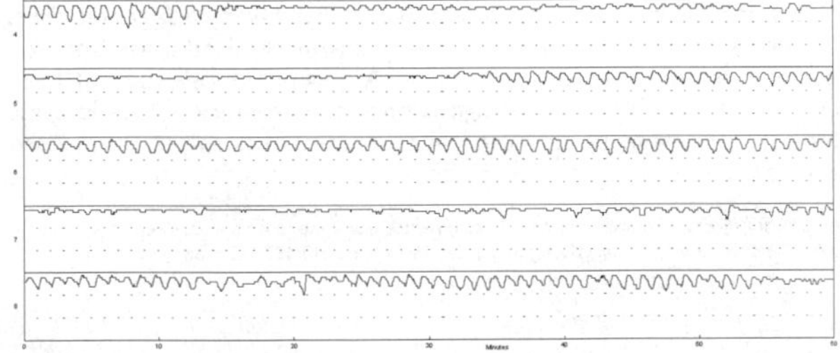

Fig. 47.4 Cheyne–Stokes ventilation. Prolonged periods of dipping, often more sinusoidal, rather than sawtooth.

OSA: driving advice to patients

In UK law, one is responsible for one's vigilance levels while driving. We know when we are sleepy and should stop driving. Driving while sleepy has been likened to driving whilst drunk, and a prison sentence can result from sleep-related accidents on the road. No one should drive while they are sleepy, and the same applies to pathological causes of sleepiness.

Advice to all patients with OSAS or suspected OSAS

Whatever the situation, do not drive while sleepy; stop and have a nap; this is common sense, regardless of the cause of the sleepiness. If the sleepiness is sufficient to impair driving ability, patients must stop driving. Patients with OSA *syndrome* (i.e. OSA with daytime hypersomnolence) should write to the DVLA who will send them a questionnaire SL1. If they admit to excessive and inappropriate daytime sleepiness, their licence is revoked. If already treated and the sleepiness has resolved, then the licence is not revoked; hence, rapid treatment is essential. It is the doctor's duty to tell the patient of the diagnosis of OSAS and of the requirement to inform the DVLA if there is sleepiness sufficient to impair driving. Patients who are not sleepy and only have OSA on their sleep study do not have OSAS and thus do not need to inform the DVLA, although the DVLA is inconsistent on this issue. According to USA epidemiological studies, at least 1/20 men have OSA on a sleep study (but, at most, only a quarter will be sleepy); thus, if all OSA were reported to the DVLA, this would rather overwhelm the DVLA and be illogical. The DVLA rules change from time to time, and reference to the latest version of their website and the *At a Glance Guide* is recommended.

The doctor can advise the patient whether they should stop driving entirely (essential if the patient is very sleepy, has had a sleepiness-related accident or near miss, and/or drives a HGV or public service vehicle—class 2 licence holders) or to continue driving only with extreme caution for short distances. The advice given to the patient should be recorded in the notes. The latest American Thoracic Guidelines are entirely sensible and useful.* Inappropriate and illogical curbing of driving privileges will push the problem underground, through fear of loss of livelihood, and is the worst of all worlds.

Driving can be restarted as soon as the sleepiness has resolved and preferably been confirmed by medical opinion, but, in the case of class 2 licence holders, the success of the treatment must be verified by a specialist clinic. This means a normal ESS and evidence of adequate CPAP usage from the hour meters built into CPAP machines. A minimum usage has not been defined, but >3h/night on average is often the arbitrary threshold used. Non-usage for even one night can lead to a return of sleepiness in some, so patients have to continue to act responsibly.

* An official American Thoracic Society Clinical Practice Guideline: sleep apnea, sleepiness, and driving risk in noncommercial drivers. *Am J Respir Crit Care Med.* 2013;**187**:1259–66.

OSA in children

OSA in children

Adult respiratory physicians interested in sleep apnoea may be asked to investigate children with OSA, due to fewer sleep services for children.

- Mainly due to enlarged tonsils and adenoids; varying degrees of OSA are present in up to 4% of children around the age of 5; prevalence tails off as tonsils atrophy
- These children present with snoring, restless sleep, and different daytime symptoms to those of adults. Obvious sleepiness is less common
- Sleep-deprived children tend to become hyperactive, with reduced attention spans, and be labelled as difficult or disruptive, or even ADHD
- Symptoms will fluctuate with the size of the tonsils, and this depends on the presence of upper respiratory infections
- Mild intermittent sleep disturbance may not matter, but every night sleep fragmentation for months interferes with development in a variety of ways
- The clinical decision is mainly whether to recommend removal of tonsils or a wait-and-see policy, remembering that there is a significant morbidity from adenotonsillectomy, and even the occasional death
- A halfway house is the use of nasal steroids, which can reduce tonsillar size sufficiently to improve symptoms until natural tonsillar atrophy occurs.

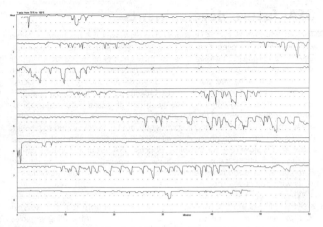

Fig. 47.5 REM sleep hypoventilation in scoliosis. Substantial dips, in bursts, compatible with the occurrence of REM periods.

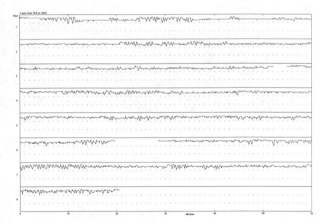

Fig. 47.6 Moderate OSA with many small, <4%, dips in SaO$_2$.

OSA: future developments

The old view that sleep PSG is required to diagnose OSA has been replaced with an evidence-based approach, using simpler and cheaper equipment. OSA is so common that diagnosis will move into general practice. Simpler ways to establish patients on CPAP have evolved. RCTs show that, with appropriate training and supervision, diagnosis and management of OSAS can be carried out in the community. Obesity surgery is improving and, in appropriate cases, may become the treatment of choice. Appetite suppressants are being developed and should greatly reduce the prevalence of obesity and hence OSA. Pharmacological agents are being developed to prevent the loss of tone in the pharyngeal dilators during sleep, although progress in this area is slow (e.g. mirtazapine reduces OSA but unfortunately causes sedation and weight gain!). New pharyngeal operations are being devised all the time, but none have been very effective when investigated properly; RCTs with objective outcome data are badly needed in this area.

Whether OSA is a significant independent risk factor for vascular diseases is still debated. Cross-sectional and non-randomized data suggest so. However, it is difficult to adequately control for confounding variables such as visceral obesity; non-randomized studies carry important bias. RCTs treating OSA with CPAP show small benefits to BP and endothelial function.

Further information

Heatley EM et al. Obstructive sleep apnoea in adults: a common chronic condition in need of a comprehensive chronic condition management approach. *Sleep Med Rev* 2013;**17**:349–55.

Loke YK et al. Association of obstructive sleep apnea with risk of serious cardiovascular events: a systematic review and meta-analysis. *Circ Cardiovasc Qual Outcomes* 2012;**5**:720–8.

Eastwood PR et al. Obstructive sleep apnoea: from pathogenesis to treatment: current controversies and future directions. *Respirology* 2010;**15**:587–95.

Chai-Coetzer CL et al. Primary care versus specialist sleep centre management of obstructive sleep apnea and daytime sleepiness and quality of life. *JAMA* 2013;**309**:997–1004.

Stradling JR. Driving and sleep apnoea. *Thorax* 2008;**63**:481–3.

Sleep Apnoea Trust, Patients Association. ℘ http://www.sleep-apnoea-trust.org.

NICE technology appraisal of CPAP for OSA. ℘ http://www.nice.org.uk/nicemedia/live/11944/40085/40085.pdf.

IMPRESS Service Specification for Investigation and treatment of OSAS. ℘ http://www.impressresp.com/index.php?option=com_docman&task=doc_download&gid=12&Itemid=69.

Cochrane database on CPAP. Continuous positive airways pressure for obstructive sleep apnoea in adults. ℘ http://onlinelibrary.wiley.com/doi/10.1002/14651858.CD001106.pub3/abstract;jsessionid=6AFDAAFA6FD5F175EF242B29324D4E96.d03t04.

Interventions to improve compliance with continuous positive airway pressure for OSA. ℘ http://onlinelibrary.wiley.com/doi/10.1002/14651858.CD001106.pub3/abstract;jsessionid=6AFDAAFA6FD5F175EF242B29324D4E96.d03t04.

American commercial website, but useful for showing the large variety of CPAP equipment. ℘ http://www.cpapman.com.

Main American Sleep Information website. ℘ http://www.sleephomepages.org.

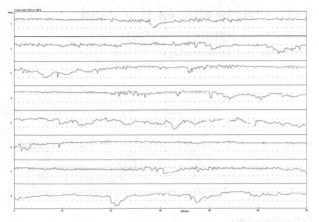

Fig. 47.7 Nocturnal hypoxia in COPD. Low baseline SaO$_2$, with more dramatic falls (often quite prolonged) during periods compatible with the occurrence of REM.

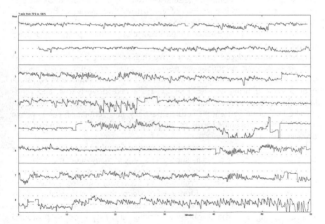

Fig. 47.8 Overlap syndrome—OSA and COPD. Low baseline SaO$_2$. Some periods with typical sawtooth-dipping; other periods with prolonged falls in SaO$_2$.

Central sleep apnoea (CSA) and nocturnal hypoventilation

Definition and epidemiology 'CSA/hypopnoea', or 'hypoventilation' or 'periodic breathing', are said to occur when there is no evidence of upper airway obstruction as the cause for the episodic reduced ventilation during sleep. Compared with OSA, it is much less common.

* *CSA* tends to be used as a term when there are actual apnoeas and referred to as Cheyne–Stokes breathing when there is regular symmetrical waxing and waning, usually in the context of left heart failure
* *Periodic breathing* is an alternative and can be used to describe regular fluctuations in breathing, with or without actual apnoeas
* The description *nocturnal hypoventilation* tends to be used when the hypoventilation and hypoxaemic dips are not particularly periodic in nature. However, these terms are imprecise and sometimes mixed indiscriminately.

Pathophysiology

CSA, or hypoventilation or periodic breathing, can occur in a number of settings with different aetiologies (see also Chapter 15, ⊃ pp. 96–8). At one end of the spectrum is pure loss of ventilatory drive, while at the other is pure reduction in the ability to expand the chest adequately, with dependence on accessory muscles of respiration. Many clinical presentations are mixtures of these two.

Patients with *reduced ventilatory drive* (e.g. following brainstem damage) can often maintain adequate, or near adequate, ventilation whilst awake, as there is a non-metabolic 'awake' ventilatory drive equivalent to about 4 or 5L/min. During non-REM sleep, this awake drive is lost, and ventilation becomes dependent on PaO_2 and $PaCO_2$. During REM sleep, an 'awake-like' drive sometimes returns partially, and ventilation can improve again (seen in congenital forms of absent drive where REM sleep can temporarily restore SaO_2 levels).

In patients with *impaired mechanical ability to ventilate*, accessory muscles of respiration become critically supportive (e.g. in many neuromuscular disorders and obstructive/restrictive respiratory conditions). However, during non-REM sleep, this reflex recruitment of accessory muscles is attenuated and hypoventilation follows. During REM sleep, the physiological paralysis of all postural muscles (REM atonia) can remove all compensatory mechanisms, leaving only the diaphragm working, and may produce profound hypoventilation or apnoea.

Chronic hypoventilation, often 2° to poor respiratory function (e.g. as evidenced by CO_2 retention in some patients with COPD or chest wall restrictive disorders), can eventually force resetting of ventilatory control mechanisms. This is an acquired blunting of ventilatory drive and leads to sleep-related changes in ventilation, similar to those described in the previous paragraphs.

Unstable ventilatory control can lead to regular oscillations in ventilation, e.g. as occurs in heart failure and at altitude. During REM sleep, it is normal to have fluctuations in ventilation, sometimes with complete apnoeas.

Sometimes, sleep studies can be misinterpreted, and apnoeas, really of obstructive origin, are mistakenly labelled as central. For example, if inspiratory muscles are very weak, their poor efforts during obstructive apnoeas may be missed on the ribcage and abdominal bands used in sleep studies but may be detectable with oesophageal pressure monitoring.

Causes and clinical features of CSA/hypoventilation

Although there are many different causes, only four relatively common clinical scenarios occur (but with overlap).

Absent or reduced ventilatory drive

Brainstem involvement from strokes, tumours, syringobulbia, surgical damage, post-polio syndrome, congenital (Ondine's curse—usually presents soon after birth, can be later, abnormalities of neural crest development due to increased number of 'alanine repeats' in one of the homeobox genes—*PHOX2B*). Presents clinically with unexplained ventilatory failure, much worse during sleep when the 'awake' drive is lost.

- *May be recognized early*, cyanosis, morning confusion, ankle oedema
- *May be recognized late*, loss of consciousness, and an emergency admission to ICU for ventilation following a chest infection or general anaesthesia.

Lung function is often normal, with no evidence of respiratory muscle weakness, indicating normal innervation from the voluntary motor system. Arnold–Chiari malformation with brainstem compression can present like this, but there is usually involvement of surrounding structures such as the lower cranial motor nuclei supplying the larynx and pharynx (with associated OSA; see ➔ p. 96).

These patients will have no apparent neuromuscular or respiratory cause for their hypoventilation but may have a previous history of brainstem stroke (or other form of brain damage). The congenital form usually presents shortly after birth when the amount of REM sleep reduces and is replaced by non-REM.

Post-polio syndrome is:

- Ill-defined syndrome—decline in function, decades after initial illness
- Return of weakness in previously affected areas (mechanism unclear)
- Late development of ventilatory failure is more likely if:
  - Inspiratory muscles were affected in the original illness
  - Additional scoliosis due to paravertebral muscle involvement (in which case VC will be reduced).

This may be due to premature ageing of the upper and lower motor neurones due to their 'overuse'. This could follow the original destruction of some of the anterior horn cells to the inspiratory muscles and the subsequent reinnervation by surviving neurones which then have to continuously supply more neurones than they were 'designed' for.

Weak or mechanically disadvantaged inspiratory muscles with/without 2° reduction of awake ventilatory drive

Neuromuscular inspiratory muscle weakness will produce diurnal ventilatory failure in its own right, particularly when the supine VC falls below 20% predicted (~1L).

With increasing inspiratory muscle weakness, other accessory inspiratory muscles are recruited to maintain ventilation. When this is lost during non-REM sleep, and more so during REM sleep, ventilation will fall much more than in normal subjects. Whilst metabolic ventilatory drive is reasonably preserved, this will result in recurrent arousals to 'rescue' the ventilation and consequent marked sleep disturbance.

As ventilatory drive becomes progressively blunted, following the hypoventilation forced on the system by weak muscles, extra sleep hypoventilation (from loss of 'awake' drive) is tolerated, and profound hypoxaemia is observed until there is finally an arousal that recovers the ventilation and SaO_2.

The above patients should have a history of a progressive neuromuscular disorder.

Chest wall restrictive diseases, such as scoliosis or post-thoracoplasty patients (see Fig. 47.5), can behave in a similar way with gradual onset of ventilatory failure, particularly when VC <1L. The muscles are not weak but operating at severe mechanical disadvantage.

The same situation occurs in **COPD**, when muscles are overloaded and accessory muscles provide important support, but this too is reduced with non-REM sleep and lost during REM sleep. Again, any 2° reduction in ventilatory drive amplifies the sleep-related falls in SaO_2.

- Chest wall restrictive patients should have an obvious restrictive disorder with reduced VC to 1L or below
- Increasing degrees of COPD will produce increasing degrees of sleep hypoventilation (see Fig. 47.7)
- If the awake SaO_2 is already low, the sleep-related falls in ventilation will produce dramatic dips in SaO_2
- COPD and OSA together (overlap syndrome; see ➲ p. 97) provoke profound nocturnal hypoxic dipping (see Fig. 47.8), and probably a more rapid progression to diurnal hypoventilation with CO_2 retention, due to extra blunting of ventilatory drive.

The diaphragm is the only respiratory muscle working during REM sleep, as all other postural muscles are profoundly hypotonic.

- If the diaphragm is paralysed, then REM sleep is a particularly vulnerable time, as there are no muscles of ventilation left working, thus producing particularly profound falls in SaO_2 during REM
- Patients with bilateral diaphragm weakness can present early, with no obvious weakness elsewhere. Diaphragm weakness is best detected with the patient supine. Inspiration, particularly on sniffing, will provoke a paradoxical indrawing of the abdominal wall. The VC will also fall on lying down, increasingly with greater degrees of paralysis (often a >30% fall in VC with complete diaphragm paralysis).

In a progressive neuromuscular disorder, such as MND, the above patterns will be variable between individuals but will gradually worsen. Predominant diaphragm weakness, as occurs sometimes in MND, spinal muscular atrophy, and particularly acid maltase deficiency, can lead to ventilatory failure at a time when the patient is still ambulant.

Cheyne–Stokes breathing associated with LVF

(See Fig. 47.4.)

The raised left atrial pressure in left heart failure increases ventilatory drive through stimulation of J receptors; this in addition to ventilatory stimulation from any hypoxaemia from pulmonary oedema.

• This ventilatory stimulation lowers the awake $PaCO_2$, producing a respiratory alkalosis
• In addition, the use of diuretics may produce a mild metabolic alkalosis, especially if there is hypokalaemia
• This extra J receptor ventilatory stimulation appears to reduce at sleep onset. This, together with the loss of the awake ventilatory drive, allows central hypoventilation or apnoea to occur
• This hypoventilation or apnoea will continue until the $PaCO_2$ builds up driving ventilation again or until the hypoxaemia provokes arousal
• The return of ventilation itself may provoke arousal too. The arousal itself then injects the increased 'wake' ventilatory drive, reducing the $PaCO_2$ again
• Sleep returns, and, once again, the low $PaCO_2$ and alkalosis cause hypoventilation or apnoea.

Thus, a cycle is maintained that involves a fluctuating sleep state with arousals, and usually a fluctuating SaO_2. As with OSA, the patient may be completely unaware of these arousals. The delayed circulatory time of left heart failure may compound this instability by introducing a time delay between any change in $PaCO_2$ in the blood leaving the lungs and its arrival at the carotid body or central chemoreceptors.

Cheyne–Stokes breathing associated with altitude

The acute hypoxia following ascent to altitude provokes increased ventilation. The degree is variable between individuals, and hence the degree of hypocapnia and respiratory alkalosis varies (see ➲ p. 242). With sleep onset, with a lessening of the hypoxic drive, and removal of the awake drive, an uncompensated alkalosis will allow hypoventilation, and even apnoea—similar to the situation described previously for Cheyne–Stokes breathing. Again, ventilation will restart, either when the $PaCO_2$ rises to a critical level or the hypoxia provokes arousal. Sleep is fragmented with complaints of insomnia, but the cause of this is rarely recognized by the sufferer.

Skiing in Colorado, altitude 2,400–3,400m (~10,000ft), is high enough to provoke significant periodic breathing in about a fifth of individuals. It seems that this fifth are the ones with the highest hypoxic ventilatory response. This gives them the largest respiratory alkalosis and hence the greatest tendency to sleep-onset hypoventilation. In addition, the tendency to arouse with the resultant extra hypoxaemia may be greater too, thus provoking large increases in ventilation on arousal and greater sleep disturbance. As the kidney excretes extra bicarbonate and produces a compensatory metabolic acidosis over a few days, the periodic breathing lessens. See also ➜ pp. 242–3 (altitude sickness).

Two pharmacological approaches have been taken to reduce this sleep-related periodic breathing at altitude.

- Pre-acclimatization with acetazolamide prior to ascent. This produces a mild metabolic acidosis and maintains the ventilatory drive at sleep onset, thus blocking the hypoventilation. RCTs show the efficacy of this approach with doses between 250 and 500mg/day, 1–3 days prior to ascent
- Hypnotics, such as temazepam, can reduce the degree of periodic breathing by reducing the tendency to arousal with each return of ventilation, and thus damping the system. Randomized trials suggest benefit for the early part of the night, with no impairment of nocturnal hypoxaemia or daytime functioning
- Of course, extra O_2 will abolish the problem.

CSA/hypoventilation: investigations

Simple PFTs will characterize weakness of inspiratory muscles. Supine VC is the best predictor of ventilatory failure, as it incorporates diaphragm weakness that is masked during erect testing. Blood gases will reveal diurnal type II ventilatory failure. If the bicarbonate/base excess is raised, with a normal $PaCO_2$ (showing therefore a mild metabolic alkalosis), then this may indicate nocturnal hypoventilation and incipient ventilatory failure. The bicarbonate has been referred to as the 'HbA1c of $PaCO_2$', as it represents an integrated response to the average raised $PaCO_2$ over the last 48h or so (in the absence of any other reason for a metabolic alkalosis such as hypokalaemia and some diuretics).

Sleep study

(For examples, see Figs 47.3, 47.4, 47.5, 47.7, and 47.8.)

Sleep studies in patients with suspected nocturnal hypoventilation or CSA confirm the diagnosis and assess the degree of nocturnal hypoxaemia. Limited sleep studies should reveal falls in SaO_2 in association with hypoventilation, but no evidence of OSA and, in particular, no snoring. Oximetry tracings alone will show a variety of patterns, often resembling OSA. The pattern in neuromuscular weakness will vary from oscillations all the time (due to recurrent arousal) to just REM sleep-related dips in SaO_2. The same will be true for chest wall restrictive disorders and COPD, with REM dips occurring initially and greater hypoxaemia once there is an element of diurnal CO_2 retention and hypoxaemia.

- In OSA, there is a slow fall in SaO_2, as O_2 levels fall in the lung, followed by a rapid rise with the first deep inspiration as the apnoea ends (so-called sawtooth pattern); see Fig. 47.2
- In Cheyne–Stokes of left heart failure, the oscillations in SaO_2 are often more sinusoidal than in OSA, as the pattern of breathing is usually more of a symmetrical waxing and waning of ventilation; see Fig. 47.4. However, if each central apnoea is terminated by an arousal, rather than a smooth return of ventilation, then the pattern will look more like OSA.

In COPD, the degree of hypoxaemia on the sleep study will depend very much on the awake SaO_2. Because of the shape of the Hb dissociation curve, a low awake SaO_2 makes it easier for the SaO_2 to fall further with a given reduction in ventilation. Thus, during non-REM, with removal of awake drive, there will be a fairly stable reduction in SaO_2, but, during REM sleep, there will be further more dramatic dips. It is important not to diagnose OSA from just an oximetry tracing on the basis of SaO_2 oscillations when there is a low baseline SaO_2 and COPD. In this situation, a fuller sleep study is required to provide evidence of additional upper airway obstruction. The combination of hypoxic COPD and OSA (one of the overlap syndromes) can produce particularly dramatic traces (see Fig. 47.8).

Management Intervention in CSA, or hypoventilation or periodic breathing, depends on symptoms. *Better control of heart failure* may improve Cheyne–Stokes breathing but often does not. Further treatment will be required for two reasons: either to prevent the cyclical breathing and restore sleep quality, or to globally improve ventilation overnight and reset the respiratory control mechanisms such that the daytime respiratory failure reverses.

In situations where the hypoxia is playing a part in the pathogenesis (e.g. heart failure), then *raising* FiO_2 can help (using O_2 via nasal prongs only during sleep). There is limited literature on other forms of treatment for the Cheyne–Stokes of heart failure, although *acetazolamide* and *benzodiazepines* have been tried. The unstable breathing in heart failure has been treated with *CPAP; however, a large RCT has not confirmed long-term benefit.* More recently, treatment has been tried with sophisticated *servo-ventilators* that are able to cut in smoothly, as ventilation wanes and backs off when it waxes, thus ironing out the oscillations without overventilating; whether these will provide better relief of symptoms than O_2 is not yet clear, but preliminary evidence suggests they might. There are some data to suggest that the recurrent arousal in Cheynes–Stokes may raise catecholamine levels and provoke deterioration of LV function. Thus, measures to reduce the arousals may improve cardiac function as well as improve daytime vigilance.

Sedatives are contraindicated with a raised $PaCO_2$, and extra O_2 may increase the hypercapnia. In these situations, then *overnight NIV*, via either nose or face mask, may be appropriate. In slowly progressive neuromuscular disorders, with either sleep fragmentation or diurnal type II respiratory failure (or both), the symptomatic and physiological response can be dramatic. The use of NIV at night in more rapidly progressive disorders has potential difficulties but is proving very useful in the palliative care of disorders such as MND. Increasing dependence on equipment, not designed to be immediately life-sustaining, is a particular issue. In scoliosis, there is rarely any question that treatment might not be appropriate, and again responses are dramatic.

Future developments

- Treatment of LVF (acute and chronic, no evidence yet for the latter) with overnight CPAP or NIV
- Introduction of overnight ventilation earlier in the course of a progressive neuromuscular disorder (such as MND) to reduce symptoms and possibly prolong life
- Use of overnight ventilation on patients with stable COPD and hypercapnia. This may reduce exacerbations, hospital admissions, and prolong life. The evidence is inadequate yet to justify its wide use in this patient group.

Further information

Oldenburg O. Cheyne-stokes respiration in chronic heart failure. Treatment with adaptive servoventilation therapy. *Circ J* 2012;**76**:2305–7.

Naughton MT. Cheyne-Stokes respiration: friend or foe? *Thorax*;**67**:357–60.

Lanfranchi PA, Somers VK. Sleep-disordered breathing in heart failure: characteristics and implications. *Respir Physiol Neurobiol* 2003;**136**:153–65.

Berry-Kravis EM *et al.* Congenital central hypoventilation syndrome. *Am J Respir Crit Care Med* 2006;**174**:1139–44.

Gray A *et al.* Noninvasive ventilation in acute cardiogenic pulmonary edema. *N Engl J Med* 2008;**359**:142–51.

Obesity-related respiratory problems

Levels of obesity (BMI >30) are rising in all 'civilized' societies. In 1983, 8% in the UK (18% in the USA) had a BMI >30. Twenty-five years later, in 2008, this was 24% in the UK (34% in the USA). This has also had many impacts on health care outside of respiratory medicine, particularly the components of the metabolic syndrome.

Obesity, particularly in conjunction with OSA and COPD, provokes ventilatory failure and cor pulmonale (see ➲ p. 97). A common clinical scenario is the obese smoker, with a history of snoring and sleepiness, arriving in A&E with hypercapnia*. Why only some obese patients develop hypercapnia is not clear, but abdominal obesity seems the most hazardous. This may be because of greater lung volume compression, thus breathing occurs nearer residual volume where airway resistance is much higher and total compliance lower, thus increasing the work of breathing considerably.

In addition to apportioning the relative contribution of obesity, COPD, and OSA to the hypercapnia, and treating accordingly, there are other obesity-related factors to consider:

• Intubation—the best predictors of a problematic intubation are neck circumference and a Mallampati score of 3 or more (see Fig. 47.9)
• Tracheostomy tubes are often too short and too curved to cope with the increased distance between skin and trachea; tubes with adjustable flanges that allow customized intra-tracheal lengths are useful here
• Percutaneous dilatational tracheostomy is more difficult and may have a higher complication rate
• Low FRCs mean that the O_2 stores are limited, leading to rapid falls in SaO_2 during apnoeas of any cause
• Abdominal loading of the diaphragm is greatly increased, but the extra embarrassment to the diaphragm can be reduced by tilting the *whole bed*, head up, by 15–25°
• Abdominal loading of the diaphragm particularly reduces basal lung expansion. Resultant basal atelectasis increases the A–a gradient, which can be improved by raising end expiratory pressure during both invasive or non-invasive ventilation
• Abdominal loading may increase perioperative risk of aspiration
• DVTs and PEs are probably more common in the obese. It is not clear if DVT prophylaxis regimes need to be modified. Some recommend higher doses of LMWH, and this higher dose is more effective in patients undergoing bariatric surgery. Weight-based regimes of LMWH for the treatment of DVT and emboli appear satisfactory in the morbidly obese (BMI >40)
• Increased likelihood of failure to wean—NIV (inspiratory pressure 12, expiratory 4cmH$_2$O) has been shown to aid weaning, e.g. post-open gastric bypass surgery for obesity
• Possible build-up of sedating anaesthetic agents in fat, leading to prolonged half-life.

* The term 'obesity hypoventilation syndrome' is used when an obese individual (BMI >30kg/m2) has a raised PaCO2 (>6kPa) with no other apparent explanation, usually in conjunction with worsening sleep-related hypoventilation, and sometimes additional obstructive sleep apnoea.

Obese patients can often have mildly raised $PaCO_2$ and bicarbonate levels for long periods, without decline or apparent problems. Once there is acute decompensation with acidosis, management is more difficult. NIV is usually effective but may require very high inspiratory and expiratory pressures that can be difficult to deliver adequately without pressure damage and ulceration to the nasal bridge. Weight loss is very effective but, as usual, is hard to achieve without bariatric surgery, which will be hazardous if NIV has not lifted the patient out of ventilatory failure. Acetazolamide is used by some in this situation, but its use is not evidence-based.

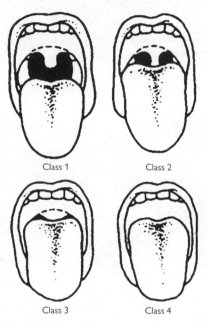

Class 1   Class 2

Class 3   Class 4

Fig. 47.9 Mallampati index. Simple scoring system for pharyngeal crowding. Affected by craniofacial shape, tongue size, and obesity. Predicts difficulty of intubation and correlates with OSA severity. Reproduced from Update in Anaesthesia; Issue 13, 2001, with kind permission from the WFSA

Further information

Chau EH et al. Obesity hypoventilation syndrome: a review of epidemiology, pathophysiology, and perioperative complications. *Anesthesiology* 2012;**117**:188–205.

El-Solh AA. Clinical approach to the critically ill, morbidly obese patient. *Am J Respir Crit Care Med* 2004;**169**:557–61.

ug-induced lung disease: clinical presentations

Introduction A vast number of drugs can damage the respiratory system, from nose to alveoli (see Box 48.1). The most up-to-date, complete, useful, and recommended list (plus references) is kept at ♒ http://www. pneumotox.com and can be queried by either drug (or drug type) or nearly 20 different clinical/radiological presentations; all agents have equal prominence but are coded with a star rating to indicate likely prevalence. This chapter describes the commoner drugs that produce respiratory problems. Often the clinical problem is to differentiate drug toxicity from other causes of ILD.

Box 48.1 Commoner presentations of drug-induced lung disease and examples of causative agents

- ILD, pneumonitis, fibrosis
  - Acute HP (nitrofurantoin, methotrexate)
  - Interstitial pneumonitis ± eosinophilia (amiodarone, ACE inhibitors, sulfasalazine)
  - Chronic OP (amiodarone, bleomycin)
  - Pulmonary fibrosis (bleomycin, amiodarone, nitrofurantoin, β-blockers)
- Airways disease
  - Bronchospasm (β-blockers, contrast media)
  - Obliterative bronchiolitis (busulfan, penicillamine)
  - Cough (ACE inhibitors)
- Pleural changes
  - Pleural effusion/thickening (β-blockers, nitrofurantoin, methotrexate, dopamine agonists)
  - Pneumothorax (bleomycin)
- Vascular changes
  - Thromboembolic disease (phenytoin)
  - PHT (dexfenfluramine, other appetite suppressants)
  - Vasculitis (nitrofurantoin, L-tryptophan)
- Mediastinal changes
  - Node enlargement (bleomycin, phenytoin)
  - Sclerosing mediastinitis (ergot)
- Pulmonary oedema (methotrexate, contrast media)
- Pulmonary haemorrhage (methotrexate, nitrofurantoin, penicillamine, contrast media).

Drug-induced lung disease: examples

Amiodarone Iodinated benzofuran used to suppress supra- and ventricular tachycardias. Lung toxicity correlates loosely with total dose and therefore usually occurs after a variable number of months. Seen in 10% of subjects on >400mg/day. Rare if <300mg/day.

Risk factors
- Daily dose >400mg
- Increasing age of patient
- Use for >2 months
- Pre-existing lung disease (although not a contraindication to its use)
- Recent surgical intervention or lung infection.

Diagnosis is usually one of exclusion and response to cessation of drug (which can take months). Infiltrative lung disease varying from acute respiratory distress (rare) through to COP (cough, pleuritic pain, fever, dyspnoea, asymmetric patchy infiltrates, effusion), and the most indolent—chronic interstitial pneumonitis (cough, dyspnoea, weight loss, diffuse, and/or focal opacities).

On *CT*, the liver, thyroid, and lungs will usually show increased attenuation, indicating a significant amiodarone load. A baseline CXR is useful.

Lung biopsies exclude other diagnoses and provide compatible findings, but there is dissent as to how diagnostic they are (except for the finding of foamy macrophages in the airspaces, filled with amiodarone–phospholipid complexes, but may occur in absence of lung toxicity). Mechanisms of toxicity are unclear, and there are features to suggest hypersensitivity and direct toxic damage.

Treatment Steroids are effective and required in severe disease. The half-life of amiodarone in the tissues is in excess of a month, and response to stopping the drug may be slow. Prognosis is good in the majority.

Anti-TNF agents (infliximab and etanercept) represent a large step forward in the treatment of RA and Crohn's disease. However, there is a small, but important, risk of reactivating TB, commonly extrapulmonary (see pp. 510–1). Pneumonia and development of antibodies are also more common; SLE develops only rarely.

Azathioprine Extensively used as an immunosuppressant but has remarkably little pulmonary toxicity other than via opportunistic lung infection. Case reports of pneumonitis only.

Bleomycin DNA-damaging glycopeptide used in the treatment of lymphomas, germ cell tumours, squamous carcinomas (cervix, head, neck, and oesophagus). Pulmonary fibrosis occurs in about 10%.

Risk factors
- Older age
- Those receiving total dose of >300,000IU (1,000IU (or 1 old/USB unit) = 1.5–2.0mg)

- Increased FiO_2, probably via increased superoxide/free radical formation. Pneumonitis may be precipitated by supplementary O_2 for some time after drug administration—warn anaesthetist if surgery planned in patients who have received bleomycin in previous 6–12 months
- Pulmonary irradiation, not just in the irradiated field
- Renal failure decreases drug elimination and thus toxicity
- Associated use of cyclophosphamide.

Symptoms (cough, dyspnoea, chest pain, fever) develop 1–6 months after bleomycin. There is hypoxia and a restrictive defect. Progressive basal sub-pleural shadowing, small lungs, and blunting of costophrenic angles.

Histology shows a dominant subpleural distribution of damage and repair with fibrosis; this appearance is non-diagnostic and common to many drugs/disorders. Toxicity is probably due to DNA damage or oxidative injury, with inter-individual variation occurring due to differing activity of the enzyme bleomycin hydrolase; only low levels of this enzyme exist in the lung (and skin). A rare acute hypersensitivity form comes on within days of administration. Other unusual presentations include pulmonary nodules or OP.

Treatment
- Bleomycin must be stopped on suspicion of damage, and some units use lung function tests (kCO) to detect early damage
- Steroids are used, but there is little evidence they alter long-term prognosis (in the acute hypersensitivity subgroup, there is a clear beneficial effect)
- Use the minimum FiO_2 to maintain an adequate SaO_2 (85–90%)
- Over 50% may experience a relentless decline in lung function.

Busulfan DNA alkylating, myelosuppressive agent mainly used to treat chronic myeloid leukaemia and prior to bone marrow transplantation, with a low rate of lung toxicity (4–10%) due to fibrosis.

Risk factors
- Cumulative doses >500mg (mostly over 120 days)
- Concurrent administration of other alkylating agents
- Pulmonary irradiation.

Presents with cough and progressive SOB, often years after exposure (usually about 4y). CXR is typically unremarkable. Reduced kCO and restrictive defect. Diagnosis is usually by exclusion. The place of steroids is unproven.

Chlorambucil DNA alkylating agent mainly used to treat CLL, lymphomas, and ovarian cancer. It has additional immunosuppressive actions and is also used in conditions such as RA. Low risk (1%) of pulmonary toxicity and confined to those who have received >2g. Similarly to busulfan, presentation may be many years later. Presents with cough, dyspnoea, weight loss, and basal crackles. CXR shows diffuse basal reticular shadowing. Non-specific histology. On suspicion, chlorambucil should be stopped; use of steroids is unproven. Prognosis is poor (50% fatal).

Cyclophosphamide DNA alkylating agent mainly used to treat CLL, SCLC, and other solid tumours. Particularly useful as an immunosuppressive agent in certain vasculitides and nephropathies. Lung toxicity is rare.

Risk factors
- Pulmonary irradiation
- O_2 therapy
- Concurrent drugs causing pulmonary toxicity, e.g. bleomycin.

Clinical presentation is usually within 6 months, with a short duration of fever, cough, and fatigue. Reticular shadowing with ground-glass appearance on CT. Later-onset progressive pulmonary fibrosis can also develop insidiously in those on therapy for many months with progressive SOB and dry cough. The histology of the more acute type can be similar to any of the acute interstitial pneumonias (e.g. COP, diffuse alveolar damage), whereas the more chronic form is indistinguishable from UIP. Cyclophosphamide is not itself toxic to the lung, but its metabolites are. There appears to be genetic variation to susceptibility, as there is no obvious dose-response relationship. Cessation of drug and steroid therapy is used successfully in the acute form, but the chronic form seems to progress inexorably, in a similar manner to UIP. Lung transplantation is an option. Note increased risk of PCP whilst taking cyclophosphamide.

Gold Used in RA, >500mg cumulative dose can produce pneumonitis (possibly COP, obliterative bronchiolitis), with cough, dyspnoea, and basal crackles. Rare (1%) but associated with certain HLA types and distinctive histological feature of alveolar septal inflammation. Good prognosis following drug cessation; poor evidence for steroids.

Methotrexate Folic acid derivative, inhibiting cell division by blocking dihydrofolate reductase and nucleic acid production. Mainly used in leukaemia and as an immunosuppressive, e.g. RA and psoriasis. Commonly (4–10%) causes a variety of lung pathologies, not associated with folic acid deficiency.

Risk factors
- Hypoalbuminaemia
- Diabetes
- Previous use of drugs that modify disease progress in rheumatoid
- Rheumatoid or other lung/pleural disease
- Not particularly dose-related; can occur at doses of <20mg/week
- Daily, rather than intermittent (weekly), therapy
- >60y.

Presents both acutely (interstitial pneumonitis, fever, and eosinophilia) and over very long time periods; however, the subacute form (within a year, dyspnoea, fever, cough, hypoxia, basal crackles, restrictive defect, and reduced kCO) is commoner. Bilateral diffuse pulmonary infiltrates or mixed pattern with alveolar shadowing on CXR, occasional effusions.

Histology More useful than in other drug toxicities, shows alveolitis, interstitial pneumonitis, epithelial cell hyperplasia, eosinophilic infiltration, and granuloma formation in the more acute hypersensitivity form and more UIP-like changes in indolent form. Mechanism of damage unknown but likely to be multifactorial.

Treatment consists of drug withdrawal and unproven use of steroids. Anecdotal reports support use of steroids in the more acute hypersensitivity form. Other methotrexate-related lung diseases include opportunistic lung infection (including PCP) and non-Hodgkin's B-cell lymphoma, which may regress with drug withdrawal and may be associated with EBV.

Nitrofurantoin is used commonly for long-term prophylaxis against urinary tract infections (UTIs). Acutely, nitrofurantoin causes a hypersensitivity vasculitis and, much less frequently, a chronic interstitial fibrosis. Most patients are women due to their much higher prevalence of chronic UTIs. The acute form presents abruptly with fever, dyspnoea, dry cough, rash, chest pain, hypoxia, crackles, and eosinophilia within a week or two of starting and is dose-independent. Lower zone diffuse patchy infiltrates and sometimes unilateral effusions on CXR. Lung biopsy reveals vasculitis, eosinophilia, reactive type II pneumocytes, focal haemorrhage, and some interstitial inflammation. Treatment consists of discontinuation, and improvement begins rapidly. Prognosis is good, with or without steroids.

O$_2$ Prolonged 80–100% O$_2$ therapy can provoke lung damage.

Penicillamine Used in the treatment of RA, penicillamine may increase the prevalence of obliterative bronchiolitis. This is dose-related but rare, with a subacute onset (after several months) of dyspnoea and cough. There is a progressive obstructive pattern without bronchodilator response; 50% mortality.

Sulfasalazine Used extensively in treatment of IBD (mainly ulcerative colitis). Rarely causes side effects but can cause new-onset dyspnoea and pulmonary infiltrates after any period of use. Cough, fever, lung crackles, and blood eosinophilia are the usual presentation. Prior allergy history, rash, and weight loss also seen with eosinophilic pneumonia, the usual pathology. Withdrawal of drugs is usually successful within weeks, and recovery can be hastened by steroids. Rare deaths when the histology is more like usual interstitial pneumonitis and may be more related to the condition requiring sulfasalazine.

Talc is commonly used for pleurodesis (see ➲ pp. 786–7). Talc particles may be small enough to enter the circulation after intrapleural instillation, being found throughout the body at post-mortem. They appear to provoke a systemic reaction with fever, raised inflammatory markers, and hypoxia, suggestive of an ARDS-like pathology. Occasional deaths after talc pleurodesis have been reported. Refined talc with fewer smaller particles seems less toxic.

Paraquat poisoning

Paraquat (Weedol®, Pathclear®, Gramoxone®) and related bipyridyl compounds are used as contact herbicides. They kill plants by inhibiting NADP reduction during photosynthesis, which involves the production of superoxide radicals. Most of the toxicity of paraquat in animals is also believed to be due to the production of damaging superoxides. Most cases of poisoning are deliberate, and the treatment should be commenced as soon as possible. Serious poisoning is usually by ingestion (although paraquat is absorbed through the skin and mucous membranes, including the conjunctiva and bronchial mucosa).

- >6g is always fatal
- <1.5g is rarely fatal
- Between 1.5 and 6g, the mortality is 60–70%
- Mouthful of 20% Gramoxone® liquid (10g/50mL) is almost certainly fatal
- <1 sachet of Weedol® granules (1.4g paraquat/57g sachet) is unlikely to cause death
- Usually fatal if blood level >0.2mg/mL at 24h.

Clinical features

- Oral and oesophageal ulceration shortly after contact, with later formation of a pseudomembrane
- Renal failure (reversible) within a few days, but delayed excretion of paraquat prevents falls in blood levels
- Pulmonary oedema early on, evolving into 'ARDS'
- Hepatic damage, jaundice, and raised transaminases
- Metabolic acidosis
- Death usually occurs within 1–2 weeks
- Pulmonary fibrosis if the patient survives, with varying degrees of recovery.

Radiation-induced pulmonary disease

Manifestations of lung injury following radiotherapy include:

Radiation pneumonitis

- Often asymptomatic although may cause dyspnoea and chronic ventilatory failure
- Radiographic abnormalities more common than clinical disease. Characteristically straight margins on CT infiltrate
- Pathological feature is of diffuse alveolar damage, with vascular intimal fibrosis
- Typically follows lung radiotherapy
- Treatment of symptomatic disease is with steroids (1mg/kg daily), although minimal evidence to support their use. Amifostine or pentoxifylline (used in the treatment of extrapulmonary manifestations of radiation-induced tissue damage) may be of benefit although unproven.

Radiation-induced organizing pneumonia

- Often presents with cough (rather than breathlessness, which is more suggestive of radiation pneumonitis)
- Characterized by migratory patchy consolidation which always extends beyond radiation field on CT
- Typically follows breast radiotherapy
- Treatment is with steroids; often long courses are needed. Macrolides may have a role.

Radiation-induced chronic eosinophilic pneumonia

- Possible association; few cases reported.

Inhalational lung injury

Definition Agents damaging the lung and airways through direct toxicity. Much of the acute damage is common to many toxic agents, including pneumonitis/pulmonary oedema, mucosal damage/sloughing/airway debris. 2° infection is common due to breached defences.

Examples of toxic agents, listed alphabetically

Aldehydes (acetaldehyde, formaldehyde)
- Chemical and plastics industry, used for disinfection
- Highly irritant to mucosal membranes
- Acute damage
  - Pneumonitis and pulmonary oedema
- Chronic effects
  - Rhinitis/asthma.

Ammonia
- Fertilizer and plastics production, used in many chemical industries
- Highly irritant to mucosal membranes
- Acute damage
  - Upper airway obstruction from secretions and mucosal oedema
  - Lung damage and 2° infection
- Chronic effects
  - Airways obstruction and bronchiectasis described.

Chlorine
- Extensive use in the chemical industry, bleaching agent
- Acute damage
  - Overwhelming toxicity, producing rapid hypoxia
  - Pneumonitis and pulmonary oedema
- Chronic effects (e.g. from repeated accidental exposure)
  - Airways obstruction; sometimes reversible.

Cocaine (when smoked)
- Pneumothorax/pneumomediastinum
- Pulmonary haemorrhage
- Pulmonary oedema
- Allergic responses (asthma, pulmonary eosinophilia, HP).

Metals and metal compounds (as fumes or nebulized solutions)
- Mainly used in the chemical industry
- Acute damage
  - Mucosal irritation
  - Pulmonary oedema
- Chronic effects
  - Pneumoconiosis
- Some specific effects such as:
  - Sarcoid-like reaction to beryllium
  - Asthma from cobalt, chromium, nickel, vanadium
  - Fibrosing alveolitis from cobalt and zinc fumes.

Methyl isocyanate (Bhopal disaster: 3,800 dead, 170,000 injured)
- Chemical industry, carbamate pesticides
- Acute damage
  - Pneumonitis and pulmonary oedema
  - 2° infection
- Chronic effects
  - Airways obstruction
  - Bronchiolitis obliterans
  - Pulmonary fibrosis.

Hydrocarbons/mineral oils
- Used as lubricant and cooling agent
- Acute damage
  - Pneumonitis
- Chronic effects
  - Pneumonitis
  - Fibrosis
  - Asthma.

Nitrogen dioxide (NO$_2$)
- Chemical industry (explosives)
- Agricultural silos
- Odourless and therefore high doses inhaled without knowing
- Acute damage (several hours after exposure)
  - Silo-fillers lung (pneumonitis/pulmonary oedema)
- Later effects
  - 2° pulmonary oedema 2–8 weeks after exposure
  - Steroid-responsive, needs 2 months therapy after exposure.

Ozone
- Bleaching agent
- Product of welding
- Similar to NO$_2$
- Both immediate and late effects of pneumonitis/pulmonary oedema.

Phosgene
- Chemical warfare, chemical industry, chlorination
- Released from heated methylene chloride (paint stripper)
- Acute damage
  - Pneumonitis and pulmonary oedema
  - Produces carboxyhaemoglobin (COHb); breath CO therefore reflects degree of exposure.

Smoke
- Most smoke injury is due to heat damage to upper airway
- Hypoxia, vaporized toxins (e.g. formaldehyde, chlorine), systemic agents (e.g. CO and cyanide)
- Acute damage
  - Mucosal oedema and sloughing with airway blockage
- Look out for:
  - Peri-oral burns
  - Black sputum

- Altered voice
- Respiratory distress
- Stridor (rapid inspiration to accentuate)
- Additional CO and/or cyanide poisoning.

Sulfur dioxide
- Used as a fumigant, and bleaching agent in the paper industry
- Very irritant as dissolves to form sulfuric acid
- Acute damage
  - Sloughing of airway mucosa
  - Pneumonitis and haemorrhagic pulmonary oedema
- Chronic effects
  - Airways obstruction.

Welding fumes
- Many agents released
- Specific examples:
  - Cadmium—pneumonitis
  - Zinc—'metal fume fever'
  - Several agents may cause airways obstruction/COPD
- Siderosis (welder's lung), non-fibrogenic pneumoconiosis
  - Iron deposits in lung, producing small rounded opacities.

Carbon monoxide poisoning

Definition and epidemiology

- CO is a colourless and odourless gas formed when carbon compounds burn in limited O_2
- It accounts for about 75 deaths per year in the UK, ~10% of which are accidental
- Accidental poisonings are commoner in the winter when faulty heating systems are in use
- Non-accidental deaths are mainly from car exhaust fumes
- Methylene chloride (industrial solvent, paint remover) is converted to CO in the liver and may present as CO poisoning
- Up to one-third die following acute high-level exposure, and another third may be left with permanent neurological sequelae
- Chronic low-grade CO exposure may present as non-specific ill health and may affect thousands of individuals.

Pathophysiology and related conditions

- CO competes avidly with O_2 (250 times greater) to bind with the iron in Hb, making it less available for O_2 carriage
- The Hb molecule is also distorted by combination with CO, making it bind more tightly to O_2, shifting the O_2 dissociation curve to the left. The PaO_2 at which the Hb is 50% saturated (P50) moves from about 3.5 down to 2kPa. This further reduces O_2 delivery to the tissues: a 50% COHb level is vastly more dangerous than a 50% anaemia
- CO also binds to extravascular molecules, such as myoglobin and some of the cytochrome chain proteins, interfering with energy production, and, in this respect, is like cyanide
- Normal levels of COHb can be up to 3%, and up to 15% in heavy smokers
- Foetal Hb combines even more avidly with CO; thus the foetus is especially vulnerable to CO poisoning of the mother.

Methaemoglobin
- Methaemoglobin is due to oxidation of Fe^{2+} to Fe^{3+} in Hb, thus preventing O_2 carriage. This is due either to inherited deficiencies of enzymes (cytochrome b5 reductase) that reduce the Fe^{3+} back to Fe^{2+}, or toxic agents (e.g. nitrites (in 'poppers'), chloroquine) that overwhelm this reversal mechanism
- Methaemoglobin is slightly left-shifted, but a 40% methaemoglobinaemia may be asymptomatic, apart from the typical grey/blue colour of the patient, often mistaken for cyanosis.

Clinical features of CO poisoning
Immediate
- Nausea, headache, malaise, weakness, and unsteadiness
- Loss of consciousness, seizures, cardiac abnormalities (ischaemia, arrhythmias, pulmonary oedema)
- No cyanosis, healthy-looking 'cherry red' colour
- Suspect if several members of household present with these features.

Delayed (~1–3 weeks, can be longer)
- Cognitive defects and personality changes
- Focal neurology and movement abnormalities.

Investigations
- Pulse oximetry will appear *normal* due to COHb having similar absorption spectra to oxyhaemoglobin. Recent developments in multiwave pulse oximetry may allow rapid COHb detection
- Arterial PaO_2 levels may be *normal*
- COHb blood levels can be measured on a co-oximeter
- Breath CO measured with devices used for smoking cessation work well
- Routine tests to rule out other diagnoses.

Future developments Isocapnic hyperpnoea may further raise the PaO_2. Alkalosis must be avoided though to prevent further left shift of the Hb dissociation curve. Can be done voluntarily with 5% CO_2 in O_2 or during intubation. Can double rate of CO elimination.

Further information

Blumenthal I. Carbon monoxide poisoning. *J R Soc Med* 2001;**94**:270–2.

Buckley NA *et al.* Cochrane review of hyperbaric O_2. ℘ http://summaries.cochrane. org/CD002041/there-is-insufficient-evidence-to-support-the-use-of-hyperbaric-O2-for-treatment-of-patients-with-carbon-monoxide-poisoning.

Plymouth Diving Disease Research Centre. ℘ http://www.ddrc.org/ (24h helpline and register of hyperbaric chambers) ☏ 01752 209999. Email info@ddrc.org.

Harper A, Croft-Baker J. Carbon monoxide poisoning: undetected by both patients and their doctors. *Age Ageing* 2004;**33**:105–9.

Kreck TC *et al.* Isocapnic hyperventilation increases carbon monoxide elimination and O_2 delivery. *Am J Respir Crit Care Med* 2001;**163**:458–62.

Roth D *et al.* Accuracy of noninvasive multiwave pulse oximetry compared with carboxyhemo-globin from blood gas analysis in unselected emergency department patients. *Ann Emerg Med* 2011;**58**:74–9.

Chapter 49

Unusual lung diseases

Introduction to unusual lung diseases

In continental Europe, there have been registers of rare lung diseases for many years. The term 'orphan' lung disease was coined because of the feeling that these diseases have, in the past, tended to be neglected because of their rarity; hence, there is limited knowledge of the conditions and limited available data on which to base clinical practice.

The previous British reporting system (BOLD) has now closed. The BTS Specialist Advisory Group on interstitial and rare lung diseases may continue this initiative in due course.

Alveolar microlithiasis

This is a rare ILD, characterized by the accumulation of numerous and diffuse calcified microliths (round calcium and phosphate hydroxyapatite bodies) in the alveolar space. There is no identifiable abnormality of calcium metabolism. A mutation in the *SLC34A2* gene that encodes a type IIb sodium-phosphate co-transporter in alveolar type II cells, resulting in the accumulation and formation of microliths rich in calcium phosphate (due to impaired clearance), is considered to be the cause of the disease. Microliths are occasionally identified in the sputum. At post-mortem, the lungs are heavy and rock hard, often needing a saw to cut them. Fewer than 200 cases are reported.

Clinical features
- Typically presents in young adults, most commonly in the third and fourth decades of life
- May be an incidental CXR finding in asymptomatic patients
- Familial tendency—probable autosomal recessive inheritance
- Equal sex distribution in sporadic cases, 2:1 ♀ preponderance in familial cases
- Usually slowly progressive, with progressive breathlessness, hypoxia, respiratory failure, and death
- CXR and chest CT show fine micronodular lung calcification, predominantly basally or around the hila. It may produce complete radiographic opacification. There is no associated lymph node enlargement. Progressive lung infiltration causes restriction of lung movement and impairs gas exchange, leading to progressive respiratory failure.

Treatment
- There is no effective medical treatment
- Lung transplantation has been successful.

Further information
Francisco F *et al.* Pulmonary alveolar microlithiasis. State-of-the-art review. *Respir Med* 2013;**107**:1–9.

Amyloidosis: pathophysiology and classification

Definition Amyloidosis is the extracellular deposition of low molecular weight protein molecules as insoluble fibrils. More than 20 such proteins have been described in different diseases and circumstances. For classification, see Box 49.1.

Pathophysiology The disease is one of abnormal protein folding and is classified by the origin of the precursor proteins that form the amyloid. For example, AL amyloid forms from the light chains of immunoglobulins. In familial forms, genetic missense mutations produce abnormal folding of the protein. Little is known of the specific genetic and environmental factors that lead to the development of this abnormal folding. Despite their different origins, these protein molecules fold into alternative forms that are very similar to each other; in the classic 'β-pleated sheet' structure, fibrils form in an ordered fashion, with uniformity of fibril structure within the sheet. Substitutions of particular amino acids at specific positions in the light chain variable region lead to destabilization of the light chains, increasing the chance of fibrillogenesis. In certain models, this abnormal folding can be initiated by the addition of 'amyloid-enhancing factor', rather like the initiation of crystal formation in a supersaturated solution. Amyloid deposits accumulate in the extracellular space, disrupting normal tissue architecture and leading to organ dysfunction, both directly, and having space-occupying effects. The fibrils may be directly cytotoxic (possibly by promoting apoptosis). The subdivisions of amyloid are largely based on the origin of the amyloid protein and shown in Box 49.1.

Epidemiology The epidemiology is difficult to define accurately, as the disease is often un- or misdiagnosed. The age-adjusted incidence is estimated to be 5–13 per million person years.

Future developments Anti-amyloid drugs are under investigation, including drugs to stabilize the amyloid precursor proteins in their normal configuration and enhance fibril degradation.

Box 49.1 Classification of amyloidosis

- 1°/light chain amyloid (AL), from immunoglobulin light chain fragments (λ or κ), usually monoclonal due to a plasma cell dyscrasia (a subtype of lymphoproliferative disorders)
  - 1 in 5,000 deaths due to this type of amyloid
  - Median survival is 6–15 months
  - Frank myeloma is present in 20%, and a subtle monoclonal gammopathy in 70% (MGUS)
  - Systemic form due to circulating monoclonal light chains, widespread organ involvement, particularly heart, liver, and kidneys
  - Localized amyloid production by local clonal B-cells; hence, heterogeneous organ involvement is seen, commonly in the upper respiratory tract and orbit, with urogenital and GI involvement—virtually any organ (except the brain) can be involved
- 2° amyloid (AA)
  - A complication of chronic disease with ongoing/recurring inflammation, e.g. rheumatoid, chronic infections
  - The fibrils are fragments of acute phase reactant, serum amyloid A
  - Commonly renal, hepatic, and lower GI involvement; rarely neurological, lung, and cardiac involvement
  - Median survival 5y
  - Only a small number of patients with chronic inflammation will develop AA amyloidosis, and the time period for the development of the disease is very variable
- Dialysis-related amyloid (DA), due to fibrils derived from β_2 microglobulin that accumulate in dialysis patients
- Inherited amyloidosis, e.g. due to abnormal pre-albumin (transthyretin, TTR), damaging neural and cardiac tissue
- Organ-specific amyloid such as Alzheimer's disease; plaques of the β protein derived from the larger amyloid precursor protein (APP). Protein presumed to be generated locally.

Amyloidosis: lung involvement 1

Clinically significant respiratory tract disease is almost always AL in type, though the presence of a strong family history or chronic inflammatory disease may suggest other types.

Laryngeal amyloidosis Amyloid causes up to 1% of benign laryngeal disease. May present as discrete nodules or diffuse infiltration and is usually localized, though can be a rare manifestation of systemic (AL) amyloid. Deposits are seen most commonly in the supraglottic larynx (presenting with hoarse voice or stridor). May present with choking and exertional dyspnoea that can be progressive or recurrent.

Tracheobronchial amyloid is rare (67 worldwide cases reported by the mid 1980s). Macroscopically, is either diffusely infiltrative or 'tumour-like'. It is associated with tracheobronchopathia osteoplastica (a disorder characterized by the deposition of calcified submucosal airway nodules). It presents after the fifth decade with dyspnoea, cough, and rarely haemoptysis. Airway narrowing can lead to atelectasis or recurrent pneumonia; solitary nodules may lead to investigation for presumed lung cancer. Symptomatic disease is usually localized.

Parenchymal amyloid is the most frequently diagnosed amyloid respiratory disease. It is usually divided radiologically into solitary/multiple pulmonary nodules (usually localized AL amyloid) or a diffuse alveolar pattern (usually a manifestation of systemic AL amyloid). Parenchymal amyloid lung nodules are usually peripheral and subpleural, may be bilateral, and are more common in the lower lobes, ranging in diameter from 0.4 to 15cm. They may cavitate or calcify. Clinical signs are non-diagnostic; PFTs may show a restrictive defect with reduced transfer factor. The differential diagnosis usually includes fibrosis. Cardiac amyloid may coexist, and distinguishing the contribution to the symptoms of the pulmonary and cardiac disease can be difficult. Median survival with clinically overt lung disease is about 16 months (similar to that of systemic amyloid).

Mediastinal and hilar amyloidosis are rarely associated with localized pulmonary amyloidosis, and their diagnosis should lead to a search for a systemic cause of amyloid. Amyloid lymphadenopathy can also represent localized AL deposition, in association with B-cell lymphoma.

Other Rare reports of:
• Ventilatory failure due to diaphragm or other respiratory muscle involvement
• Sleep apnoea from macroglossia due to amyloid
• Exudative pleural effusions.

Clinical features
• Dyspnoea and cough
• None—parenchymal disease may be an incidental finding on routine radiography
• Consider the diagnosis particularly in patients with odd upper airway symptoms and parenchymal involvement or those with unexplained CCF or nephrotic syndrome.

Diagnosis Histological confirmation is usually required. Congo red stain producing 'apple green' birefringence in crossed polarized light is the gold standard. Positive histology must lead to immunohistochemistry to determine the fibril type.

- *Histology* TBB or occasionally open or VATS biopsy (more likely if investigation for solitary pulmonary nodule)
- *123I-labelled scintigraphy* Radiolabelled serum amyloid P (SAP) localizes to amyloid deposits in proportion to the quantity of amyloid present, therefore allowing identification of the distribution and burden of disease. It is most sensitive for solid organ disease though, in lung disease, is useful for determining the extent of disease in other organs. It is, however, expensive and carries an infection risk, as the SAP component is currently obtained from blood donors
- *HRCT* may show nodules or parenchymal disease
- *Laryngoscopy and bronchoscopy* may be needed to obtain samples for histology, depending on the clinical presentation
- *PFTs* to assess the effect of disease on respiratory function. May show reduced transfer factor and a restrictive pattern. Tracheobronchial involvement may lead to abnormal flow–volume loops due to larger airway obstruction
- Systemic disease:
  - FBC, biochemistry, and urinalysis (?renal involvement)
  - Investigate for underlying blood cell dyscrasia, e.g. myeloma, Waldenström's macroglobulinaemia (bone marrow examination, and search for urine and serum monoclonal protein by immunofixation—the clonal proliferation underlying systemic AL amyloid is usually very subtle, and its identification may be difficult)
  - Echo for associated cardiac involvement (when CCF is present; survival is 4–6 months)
  - Thyroid/adrenal function is impaired in up to 10%.

Amyloidosis: lung involvement 2

Treatment There are limited clinical trials with which to guide management of respiratory tract amyloid. Management decisions are therefore often made empirically.

- No treatment may be needed
- Local measures may be warranted for endobronchial disease, e.g. symptomatic laryngeal disease—endoscopic excision, CO_2 laser evaporation (useful for small recurrent lesions), stenting. Steroids have no effect on laryngeal amyloid
- Tracheobronchial amyloid—management depends on symptoms, and treatment may involve repeated endoscopic resection, YAG (yttrium–aluminium–garnet) laser therapy, and surgical resection. Repeated endoscopic procedures are thought to be safer than repeated open surgery
- Chemotherapy may be warranted for diffuse parenchymal amyloid if there is objectively measurable disease (prednisolone and melphalan to suppress the underlying blood cell dyscrasia). More intensive chemotherapy has a better clinical response, but there are few trials.

Further information

Blancas-Mejia LM, Ramirez-Alvarado M. Systemic amyloidoses. *Annu Rev Biochem* 2013;**82**:745–74.
Gillmore JD, Hawkins PN. Amyloidosis and the respiratory tract. Rare diseases. *Thorax* 1999;**54**:444–51.

Hereditary haemorrhagic telangiectasia

(HHT; also referred to as Osler–Weber–Rendu syndrome)
Prevalence: 1 in 5,000–8,000.

Definition

An autosomal dominant disorder, >80% of all cases of HHT are due to mutations in either *ENG* or *ACVRL1* (endoglin and activin, both TGF-β1 receptors). A total of over 600 different mutations is known. It is characterized by the development of abnormal dilated vessels in the systemic circulation, which may bleed, leading to:

- Recurrent epistaxis
- GI bleeding
- Iron deficiency anaemia
- Other organ involvement, e.g. hepatic (in 30%, commonly asymptomatic), renal, pulmonary, and spinal AVMs.

Screening Careful questioning of family members (does anyone in the family have frequent nose bleeds?) and examination for telangiectasia should reveal those in whom screening should occur.

All those with HHT should be screened for pulmonary AVMs (PAVMs; see ➔ pp. 636–7), and all of their offspring post-puberty and pre-pregnancy. There is increasing penetrance with increasing age (62% at age 16, 95% at age 40). Similarly, the detection of PAVMs in a patient should lead to screening for HHT in family members.

There is no consensus regarding the best screening method, but a combination of the following tests may be used:

- CXR
- Supine and erect oximetry
- CT chest
- Shunt quantification techniques, e.g. contrast echo, 100% O_2 rebreathing.

Screening should continue throughout life (every 5–10y) and during times of enlargement or development of AVMs—post-puberty and pre-pregnancy.

Management

- Usually involves liaison with ENT and gastroenterology colleagues for symptomatic treatment
- Iron replacement, transfusions
- Asymptomatic hepatic AVMs—no treatment usually required
- Cerebral AVMs (in 15% of HHT patients)—some specialists argue these should be treated prophylactically due to the risk of rupture and bleeding (2%/y, often fatal).

Further information

Shovlin CL, Letarte M. Hereditary haemorrhagic telangectiasa and pulmonary AVMs: issues in clinical management and review of pathogenic mechanisms. *Thorax* 1999;**54**:714–39.

Idiopathic pulmonary haemosiderosis

A rare disease of undetermined aetiology, characterized by recurrent episodes of alveolar haemorrhage and haemoptysis (in the absence of renal disease), usually leading to iron deficiency anaemia.

Pathophysiology The alveolar space and interstitium contain haemosiderin-laden macrophages, with variable degrees of interstitial fibrosis and degeneration of alveolar, interstitial, and vascular elastic fibres, depending on the chronicity of the condition. Electron microscopy shows damage to the endothelial and basement membranes, but no consistent or diagnostic features have been recognized.

No antibodies have been identified, though serum IgA levels are sometimes raised. With recurrent alveolar haemorrhage, the alveolar blood provokes a fibrotic reaction, with the development of diffuse pulmonary fibrosis.

Iron turnover studies show that the accompanying iron deficiency anaemia is due to loss of iron into the lung through haemorrhage.

Aetiology is uncertain but likely to be multifactorial. Possible associations include toxic insecticides (epidemiological studies in rural Greece), premature birth, and fungal toxin exposure. The disease has an equal sex incidence in childhood, with twice as many men affected in adulthood.

Most patients present in childhood, with 85% of cases having onset of symptoms before 16y. The actual prevalence is unknown, but a cohort study of Swedish children in the 1960s described an incidence of 0.24 per million children. Familial clustering is reported.

Pulmonary haemosiderosis is associated with RA, thyrotoxicosis, coeliac disease, and autoimmune haemolytic anaemia, suggesting a potential autoimmune mechanism.

Clinical features The clinical course is very variable and ranges from continuous low-level bleeding to massive pulmonary haemorrhage. The latter may be fatal but is fortunately rare.
- Continuous mild pulmonary haemorrhage leads to a chronic non-productive cough with haemoptysis, malaise, lethargy, and failure to thrive in children
- Iron deficiency anaemia is common, as are positive faecal occult blood tests (due to swallowed blood)
- Generalized lymphadenopathy and hepatosplenomegaly are recognized
- With an acute bleed, cough and haemoptysis may worsen, and dyspnoea, chest tightness, and pyrexia may develop
- Chronic bleeding leads to chronic disabling dyspnoea, chronic anaemia, and clubbing (in 25%). Cor pulmonale 2° to pulmonary fibrosis and hypoxaemia may develop.

Examination may be normal. Clubbing, basal crepitations, and cor pulmonale are all recognized, depending on the severity of the resulting lung disease.

Investigations The diagnosis is one of exclusion, with no evidence of other organ involvement. The main differential diagnosis is Goodpasture's syndrome, GPA, SLE, and microscopic polyarteritis.

- *Blood tests* Microcytic, hypochromic anaemia, with low iron levels. ANCA, dsDNA, and anti-GBM antibodies should be negative
- *CXR* May show transient patchy infiltrates, which worsen during an acute bleed. The apices are usually spared. Progressive disease leads to the development of reticulonodular infiltrates and a ground-glass appearance that is typically perihilar or in the lower zones. Hilar lymphadenopathy may be seen
- *PFTs* kCO is transiently elevated during bleeding episodes ($\geq$130% is abnormal), but this is only useful acutely. A restrictive defect with reduced kCO may develop with chronic disease
- *CT chest* The changes seen are fairly non-specific, showing a diffuse bilateral infiltrate, with patchy ground-glass change
- *BAL* (if done) contains haemosiderin-laden macrophages.

Management

There is no specific treatment.

- Steroids and immunosuppressive drugs (e.g. cyclophosphamide) may be of benefit during acute bleeding episodes but do not appear to affect the long-term outcome. There are no published data to guide the optimal timing of treatment during the course of disease
- The iron deficiency anaemia responds to replacement therapy, and blood transfusion may be needed in severe bleeds
- Lung transplant has been tried.

At routine clinic appointments
- Check spirometry
- Measure Hb and serum iron levels
- Ask about increases in SOB or haemoptysis.

Prognosis The prognosis is very variable, with some patients showing spontaneous remission, others progressing to death. The duration of disease in the literature ranges from death within days, following an acute severe illness, to survival with cor pulmonale associated with chronic disease after 20y.

Langerhans cell histiocytosis

Definition Pulmonary Langerhans cell histiocytosis (LCH; previously termed pulmonary histiocytosis X or pulmonary eosinophilic granuloma) is a rare condition characterized by infiltration of the lung with histiocytes (Langerhans cells). Pulmonary LCH overlaps with a number of other conditions with similar pathological findings but diverse clinical features. These range from localized infiltration of a single organ (e.g. eosinophilic granuloma of bone) to systemic diseases affecting multiple organs (Letterer–Siwe disease, a multi-organ disease affecting infants and elderly, associated with poor prognosis; also Hand–Schueller–Christian syndrome). Although the isolated pulmonary form most commonly presents to chest physicians, pulmonary manifestations also commonly occur in the systemic forms of the disease.

Epidemiology Rare, it tends to affect young adults aged 20–40y. The vast majority of cases occur in current smokers, usually heavy smokers (tobacco and cannabis). May be more common in men, who tend to present at a younger age than women.

Pathogenesis Langerhans cells are involved in antigen presentation and are characterized by the presence of well-demarcated cytoplasmic organelles called Birbeck granules on electron microscopy. The Langerhans cells seen in LCH appear to be monoclonal, although it is unclear if this represents a true neoplastic process. The antigen stimulus for activating Langerhans cells in the lung is unknown, although cigarette smoke is a possible candidate. Langerhans cells are typically organized into granulomata that are located in bronchiolar walls and subsequently enlarge and invade adjacent structures. This results in the radiological appearance of nodules that, at first, cavitate and then become cystic.

Clinical features Typically exertional breathlessness and cough, sometimes with systemic symptoms (e.g. fever, weight loss). Pneumothorax occurs in at least 10% of patients and may be the presenting feature. Rib lesions may also give rise to chest pain. Around 25% of patients are asymptomatic. Examination is usually normal.

Investigations

- *CXR* Typically diffuse reticulonodular shadowing, sometimes with cystic change; upper and middle lobe predominance. May be normal
- *HRCT* Diffuse centrilobular nodules, sometimes with cavitation, and thin- and thick-walled cystic lesions, reflecting lesions of varying age. These are interspersed with normal lung. Upper and middle lobe predominance; costophrenic angles are typically spared. Purely nodular or purely cystic appearances may occur. Unusual manifestations, such as single nodules or large airways involvement, are also described
- *PFTs* Variable, ranging from normal to obstructive, restricted, or mixed patterns. Reduced gas transfer and exertional hypoxia are common
- *TBB* may yield diagnostic material although is often unhelpful; risk of pneumothorax is unknown although may be increased. Surgical lung biopsy is often preferable

- *BAL* Increased total cell counts and pigmented macrophages, reflecting simply the presence of cigarette smoking. Use of antibodies (e.g. OKT6) to detect Langerhans cells in BAL fluid is limited by poor sensitivity
- *Extrathoracic biopsy* of involved sites (e.g. bone) may be diagnostic.

Diagnosis Usually based on the combination of clinical and HRCT findings: typically a young adult smoker with cysts and nodules on HRCT. Confirmation by surgical lung biopsy may be considered in atypical presentations such as the finding of solely nodular or cystic disease on HRCT. The appearance of purely cystic disease on HRCT may be confused with emphysema (where cysts lack walls) or LAM (where cysts are present uniformly in all regions of lung, including the costophrenic angles).

Associations

- Severe PHT—may be seen in the absence of significant parenchymal lung involvement; direct disease involvement of pulmonary vessels has been described
- Manifestations of systemic LCH—particularly diabetes insipidus from pituitary disease, skin involvement, lytic bony lesions, and rarely cardiac or GI disease
- Lymphoma—may precede, complicate, or coexist with pulmonary LCH
- Lung cancer—more common, probably as a result of cigarette smoking.

Management Treatment, other than smoking cessation, is often not required and may be entirely successful with resolution of radiographic abnormalities. Oral corticosteroids may be tried in symptomatic disease, although there is little evidence to support their use; they are usually administered for at least 6 months. Lung transplantation should be considered in patients with severe respiratory failure or PHT. Pulmonary LCH may recur in transplanted lungs. Experimental treatments, such as the use of IL2 and anti-TNF-α, may be of benefit in the systemic forms of LCH seen in children.

Prognosis is variable. Spontaneous improvement is common, although later reactivation of disease may occur. A minority of patients deteriorate rapidly, with respiratory failure and death within months. Overall life expectancy is reduced, with median survival 12–13y from diagnosis. Death is most commonly due to respiratory failure. Poor prognostic factors include reduced FEV_1, increased RV, and reduced gas transfer.

Further information

Sundar KM *et al.* Pulmonary Langerhans cell histiocytosis. *Chest* 2003;**123**:1673–83.
Patient support group. ℘ http://www.hrtrust.org.

Lymphangioleiomyomatosis (LAM): clinical features

Definition and aetiology A rare disorder characterized by abnormal proliferation of smooth muscle cells, affecting women of childbearing age, usually in their 30s. The disease is hormone-dependent so can occur in post-menopausal women on oestrogen replacement therapy.
- Incidence of 1 in 1.1 million population
- 40% of adult women with tuberous sclerosis (learning difficulties, subungual fibromas, seizures, facial angiofibromas, autosomal dominant inheritance or spontaneous mutation) develop pulmonary changes identical to those of LAM.

Pathology Abnormal proliferation of atypical smooth muscle cells (LAM cells) throughout the lung, airways, blood vessels, and lymphatics. There is nodular infiltration, which is initially subtle. Progressive growth causes lymphatic and airway obstruction, leading to cyst formation throughout the lungs. The infiltrating cells stain with antibodies to smooth muscle actin and desmin with HMB-45, an antibody that recognizes an epitope within the protein gp-100 in the melanogenesis pathway. LAM is caused by mutations in the tuberous sclerosis (*TSC*) genes, resulting in activation of the mTOR complex 1 signalling network. Inactivation of both alleles of *TSC2* seems to be necessary.

Clinical features

Common
- 2° pneumothorax (in two-thirds of patients; occurs due to lung cystic change; recurrence is common)
- Dyspnoea (in 42%) and cough (in 20%)
- Haemoptysis (in 14%)
- Chylothorax (in 12%, thoracic duct leakage as a result of lymphatic obstruction by LAM cells, may be bilateral).

Less common
- Pleural effusion
- Chest pain
- Pulmonary haemorrhage (due to blocked blood vessels and increased intraluminal pressure).

Other organs affected

Kidney Angiomyolipoma, a benign tumour, occurs in 50% of LAM patients. Usually diagnosed on CT, these are mostly small and single but can be multiple and larger in tuberous sclerosis. Smaller tumours are usually asymptomatic, but larger ones can cause flank pain and bleeding into the renal tract. Treatment options include tumour resection or embolization. Nephrectomy is not usually required. Screening for these lesions is important, as it allows careful treatment planning in case they become symptomatic.

Abdomen Lymphadenopathy due to lymphatic obstruction. Occurs in one-third of patients and is usually asymptomatic.

Pelvis Lymphangioleiomyoma—a cystic mass that enlarges during the day and causes fullness and bloating.

Chylous ascites can occur in the absence of chylothorax.

Skin Cutaneous swellings, likely due to localized oedema.

Examination May be normal. There may be pulmonary crepitations or signs of pleural effusion. Palpable abdominal masses may be present.

Investigations

- *PFTs* may be normal or show a predominantly obstructive pattern. Rarely restrictive. Decreased TLCO, with a normal or increased TLC
- *CXR* may be normal. Lungs may appear hyperinflated, with reticular shadowing and septal lines due to obstructed lymphatics. There may also be a diffuse interstitial infiltrate
- *HRCT* shows a characteristic appearance, with multiple cysts throughout the lung of varying size, which are usually small (<1cm) and thin-walled. The adjoining lung parenchyma is normal. There may be pleural effusions
- *CT abdomen* to examine for presence of angiomyolipomas and other lymphatic involvement.

LAM: diagnosis and management

Diagnosis Consider particularly in young or middle-aged women with:
• Recurrent pneumothoraces, especially those with pre-existing dyspnoea or haemoptysis
• Cystic lung disease, airflow obstruction, or chylous pleural effusions
• Angiomyolipomas or other retroperitoneal tumours
• Tuberous sclerosis and respiratory symptoms.

The disease is easily missed in its early stages. The diagnosis can be made on the characteristic CT appearances or with open lung biopsy. TBBs may not be diagnostic. Large retroperitoneal abdominal lymph nodes can also be biopsied.

Management The course of LAM is variable. Treatment should be aimed at those who are symptomatic and declining.
• Refer to a specialist centre (Nottingham City Hospital in the UK).
• *Diet* Low-fat diet with medium-chain triglyceride supplementation may prevent chylothorax recurrence; no strong evidence for this, difficult diet to follow
• *Bronchodilators* may improve airflow obstruction
• *Sirolimus* shown to stabilize lung function and improve QoL and is recommended treatment
• *Hormonal manipulation* with progesterone has been tried. It may be beneficial in reducing the decline in FEV_1 and TLCO, particularly in patients with progressive disease, but there are no large studies. Tamoxifen and oophorectomy have also been tried
• *Avoid oestrogens*, i.e. the OCP and HRT
• *Contraception* An increase in symptoms and accelerated disease decline are reported in pregnancy. Use the progesterone-only pill
• *Pleural aspiration* when required for pleural effusions. For recurrent effusions or chylothoraces, thoracic duct ligation or pleurectomy may be effective. Pleurodesis can be performed, but this is relatively contraindicated if future lung transplant is an option
• *Recurrent pneumothoraces* Advise regarding flying and diving. Thoracic surgery may be necessary
• *Avoid air travel*, if possible, due to risk of pneumothorax
• *Transplant* Single (usually) or double lung, or heart-lung. LAM can recur in the transplanted lung
• *Stop smoking*, as this accelerates the rate of decline
• Influenza vaccine.

Prognosis is very variable. The condition usually slowly progresses to respiratory failure. At 10y, 55% of patients have MRC grade 3 dyspnoea, 23% are on LTOT, and 10% are housebound. Survival: 70% of patients are alive at 10y, 33% are alive at 15y, and 25% are alive at 20y.

Further information

Henske EP, McCormack FX. Lymphangioleiomyomatosis—a wolf in sheep's clothing. *J Clin Invest* 2012;**122**:3807–16.
Patient support group. ℘ http://www.lamaction.org.

Primary ciliary dyskinesia (PCD)

Clinical features

Confirm the diagnosis

Primary ciliary dyskinesia (PCD)

A rare genetic cause of chronic respiratory disease, usually encountered in adult respiratory clinics as a cause of bronchiectasis. Cilia are found in:
* The whole length of the upper respiratory tract
* Brain ventricles
* Fallopian tube/ductus epididymis.

They are made up of dynein arms, with outer and inner connecting rings, and beat at 14 beats/s. Many gene defects have been identified in PCD, causing a number of cilial abnormalities.

Abnormal cilia do not beat normally, leading to reduced mucociliary clearance, microbiological colonization (which further inhibits cilial action), chronic infection, and the development of bronchiectasis.

The main aim following diagnosis in childhood is the prevention of chronic respiratory disease and bronchiectasis.

Clinical features
* Autosomal recessive, >200 phenotypes
* May present with neonatal respiratory distress
* Situs inversus (in about 30%, as cilia determine the side of the organs. Random organ siting occurs with cilial dysfunction, hence the situs inversus of Kartagener's syndrome)
* Nasal blockage/rhinitis
* Persistent wet cough in childhood
* Hearing problems/history of glue ear/grommets in childhood
* Clubbing and signs of chest disease are rare in childhood
* Wheeze in 20%
* Infertility due to immotile sperm (sperm tails have same morphological defect as the cilia and do not beat correctly)
* In adults, the disease usually presents with the clinical signs of bronchiectasis: cough productive of purulent sputum, recurrent chest infections, intermittent haemoptysis.

Diagnosis Saccharin test (see ➲ pp. 156–7). Nasal NO is very low in PCD (possibly because NO mediates ciliary function); this is the most sensitive and specific screening test. Cilial biopsy via the nasal route. Cilia are examined by high-speed digital video where their beat frequency and pattern can be assessed, confirming the diagnosis. Most cases of PCD are diagnosed in childhood. There is an increased frequency in the children of consanguineous marriages.

Consider the diagnosis in:
* Bronchiectasis
* Situs inversus
* Persistent upper and lower respiratory infection from early childhood
* Infertility—♂ may present in infertility clinics.

Management

A national service for the diagnosis of PCD was set up in 2007, with three centres—London (Royal Brompton), Southampton, and Leicester.

In adults, this includes the treatment of 2° bronchiectasis (see ➡ pp. 158–9), with:
- Antibiotics
- Physiotherapy
- Vaccinations
- Management of haemoptysis.

Further information

Bush A, Hogg C. Primary ciliary dyskinesia: recent advances in epidemiology, diagnosis, management and relationship with the expanding spectrum of ciliopathy. *Expert Rev Respir Med* 2012;6:663–82.
Patient support group. ℰ http://www.pcdsupport.org.uk.

Pulmonary alveolar proteinosis (PAP): pathophysiology and clinical features

PAP, also referred to as alveolar lipoproteinosis, is a rare alveolar filling defect affecting around 3 per million people. There is a limited published literature: five reported case series of ≥10 cases, and only 410 total cases reported.

Pathophysiology PAP is due to failure of alveolar macrophages to clear spent surfactant, leading to the filling of alveoli with a phospholipid proteinaceous material. It is thought that the defect has an autoimmune basis and, in the idiopathic form, is due to the presence of antibodies to granulocyte-macrophage colony-stimulating factor (GM-CSF), which cause inhibition of normal alveolar macrophage function, leading to abnormalities of surfactant homeostasis. Defects in GM-CSF signalling have been identified in animal models. Congenital disease is thought to be due to mutations in surfactant gene proteins. Other mechanisms for surfactant accumulation have also been identified:

- *Heavy dust exposure* leads to surfactant hypersecretion, which exceeds the lungs' normal clearance mechanism. Animal models have shown that this condition develops from endogenous lipoid pneumonia, with the accumulation of lipid-laden macrophages, which break down to release surfactant
- *Amphiphilic drugs*, e.g. amiodarone, chlorphentermine
- *Lymphoma, leukaemia, and immunosuppression* The mechanism is uncertain, but it is thought that the lipoprotein may be generated from degenerating alveolar cells.

Appearances similar to alveolar lipoproteinosis may also be seen in endogenous lipoid pneumonia resulting from bronchial obstruction and are described in surfactant-secreting alveolar cell carcinoma.

Histology The alveoli are filled with a granular acellular eosinophilic PAS (periodic acid–Schiff)-positive deposit. Cholesterol clefts and large foamy macrophages may also be seen. The alveolar architecture is usually well preserved. Surfactant protein can be identified using immunohistochemistry. Electron microscopy shows multiple osmiophilic bodies, consistent with denatured surfactant.

Epidemiology

- Presents aged 30–50 (case reports in children and the elderly)
- ♂:♀ ≈ 4:1
- Increased incidence in smokers
- Rare familial cases reported.

Clinical features

- Typically presents with breathlessness and a non-productive cough. Examination may be normal, or crackles may be heard on auscultation. Clubbing in one-third
- May present with superadded infection, causing an apparent acute onset of symptoms, in association with fever
- Median duration of symptoms before diagnosis is 7 months
- Opportunistic infection is the major complication, most commonly *Nocardia* species, fungi, and mycobacteria. This occurs due to impaired macrophage function and impaired host defence due to surfactant accumulation.

PAP: diagnosis and treatment

Diagnosis is usually made on the basis of a characteristic CT appearance, although other tests may also be useful.

- Raised serum LDH
- *ABGs* Hypoxia and increased A–a gradient
- *PFTs* Restrictive defect, with reduced lung volumes and transfer factor
- *CXR* Bilateral consolidation with thickened interlobular septa. Usually bilateral. The pattern is very variable and, in up to 50%, may be perihilar (bat-wing appearance)
- *CT* appearance is characteristic, with airspace shadowing in a geographical distribution, alternating with areas of normal lung, the so-called 'crazy paving' pattern. This CT appearance is not specific to alveolar proteinosis but is also seen in lipoid pneumonia and bronchoalveolar cell carcinoma
- *BAL* reveals milky washings. Identification of antibodies to GM-CSF in BAL washings is diagnostic. Cytological examination shows a granular extracellular deposit with foamy macrophages and cellular debris
- *Transbronchial/open lung biopsies* when CT is not characteristic.

Treatment of choice is repeated therapeutic whole lung lavage, which should be performed at a specialist centre. There are no RCTs of this treatment, but there is evidence of efficacy in terms of subsequent improvement of symptoms, physiology, and radiology.

- The indication for whole lung lavage is usually breathlessness, limiting activities of daily living
- The procedure is done under general anaesthesia using 100% O_2 and one-lung ventilation using a double-lumen tube. Repeated warm saline lavage using a closed circuit continues until the bronchial washing returns are clear—this may take up to 40L lavage. One or both lungs may be treated at a time
- The response is variable—some patients need only one treatment; others may need multiple treatments, and about 10% fail to respond
- May be done on bypass if the patient is very hypoxic
- Characteristic milky lavage fluid is obtained
- Granulocyte colony-stimulating factor (SC injections) is a novel treatment option (only phase II studies, no RCT yet), which may prevent progression of disease
- There is no benefit from treatment with steroids, and they may exacerbate opportunistic infections.

Prognosis with whole lung lavage is generally good. Spontaneous remission occurs in one-third; one-third remains stable, and one-third progresses to respiratory failure and death. There are reports of progression to pulmonary fibrosis (which may be a coincidental occurrence).

Further information

Patel SM et al. Pulmonary alveolar proteinosis. *Can Respir J* 2012;**19**:243–5.
Patient website. ℅ http://www.papfoundation.org (USA).

Pulmonary arteriovenous malformations (PAVMs): aetiology and diagnosis

Aetiology

- PAVMs are abnormal blood vessels replacing normal capillaries, making a direct low-resistance connection between the pulmonary arterial and systemic venous circulations. They vary in size, from tiny clusters of vessels (telangiectasia) to larger, more complex aneurysmal-type sacs
- The disorder is rare, affecting 1 in 15,000–24,000
- Several genetic susceptibility loci have been identified on Chr 9 and Chr 12. One identified mutation is in the endoglin gene. This modulates signalling via the TGF-β family of growth factors. This gene is also implicated in the development of PPH
- Subjects with significant PAVMs have low pulmonary vascular resistance, a low mean PAP, and a high cardiac output—due to long-standing adaptive mechanisms to the effects of the shunt, in addition to vascular remodelling effects
- Most patients present post-puberty, as AVMs probably develop at this time. They probably grow throughout life, especially during puberty and in pregnancy. They may rarely regress spontaneously.

Diagnosis

- Most patients present with an abnormal *CXR*, classically showing a smooth, rounded intrapulmonary mass, with draining or feeding vessels
- Mild *hypoxaemia* An AVM is a direct communication between the pulmonary artery and pulmonary vein. Blood therefore bypasses the pulmonary capillary bed, with reduced oxygenation, which poorly corrects with supplementary O_2
- *Orthodeoxia* is desaturation on standing, due to an increase in blood flow in the dependent lung areas. 70% of PAVMs are basal, hence the desaturation seen
- *CT* identifies all AVMs and can determine those suitable for embolization. Contrast is not required
- Patients may present with the complications of a PAVM, particularly bleeding or peripheral abscess formation. The absence of a normal filtering capillary bed means small particles can reach the systemic circulation, leading to sequelae, particularly in the cerebral circulation—strokes and cerebral abscesses. These abnormal vessels are also at risk of rupture.

Shunt quantification

- *100% O_2 rebreathing study*, a non-invasive method of shunt quantification
- *^{99m}TC perfusion scan*, a tracer study; the size of the shunt can be assessed from the proportion of radiolabelled macro-aggregates reaching the systemic circulation, compared with the total number injected. In a normal study, aggregates accumulate in the kidneys
- *Contrast echo* to measure the circulatory transit time of injected echo contrast

- *Angiography* at specialist centre only
- In normal individuals, the anatomical shunt is <2–3.5% of the cardiac output (due to post-pulmonary drainage of bronchial veins into pulmonary vein and drainage into the left atrium).

Clinical features

- Asymptomatic (50%)
- Dyspnoea
- Haemoptysis (10%), probably due to additional bronchial telangiectasia, which can also cause haemorrhage into bronchi or the pleural cavity
- Chest pain (12%); aetiology is uncertain
- Clubbing
- Cyanosis
- Orthodeoxia
- Vascular bruits
- Telangiectasia; 80% of PAVM patients have HHT, and their families should be screened because of the risk of stroke (see p. 621)
- May present with acute stroke, with focal neurological signs.

PAVMs: management and complications

Management

Embolization is usually done with coils, which generate local thrombin, leading to cessation of blood flow in AVM feeding vessels. This results in a reduction in the right-to-left shunt and improvement in hypoxaemia and should be done by an expert in a specialist centre only. The small risk of neurological sequelae and angina/arrhythmias is reduced with operator experience.

60–70% of patients are left with a small persisting shunt following treatment and retain a small risk of abscess formation. Patients are therefore given prophylactic antibiotics for dental and surgical procedures (ensure the patient has a MedicAlert card).

Surgical resection may be more appropriate than embolization in some cases.

Antiplatelet therapy (rarely) in individual cases, if ongoing transient ischaemic attacks.

Transplantation is not advised, as there is no increased survival benefit over medical treatment.

Screening—the majority of patients with PAVMs have HHT, and so screening of family members is important.

Follow-up—all patients need regular follow-up, with shunt assessment post-surgical resection or embolization, as removal of one shunt may unmask or provoke the development of others.

♀ *patients* should be advised to defer pregnancy until completion of formal assessment because of the risks of growth and rupture of PAVMs in pregnancy (see Complications).

Complications

- PAVM patients never die of respiratory failure in the absence of additional respiratory disease
- All patients are at risk of stroke and cerebral abscesses
- Transient ischaemic attack/stroke (in 25%) due to rupture of abnormal capillaries in aneurysms
- Abscess (in 10%) due to paradoxical emboli, through the right-to-left shunt, and the absence of a filtering capillary bed.

Pregnancy is associated with an increase in size of AVMs, and new ones may develop, with potentially catastrophic consequences. Careful shunt assessment is therefore needed prior to pregnancy, with contraceptive advice prior to specialist assessment. Close liaison between the specialist centre and obstetric team is paramount. AVMs may need embolization in the third trimester to allow safe delivery.

Further information

Shovlin CL. Hereditary haemorrhagic telangiectasis: pathophysiology, diagnosis and treatment. *Blood Rev* 2010;24:203–19.

Recurrent respiratory papillomatosis

These are essentially warts of the upper respiratory tract, caused by the human papillomavirus (HPV 6 or 11). The virus infects epithelial cells and mucous membranes, similar to that seen in cutaneous and anogenital infection. The infection is most commonly acquired during ororespiratory exposure from the mother during vaginal delivery and typically presents in childhood from 6 months onwards, with signs and symptoms of URTI. It may also present for the first time in adulthood. It is associated with HLA-DR3 and with sexual transmission in adults. Recurrent respiratory papillomatosis is rare (2 per 100,000), but oral HPV infection is common.

Clinical course

This is variable.
- May remit spontaneously
- Progressive voice loss and airway obstruction
- Most cases are confined to the larynx, although up to 25% of patients subsequently develop extralaryngeal spread to the bronchial tree
- 1% have malignant change to squamous cell carcinomas.

Management

- Surgical excision to maintain airway patency
- Laser therapy—but potential problems of thermal injury, stricture formation, and spread of papillomas
- PDT reduces recurrence rate, using oral or IV photosensitizing agent, then a laser to destroy photosensitive tissue
- Microdebrider is now used more commonly
- Medical treatment—interferon, aciclovir, ribavirin, isotretinoin, and methotrexate have all been tried
  - *Interferon alfa* as a daily SC injection leads to complete remission in 30–50%, and partial resolution in 30%. One-third recur when treatment is stopped. Adverse reactions are common: flu-like symptoms, deranged LFTs, leucopenia, and alopecia
  - *Cidofovir* is a nucleoside monophosphate analogue and inhibits viral polymerase. It is given as an intralesional injection. Theoretical side effects include nephrotoxicity and neutropenia but have not been seen in practice.

Further information

Pian T et al. Safety of intralesional cidofovir in patients with recurrent respiratory papillomatosis. *Eur Arch Otorrhinolaryngol* 2013;**270**:1679–87.

Chapter 50

Upper airway diseases

Acute upper airway obstruction

Presentation Sudden respiratory distress with cyanosis and aphonia. Airway obstruction can occur at any level within the airway. Partial airway obstruction leads to noisy breathing, with stridor, gurgling, or snoring. Complete airway obstruction is associated with distress and marked respiratory effort, with paradoxical chest and abdominal movement ('seesaw breathing') and use of accessory muscles of respiration. This may be followed by collapse with loss of consciousness and progress to cardiorespiratory arrest. Look for chest and abdominal movements, and listen and feel for airflow at the nose and mouth.

Causes

- Pharyngeal occlusion by tongue and other upper airway muscles, 2° to loss of muscle tone. This may be 2° to drugs, alcohol, a neurological event, or cardiorespiratory arrest
- Vomit or blood
- Inhaled foreign body, which may also cause laryngeal spasm
- Laryngeal obstruction due to oedema from burns, inflammation, or anaphylaxis
- Excessive bronchial secretions, mucosal oedema, bronchospasm: may cause airway obstruction below the larynx
- Infection such as epiglottitis
- Any cause of chronic airway obstruction, such as an airway tumour or extrinsic compression due to tumour or lymphadenopathy, may deteriorate precipitously.

▶▶ Management of upper airway obstruction

Call for senior anaesthetic help early

- Open the airway with backwards head tilt, chin lift, and forward jaw thrust. In cases of trauma, do not tilt the head in case of cervical spine injury, but perform a jaw thrust only
- If unsuccessful at restoring normal respiration, visually inspect the mouth for obvious obstruction, and remove it with a finger sweep. Leave well-fitting dentures in place
- If there is a witnessed history of choking, consider performing the Heimlich manoeuvre to dislodge the particle (firm and rapid pressure applied beneath the diaphragm in an upwards movement), or directly visualize the airway with a laryngoscope, and use McGill's forceps to remove the particle or with bronchoscope and the use of biopsy forceps
- If the patient is breathing, consider inserting an airway to maintain patency: oropharyngeal (Guedel) or nasopharyngeal. Maintain oxygenation, using mask with reservoir bag, delivering 10–15L/min. If there is no spontaneous respiratory effort, insert a laryngeal mask or endotracheal tube, and deliver O_2 via self-inflating bag with supplemental O_2 10 L/min and reservoir bag. If not breathing and cannot be ventilated, a cricothyroidotomy may be necessary (see ➲ pp. 770–1)
- Suction out secretions
- Maintain circulation with cardiac compression, if necessary
- Seek definitive treatment for the cause of airway obstruction, as appropriate.

Heliox Helium–O_2 mixtures can be used for patients with airway obstruction, often due to tumour compression or invasion. Helium has a lower density than nitrogen and can improve airflow, and, when used with O_2, ventilation rapidly improves and work of breathing is decreased. It can be used as an interim measure until more definitive management is available, such as radiotherapy, or to allow time for radiotherapy to take effect. The evidence relating to its use is mainly case studies, with no RCTs. Doses used = 80:20 or 70:30 helium to O_2 ratio; optimum dose unclear. Use the highest helium ratio which keeps O_2 saturations >90%. If it works, it will be effective within minutes.

Nebulized adrenaline may also be helpful in upper airway obstruction, especially laryngeal oedema (dose 1mL of 1:1,000 made up to 5mL with NaCl 0.9%). This is only a stabilizing measure to buy time until definitive treatment is available.

Anaphylaxis

▶▶ *This is a life-threatening medical emergency. Call for help.*

Causes IgE-mediated type I hypersensitivity reaction to allergen. Histamine release causes the clinical syndrome. Typical allergens include bee or wasp sting, peanuts, fish, drugs, foods, latex, contrast media, muscle relaxants, anaesthetic agents. Incidence of anaphylaxis is increasing.

Presentation Typically a rapid onset of symptoms of varying severity:
• Angio-oedema
• Urticaria
• Dyspnoea
• Wheeze
• Stridor
• Hypotension
• Arrhythmias
• Also rhinitis, abdominal pain, vomiting, diarrhoea, sense of impending doom.

Symptoms typically resolve within minutes to hours. It is not clear what determines severity of anaphylaxis in individuals. Asthma and cardiovascular disease are important comorbidities that carry a worse prognosis in anaphylaxis. Patient may have had previous episodes of severe allergic-type reactions. May need in-hospital observation for 6–12h.
• *Biphasic anaphylaxis* is a further episode, typically within 10h, after the initial anaphylaxis seems to have resolved, without further allergen exposure
• *Protracted anaphylaxis* lasts for hours or days.

▶▶ Management of anaphylaxis
• Remove likely allergen
• Cardiopulmonary resuscitation if necessary
• *Airway and breathing* Administer high-flow O_2 through non-rebreathe mask. If airway obstruction present, consider tracheal intubation. Airway swelling may make this difficult, and cricothyroidotomy may need to be performed (see ➲ pp. 770–1)
• *Circulation* Give adrenaline (epinephrine) IM 1:1,000 solution 0.5mL (500 micrograms). Repeat after 5min if no improvement or deterioration
• In those with profound shock and immediately life-threatening anaphylaxis, such as during anaesthesia, or those with no pulse, IV adrenaline can be given slowly, 100 micrograms/min or 1mL of 1:10,000 solution/min. Stop as soon as there is a response. This can be hazardous and needs cardiac monitoring
• IV fluids if hypotension persists: 1–2L rapidly infused
• Antihistamines, such as chlorphenamine 10mg slow IV or IM, for itch and urticaria
• Consider steroids: 100mg hydrocortisone slow IV or IM
• Consider nebulized salbutamol or adrenaline if bronchospasm
• On discharge, provide IM self-administered adrenaline and advise on future episodes, medicalert bracelet, and card
• Offer allergy service/immunology referral
• Consider C1 esterase inhibitor deficiency, especially if repeated episodes.

Subcutaneous allergen immunotherapy (SCIT) aims to desensitize a person to an allergen to which they are sensitive, thus minimizing their allergic reaction. Suitable for people with allergic asthma and/or allergic rhinitis, with specific IgE to the allergen identified as causing symptoms. Useful in those who cannot avoid allergen exposure. Small amounts of a single or multiple allergens are injected once or twice weekly, with slowly increasing dose strengths until the maximum dose of the allergen is administered, which can take up to 12 months. Mechanism unknown but probably related to increased IgG binding to the allergen, falling allergen-specific IgE levels, and decreased amount of circulating inflammatory cytokines. Can protect against anaphylaxis for 3–5y, but 'top-up' doses necessary. Effective for dust, grass, tree and weed pollen, mould spores, latex, and insect venom, as well as some animal allergens. Side effects of administration: anaphylaxis, bronchoconstriction, local reaction. Some centres may not perform in people with severe or unstable asthma because of the risk of death.

Future developments A diagnostic test to accurately identify anaphylaxis will be useful, as current tests involving measurement of serum or plasma tryptase or plasma histamine are not perfect. Tryptase levels need to be checked as soon as possible after emergency treatment has started, with a second sample 1–2h later but within 4h of the anaphylactic episode. They may not be raised. Histamine levels have usually returned to baseline within 60min, and therefore measurement may not be helpful.

Further study of biphasic reactions is needed, along with work on the ideal duration of observation post-anaphylaxis and the effect of specialist allergy services on health care-related QoL.

Further information

Abramson M et al. Allergen immunotherapy for asthma. *Cochrane Database Syst Rev* 2003;4:CD001186.

Resuscitation Council (UK). Emergency treatment of anaphylactic reactions. Guidelines for healthcare providers. ℛ http://www.resus.org.uk.

NICE CG134. Initial assessment and referral following emergency treatment for anaphylactic episode, 2011.

Kannan JA, Epstein TG. Immunotherapy safety: what have we learned from surveillance surveys? *Curr Allergy Asthma Rep* 2013;**13**:381–8.

Upper respiratory tract infections 1

Acute URTIs include rhinitis, pharyngitis, tonsillitis, and sinusitis.

URTIs are the commonest cause of time off work in the UK. The majority are managed by GPs and will not reach a respiratory specialist. They are usually self-limiting and often do not require specific treatment.

Acute rhinitis Nasal congestion with rhinorrhoea, mild malaise, and sneezing. Most commonly due to viral infection (the common cold). Topical decongestants may be useful. There is no evidence for the use of antibiotics or antihistamines.

Candidiasis Oral *Candida* infection is common in those who have received antibiotics, are immunosuppressed, or are on oral or inhaled steroids. Seen as white plaque-like lesions on the tongue and pharyngeal mucosa. Treat with oral nystatin or amphotericin lozenges, and with oral hygiene. Severe infection can be debilitating, leading to difficulties with eating, especially in the elderly. Exclude underlying immunocompromise (e.g. HIV, leukaemia) in those with persisting infection despite treatment.

Acute epiglottitis (supraglottitis) is infection mainly localized to the epiglottis and surrounding supraglottic structures. It is commoner in children than adults, but a mortality of up to 7% is reported in adults. This is due to upper airways obstruction from grossly oedematous upper airway tissue and can be life-threatening.
- *Haemophilus influenzae*, streptococci, and staphylococci are causative organisms
- Acute epiglottitis typically presents with a sore throat, fever, drooling, hoarseness. Inspiratory stridor is less common, but it can also present with acute upper airway obstruction and CXR infiltrates consistent with pulmonary oedema (due to high negative intrathoracic pressure)
- Diagnosis is made by visualizing epiglottis (direct or indirect laryngoscopy), but this may not be possible
- May need airway protection with an endotracheal tube or tracheostomy: liaise with ENT/anaesthetic colleagues early
- In severe infection, epiglottic swabs may be of diagnostic use, but beware of precipitating airway obstruction. Treat with third-generation cephalosporin for 2 weeks (to cover β-lactam-producing *H. influenzae*). Change to amoxicillin if sensitive.

Rhinosinusitis The sinuses are normally sterile. The paranasal sinuses communicate with the nose and are therefore susceptible to infection from this route. All the sinuses drain by means of the mucociliary escalator. Blockage of free sinus drainage is a predisposing factor for bacterial infection. Sinusitis is a common cause of persistent cough (see ➔ pp. 18–9). Dental sepsis may lead to maxillary sinusitis by direct spread.

Acute rhinosinusitis complicates 1 in 200 URTIs and usually presents with fever, nasal congestion/purulent discharge, maxillary tooth pain, and sinus pain which is worse on leaning forward. It may be associated with systemic upset. Respiratory viral infection interrupts normal defences of the mucosal lining, producing mucous exudates, with 2° bacterial infection. *S. pneumoniae* and *H. influenzae* are the commonest pathogens. *S. aureus* and *S. pyogenes* are also causes, with Pseudomonas in CF. Mixed infections with anaerobes are seen in 10%. Specific diagnostic tests are not usually needed. Antibiotic treatment may be indicated if symptoms persist longer than 10 days, or severe symptoms of fever, facial pain, and purulent discharge at onset lasting >3 days.

Chronic rhinosinusitis by definition, if present for >3 months. The ciliated epithelial sinus lining is replaced by thickened stratified squamous lining, with absent cilia, due to repeated infection. Anaerobic infection is more common. Fungal infection is more common in atopic people with nasal polyps. Sinus mycetoma is a rare complication in neutropenic patients, diabetics, and the immunocompromised.

Presents with frontal headache (frontal sinusitis), maxillary pain, pain over bridge of nose (ethmoidal sinusitis), retro-orbital headache (sphenoidal sinusitis), with purulent nasal discharge and blockage. GPA (Wegener's) may mimic the symptoms of sinusitis.

Investigations are not usually warranted, but a sinus radiograph may show an air-fluid level, with thickened mucosal lining, or sinus opacification. CT is more sensitive but not usually warranted unless surgical intervention planned or malignant disease suspected.

Treatment—analgesia, topical decongestants, antibiotics if severe infection.

Surgery may be warranted if prolonged infection, anatomical abnormality, or other complications, e.g. if infection has spread to the cranial cavity or orbit. Spreading infection is uncommon if there has been prior antibiotic treatment.

Upper respiratory tract infections 2

Acute pharyngitis and tonsillitis 80–90% are caused by viruses, most commonly adenoviruses, coronaviruses, rhinoviruses, and influenza viruses. Group A streptococci, *Streptococcus pneumoniae*, and *Haemophilus influenzae* may cause 2° infection. *Mycoplasma* and *Chlamydia* are seen less commonly.

- Pharyngitis and tonsillitis present with a sore throat, which is usually self-limiting. May be associated with fever, malaise, lymphadenopathy, conjunctivitis, headache, nausea, and vomiting
- Infectious mononucleosis (EBV) is associated with pharyngitis in 80% of cases. Diagnose with Paul Bunnell test for heterophil antibodies and atypical mononuclear cells in peripheral blood
- Coxsackie A and herpes simplex cause 'herpangina syndrome'— ulcerating vesicles on the tonsils and palate
- CMV can also cause pharyngitis associated with lymphadenopathy and splenomegaly
- Lemierre's syndrome (jugular vein suppurative thrombophlebitis) is a rare anaerobic pharyngeal infection (see ➲ p. 351).

Other causative agents
- *Corynebacterium diphtheriae* in unvaccinated populations. A pharyngeal membrane may form, with systemic symptoms, and 'bull neck' due to cervical lymphadenopathy. Low-grade fever, with a relatively high pulse rate. Treat urgently with diphtheria antitoxin
- Vincent's angina is anaerobic infection in those with poor mouth hygiene. Caused by Gram-negative *Borrelia vincenti* and other anaerobic infections. Treat with penicillin
- Group A *Streptococcus* may cause a more unpleasant illness, with systemic upset and dysphagia, due to pharyngotonsillar oedema.

Treatment is usually supportive, but anti-streptococcal antibiotics may be warranted if there is severe infection (fever, tonsillar exudates, tender anterior cervical lymphadenopathy, no cough). There is no evidence that antibiotics reduce the duration of symptoms, but they may reduce complications (e.g. sinusitis, quinsy, and rheumatic fever, which is rare in the Western world). Oral penicillin is the first-line treatment (or a macrolide if penicillin-allergic). Amoxicillin can cause a rash in infectious mononucleosis and so should be avoided. Throat swabs for group A *Streptococcus* may be helpful in directing treatment.

Complications of untreated infection include peritonsillar abscess (quinsy), retropharyngeal abscess, and cervical abscess. Treat with appropriate antibiotics. Surgical drainage is occasionally required.

Laryngitis This is usually part of a generalized URTI. Often viral, but *Moraxella catarrhalis*, *Haemophilus influenzae*, and *Streptococcus pneumoniae* are also causative. It may cause a hoarse voice or aphonia.

Other causes include inhaled steroids, occupational exposure to inhaled chemicals, and GORD. If a hoarse voice persists in a smoker, a laryngeal or lung cancer (with recurrent laryngeal nerve involvement) must be excluded.

Other causes include tuberculous infection, HSV, CMV, diphtheria, fungal infections, and actinomycoses.

Treatment—usually no specific treatment is required, as the illness is typically self-limiting.

Acute bronchitis, tracheitis, and tracheobronchitis

Inflammation due to infection can occur in any part of the tracheobronchial tree and is termed tracheitis, tracheobronchitis, or bronchitis, depending on the anatomical site. It usually follows viral infection, especially of the common cold type, and is commoner during influenza epidemics. 2° bacterial infection is common, with *H. influenzae* and *S. pneumoniae* commonest. There is increased prevalence in the winter months.

Presents with a productive cough, small-volume streaky haemoptysis, and fever. Breathlessness and hypoxia are uncommon, unless there is coexistent cardiorespiratory disease or a concomitant pneumonia. Retrosternal chest pain is common in tracheitis. Examination is often normal.

Diagnosis is usually on the basis of the history. A persisting cough, especially in a smoker, may warrant further investigation.

Treatment is usually symptomatic, particularly in the previously well. Use antibiotics for persistent cough productive of mucopurulent sputum or if there is coexistent cardiopulmonary disease.

Acute bronchitis, tracheitis, and tracheobronchitis

Vasculitis and the lung

Classification

These are rare conditions but are often seen in the specialist chest clinic (see ➲ p. 28 for an approach to diffuse alveolar haemorrhage). Clinical features can be non-specific and similar to those seen in other diseases, and diagnosis can therefore be difficult. Vasculitides are great 'mimickers' of other diseases, such as lung cancer or ARDS, and have a high untreated mortality. There is considerable overlap between the different vasculitides, which can make definitive diagnosis difficult. Suspect a diagnosis of vasculitis if:

• Weight loss
• Low-grade fever
• Raised inflammatory markers
• Chest disease is not improving or responding to treatment as expected:
  • Unexplained dyspnoea
  • Hypoxia
  • Unexplained desaturation on exercise
  • Haemoptysis
  • Sinus or nasal disease
  • Wheeze
  • CXR abnormalities/infiltrates
  • Abnormal kCO
• Associated renal impairment or positive urine dip for blood or protein
• Raised autoantibodies
• No other clear diagnosis.

The 1° pathology in vasculitis is inflammation and necrosis of differing sized blood vessels. The pulmonary vessels are involved as part of a multi-systemic vasculitis process.

Small-vessel vasculitides are the most common to involve the lung. Arterioles, capillaries, and venules located within the lung interstitium are affected. Neutrophil infiltration and subsequent fibrinoid necrosis cause vessel wall destruction. Necrotizing pulmonary capillaritis can also occur, characterized by a marked neutrophilic infiltration of the interstitium. Interstitial capillaries become damaged, allowing red blood cells to enter the alveolus; thus, alveolar haemorrhage is a feature of many of the small-vessel vasculitides.

New nomenclature for the vasculitides was released by the International Chapel Hill Consensus Conference in 2012, revising that of 1994 (see Table 51.1).

Further information

2012 revised International Chapel Hill Consensus Conference Nomenclature of Vasculitides. *Arthritis Rheum* 2013;**65**:1–11.

Bosch X *et al*. ANCA. *Lancet* 2006;**368**:404–18.

Schwarz M, Brown K. Small vessel vasculitis of the lung. Rare diseases 10. *Thorax* 2000;**55**:502–10.

Table 51.1 Classification of vasculitis, based on the Revised International Chapel Hill Consensus, 2012

1° vasculitis	Lung involvement	ANCA
Small vessel		
ANCA-associated vasculitis (AAV)		
- Microscopic polyangiitis (MPA)	Frequent	c/p-ANCA
- GPA (Wegener's)	Frequent	c-ANCA in 75%, p-ANCA in 15%
- EGPA (Churg–Strauss)	Frequent	p-ANCA in 70%
Goodpasture's disease	Frequent	p-ANCA in 10–20%
Medium-sized vessel		
Polyarteritis nodosa (PAN)	Rare	Negative
Large vessel		
Giant cell arteritis	Rare	Negative
Takayasu's arteritis	Frequent	Negative

ANCA

ANCAs react with cytoplasmic granule enzymes in neutrophils and stain them in one of two ways:
• Diffusely cytoplasmic pattern or *c-ANCA*
• Perinuclear pattern or *p-ANCA*.

These autoantibodies may have a direct role in pathogenesis as well as being disease markers.

ANCA have two major specificities:
• Antiproteinase 3 antibodies (anti-PR3)—associated with c-ANCA pattern
• Antimyeloperoxidase antibodies (anti-MPO)—associated with p-ANCA pattern.

c-ANCA (anti-PR3) targets PR3 and may suggest GPA (75% of cases are c-ANCA positive). Levels correlate with disease activity and extent. Also found in patients with MPA (45% of those with clinical disease will be c-ANCA positive).

p-ANCA (anti-MPO) targets MPO and has a wider range of disease associations, including other vasculitides and autoimmune diseases, HIV, lung cancer, pulmonary fibrosis, and PEs.

Granulomatosis with polyangiitis (Wegener's): presentation and diagnosis

Definition and epidemiology Necrotizing vasculitis affecting small and medium-sized vessels, especially in the upper and lower respiratory tract and also the kidneys. Associated granulomata. Renamed in 2011.
• Unknown cause
• ♂ = ♀
• 3/100,000, 80–97% Caucasian
• Any age, but most common between 40 and 55y.

Clinical features
• *ENT* In 90%, upper airways involvement will be the first presenting sign. Nasal congestion and epistaxis, with inflamed, crusty, ulcerated nasal mucosa. Nasal septum perforation. Late sign is a saddle nose deformity. Sinusitis is common and may be painful. Otitis media. Subglottic stenosis, causing upper airway obstruction, dyspnoea, voice change, and cough. Abnormal flow–volume loops
• *Lung* Affected in 85–90% of patients. Haemoptysis, cough, dyspnoea. Pleuritic chest pain
• *Kidney* Affected in 77% of patients. Haematuria, proteinuria, and red cell casts. Only 10% have renal impairment initially, but 80% will have involvement during their disease course. Characteristic progressive deterioration of renal function
• *Systemic* Fever and weight loss
• *Other organ systems (skin, eyes, joints, CNS)* Vasculitic skin rash, with granulomatous involvement in 46%. Muscle and joint pains. Conjunctivitis, scleritis, proptosis, eye pain, visual loss. Mononeuritis multiplex and CNS disease.

Investigations
Consider:
• *CXR* Flitting cavitating pulmonary nodules, consolidation, or pulmonary infiltrates, alveolar haemorrhage, parenchymal distortion, large and small airway disease, pleural effusion, bronchiectasis. Can look like neoplasms, infection, or fluid overload
• *HRCT* of chest
• *O_2 saturations*
• *FBC, U&E, CRP, ESR*
• *Serum ANCA*, especially c-ANCA, is sensitive and fairly specific. Present in 90% of patients with extensive GPA and 75% with limited. p-ANCA positive in 5–10% of patients with GPA. Combining indirect immunofluorescence with specific immunoassays for antibodies to PR3 and MPO increases sensitivity and specificity for GPA and MPA to over 90%. **Remember ANCA can be negative, especially in disease confined to the respiratory tract.** ANCA titres rise prior to a relapse and are higher when disease is active, and this can act as a guide to

starting treatment. However, high ANCA levels in the absence of clinical symptoms or signs may not represent active disease, and, therefore, ANCA levels should not be used in isolation to determine treatment. Also consider CRP ± ESR

- *Urine dipstick and microscopy* Red cell casts
- *PFTs, including kCO*
- *Image sinuses* Bony destruction makes GPA likely
- *Bronchoscopy* May show inflammation and ulceration of larynx, trachea, and bronchi. Scarring and stenosis may be seen. BAL is neutrophilic, also with eosinophils and lymphocytes. TBB is unlikely to be diagnostic
- *Biopsy*
  - *Respiratory tract and nose*—granulomata in association with medium- and small-vessel necrotizing vasculitis and surrounding inflammation. Nasal biopsies are often non-specific and may not be diagnostic
  - *Renal biopsy*—focal segmental or diffuse necrotizing glomerulonephritis. Pauci-immune and granulomata rare. Not specific for GPA
  - *Skin biopsy*—leukocytoclastic vasculitis ± granulomata.

Diagnosis Biopsy and ANCA are key to diagnosis. Biopsy whichever site is affected. May be nasal, lung (open or thoracoscopic), skin, or renal. If there is evidence on urine dip of renal vasculitis, this may be the best and easiest biopsy site. Disease may be patchy in nature, requiring repeat biopsies if the first is negative. High c-ANCA and anti-PR3 is highly suggestive of GPA.

Differential diagnosis of GPA

Malignancy, TB, sarcoidosis, ABPA, Goodpasture's disease (anti-GBM disease with pulmonary haemorrhage and nephritis), SLE, MPA, connective tissue disease.

Granulomatosis with polyangiitis (Wegener's): management

Involve the renal team, and share care of the patient. See Chapter 54 for immunosuppressive drug details.

- Standard regimen for *generalized or organ-threatening disease* (e.g. active/ progressive pulmonary or renal disease or CNS disease):
  - Induce remission with oral prednisolone (1mg/kg/day, tapering weekly to a dose of 15mg or less daily by 3 months) and cyclophosphamide, orally (2mg/kg/day, up to 200mg/day) or IV (pulses at 2- or 3-week intervals, 15mg/kg), for 3–6 months. Reduce cyclophosphamide dose in elderly (e.g. reduce oral dose by 25% if >60y and by 50% if >75y) and in setting of renal impairment. Taper cyclophosphamide dose to maintain WCC >4 × 10^9/L and neutrophils >2 × 10^9, to reduce infection risk (see ➜ p. 679 for more detail)
  - The aim is to prevent irreversible tissue necrosis. There is evidence that this regime induces remission in 80% of patients at 3 months and 90% at 6 months
  - After induction of remission (at 3–6 months), consider switch from cyclophosphamide and prednisolone to maintenance therapy with prednisolone and either azathioprine (2mg/kg/day for 12 months, then reduce to 1.5mg/kg/day; check TPMT levels; see ➜ pp. 676–7) or methotrexate (15mg once/week, increase to maximum of 20–25mg once/week by week 12; see ➜ p. 678). This avoids the morbidity associated with long-term cyclophosphamide use. Both azathioprine and methotrexate have been demonstrated to maintain remission, although the evidence favours use of azathioprine
  - Restart the regime if the patient relapses—this may occur in 50%
- For *severe life-threatening disease* (e.g. rapidly progressive renal failure or massive pulmonary haemorrhage):
  - Plasma exchange/plasmapheresis (7 × 4L exchanges over 2 weeks) has been shown to be more effective than methylprednisolone in the treatment of GPA. In patients with severe pulmonary haemorrhage, it is also effective and can be given along with fresh frozen plasma
  - In addition, treat with pulsed methylprednisolone (500–1,000mg/ day, depending on body weight for 3 days) and IV cyclophosphamide (15mg/kg, reduce if elderly or renal impairment)
  - Dialysis for renal failure
  - After induction of remission (over 3–6 months), switch from cyclophosphamide to azathioprine or methotrexate with prednisolone as maintenance therapy

- For *localized disease or early systemic disease* (without threatened organ involvement):
  - Prednisolone with either methotrexate or oral/ pulsed cyclophosphamide. Use of methotrexate avoids cyclophosphamide-related toxicity but may be associated with a higher relapse rate. Localized disease may still be serious (e.g. retro-orbital involvement), and, in these situations, cyclophosphamide should be considered
- *Duration of treatment* Maintenance therapy is recommended to continue for at least 24 months after initial disease remission, as relapses are common. Some recommend continuing treatment for up to 5y, particularly if the ANCA remains positive
- PCP prophylaxis with co-trimoxazole is recommended (960mg 3×/ week) in patients receiving cyclophosphamide and prednisolone. There is some evidence that co-trimoxazole alone may be effective in the treatment of especially limited GPA, although the reasons for this are not clear—it may be due to suppression of nasal *Staphylococcus aureus* carriage, the presence of which is associated with an increased risk of relapse
- Osteoporosis prophylaxis should be considered
- *Follow-up* monthly for 3 months, then 3–6-monthly. Monitor FBC, U&E, CRP, LFT, ANCA, CXR, and kCO. Rising ANCA titres are a poor predictor of relapse; in the absence of other features of a relapse, follow up more closely, but do not increase immunosuppression solely on this basis. Withdrawal of immunosuppression in the setting of a persistently positive ANCA is associated with relapse, however
- *Relapses* Treat minor relapses with an increase in the prednisolone dose. Treat major relapses with cyclophosphamide and increasing prednisolone; consider IV methylprednisolone, plasma exchange
- *Refractory disease* Liaise with specialist; consider alternative therapies such as infliximab, high-dose IV immunoglobulin, rituximab, anti-thymocyte globulin, or CAMPATH 1H (alemtuzumab, anti-CD52). Mycophenolate or leflunomide are alternatives to azathioprine or methotrexate. Exclude underlying infection, malignancy, and non-compliance.

Prognosis *Limited disease* with pulmonary, but no renal, involvement and an often negative c-ANCA test has a better prognosis. However, this can progress over time to *extensive disease*, with classical destructive sinusitis, nephritis, and vasculitis and strong c-ANCA positivity, and is associated with higher mortality. Untreated, 80% of people with extensive GPA will die in 1y. Overall, 75–90% of patients can be brought into remission with treatment, although 50% relapse in 5y, and long-term follow-up is required.

Microscopic polyangiitis

At least as common as GPA and may be hard to distinguish. Managed in the same way.

- *Incidence* ♂ = ♀, mean age 50, mainly Caucasians
- *Kidneys* Main organ affected by a small-vessel necrotizing vasculitis, causing proteinuria and haematuria. Renal biopsy shows focal segmental glomerulonephritis with fibrinoid necrosis and sparse immune deposits
- *Pulmonary involvement* occurs in 30–50% of patients, with pleurisy, asthma, haemoptysis, and pulmonary haemorrhage. CXR may be suggestive of pulmonary haemorrhage
- *p-ANCA* positive, often c-ANCA also.

Treatment with immunosuppression: steroids and cyclophosphamide (see ➲ pp. 656–7).

Future developments

It had been thought that *anti-TNF-α agents* were likely to have a role in acute vasculitis and seemed to work best in granulomatous disease. An RCT of etanercept plus standard therapy for GPA showed no significant effect on remission rates (*N Engl J Med* 2005;**352**:351–61). Further studies are ongoing of other anti-TNF-α agents.

B-cell depletion with the monoclonal anti-CD20 antibody rituximab. This is used for non-Hodgkin's lymphoma, SLE, RA. Encouraging results in small studies of ANCA-positive vasculitis, but no RCT as yet.

Mycophenolate for immunosuppression in vasculitis to induce remission. Used post-transplant. A large study vs azathioprine is underway.

Further information

Lapraik C et al. British Society of Rheumatology and British Heath Professionals in Rheumatology guidelines for the management of adults with ANCA associated vasculitis. *Rheumatology* 2007;**46**:1615–16.

Langford C, Hoffman G. Wegener's granulomatosis. Rare diseases 3. *Thorax* 1999;**54**:629–63.

Frankel SK et al. Update in the diagnosis and management of pulmonary vasculitis. *Chest* 2006;**129**:452–65.

Goodpasture's disease

Definition and epidemiology Linear deposition of IgG on the basement membranes of alveoli and glomeruli, which damages collagen and in the lungs allows leakage of blood.
- Anti-GBM antibodies are detectable in blood
- Alveolar haemorrhage and glomerulonephritis
- Important differential diagnosis of pulmonary-renal syndrome
- Annual incidence of 1 case per million
- ♂:♀ = 4:1
- Commonest age 20–30y
- Second peak when women in their late 60s are affected by glomerulonephritis alone
- Cause unknown. Often a preceding viral infection. Smokers at greater risk of pulmonary haemorrhage, but not of Goodpasture's disease
- HLA-DR2 association in 60–70%.

Clinical features
- Haemoptysis in 80–90%—more common in smokers
- Cough, dyspnoea, fatigue, and weakness
- Examination: inspiratory crackles common.

Investigations
- *Serum electrolytes* show impaired renal function and often renal failure
- *FBC* Iron deficiency anaemia
- *Urine dip and microscopy* Haematuria, proteinuria, granular and typically red blood cell casts. Occasionally macroscopic haematuria
- *Anti-GBM* and autoantibody screen
- *CXR± CT* Diffuse bilateral patchy airspace shadowing in mid- and lower zones. May see air bronchograms
- *PFTs* Restrictive defect with raised kCO if alveolar haemorrhage present.

Diagnosis Renal biopsy usually shows diffuse crescentic glomerulonephritis. Linear IgG deposition detected by immunofluorescence or immunoperoxidase. Lung biopsy shows active intra-alveolar haemorrhage, with collections of haemosiderin-laden macrophages. These are not specific changes but may also show linear immunofluorescence staining of IgG.

Differential diagnosis GPA, other pulmonary renal syndromes.

Management
- Involve the renal team, and share care of the patient
- Plasma exchange improves the speed of response to immunosuppression
- High-dose steroids and cyclophosphamide
- May need dialysis. Renal function may not improve, and renal transplant is only an option later if anti-GBM antibody levels become low
- Recurrence is uncommon once disease is controlled. It usually responds to further immunosuppression. Residual defects in PFTs frequent.

Prognosis Rapidly progressive pulmonary haemorrhage and renal failure. Usually fatal if not treated.

Churg–Strauss syndrome/eosinophilic granulomatosis with polyangiitis

Definition and epidemiology Asthma, blood eosinophilia, and an eosinophilic granulomatous inflammation of the respiratory tract, with necrotizing vasculitis affecting small and medium-sized vessels.
- Rare, 2.4 per million population, but 64 per million of an asthmatic population (who may have been misdiagnosed with asthma)
- Middle-aged adults
- ♂:♀ ≈ 2:1
- Unknown cause. Montelukast was postulated as a possible cause, but this is now thought unlikely. Development of Churg–Strauss syndrome/ EGPA in people on montelukast probably related to their decreased steroid dose 'unmasking' Churg–Strauss syndrome/EGPA, or as part of an increasing treatment regime in those with uncontrolled asthma, later diagnosed as Churg–Strauss syndrome/EGPA.

Clinical features A diagnosis of Churg–Strauss syndrome/EGPA can be made if four of the following six criteria are present:
- Asthma—may have had for years, often maturity onset, difficult to control, associated with rhinitis and nasal polyps
- Blood eosinophilia >10%
- Vasculitic neuropathy such as mononeuritis multiplex (occurs in 75%)
- Pulmonary infiltrates
- Sinus disease
- Extravascular eosinophils on biopsy findings.
(American College of Rheumatology criteria, 1990)
- Also may have:
  - Myositis and cardiac failure, cardiomyopathy, coronary artery inflammation, pericardial effusion
  - Eosinophilic infiltration of mesenteric vessels, causing GI disturbance
  - Alveolar haemorrhage
  - Rarely, proteinuria caused by renal disease with focal segmental glomerulonephritis. Renal failure is rare
  - Skin nodules and purpura
  - Myalgia and arthralgia
  - Fever and weight loss.

Typical pattern of disease has three phases: beginning with asthma, then developing blood and tissue eosinophilia, then going on to systemic vasculitis. The asthma precedes the vasculitis, often by years (mean 8y).

Investigations
- *CXR* Fleeting peripheral pulmonary infiltrates and bilateral multifocal consolidation
- *HRCT* Ground-glass inflammation, pulmonary nodules, bronchial wall thickening, or alveolar haemorrhage
- *Bronchoscopy* BAL Marked eosinophilia

- *Pathology* Extravascular tissue eosinophilia, necrotizing angiitis, granulomata
- *Serum markers* Peripheral blood eosinophilia. p-ANCA and anti-MPO positive in two-thirds. ANCA levels may not correlate with disease activity, but blood eosinophilia is a good guide.

Diagnosis Predominantly a clinical diagnosis. Pathological confirmation of eosinophilic tissue infiltration or vasculitis desirable. Biopsy easiest site affected, such as skin, kidney, or open or thoracoscopic lung biopsy.

Differential diagnosis ABPA, sarcoidosis, drug and parasitic causes of eosinophilic pneumonias, HP, hypereosinophilic syndrome.

Management Depends on severity of disease at presentation.
- *If isolated pulmonary disease*, oral prednisolone 1mg/kg (max 60mg/day) for 1 month or until no evidence of disease, then slowly decrease over 1y, with increases if symptoms recur
- *If unwell or with alveolar haemorrhage*, pulsed methylprednisolone IV for 3 days, followed by high-dose oral steroids, with or without cyclophosphamide (see ➡ pp. 656–7)
- *In cardiac or GI disease, relapse, or life-threatening situations*, such as requiring organ support, cyclophosphamide should be added (see ➡ pp. 656–7)
- Plasma exchange is of no benefit
- Treatment is aimed at reversing organ damage and reducing relapse rate
- *To maintain remission*, prednisolone and one other immunosuppressant drug are usually required. Cyclophosphamide is often changed to azathioprine after 4–6 months
- Prophylactic co-trimoxazole should be given (960mg 3×/week), and consider bone protection for steroids
- *Follow up* regularly, with checks on FBC and eosinophil count, CXR.

Prognosis Good prognosis if isolated pulmonary disease. Good response to steroids. May continue to have asthma, despite control of vasculitis, which can be severe and difficult to control. Poor prognosis associated with cardiac disease and severe GI disease, causing bleeding, perforation, or necrosis. Untreated, 5y survival rate is 25%. Also associated with worse prognosis: proteinuria >1g/24h, renal insufficiency, CNS involvement. Cardiac disease is the main cause of death.

Further information

Noth I et al. Churg–Strauss syndrome. *Lancet* 2003;**361**:587–94.
🔊 http://www.vasculitis-uk.org.
🔊 http://www.vasculitis.org.

Rare pulmonary vasculitides

Polyarteritis nodosa

- Similar to MPA but affects medium-sized vessels
- May exist as an 'overlap' disorder with GPA or Churg–Strauss/EGPA
- Lung involvement is rare
- Sometimes associated with previous hepatitis B or rarely hepatitis C infection.

Takayasu's arteritis

- Predominantly young women, often Asian
- Vasculitis affecting the aorta and its major branches. Large and medium-sized pulmonary vessels affected, but involvement is usually silent. Pulmonary artery stenosis and occlusion common, occasionally with mild PHT
- *Presents* with fevers and weight loss. Absent or weak upper limb peripheral pulses, particularly on left (as left axillary artery comes off aortic arch), and arterial bruits
- *Diagnosis* made by angiography
- *Treatment* Steroids may reduce symptoms but do not affect mortality. Angioplasty and surgical procedures may reduce the complications. Spontaneous remissions may occur.

Giant cell arteritis

- Commonest form of systemic vasculitis affecting large and medium-sized vessels
- 24 cases per 100,000. Predominantly elderly ♀
- *Presents* with non-specific symptoms of fever and weight loss; also headache, scalp tenderness, and jaw pain. Amaurosis fugax and visual loss due to optic neuritis
- *Pulmonary complications* occur in 9–25% of cases. They are relatively minor, with cough, sore throat, and hoarseness. PFTs and CXR normal
- *Diagnosis* High ESR, temporal artery biopsy showing pan-arteritis and giant cell formation
- *Treatment* Good response to oral steroids. Continue for 1–2y.

Part 3

Supportive care

Ethical issues

Background

Respiratory physicians are often involved in making difficult decisions about the appropriateness of treatment and the prolongation of life in patients with chronic underlying lung disease. Some common clinical scenarios encountered are discussed here. Sometimes, artificial ventilation may prolong the dying process; life has a natural end, and the potential to prolong life in the ICU can sometimes cause dilemmas. In other cases, these interventions are valuable at prolonging life with a reversible complication.

The General Medical Council (GMC) states that doctors have an obligation to respect human life, protect the health of their patients, and put their patients' best interests first. This means offering treatments where the benefits outweigh any risks and avoiding treatments that carry no net gain to the patient. If a patient wishes to have a treatment that, in the doctor's considered view, is not indicated, the doctor and medical team are under no ethical or legal obligation to provide it, but the patient's right to a second opinion must be respected.

Discussions about resuscitation and invasive ventilation are rarely easy but should ideally be held with the patient, their next of kin, and nursing staff, in advance of an emergency situation. Clearly, this is not always possible. Ideally, all decisions regarding resuscitation and the ceiling of treatment (particularly relating to ventilation) should be documented in advance and handed over to on-call teams. Most possible outcomes can be anticipated.

Where it has been decided that a treatment is not in the best interests of the patient, there is no ethical distinction between stopping the treatment or not starting it in the first place (though the former may be more difficult to do), and this should not be used as an argument for failing to initiate the treatment in the first place.

Lasting power of attorney (LPA) allows an appointed attorney to make decisions about personal welfare, including giving or refusing consent to treatment, if the patient loses their capacity as defined by the Mental Capacity Act 2005. Neither the next of kin nor those with LPA have the legal right to determine any treatment; the responsibility remains with the doctor and MDT, occasionally involving the courts of law.

Advance decisions (also known as living wills and formerly advance directives) are statements documenting what treatment the individual would want in the future or would want to refuse in specific circumstances, should they lack capacity. They are legally binding in England and Wales, and doctors giving treatment against the patient's wishes expressed in a directive could be prosecuted. In Scotland and Northern Ireland, advance decisions are governed by common law, rather than legislation. If there are concerns about the validity of the document, doctors should seek input from senior colleagues or the hospital medical director. Advance decisions do not have to be written down, signed, and witnessed, unless they include decisions about resuscitation and other potential life-prolonging treatments. The patient must understand the implications of his/her decision, although, if they have capacity, their word can override their advance directive or their legal representative.

Advance statements are written by the patient about their preferences, wishes, beliefs, and values but are not legally binding. They provide a guide for others to make decisions in the patient's best interests if they lose capacity in the future.

COPD

COPD is the 4th commonest cause of death in America, and most patients die of respiratory failure during an exacerbation. A commonly encountered clinical situation is where a patient with COPD is admitted with an exacerbation and is in type II respiratory failure. Standard treatment does not improve the respiratory acidosis, so NIV is commenced. Before starting NIV, a decision must be clearly documented as to whether or not NIV is the ceiling of treatment. It may be, especially if the patient has severe or end-stage COPD.

Invasive ventilation in the ICU may be appropriate in certain specific situations, for example:

- In a relatively young patient (i.e. <65y)
- A patient with a relatively new diagnosis of COPD, in whom the episode is the first or second admission
- In the patient in whom there is a very obviously potentially reversible cause for the exacerbation, e.g. pneumonia.

Sometimes, in this situation, a defined time period for intensive care input may be decided, e.g. ventilation for 48h (to allow treatments to work and to allow time to assess for any improvement), with extubation after that time period if no improvement has been made.

Decisions about intubation/ventilation and intensive care admission can only be made knowing the patient's usual level of functioning and previous QoL. The difficulty is that QoL is a very subjective measure. Objective measures of usual functioning, e.g. measures of daily activity, usual exercise tolerance, and whether home care or assistance with activities of daily living is required, are often more useful in guiding the appropriateness of escalating therapy. With reference to the patient with COPD, the number of hospital admissions and exacerbations and the need for home O_2 or nebulizers will also be useful. Helpful information may be obtained from the GP, especially if the previous hospital notes are unavailable. Where limited information is available about the patient and therefore uncertainty exists about the appropriateness of ventilation, it should be started until a clearer assessment can be made. This may be relevant for a patient attending the emergency department where little information is available. The above point concerning the withdrawal of therapy, should it subsequently be found to be inappropriate, also holds.

There are downsides to invasive ventilation: the risk of pneumothorax is increased in those with end-stage emphysema, and the risk of VAP increases with time ventilated (see ➔ p. 438). Knowledge of the risk of these adverse events helps the medical team to balance the argument and make a decision about whether the risks of ventilation are likely to outweigh its benefits. The issue of limited resources should not influence a decision about formal ventilation or ICU admission.

The average length of intubation of patients with COPD admitted to ICU is 3.2 days. These patients have a 20–25% in-hospital mortality, with 50% of patients surviving 1y post-ICU discharge. About 50% will be living independently 1y post-hospital discharge. Clearly, only a very selected subgroup of patients are admitted to ICU, but concerns about prolonged periods of ventilation in this group of patients seem to be unfounded. Patients in whom a clear cause for the exacerbation can be identified (e.g. pneumonia) tend to do better, as there is a treatable cause for the exacerbation, and not just progression of the underlying disease.

Lung cancer and neurological disease

Lung cancer The use of antibiotic treatment for pneumonia in a patient with advanced lung malignancy may be inappropriate in some circumstances. The patient's wishes and QoL, stage and extent of disease, response to other treatments (e.g. chemotherapy) are all paramount. This is another situation in which it might be appropriate to define at the outset the treatments that are appropriate, e.g. 10 days total of IV and oral antibiotics. Note that treatments, such as antibiotics, can lead to improvement in symptoms (e.g. by reducing fever), without necessarily prolonging life, and it may be kinder to continue antibiotics in this situation.

Progressive neurological disease The decision about NIV in a patient with a progressive neuromuscular disease can be difficult. There is now strong RCT evidence that NIV in patients with some neuromuscular diseases (Duchenne muscular dystrophy, MND, neuromuscular and chest wall disease), improves QoL and survival. Decisions about the requirement and timing of NIV need to be made by specialists in neuromuscular disease, in conjunction with home ventilation teams. Clinical deterioration can usually be anticipated, with serial measurements of spirometry and overnight O_2 or CO_2. Discussions should take place early on (unless the patient presents in respiratory failure, e.g. due to pneumonia, and subsequent ventilator weaning is difficult). Clinicians, patients, and their relatives may differ in their approaches to NIV in the face of progressive neuromuscular disability, but, of all the palliative options available, NIV can be particularly useful. Further decisions about withdrawal of treatment with progression of the underlying neurological disease of course will still be needed. These can be difficult and require multidisciplinary input. Actual practical NIV withdrawal can also be hard, requiring specialist assistance, but it usually done gradually with sedation cover.

Further information

General Medical Council 2010. *Treatment and care towards the end of life: good practice in decision making.*

Chapter 53

Financial entitlements

General points

Patients with chronic lung disease and their carers may be eligible for financial support. There are a large number of potential benefits that can be claimed, and the process is often time-consuming and complicated. The best sources of information are:

- Benefits Enquiry Line ☎ 0800 882200 (☎ 0800 220674 in Northern Ireland)
- Websites:
  - ☞ http://www.gov.uk/financial-help-disabled/overview (useful guide)
  - ☞ http://www.gov.uk/browse/benefits (various online tools)
  - The Citizens Advice Bureau ☞ http://www.citizensadvice.org.uk
- The ward social worker is usually a good source of information.

Available financial support

Patients who are unable to work may be eligible for:

Statutory sick pay (SSP) A doctor's certificate ('fit note' = Med 3) is usually required for >1 week's SSP. Paid up to 26 weeks. New rules now make the doctor's certificate the responsibility of the hospital consultant under whom the patient was admitted, and it should be completed on discharge to cover the advised period off work. This also applies to patients needing time off work but not admitted to hospital. Nursing staff usually complete the forms for the period during which the patient was in hospital.

Employment and Support Allowance (ESA) (replaces Incapacity Benefit and Severe Disablement Allowance). Has two phases: (1) assessment phase, in which patients must get Med 3s for first 13 weeks of claim and complete a medical questionnaire (ESA50), (2) work capability assessment phase, during which patients attend a face-to-face assessment to determine ongoing need and set a date for further assessment. For patients who are terminally ill (<6 months' life expectancy), doctors complete a DS1500 form, and such patients normally avoid requirement for face-to-face assessment.

Personal Independence Payment (PIP) for those <65 (replacing Disability Living Allowance) or *Attendance Allowance (AA)* for those >65. These are benefits for the extra costs of disability and are designed for help with personal care or mobility. For PIP, patients have to satisfy a 3-month qualifying period and have a prospective estimate of disability lasting at least 9 months. 'Special rules' allow terminally ill people (<6 months' life expectancy) to claim PIP/AA quickly, using a DS1500 form completed by doctors.

Direct payments These are payments from Social Services to allow patients to buy care services for themselves.

Carer's Allowance Those who care for someone receiving allowances, including PIP/AA, for at least 35h/week are eligible.

Income Support ± Disability Premiums For those on a low income, with extra support for disability.

Working Tax Credit (with extra credit for disability) This is not a benefit as such, but a tax credit from the HMRC (paid in addition to benefits).

Disabled Students' Allowance (DSA) Available for higher education students in England with disability or long-term health conditions.

Access to Work Grant Financial support to help disabled people to undertake their job, giving money for, e.g. specialist equipment, travel when unable to use public transport.

Disabled Facilities Grant Available from local councils to allow essential household modifications (e.g. widen doors, stairlifts).

Other transport assistance, e.g. Blue Badge, exemption from paying vehicle tax, disabled person's bus pass/railcard.

Industrial Injuries Disablement benefit (see Chapter 36 on pneumoconioses, ➲ pp. 362–3, and Chapter 17 on asbestosis, ➲ pp. 122–3). Patients can additionally claim *Constant Attendance Allowance* if require daily care and attention because of a disability.

Reduced earning allowance For those suffering from disability caused by a work-related accident or disease that happened before 1 October 1990.

Further information

There are a number of charities who give grants/aid towards the cost of buying equipment.

🔊 http://www.charityfinancials.com.

🔊 http://www.charity-commission.gov.uk.

Chapter 54

Immunosuppressive drugs

Patient advice and monitoring

Immunosuppressive drugs are used mainly in the management of pulmonary vasculitis, but also in asthma, sarcoidosis, and ILD. Centres differ in their use of these drugs, and local guidelines are often available. A summary of tests to perform before and during immunosuppressive drug treatment is shown in Table 54.1.

General advice for patients on immunosuppressive drugs

- Increased risk of infections and increased likelihood of severe infections. Check FBC if develop febrile illness
- May have atypical presentation of infections and atypical pathogens
- Avoid live vaccines such as measles, mumps, rubella, BCG, yellow fever, oral typhoid, oral polio
- If never had varicella-zoster:
  - Avoid contacts with chickenpox or shingles
  - Consider passive immunization
  - Immunoglobulin therapy if exposed
  - Hospital treatment, with close monitoring, if develop chickenpox
- Avoid measles exposure. Prophylaxis with immunoglobulins if exposed.

Table 54.1 Summary of tests to perform before and during immunosuppressive drug treatment of respiratory disease

Drug	Check before starting	Follow-up
Corticosteroids	BP, glucose Consider bones/osteoporosis	BP, glucose if symptoms of diabetes
Azathioprine	FBC, LFT, TPMT test (see text)	FBC every 2 weeks for 3 months, then monthly LFT monthly
Methotrexate	FBC, U&E, LFT CXR Folic acid	Bloods every 2 weeks for 3 months, then monthly
Cyclophosphamide	FBC, U&E, LFT Urine dip Semen store	Check all every week for 1 month, then every 2 months

Corticosteroids and azathioprine

Corticosteroids

- First-line treatment for suppressing inflammation. At high doses, also cause immunosuppression. Ineffective as sole therapy for induction of remission in systemic vasculitis
- IV methylprednisolone (500–1,000mg/day) for 3–5 days can be used for aggressive induction of remission, e.g. GPA, followed by maintenance oral steroids (prednisolone 30–40mg/day)
- Usually taken in the morning, as they may disturb sleep
- Dose should be slowly reduced when control of the disease is achieved. Gastric and bone protection may be necessary, as the patient will be on high doses for some months. Also ensure BP and glucose are controlled
- Ensure patients have steroid treatment card

Side effects include skin and hair thinning, obesity, cataracts, diabetes, and aseptic bone necrosis. Inform patient of these, and document. PCP infection can occur 2° to steroid treatment, particularly with high doses for prolonged periods. Some centres use PCP prophylaxis.

Steroids and osteoporosis

Current guidelines suggest patients being started on long-term steroids, with one other osteoporosis risk factor (such as being over 65 or having had a previous osteoporotic fracture), should also start on a bisphosphonate.

In other patients who will be on 7.5mg/day or more for >3 months, consider checking bone mineral density via DEXA scan of hip and spine, and offer lifestyle advice and bisphosphonates if this is reduced (T score –1.5 or lower).

(See Royal College of Physicians guidelines, available at ℞ http://www.rcplondon.ac.uk, and National Osteoporosis Society at ℞ http:www.nos.org.uk.)

Azathioprine

- Mainly used as a steroid-sparing agent or when vasculitis is under control to enable cyclophosphamide to be stopped. Is a pro-drug for 6-mercaptopurine. Takes ~4 weeks to work
- Cytotoxic drug, less effective than cyclophosphamide. May be reasonable alternative if side effects of cyclophosphamide are unacceptable
- Maximal effect on disease may not be evident for 6–9 months but can be used long term
- TPMT testing should be performed prior to commencement. TPMT breaks down azathioprine to an inactive product. 90% of the population have normal TPMT levels and 10% have intermediate activity, so azathioprine should be given with caution; 0.3% have no TPMT activity, and azathioprine should be avoided
- For vasculitis, start with 2mg/kg/day after cyclophosphamide. Maximum dose usually around 150–200mg/day

- As steroid-sparing regime: could start 50mg od for 2 weeks, increasing to 100mg od for 2 weeks if FBC satisfactory, and increasing to 150mg od (or 75mg bd) after further 2 weeks if FBC satisfactory. Reduce prednisolone by 5mg every 4 weeks
- *Check FBC* every 2 weeks for 6 weeks, then at 2 and 4 weeks after each dose increase, and thereafter monthly. *Check LFTs* monthly. Stop treatment if WCC <3, platelets <100, or ALP and transaminases 3× normal. Restart when they recover.

Side effects include sore mouth, ulcers, nausea and vomiting, diarrhoea, skin rash, alopecia (rare). Most respond to stopping the drug and restarting at a lower dose. If taken for a number of years, then increased risk of some types of cancers, including skin. Advised to contact doctor if any concerns about new skin problems. Interacts with allopurinol and leads to increased toxicity.

Methotrexate and cyclophosphamide

Methotrexate

- Can be used as a second-line treatment
- Dose: 7.5–25mg once/week. Usual starting dose is 10mg. Can increase after 6 weeks to 15mg, in increments of 2.5mg weekly
- Baseline CXR. Monitor FBC, U&E, and LFTs every 2 weeks for 3 months, then monthly. Give folic acid 5mg 3–4 days after dose to reduce toxicity.

Side effects include mouth ulcers, skin rashes, nausea, macrocytosis, myelosuppression, pneumonitis (dyspnoea and dry cough). Avoid if significant renal or hepatic impairment, or if pleural effusions or ascites, as it can accumulate in these fluids. Stop if WCC <3, platelets <100, transaminases 3× normal, pneumonitis.

Cyclophosphamide

- The 1° cytotoxic drug used for treating systemic vasculitis
- Causes immunosuppression without anti-inflammatory effects
- Used particularly if there are life- or organ-threatening features, e.g. ventilation for lung vasculitis, systemic features, renal involvement
- Takes 12–14 days to work; hence is combined with high-dose steroids at the beginning of treatment. When combined with steroids, it induces remission of vasculitis in 90% of patients
- Perform a baseline urine dip for blood prior to treatment (although note microscopic haematuria is common with active vasculitis). Check routinely for macroscopic haematuria in patients receiving IV cyclophosphamide, and, if it is present, stop drug and arrange cystoscopy (rare if mesna is used and rare with oral cyclophosphamide regimes)
- PCP prophylaxis with co-trimoxazole is recommended (960mg 3×/week) in patients receiving cyclophosphamide and prednisolone
- Semen storage for men prior to starting treatment.

Usual treatment duration of cyclophosphamide is 3–6 months. Courses longer than 6 months should generally be avoided; they are no more effective and carry the risk of side effects from the cumulative dose. Induce remission with cyclophosphamide and prednisolone, and maintain remission with prednisolone and another immunosuppressant (azathioprine or methotrexate) for at least 2y.

Side effects Haemorrhagic cystitis is a potentially serious side effect of cyclophosphamide therapy. Risk of bladder cancer is increased (and is greater with increasing cumulative dose), and indefinite monitoring of urinalysis 3–6-monthly after treatment with cyclophosphamide is recommended. Other side effects include nausea, vomiting, infection (including PCP), hair thinning or alopecia (reversible), bone marrow suppression (2%), leucopenia, infertility, lymphoma (0.7%) and leukaemia, pulmonary and bladder fibrosis. Risk of cervical cancer may be higher—recommend annual cervical smear for 3y and thereafter, as per population screening programme. Should not be taken in pregnancy or if breastfeeding. Men and women should avoid starting a family during, and for 6 months following, treatment with cyclophosphamide.

Cyclophosphamide regimes

Oral cyclophosphamide is used, if possible, in active vasculitis at a dose of 2mg/kg (up to 200mg/day). Reduce dose in elderly (by 25% if >60y and by 50% if >75y) and in setting of renal impairment.

Monitoring Check FBC and renal function weekly for the first month, 2-weekly for 2nd and 3rd months, and monthly thereafter.

- If WCC <4 × 10^9/L, neutrophils <2 × 10^9/L, stop oral cyclophosphamide, and restart with dose reduced by at least 25mg when WCC recovered, and then monitor weekly for 4 weeks
- If prolonged (WCC <4 × 10^9/L, neutrophils <2 × 10^9/L for >2 weeks) or severe (WCC <1 × 10^9/L, neutrophils <0.5 × 10^9/L) leucopenia/ neutropenia, stop cyclophosphamide, and restart at 50mg daily when WCC recovered; then increase to target dose weekly, WCC permitting
- If WCC is falling (<6 × 10^9/L and fall of >2 × 10^9/L since previous count), reduce dose by 25%.

Pulsed IV cyclophosphamide is given if patients cannot take oral preparations, using doses of 15mg/kg (reduced for age and renal function, maximum dose 1,500mg) every 2 weeks for the first three pulses, and then at 3-weekly intervals. The lowest WCC occurs 10 days after a pulse. A randomized study has shown that pulsed doses give a lower cumulative dose than oral regimes, but there is no difference in remission rates between the two. The infection rate is higher with oral regimes (European Vasculitis Study Group).

If giving IV cyclophosphamide, patients should be well hydrated before (1L normal saline) and after (3L/day oral fluids for 3 days) and given mesna, which chelates with the urotoxic cyclophosphamide metabolite acrolein. Dose varies according to the cyclophosphamide dose and is available on product literature. Give during cyclophosphamide infusion and also 4 and 8h after. Prescribe anti-emetics.

Monitoring Check FBC and renal function on day of pulse or previous day.

- If WCC <4 × 10^9/L, neutrophils <2 × 10^9/L, postpone pulse until WCC >4 × 10^9/L, neutrophils >2 × 10^9/L, whilst checking FBC weekly, and reduce dose by 25%
- After first pulse, check FBC between days 10 and day of next pulse: reduce dose of next pulse by 40% of previous dose if WCC nadir 1–2 × 10^9/L or neutrophil nadir 0.5–1.0 × 10^9/L
- Reduce dose of next pulse by 20% of previous dose if WCC nadir 2–3 × 10^9/L or neutrophil nadir 1–1.5 × 10^9/L
- Thereafter, check FBC on day of pulse or previous day, unless dose adjustment when checked additionally at day 10.

Further information

Lapraik C *et al.* British Society of Rheumatology and British Heath Professionals in Rheumatology guidelines for the management of adults with ANCA associated vasculitis. *Rheumatology* 2007;**46**:1615–16.

Chapter 55

Inhalers and nebulizers

Background

Inhalers

- There are many different inhaler devices that deliver drugs directly to the airways, but essentially two basic types MDIs and dry powder inhalers (DPIs). New devices are being introduced all the time, with one or two (or even three) drugs delivered simultaneously. Check what is available through your local formulary (see Table 55.1)
- Ideally patients should try a range of devices to choose the most appropriate for them
- Patients should receive advice and a demonstration on inhaler technique and use (see Table 55.2)
- Technique should be checked regularly, and, if patients cannot manage a particular device, they should be switched to another
- Many pharmacists have been trained to assess inhaler technique
- The percentage of a drug delivered to the airway varies for each device (from 15% to 60%, according to the manufacturers) and depends on good technique
- Spacer devices improve the delivery with MDIs and are particularly useful for the elderly, children, and those who find it difficult to coordinate inhaler administration with breathing. They reduce unwanted oropharyngeal deposition of steroids
- Try to use the same type of inhaler device for all the drug classes used by a patient
- Advise the patient how to recognize when a device is empty: some have dose counters; others are shaken to hear if they still have contents
- Titrate inhaler doses with clinical response, using the minimum possible. Inhaled steroids do have side effects, and the dose should be kept to a minimum.

Different inhaler types and instructions for their use

Table 55.1 Different medications available for inhalers (not exhaustive; new ones come on the market regularly; check with your local formulary)

Generic name of drug (with product names)	Mechanism of action	Usual inhaler colour
Salbutamol (Ventolin®, Asmasal®, Pulvinal®, Salbutamol, Salamol®, Salbutamol Cyclocaps®, Airomir®, Asmasal Clickhaler®, Salamol Easi-Breathe®)	Short-acting β₂ agonist Duration 3–5h	Blue
Terbutaline (Bricanyl®)		
Salmeterol (Serevent®)	LABA	Green
Formoterol (Foradil®, Oxis®, Atimos Modulite®)	Duration 12h	Green/turquoise
Indacaterol maleate (Onbrez Breezhaler®)	Duration 24h	White/blue
Ipratropium bromide (Atrovent®)	Short-acting anticholinergic	White/grey
Ipratropium and salbutamol (Combivent®)		
Tiotropium (Spiriva®)	Long-acting anticholinergic	Grey Handihaler®, Respimat®
Aclidinium bromide (Eklira Genuair®)	Duration 12h	White/green
Glycopyrronium bromide (Seebri Breezhaler®)	Duration 24h	White/orange
Beclometasone dipropionate (Pulvinal®, Beclometasone, AeroBec®, AerobecForte®, Asmabec Clickhaler®, Qvar®, Pulvinal®)	Corticosteroid	Brown
Budesonide (Pulmicort®, Novolizer®)		Brown
Fluticasone propionate (Flixotide®)		Red
Mometasone furoate (Asmanex®)		Red
Ciclesonide (Alvesco®)		Red
Salmeterol and fluticasone (Seretide®)	Combined steroid and bronchodilator	Purple
Eformoterol and budesonide (Symbicort®)		Red/white
Formoterol and beclometasone (Fostair®)		White/orange
Fluticasone and formoterol (Flutiform®)		White/grey/orange
Sodium cromoglicate (Intal®)	Unknown, stabilize mast cells	Yellow/white
Neocromil sodium (Tilade®)		

Table 55.2 Instructions for use of different inhaler types

Type of device	Instructions for use
Pressurized aerosol MDI (e.g. aerosol Evohaler®)	Remove the mouthpiece, and shake the inhaler well. Hold the inhaler upright, with the thumb on the base below the mouthpiece and the first finger on the metal canister. Breathe out as far as is comfortable, then place the mouthpiece between the teeth, and close lips around it. Do not bite it. As you start to breathe in through the mouth, press on the top of the inhaler to release the medication whilst still breathing in steadily and deeply. Hold your breath; take the inhaler from your mouth, and continue holding your breath for up to 10s, if possible. Wait 30s prior to taking 2nd puff. Use with spacer device to improve drug delivery.
	CFC-free inhalers need washing every 2–3 weeks, as they can block.
Spacer Nebuhaler® Nebuchamber® Volumatic® Aero Chamber® Able Spacer® PARI Vortex Spacer® Pocket Chamber® OptiChamber® OptiHaler®	Ensure spacer is compatible with patient's inhaler. Remove cap of inhaler, and shake it. Insert it into end of spacer device. Place the other end of the spacer in the mouth. Press the inhaler canister once to release one dose of the drug. Take one long, slow breath in and hold, or take 3–4 steady breaths in and out. Repeat as indicated. In some, the valve should click.
	Clean the spacer once a month with mild detergent; rinse, and air-dry. Replace after 6–12 months. Some spacer devices will whistle or sound if you breathe in too fast.
Breath-actuated devices Autohaler® Easi-Breathe®	If an **Autohaler®**, remove the cap and lift the red lever. Insert device into mouth. Inhale slowly and deeply. Continue inhaling when the device 'clicks'. Hold breath for up to 10s, if possible. Slowly breathe out. To take a 2nd inhaled dose, lower the red lever and lift again. If an **Easi-Breathe®**, open the hinged cap. Insert device into mouth. Inhale slowly and deeply. Continue inhaling when the device 'clicks'. Hold breath for up to 10s, if possible. Slowly breathe out. Close the cap, and reopen for further doses. If **Easi-Breathe®** spacer used, it will need to be removed between each inhalation so that cap can be opened and closed.

(Continued)

Table 55.2 (Continued)

Type of device	Instructions for use
Dry powder devices Accuhaler® Breezhaler® Turbohaler® Dischaler® Clickhaler® Genuair® Handihaler® Inhaler Pulvinal® Twisthaler® Easyhaler® Cyclohaler® Aerocaps® Novolizer®	Prime the device. **Turbohaler®**: hold upright; remove the cap; twist the base as far as possible until the click is heard, and then twist back again. **Clickhaler®**: shake the device; remove the cap; click the top down and release, dose ready. **Twisthaler®**: remove the cap by twisting and the dose ready. **Accuhaler®**: open inhaler cover, mouthpiece facing you, and push lever down to pierce the blister containing dose. **Diskhaler®**: insert disc into device by opening and pulling out mouthpiece section. To prepare dose, lift up back of lid to 90° until the blister is pierced, then lower the lid. **Handihaler®** and **Breezhaler®**: open devices; insert capsule into chamber; close mouthpiece section; pierce capsule by firmly pressing side button(s). To use all the devices, hold them level; exhale fully; place the mouthpiece into mouth between teeth, and inhale deeply and forcefully. Hold your breath, and remove the inhaler. For a 2nd dose, repeat the above actions.
Respimat® for Spiriva® and Combivent®	To load cartridge, remove clear base; insert cartridge until flush with device; replace clear base. Hold inhaler upright, with cap closed. Turn the transparent base until it clicks. Open the cap. Breathe out slowly, and insert the mouthpiece and seal with lips. Point towards the back of the throat. While taking a deep breath, press the button and continue to breathe in. Hold your breath for 10s, if possible, and breathe out slowly.

There are many YouTube videos showing how to use most of these inhalers.

These lists (see Tables 55.1 and 55.2) are up to date at time of writing. Some inhalers are only licensed for asthma or COPD.

Nebulizers are used when they bring greater relief than inhaled therapy, either during acute respiratory illnesses, because of disease severity, or because they are unable to use inhalers. Patients for possible nebulizer therapy should be referred to a respiratory physician. Nebulized antibiotics need a more powerful pump and special neb-set.

How to use Open the ampoule containing the drug solution, and squirt the solution into the nebulizer chamber. Salbutamol and ipratropium bromide can be taken together, but nebulized budesonide or antibiotics should be used separately. If ipratropium bromide only is being used, this should be delivered via a mouthpiece, as it can lead to glaucoma if used via a mask (atropine-like constricting effects on the pupil). Re-attach the chamber to the nebulizer mask or mouthpiece. Put the mask over nose and mouth, or position mouthpiece between the lips fully in the mouth. Switch the compressor on. Breathe slowly in and out. Continue until all the solution is gone. Switch off the machine. Rinse the nebulizer chamber with hot water (and very dilute washing-up liquid) after each use. If nebulization takes >10min, change the neb-set (mask, chamber, tubing last 1–3 months). If no improvement, consider servicing the machine. If the patient is using O_2, this can still be used during nebulization, either via nasal prongs under the nebulizer mask or by using O_2 tubing attached directly to the nebulizer chamber to drive the nebulization; at home, most cylinders do not provide sufficient flow rates to allow this. Nebulizer machines should be serviced annually.

Chapter 56

Intensive care unit (ICU)—when to involve

General points

Ideally, communicate with ICU early, as it is much better that they know about a potentially sick patient who may need ICU input than to find your patient (and you!) in difficulty later on, with no ICU bed.

Scoring systems for the early recognition of sick patients are in use in many hospitals, enabling doctors and nursing staff to readily identify and assess a deteriorating patient, including response to treatment. An example is shown in Table 56.1.

The common situations in which ICU input may be required in relation to respiratory disease are principally those relating to decisions about intubation and ventilation. Most commonly these will be:

- Respiratory failure (either type I or type II)
  - Exacerbation of COPD (usually type II failure). Patients with COPD admitted to ICU have a hospital mortality of 20–25%. Poor prognostic factors include low baseline FEV_1, long-term O_2 use, low sodium and albumin, low BMI, poor functional status, and comorbid disease. Age does not add prognostic information
  - Pneumonia (to maintain an adequate pO_2—usually type I failure). In this situation, ICU input may not necessarily lead to intubation, as adequate oxygenation may be achieved by the proper use of a non-rebreathe mask, Optiflow (humidified high-flow nasal O_2), or CPAP, with the additional benefits of one-to-one nursing. Altered mental state and difficulty clearing secretions may make invasive ventilation necessary
- Upper airway emergencies
- ≥1 organ failure (not necessarily with respiratory failure)
- Sepsis requiring organ support, particularly circulatory support requiring vasoactive drugs

Many factors are considered when assessing suitability for ICU admission including: diagnosis, illness severity, coexisting disease, physiological reserve, prognosis, availability of suitable treatment, response to treatment to date, anticipated QoL, patient's wishes.

National Early Warning Score (NEWS)

This is an example of a ward-based patient illness severity scoring system. It is used to assist medical and nursing staff in the early identification of sick patients, to enable prompt and appropriate HDU/ICU liaison (see Table 56.1).

Table 56.1 Scoring system for the early recognition of sick patients

Score	3	2	1	0	1	2	3
HR/min	≤40		41–50	51–90	91–110	111–130	≥131
SBP	≤90	91–100	101–110	111–219			≥220
RR/min	≤8		9–11	12–20		21–24	≥25
Temp/°C	≤35		35.1–36	36.1–38	38.1–39	≥39.1	
SaO₂	≤91	92–93	94–95	≥96			
Supplemental O₂		Yes		No			
Conscious level				A			V, P, or U

A = alert; V = responds to voice; P = responds to pain; U = unresponsive.

Calculate the NEWS total by the addition of the scores in each column.

Total score 1–4: increase observations to 4–6-hourly.

Total score ≥5 (or 3 in any parameter): increase observations to hourly; contact doctor for urgent review.

Total score ≥7: continuous monitoring of vitals; contact senior doctor for immediate review, including assessment by critical care team.

Respiratory rate is the most sensitive marker of illness severity.

Chapter 57

Non-invasive ventilation

Terminology

Ventilatory support may be invasive (via endotracheal tube or tracheostomy) or non-invasive (via nasal mask or face mask). NIV may be subdivided into positive or negative pressure ventilation (rarely used now).

Positive pressure ventilators (also called NIV, bi-level, BiPAP (trade name)) deliver volume or pressure support; many different types are available. Bi-level pressure support devices are used extensively and provide ventilation with a higher inspiratory positive airway pressure than expiratory pressure (IPAP and EPAP, the difference in pressure between the two is also called pressure support), selected by the prescriber. They function in several modes, but usually patient-triggered inspiratory support, with provision of an underlying back-up rate that will cut in if the patient fails to breathe. Non-invasive positive pressure support may be provided by specialized portable ventilators or by standard critical care ventilators.

New 'intelligent' non-invasive ventilators are becoming available that adjust the ventilation on a breath-to-breath basis. Servo-ventilators (adaptive servo-ventilation, ASV) for Cheyne–Stokes breathing 'learn' this ventilation pattern and can increase the pressure support during the hypoventilation phase and decrease it during the hyperventilation phase, effectively 'ironing out' the oscillations without leading to over-ventilation and hypocapnia. Volume-assured pressure support ventilation (VAPSV) is where tidal volumes and minute ventilation are monitored and the inspiratory pressure is adjusted to maintain the previous 'learned' ventilation. The role of these new ventilators is still being assessed, and they may only be appropriate for certain clinical situations.

Negative pressure ventilators assist inspiration by 'sucking out' the chest wall; expiration occurs through elastic recoil of the lungs and chest wall. Includes devices such as tank ventilators and chest 'cuirasse' or 'shell' ventilators. The Hayek oscillator is a high-frequency version of the negative pressure cuirasse ventilator. Other devices, such as the rocking bed and 'pneumobelt', displace abdominal contents to aid diaphragmatic contraction. Used extensively in the polio epidemics of the 1950s, they are now only very rarely used to manage chronic respiratory failure.

CPAP supplies constant positive pressure during inspiration and expiration and is therefore not a form of ventilation but is sometimes mistakenly referred to as such. It provides a 'splint' to open the upper airway and collapsed alveoli (thus improving V/Q matching). CPAP is used extensively in the community to treat OSA but also has a role in improving oxygenation in selected patients with acute respiratory failure, e.g. patients with cardiogenic pulmonary oedema, pneumocystis pneumonia (see pp. 472–3), and the obese (see pp. 594–5).

Abbreviations

- NIV: non-invasive ventilation, also referred to as non-invasive mechanical ventilation (NIMV)
- NIPPV: non-invasive positive pressure ventilation; confusingly, it is also sometimes interpreted as nasal intermittent positive pressure ventilation and sometimes referred to as 'NIPPY', after the name of a particular type of ventilator
- IPAP: inspiratory positive airways pressure
- EPAP: expiratory positive airways pressure, also referred to as positive end expiratory pressure (PEEP)
- BiPAP: bi-level positive airway pressure (IPAP > EPAP), refers to a commercial product but now mistakenly used to refer to similar machines
- CPAP: continuous positive airway pressure (IPAP ≈ EPAP)
- VAPSV : volume-assured pressure support ventilation
- ASV: adaptive servo- (or support) ventilation.

Further information

Mehta s, Hill NS. Noninvasive ventilation. *Am J Respir Crit Care Med* 2001;**163**:540–77.

Antonescu-Turku A, Parthasarathy S. CPAP and bi-level PAP therapy: new and established roles. *Respir Care* 2010;**55**:1216–29.

Harris N, Javaheri S. Advanced PAP therapies, in *Fundamentals of sleep technology, 2nd edn*, Lippincott, Williams and Wilkins, Philadelphia 2012; pp. 444–52.

Indications

NIV may be used in an attempt to avoid invasive ventilation and its complications (e.g. upper airway trauma, VAP); alternatively, NIV may represent the 'ceiling' of treatment in patients deemed unsuitable for intubation. NIV is *not* an alternative to invasive ventilation in patients who require this definitive treatment, as it is not sufficiently secure.

Acute exacerbation of COPD

- Consider NIV in patients with an acute exacerbation of COPD who have a respiratory acidosis (pH <7.30) despite initial medical treatment and controlled O_2 therapy
- Still often required to rescue patients who have been given too high a concentration of O_2 to breath, reduced hypoxic drive, and have become hypercapnic and acidotic; response to NIV can be rapid
- Benefits include reduced mortality and need for intubation, more rapid improvement in physiological outcomes (RR, pH), and symptomatic relief from breathlessness, when compared with standard medical treatment
- NIV only assists ventilation; the pressures used are not enough to take over ventilation due to the high airways resistance
- Invasive ventilation, if deemed appropriate, should be considered, particularly in patients with a severe respiratory acidosis (pH <7.25), as this is associated with treatment failure and increased mortality with NIV alone
- High expiratory pressures (e.g. 6–8cmH$_2$O, PEEP) may help reduce the work of breathing by offsetting intrinsic PEEP but will lessen the IPAP–EPAP difference (thus reducing the ventilation component), unless inspiratory pressures are further increased.

Acute cardiogenic pulmonary oedema

- Use of CPAP via face mask is effective and should be considered in patients who fail to improve with medical management alone
- Bi-level NIV has not been shown to be superior to CPAP, and there is a suggestion of increased MI rates following its use. It may, however, have a role in patients who do not respond to CPAP.

Decompensated OSA

NIV is effective in the treatment of OSA and the overlap syndrome (i.e. raised $PaCO_2$, typically with associated obesity hypoventilation or COPD; see pp. 594–5) when CPAP alone fails to reverse the CO_2 retention. NIV is generally recommended as the first choice over CPAP when an acute respiratory acidosis is present, but conversion to CPAP later may be possible when the ventilatory failure has been reversed.

Respiratory failure from neuromuscular weakness

- NIV is the treatment of choice for ventilatory failure resulting from neuromuscular weakness or chest wall deformity
- The pressures used may be adequate to fully take over ventilation, because the chest and lung compliance are often little impaired.

Immunocompromised patients

- Immunocompromised patients who develop acute respiratory failure have an extremely high mortality following endotracheal intubation and ventilation
- In immunocompromised patients with pulmonary infiltrates, fever, and hypoxaemic acute respiratory failure, intermittent NIV results in lower intubation rates and hospital mortality when compared with standard treatment
- CPAP is effective in the treatment of pneumocystis pneumonia.

CAP

- Use of NIV may result in a reduction in need for intubation, compared with standard medical treatment, although no significant differences in hospital mortality or length of hospitalization have been shown
- CPAP may have a role in improving oxygenation in severe pneumonia
- In patients who would potentially be candidates for intubation, use of NIV or CPAP should not inappropriately delay invasive ventilation and so should only be attempted in an ICU setting.

Other conditions

- There is no evidence to support use of NIV in acute severe asthma, and it should not be used; if ventilation is required, then it should be invasive
- No strong evidence to support use of NIV in exacerbations of bronchiectasis or CF; NIV often used, improving symptoms, and may be useful as a 'ceiling' of treatment in patients with severe underlying disease who would not be considered candidates for invasive ventilation
- Bi-level NIV or CPAP may have a role in improving gas exchange following trauma or surgery
- NIV is being increasingly used to aid weaning after invasive ventilation.

Contraindications

Contraindications (some relative) to the use of NIV should be considered in the context of individual patients, e.g. severe hypoxaemia may not be considered a contraindication for NIV in a patient who is unsuitable for invasive ventilation.

Contraindications to NIV

- Cardiac or respiratory arrest
- Impaired consciousness or confusion (relative)
- Severe hypoxaemia
- Copious respiratory secretions
- Haemodynamic instability (relative)
- Facial surgery, trauma, burns, or deformity
- Upper airway obstruction (except from pharyngeal or laryngeal OSA)
- Undrained pneumothorax
- Inability to cooperate or to protect the airway
- Vomiting, bowel obstruction, recent upper GI tract surgery, oesophageal injury.

Further information

Plant PK *et al.* Early use of non-invasive ventilation for acute exacerbations of chronic obstructive pulmonary disease on general respiratory wards. *Lancet* 2000;**355**:1931–5.

Royal College of Physicians, BTS, and Intensive Care Society guidelines. Non-invasive ventilation in chronic obstructive pulmonary disease: management of acute type 2 respiratory failure. ℜ http://www.rcplondon.ac.uk/sites/default/files/concise-niv-in-copd-2008.pdf.

NIV in acute respiratory failure: practical use

The decision to start NIV should follow a period of initial standard medical treatment, including appropriate supplementary and controlled O_2 therapy; a proportion of patients will improve and will no longer require ventilation. Prior to commencing NIV, a senior doctor should make a decision with the patient and their family regarding suitability for invasive ventilation, should NIV fail, and document this clearly in the medical notes. *If the patient is a candidate for invasive ventilation, care must be taken to avoid inappropriate delays in intubation through the use of NIV or CPAP. Liaise with ICU staff early.*

Setting up NIV

1. Select an appropriate mask type and size for the patient. Masks may be nasal or oronasal (full face). Nasal masks require clear nasal passages but often allow mouth leaks, particularly in the acutely breathless patient, but may be more comfortable. Full-face masks avoid mouth leakage and are now generally favoured for ventilatory failure

2. Allow the patient to hold the mask to their face prior to attaching the head straps—this may increase confidence and compliance. Mask adjustments are often necessary to minimize air leaks, although some leakage may have to be accepted. Avoid excessive strap tension; one or two fingers should be able to fit under the strap

3. Set up the ventilator. Typical initial pressures for ventilating a patient with hypercapnic respiratory failure due to an exacerbation of COPD would be EPAP 4cmH_2O and IPAP 12cmH_2O, with a back-up rate of 15/min and inspiratory:expiratory ratio of 1:3 in spontaneous/timed mode. Increase the IPAP in increments of 2cmH_2O to a maximum of 20, as tolerated by the patient. Similar settings can be used for patients with hypercapnic respiratory failure resulting from neuromuscular weakness. Increase the EPAP (e.g. to 8 or 10cm) in obese patients with an 'overlap' syndrome of COPD and OSA to maintain airway patency during inspiration to allow triggering.

   Pressure support ventilators can also be set to provide CPAP by equalizing the IPAP and EPAP; typical pressures range from 5 to 12.5cmH_2O. CPAP may improve oxygenation in selected patients with cardiogenic pulmonary oedema or pneumonia.

4. Supplementary O_2 concentration (FiO_2) should be guided by the underlying disease process and by oximetry monitoring. For many hypercapnic patients with COPD, aiming for O_2 saturations between 88% and 92% effectively balances the risks of hypoxia vs hypercapnic respiratory acidosis. By adding O_2, you are potentially masking gradual ventilation failure (by deceptively achieving adequate oxygenation) and thus hypercapnia, hence more careful blood gas monitoring will be required. If at all possible, use no, or very little, added O_2

5. Patient monitoring should involve assessment of comfort, RR, synchrony with the ventilator, mask leaks, pulse rate, BP, and O_2 saturations

6. Arterial or capillary blood gas analysis should be performed after no more than 1h, and again after within an hour if there has been no improvement. Improvement in acidosis and decline in RR after 1 and 4h

of treatment are associated with a better outcome. Repeat the blood gas analysis if the clinical condition changes

7. Lack of response may be indicated by a worsening acidosis or persistently abnormal ABGs, or by a reduced conscious level and clinical deterioration. Consider invasive ventilation, if appropriate. The decision to halt NIV depends on the circumstances of the individual patient and should be made by a senior doctor

8. Subsequent management depends on the patient's response. Optimal duration of NIV is unclear, but it is typically administered for about 3 days in acute respiratory failure. NIV does not need to be continuous; the patient may have breaks for meals and nebulizers. Weaning should be gradual and achieved by increasing the period off NIV, with nocturnal use withdrawn last.

There is no substitute for personally assessing the efficacy of NIV (see Table 57.1). For example, failure to see the lungs inflating can be due to head position (best head position is the so-called 'sniffing the morning air' position; produces least pharyngeal resistance). Leaks can be heard. Adjustments can be made; immediately observe the effect. Sometimes, the presence of intrinsic PEEP means significant inspiratory effort is being made (visible intercostal movement) before the ventilator senses inspiration and triggers, thus increasing work of breathing. This can be seen and the EPAP gradually raised, until there is no delay between patient inspiratory effort and the triggering of the ventilator.

Table 57.1 Troubleshooting

Problem	Possible solution
Clinical deterioration or worsening respiratory failure	Ensure optimal medical therapy
	Consider complications, e.g. pneumothorax, aspiration, sputum retention
	Does the patient require intubation, if appropriate?
pCO_2 remains high (persistent respiratory acidosis)	Exclude inappropriately high FiO_2 (producing SaO_2 >92%)
	Check mask and circuit for leaks
	Check for patient–ventilator asynchrony
	Check expiration valve or blow off is patent
	Consider increasing IPAP
pO_2 remains low (<7kPa), with pCO_2 OK	Consider increasing FiO_2
	Consider increasing EPAP
Irritation or ulceration	Adjust strap tension of nasal bridge
	Try cushion dressing
	Change mask type
Dry nose or mouth	Consider humidifier
	Check for leaks
Dry sore eyes	Check mask fit
Nasal congestion	Decongestants, e.g. xylometazoline
Hypotension	Reduce IPAP (or EPAP if already high)

NIV in chronic respiratory failure

Chest wall deformity and neuromuscular weakness
(see ⊃ pp. 592–3)

- NIV has a well-established role in the management of chronic respiratory failure due to chest wall deformity or neuromuscular weakness and has been shown to improve symptoms, gas exchange, and mortality

- Common underlying diagnoses include chest wall deformity and scoliosis, post-polio syndrome, MND, spinal cord injury, neuropathies, myopathies, and muscular dystrophies. The nature of the underlying disease must influence the appropriateness of initiating ventilation; progressive conditions, such as MND, often result in increasing dependence on the ventilator, and the patient and their caregivers should be made aware of this

- NIV is administered at home overnight, and this improves daytime gas exchange. The mechanism for this is unclear; it probably resets the central respiratory drive, although respiratory muscle rest and improved chest wall and lung compliance may also play a part

- Small portable positive pressure ventilators, with either face (usual) or nasal (less often) masks, are used in the majority of cases; negative pressure or abdominal ventilators rarely have a role these days, and their use may be limited by upper airways obstruction

- The decision to introduce overnight NIV is difficult and is based on both symptoms (morning headaches, hypersomnolence, fatigue, poor sleep quality) and evidence of ventilatory failure (daytime hypercapnia (pCO_2 >6.0kPa, and/or base excess >3) and/or nocturnal hypoventilation (with O_2 saturations <88% on overnight oximetry). Daytime ventilatory failure, however, is often a late feature and is typically preceded by hypoventilation during sleep

- A study in patients with myopathies demonstrated supine inspiratory VC (more sensitive to any diaphragm weakness than sitting or standing) to be an accurate predictor of respiratory reserve; supine inspiratory VC <40% predicted was significantly associated with hypercapnic hypoventilation, and such patients should be considered for treatment with NIV. Supine inspiratory VC <20% was typically associated with daytime respiratory failure, whereas supine inspiratory VC >60% indicated a minimal risk of respiratory complications. Other factors include signs of cor pulmonale or hospital admission with respiratory failure

- Patients with excessive secretions may not be suitable for NIV, although face mask ventilation is possible, even in the setting of bulbar weakness

- Regular follow-up of patients on overnight ventilation is important. Ask about symptoms and compliance, and repeat arterial or capillary blood gas analysis, if indicated. Lack of improvement in gas exchange may reflect non-compliance, excessive air leakage, inadequate pressure support, or progression of underlying disease; consider repeating nocturnal oximetry monitoring on the NIV. Patients with persisting

severe hypoxia may benefit from long-term supplementary O_2, although this may worsen CO_2 retention
• There are significant issues of risk management when prescribing home NIV, particularly rapid access to replacement ventilators, battery back-up facilities, careful reassessment when there is evidence of a deterioration, and appropriate training of both the patient and their carer(s).

Sleep apnoea
(see ➲ pp. 592–3)
Overnight NIV can have a role in patients with central hypoventilation, opiate-induced central apnoea, Cheyne–Stokes respiration, obesity hypoventilation, overlap syndromes of OSA with coexisting COPD or obesity. There is the prospect of further developments in 'smart' ventilators, beyond ASV and VAPSV where not only is the pressure support monitored and adjusted, but the level of EPAP required to hold open the pharynx is also adjusted; additional forced oscillation is superimposed on the airflow from the ventilator, and the resultant pressure oscillations enable obstructive episodes (both apnoeas and hypopnoeas) to be distinguished central events. Thus, appropriate inspiratory and expiratory pressures are automatically selected. It is not clear if these new devices work consistently across all aetiologies.

CF
(see ➲ p. 223)
Overnight NIV may have a useful role as a 'bridge' to transplantation in patients with CF and chronic respiratory failure.

COPD
(see ➲ pp. 174–5)
Use of NIV in the management of chronic stable COPD is controversial. Trials have shown conflicting results, although there is some possible benefit in a subgroup of patients with severe hypercapnia, extra nocturnal hypoventilation, and recurrent admissions for worsening ventilatory failure. A recent RCT suggested no overall benefit but may have used suboptimal pressures and interfaces. Further RCTs in this area are ongoing, and the use of the new 'smart' ventilator technology may improve the success rate.

Further information
Elliott MW. Domiciliary non-invasive ventilation in stable COPD? *Thorax*; 2009;**64**:553–6.

Ragette R et al. Patterns and predictors of sleep disordered breathing in primary myopathies. *Thorax* 2002;**57**:724–8.

De Backer L et al. The effects of long-term noninvasive ventilation in hypercapnic COPD patients: a randomized controlled pilot study. *Int J Chron Obstruct Pulmon Dis* 2011;**6**:615–24.

McEvoy RD et al. Nocturnal non-invasive nasal ventilation in stable hypercapnic COPD: a randomized controlled trial. *Thorax* 2009;**64**:561–6.

O'Donaghue FJ et al. Effect of CPAP on intrinsic PEEP, inspiratory effort, and lung volume in severe stable COPD. *Thorax* 2002;**57**:533–9.

Marinii JJ. Dynamic hyperinflation and auto-positive end-expiratory pressure. *Am J Respir Crit Care Med* 2011;**184**:756–62.

Simonds AK. Risk management of the home ventilator dependent patient. *Thorax* 2006;**61**:369–71.

Chapter 58

Oxygen therapy

Emergency O_2 therapy

O_2 therapy is either 'controlled' or 'uncontrolled'.
- *Uncontrolled* and highest levels thought to be important, e.g.:
  - Shock, sepsis, major trauma
  - Cardiac arrest and during resuscitation
  - Anaphylaxis
  - CO or cyanide poisoning
  - Pneumothorax
- *Uncontrolled* and SaO_2 values between 94 and 98% are thought best. Use when extra O_2 is required to raise the SaO_2 *and* where there are no concerns that high PaO_2 values will depress ventilatory drive to the point that $PaCO_2$ will rise and pH fall dangerously, e.g.
  - Pneumonia
  - Asthma
  - Acute heart failure
  - PE
- *Controlled* Use when extra O_2 is required, but ventilation critically depends on hypoxic drive (BTS recommends 88–92%), e.g.:
  - Exacerbations of COPD (particularly when there has been a chronically raised $PaCO_2$, as evidenced by a significant base excess)
  - Exacerbations of CF
  - Exacerbations of ventilatory failure due to obesity hypoventilation syndrome
  - Exacerbations of chronic ventilatory failure due to scoliosis, neuromuscular disease, and any other cause of 'pump' failure.

With stable type II ventilatory failure, ventilation still seems to be dominantly driven by $PaCO_2$/pH, but, in exacerbations (when PaO_2 usually falls), peripheral chemoreceptor drive from low PaO_2 becomes dominant. Thus, O_2 therapy must not raise PaO_2 above 8kPa ($\approx$ 92% SaO_2), as this will 'turn off' ventilatory drive, allowing hypoventilation, hypercapnia, acidosis, and potentially death. There is some evidence that high alveolar PO_2 also 'turns off' hypoxic pulmonary vasoconstriction. This allows an increase in pulmonary blood flow to poorly ventilated areas and reduces CO_2 excretion (accounts for ~20% of the $PaCO_2$ rise following excessive FiO_2 in COPD exacerbations).

There is increasing evidence that indiscriminate use of O_2 in some medical emergencies may actually be *harmful* and should only be used if the patient is hypoxaemic (<94% and then to achieve no higher than 98%), e.g.:
- Ischaemic heart disease, including MI
- Post-cardiac arrest, once stable
- Sickle cell crisis
- Obstetric emergencies
- Most poisonings (other than CO or cyanide)
- Metabolic or renal acidosis with SOB.

High O$_2$ levels can be toxic through release of free radicals, and this may be the mechanism of damage in some of the above situations. Following lung injury, particularly from paraquat and bleomycin, high O$_2$ concentrations are clearly damaging to the lung; thus, a degree of controlled hypoxia may be preferable.

Delivering uncontrolled O$_2$ This can be done in many ways, essentially by blowing O$_2$ over the face, whilst limiting inhalation of surrounding air, or exhaled CO$_2$.

- Standard O$_2$ face masks (sometimes called high-flow masks). Set the O$_2$ regulator to at least 4L/min, much more if very breathless (to prevent dilution by air drawn into mask by high inspiratory flows via exit holes). Can deliver about 50–60% O$_2$
- Nasal cannulae/prongs/catheters are *uncontrolled* and deliver unpredictable levels of O$_2$ (depending on flow rate, minute ventilation, and oral vs nasal breathing). Titrate using an O$_2$ saturation monitor
- Non-rebreathe reservoir masks can deliver FiO$_2$ values over 60% by means of a soft plastic bag between the end of the tubing and mask, plus one-way valves between the bag and mask and on the mask exit ports. This mechanism ensures that most of the inspired air is pure O$_2$. The ability of the reservoir to empty on inspiration briefly allows higher inspiratory flows than the actual O$_2$ regulator setting, and the bag valve prevents inhalation of very much exhaled CO$_2$; the mask exit valves close, preventing air inhalation. The usual problem is kinking of the junction between the mask and bag when the head tilts forward, reducing the effectiveness of the reservoir
- Very high FiO$_2$ requires a tight seal and is generally delivered with CPAP masks (using pressures of about 5–7cmH$_2$O). This ensures no air is entrained through blow-off vents or leaks, as well as improving V/Q matching by recruiting collapsed alveoli.

Delivering controlled O$_2$ therapy This requires the ability to reliably control the FiO$_2$ in order to keep the patient's SaO$_2$ ≤92% (some prefer ≤90%), but high enough to prevent anaerobic metabolism. This lower acceptable level is debatable: 88% is generous; 85% is likely to be adequate, and 80% may be acceptable if cardiac output is adequate and patient's usual levels are around this figure.

- FiO$_2$ is controlled through Venturi masks—O$_2$ is directed through a narrow nozzle and exits at speed, lowering the air pressure at this point. This draws in surrounding air, diluting the O$_2$
- A proper Venturi mask mixes O$_2$ and air in the same proportion, *regardless of the O2 flow*
- The minimum flow setting of the regulator, written on the nozzle, ensures adequate overall flow to prevent diluting air being drawn through the exit holes during inhalation, e.g. a 28% ventimask has a 1:10 entrainment ratio—1L/min O$_2$ entrains 10L/min air (total flow 11L/min); 2L/min O$_2$ entrains 20L/min air (total flow 22L/min), etc.

- Nasal cannulae are definitely not controlled O_2 therapy and are, in fact, the opposite. If nasal cannulae do deliver too high an FiO_2 and ventilation decreases as a consequence, the proportion of the minute ventilation containing the fixed flow nasal O_2 will rise, increasing the FiO_2 and hence PaO_2 still further—a vicious cycle
- Controlled O_2 via low flows is also needed sometimes with NIV but rarely requires >1L/min to be entrained; again it should be titrated using the SaO_2
- When the patient on NIV is still required to trigger inspiration, again added O_2 should be kept to a minimum so as not do depress ventilatory drive
- When adding too much O_2, it is easy to be lulled into a false sense of security by an SaO_2 value >92%, while the $PaCO_2$ gradually rises undetected.

O_2 **alert card** should be given to all patients with a previous episode of hypercapnic respiratory failure (see Fig. 58.1). This alerts ambulance crews and medical staff to the potential risk of hypercapnia with high-flow O_2 and documents usual resting baseline SaO_2. However, some ambulance staff protocols are sufficiently rigid that they may not be allowed to override them. In some areas, letters from the patient's consultant and head of the ambulance service must be with the patient.

Patient details	Carry the card with you at all times
Sticky label	**If you need to call the ambulance service or attend the hospital accident and emergency department, show this card to the GP, paramedics, doctor, or emergency department staff looking after you, as it provides them with essential information regarding your personal oxygen needs.**
Introduction If you have a sudden worsening of your lung disease (usually due to a chest infection) it is essential that you do not receive too much or too little oxygen, either can be dangerous. Too much oxygen can cause a rise in the level of carbon dioxide in your blood and this can make you drowsy and slow your breathing. Too little oxygen can also be dangerous.	**Latest blood gas recordings:** **Date:**____/ ____/_____ **On:** Air, or % oxygen ____% **pH:** ____ pCO$_2$____pO$_2$____ **Oxygen saturation:** _____ %
Purpose of this card The purpose of this oxygen alert card is to make sure that the doctors or ambulance staff involved in your care are made aware of your special needs regarding oxygen therapy. The card recommends the appropriate amount of oxygen therapy for you based on your previous blood gas tests.	You should receive enough oxygen to achieve a % O2 saturation of no higher than 92%, but higher than 86%, if possible. This is usually done with either a 24% or 28% Venturi mask. Signed .... Name........................ Designation..

Fig. 58.1 Example of an O_2 alert card.

Further information

BTS guideline for emergency O_2 use in adult patients. *Thorax* 2008;**63**(suppl V):1–68.
O'Driscoll R. Emergency O_2 use. *BMJ* 2012;**345**:39–43 (much more readable than the BTS guidelines).
Gooptu B et al. O_2 alert cards and controlled O_2: preventing emergency admissions at risk. *Emerg Med J* 2006;**23**:636–8.

Home O₂ therapy

Home O_2 therapy was originally prescribed under three clear headings: (1) long-term (LTOT, treatment of chronic hypoxia in COPD, requiring >15h/day, with the evidence base from two randomized trials), (2) short-burst O_2 (SBOT, to cover periods of SOB such as after exercise), and (3) ambulatory to allow activity with less dyspnoea. The distinctions became blurred, and short-term use of O_2 for transient SOB was shown in most cases to be of little more value than a fan; the value of LTOT beyond COPD has been extended into other causes of hypoxia (without very much evidence of benefit), and ambulatory O_2 is now more available with increasing usage.

The BTS Standards of Care Subcommittee have recently produced useful advice on O_2 services (see Further information ➡ p. 713).

LTOT

Background and indications

Two landmark trials of LTOT in the 1980s—the British MRC Working Party trial and the American Nocturnal O_2 Therapy Trial (NOTT) established the value of LTOT. The *MRC trial* compared COPD patients receiving O_2 for 15h/day with controls receiving no O_2. The *NOTT trial* compared continuous daily O_2 (average 17.7h/day) with overnight O_2 (average 12h). The patients in the MRC trial were on average hypercapnic (mean $PaCO_2$ 7.3kPa), whereas those in the NOTT trial were on average normocapnic (mean $PaCO_2$ 5.7kPa). The main outcome in both trials was improved survival in those patients receiving O_2 for at least 15h/day, though this improved survival was not seen in the MRC trial until after a year of O_2 therapy.

The *NOTT trial* showed a reduced exercise PAP after 6 months of continuous or nocturnal O_2 therapy. The 8y survival was related to the fall in mean PAP during the first 6 months of continuous O_2 use.

The *MRC trial* failed to show a fall in mean PAP with LTOT, but the mean annual increase in PAP (3mmHg) in patients in the control arm was not seen in the O_2 treated group.

The reason for the improved survival with LTOT is not clear and is unlikely to relate to the small changes in pulmonary haemodynamics seen.

COPD is the disease for which LTOT is most commonly prescribed and the disease in which the original studies were completed. Subsequent O_2 studies have shown improved exercise endurance in COPD patients breathing supplemental O_2, with improved walking distance and ability to perform daily activities. FEV_1 is the strongest predictor of survival in COPD; LTOT does not influence the decline in FEV_1.

Additional benefits of LTOT include:

- Reduction of 2° polycythaemia
- Improved sleep quality by reducing hypoxia-associated brain arousals
- Reduced cardiac arrthymias, and potentially reducing the risk of nocturnal sudden death
- Reduced sympathetic outflow, leading to improved renal function, with increased salt and water excretion, and reduced peripheral oedema.

Indications for LTOT

LTOT is the provision of O_2 therapy to patients with a chronically low PaO_2 (≤7.3kPa, or ≤55mmHg, or SaO_2 ≤/≈88%) for ≥15h a day (to include the night, when usually most hypoxic), with the aim of achieving an awake PaO_2 >8kPa, or >60mmHg, or SaO_2 >/≈91%. $PaCO_2$ levels can be normal or raised.

The indications to which LTOT now covers are:
• COPD
• Severe chronic asthma
• LD
• CF
• Bronchiectasis
• Pulmonary vascular disease
• PPH
• Pulmonary malignancy
• Chronic heart failure.

LTOT can also be prescribed if the PaO_2 is between 7.3 and 8kPa, if associated with 2° polycythaemia or PHT. PaO_2 values above 8kPa should not lead to a prescription for LTOT.

In addition, it can be prescribed for nocturnal hypoventilation, usually in conjunction with NIV or CPAP, e.g. in:
• Obesity
• Neuromuscular or other restrictive disorders
• OSA treated with CPAP therapy but with continuing hypoxia.

This is entirely non-evidence-based (with no guidance on thresholds, etc.) and should only happen following assessment in a specialist unit and following optimization of the NIV or CPAP.

There are exceptional uses such as nocturnal O_2 for the Cheynes–Stokes of heart failure (despite adequate awake levels) which can improve sleep quality.

Finally, it is accepted that, in certain terminal diseases, hypoxia-induced dyspnoea can be usefully relieved with LTOT.

Assessment for LTOT
• Should occur when patients are stable and >5 weeks have passed since any exacerbation of their condition
• Fully optimized treatment
• Two sets of arterial gases are taken at least 3 weeks apart to ensure that the patient remains sufficiently hypoxic to merit LTOT
• Blood gases are also taken after 30min on supplemental O_2 to ensure the target PaO_2 has been reached.

Given the day-to-day fluctuation in blood gases and the relatively arbitrary nature of the cut-offs for qualifying for LTOT, it is very likely that oximetry would be equally precise (or imprecise) as arterial PaO_2. However, this is not currently recommended.

Arterial gases, rather than oximetry, may still be preferable when CO_2 retention is a possibility, but this can occur overnight follwing LTOT and not be evident during a 30min test. Thus, patients need to be warned about the symptoms of CO_2 retention and told to reduce or stop the supplemental O_2 if they occur.

Ambulatory O_2

Provision of supplemental O_2 during exercise and activities of daily living. This may be on its own or in addition to LTOT. The conditions provoking exercise hypoxia are of course similar to the conditions mentioned previously.

The requirement for O_2 in these circumstances depends on the degree of activity the patient is likely to achieve. If already on LTOT, then it is likely that ambulatory O_2 will be needed when away from home, should there be significant dyspnoea without it. Such patients are often housebound and would only require it for only short periods.

The patient must understand that they need to use the O_2 during the exercise/activity, not for recovery afterwards.

Greater use should require actual proof that there is significant exercise hypoxia and dyspnoea and that O_2 relieves these.

A 2-month assessment is usually required to determine the likely number of hours of use. A reasonable initial prescription might be for 1–2h/day. Ideally, usage should be regularly reviewed and withdrawn if of no benefit or not being used.

There are now many different options available for supplying portable O_2, e.g. conserver devices (delivering pulsed O_2 during inspiration only), self-fill cylinders, transportable or portable concentrators, lightweight cylinders, and liquid O_2 systems.

SBOT

Short-burst O_2 is now rarely justifed. It may be required for transient situations, such as during exacerbations, but usually either the patient is sufficiently hypoxic to require LTOT or they are not. If it is considered, then proof of efficacy should be sought, particularly given its expense.

Practical issues

- Home O_2 should not be supplied to patients who still smoke, due to added fire risk and probable reduced efficacy due to ↑ COHb
- LTOT is provided by an O_2 concentrator, set between 0.5 and 8L/min. Some concentrators can deliver 8L/min. Concentrators contain a molecular sieve of zeolite, which traps gas molecules, depending on size and polarity. Can produce up to 96% O_2, depending on flow (the argon is also concentrated to 4%)
- Patients may have a higher flow rate for use during activities
- Patients can use nasal prongs or a fixed concentration mask (uncontrolled or controlled O_2, e.g. 24% and 28%), depending on physiological requirements and their preference. A back-up cylinder should be prescribed in case of power cuts
- O_2 humidification (cold) is possible but rarely necessary or effective. Tube lengths of <1.5m recommended
- LTOT should be used for ≥15h/day in patients with COPD, although survival improves when used for longer; therefore, use should not be restricted to 15h/day
- Patient education in the use of LTOT and machine maintenance is important. Specialist respiratory nurses should be involved with this
- If using SBOT at >3 O_2 cylinders/week, an O_2 concentrator is more economical.

How to organize home O_2

- The UK-wide integrated O_2 service (2005) ensured provision of all modalities of domiciliary O_2 from one contractor in each area
- The prescriber completes *and signs* a Home Oxygen Order Form (HOOF), providing the supplier with the patient's details, an exact prescription of the O_2 required, including modality, and details of numbers of each piece of equipment needed (e.g. numbers of O_2 cylinders)—the supplier may be able to help advise on this (see Box 58.1)
- The HOOF is used for the prescription of all forms of O_2; must include details of the O_2 flow rate, % O_2, and delivery device/mask required
- HOOF part A can be used by non-specialists (e.g. GPs, out-of-hours services, palliative care) to temporarily prescribe static O_2 concentrators or static cylinder, pending specialist assessment
- HOOF part B is completed by specialist respiratory services after formal clinical assessment and provides access to the full range of O_2 services
- The O_2 supplier will invoice the local commissioning group; it is vital that the above information is completed, otherwise the HOOF will be returned unfilled
- A Home Oxygen Consent Form (HOCF) must be signed by the patient, consenting for the disclosure of relevant medical information, address, telephone number to the O_2 supplier and fire brigade
- The HOOF is faxed to the O_2 supplier, with copies to the local commissioners, GP, and clinical lead for home O_2 services

- The standard response time for delivery of O_2 services is 3 days although can be ordered as urgent (4h) or next day. The 4h option is more expensive
- The South West (Air Liquide) is currently using a single HOOF.

Follow-up is needed to ensure:
- Compliance; withdraw if not using despite support and explanation. Home visit within 4 weeks by specialist nurse recommended
- Confirm the ongoing requirement for LTOT. Some patients improve and no longer need LTOT. ABG tensions at 3 months and then yearly monitoring (may be performed by specialist nurses)
- Cancellation with the O_2 company as soon as a patients dies
- Inform O_2 company of any changes in flow rates/%O_2
- Inform O_2 company of any changes in patient address, etc.

Box 58.1 O_2 supplier 24h contact details

Air Liquide: covers
☎ 0808 143 9991 for **London**
☎ 0808 143 9992 for **North West**
☎ 0808 143 9993 for **East Midlands**
☎ 0808 143 9999 for **South West**
Call the prescribers helpline on ☎ 0808 2022 099.

Baywater Healthcare: covers **Yorkshire** *and* **Humberside, West Midlands** *and* **Wales.** Call them on ☎ 0800 373 580.

BOC: covers the **East** and **North East of England.** Call them on ☎ 0800 136 603.

Dolby Vivisol: covers the **South of England.** Call them on ☎ 0500 823 773.

Further information

The BTS standards of care subcommittee, home O_2 services sub-committee report. ⌕ http://www.brit-thoracic.org.uk/Portals/0/Clinical%20Information/Home%20Oxygen%20Service/clinical%20adultoxygenjan06.pdf.
Full BTS guidelines in preparation for 2014.
Patient information. ⌕ http://www.nhs.uk/conditions/home-oxygen/pages/introduction.aspx.

Chapter 59

Palliative care

General points

Palliative care is defined by the World Health Organization (WHO) as an approach that improves the QoL of patients and their families facing the problems associated with life-threatening illness, through the prevention and relief of suffering by means of early identification, impeccable assessment, and treatment of pain and other problems, physical, psychosocial, and spiritual. Palliative care is moving away from being involved just at the end of life, especially in developing countries when curative possibilities are less readily available and palliative treatments may be the only option. In the UK, patients may be under palliative care teams intermittently for symptom control, respite care, etc. and may not see the service again for months or years.

Within chest medicine, palliative care is most commonly considered for patients with lung cancer and mesothelioma; many other patients with progressive end-stage respiratory disease (such as COPD, CF, and fibrotic lung disease) also benefit from specific palliative interventions. These two areas are discussed separately in this chapter, although there is much overlap in the management.

Lung cancer and mesothelioma

- Involve the specialist palliative care team early
- Treat symptoms promptly
- An open discussion of patients' fears is often helpful, as is a calm and explicit logical approach to symptom management
- Recognize problems are often mixed, complex, and multiple
- Recognize that delirium, dyspnoea, and decreased mobility often herald the terminal phase of cancer.

Pain

- Aim to determine cause, type, and site
- Start with simple analgesia, and increase according to the WHO analgesic ladder, moving from non-opioid analgesia (paracetamol, NSAIDs) through weak opioids (codeine, tramadol) to strong opioids (morphine, diamorphine, fentanyl, etc.), while also considering adjuvant therapy (e.g. antidepressants, antiepileptics). Reassess repeatedly and regularly
- If moving to morphine from a weak opioid, 40–60mg morphine daily should be adequate (given either 4-hourly immediate release or 12-hourly modified-release preparations). 60mg codeine qds is equivalent to 24mg total daily morphine. If the first dose of morphine is no more effective than previous analgesia, increase next dose by 50%
- Prescribe analgesia as required for breakthrough pain (see Box 59.1)
- Give drugs a chance to work at appropriate doses, particularly if they have not had strong opioids before. Allows assessment of analgesic effect and side effects. Usually increase every 3rd day if required
- Once pain is reasonably controlled, morphine dose can be converted to slow-release morphine by dividing total daily amount by two and giving that dose as modified-release morphine 12-hourly (see Box 59.2). The *additional* breakthrough dose is 1/6 of the total 24h dose (e.g. if using 15mg *modified*-release morphine bd, then use an additional 5mg *immediate*-release morphine sulfate for breakthrough pain)
- Treat drug side effects, e.g. constipation, nausea. Prescribe prophylactic laxatives with morphine. Warn people they may feel more drowsy if starting morphine or having dose increase, but this usually settles within a few days
- Patients with renal failure are more likely to develop opioid toxicity (drowsiness, confusion, myoclonus), as they have difficulty excreting morphine metabolites. They may need alternatives to morphine (e.g. oxycodone, methadone, alfentanil, fentanyl) if their pain is not controlled on low-dose morphine
- The addition of an anti-inflammatory drug or steroids can be effective for bone pain and for liver capsule pain if there are hepatic metastases
- Consider radiotherapy for localized pain in the chest related to cancer
- *Pleuritic pain* Consider PE; treat any infection. Consider NSAID ± intercostal nerve block

- *Bone metastases causing local tenderness* Start a strong opioid. If there is no improvement after three dose increases, add an NSAID for a 1-week trial. If single site, consider radiotherapy or intercostal nerve block. If multiple sites, consider bisphosphonates (provided not hypocalcaemic), e.g. 90mg of pamidronate IV every 4 weeks
- *Neuropathic pain* can be treated with tricyclic antidepressants (e.g. amitriptyline started at 10–25mg nocte or nortriptyline) or antiepileptics (e.g. pregabalin started at 75mg bd or gabapentin). In some cases, there may be a role for lidocaine patches or capsaicin cream
- *Pain from chest drain tract metastases* Use analgesia, and refer for radiotherapy
- Consider referral to pain clinic or specialist centre for further intervention such as a intercostal nerve block, transcutaneous electrical nerve stimulation (TENS), cervical cordotomy, or complementary therapies.

Box 59.1 Treatment of breakthrough pain

- *If already on non-opioid analgesic* Give one extra dose of the regular analgesic
- *If already on a regular oral opioid* Give 4-hourly oral dose (= 1/6 of total 24h dose), e.g. 60mg/day = 10mg dose
- *If already on continuous SC infusion of morphine/diamorphine* Give 4-hourly dose, e.g. 30mg/24h = 5mg dose SC.

Consider increasing regular analgesic dose if the breakthrough pain occurs before the next regular dose.

If there is no response to the additional breakthrough pain treatment, repeat after 4h if non-opioid or 1h if opioid, with same dose. If still no response, consider changing from non-opioid to weak opioid, or weak opioid to strong opioid.

Box 59.2 Conversions between opioids

Different opioids at equivalent doses do not provide greater analgesic efficacy but offer alternative routes for administration to ensure adequate absorption and minimize side effects (usually toxicity and confusion).

- *Oral morphine to SC morphine* Conversion factor is ÷ 2, e.g. 60mg/24h oral morphine = 30mg SC morphine
- *Oral morphine to diamorphine infusion* Conversion factor is ÷ 3, e.g. 60mg/24h oral morphine = 20mg/24h SC diamorphine
- *Oral morphine to 72h transdermal fentanyl patch* See *British National Formulary (BNF)*.

Dyspnoea

- Consider possible causes (see Box 59.3). Dyspnoea may be due to the underlying lung disease or due to an additional pathology
- Dyspnoea is frightening and made worse by anxiety and panic. Explain to patient that alleviation of dyspnoea is possible for most patients with appropriate treatment
- Lung cancer and pulmonary metastases are associated with the sensation of SOB, often due to stimulation of receptors by malignant infiltration or lymphangitis carcinomatosis
- Optimize treatment of any underlying lung disease with bronchodilators and steroids, if appropriate
- Treat concurrent chest infection
- Give advice on planning and adapting daily activities to conserve energy
- Fan blowing cool air onto the face/open window can be helpful
- Consider patient positioning when in bed—upright posture assists diaphragmatic excursion; lying tilted may help with copious secretions
- Opioids (e.g. 2.5–5mg morphine sulfate solution 4-hourly) relieve the sensation of dyspnoea without affecting respiratory function
- O_2 cylinders/concentrator for intermittent short-burst/prn use may help symptoms but may be associated with psychological dependence, may restrict daily activities, and may dry the upper airways
- Consider the need for external beam radiotherapy, endobronchial tumour debulking, or airway stenting in a patient with lung cancer experiencing dyspnoea due to bronchial obstruction or compression with tumour
- If PE diagnosed, consider treatment with LMWH, instead of warfarin (avoids need for repeated blood tests and has a potential anti-mitotic effect)
- SC opioid infusion may relieve symptoms as death approaches; use with haloperidol, midazolam, or levomepromazine.

Box 59.3 Causes of breathlessness in patients with lung cancer

- Pneumonia
- Underlying chronic lung disease (e.g. COPD, pulmonary fibrosis) or concomitant cardiac disease
- Lobar collapse
- Pleural effusion
- Pneumothorax
- SVCO
- Upper airway obstruction
- PEs
- Lymphangitis carcinomatosis
- Chest wall infiltration
- Phrenic nerve paralysis
- Pericardial effusion
- Respiratory muscle weakness due to cachexia, paraneoplastic syndromes, steroid myopathy
- Anaemia
- Depression
- Anxiety and panic.

Other symptoms

Anxiety

- Leads to dyspnoea, which, in turn, worsens anxiety
- Reassure patients they will not suffocate; symptoms will pass
- Benzodiazepines (such as short-acting lorazepam 0.5–1mg sublingually 8–12-hourly) are effective for respiratory panic. Longer-acting diazepam 2–5mg nocte/bd may be helpful for severe anxiety or at night when dyspnoea and panic disturb sleep
- Acute panic may be helped by midazolam 2.5mg IV, increased in increments of 1mg, given in a controlled environment with O_2
- Amitriptyline or citalopram may be effective longer-term treatments
- Cannabinoids, such as nabilone, may be useful for patients who have continuous dyspnoea, anxiety and who do not tolerate other agents
- Relaxation exercises, diaphragmatic breathing training, and complementary therapies may help some patients.

Cough

- Treat the underlying cause
- Try simple or codeine linctus
- Nebulized saline may help expectoration
- Codeine 30mg qds (or even morphine sulphate solution) may be of use for intractable cough
- Methadone linctus 1–2mg nocte or bd may be used but has a long duration of action and may accumulate
- Nebulized local anaesthetic may help, e.g. 5mL 2% lidocaine 6-hourly or bupivacaine 5ml 0.25% 8-hourly (avoid in asthmatics, as it causes bronchospasm). Pharyngeal numbness is likely to occur, so avoid fluids for 1–2h afterwards
- Consider radiotherapy if haemoptysis due to lung cancer. Consider discontinuing antiplatelet drugs or anticoagulants
- If massive haemoptysis, consider tranexamic acid, plus emergency supply of opioids and benzodiazepines to ensure pain control and reduction of fear by decreasing awareness.

Pleural effusion

- Drain if symptomatic, and pleurodese early if recurrent, although not if prognosis is poor (<3 months)
- Consider IPC to drain fluid if effusion is symptomatic and talc pleurodesis has failed or with completely trapped lung. RCT evidence suggests also reasonable to use IPC for 1° therapy (in place of talc pleurodesis), but patient choice key (see p. 767).

Poor appetite

- Common symptom; may be 1°, due to cachexia-anorexia syndrome, or 2° due to mouth problems (such as candidiasis), nausea, hypercalcaemia, drugs, or depression
- May be improved in the short term (about 6 weeks) by a course of oral steroids such as dexamethasone 4mg bd or prednisolone 20mg daily
- Cachexia leads to decreased respiratory muscle strength and increased SOB
- Consider nutritional supplements.

Brain metastases

- Steroids relieve the cerebral oedema associated with brain metastases, e.g. dexamethasone 8mg bd (8 a.m. and 2 p.m.) initially and then decrease
- Avoid steroid dosing in the evening, as sleep is affected
- Palliative whole brain radiotherapy should be considered for patients with performance status 0/1 or if there is a good response to steroids.

Recurrent laryngeal nerve palsy

- Affects 10% of patients with lung cancer, causes hoarse voice
- Patients with troublesome hoarseness should be referred to ENT for consideration of Teflon® stiffening of vocal cord to prevent paradoxical movement.

Non-malignant respiratory disease (COPD, CF, fibrotic lung disease)

The main problems associated with severe non-malignant respiratory disease are dyspnoea, hypoxia, immobility, and psychosocial problems, including depression. End-stage COPD patients may have very frequent exacerbations for some years before a final terminal event. One study has shown those with end-stage COPD are more likely to have depression ± anxiety than those with terminal cancer, but they are less likely to receive specific treatment for their emotional problems or any targeted palliative care. It may be appropriate therefore to shift the focus in patients with severe end-stage respiratory disease away from management of acute exacerbations towards a more palliative approach to care.

Dyspnoea

- Dyspnoea is frightening and made worse by anxiety and panic
- Patients may decrease their mobility to avoid dyspnoea and subsequently become more deconditioned
- Dyspnoea may be due to the underlying lung disease or an additional pathology (PE, infection, pneumothorax, cardiac failure)
- Sitting upright reduces airway obstruction and optimizes ventilation. Relaxing and dropping the shoulders can improve ventilation when anxiety has caused patient to 'hunch up'
- Calm gentle reassurance can decrease anxiety and reduce dyspnoea
- Fan blowing cool air onto the face/open window can be helpful
- Optimize treatment of any underlying lung disease with bronchodilators and inhaled steroids, if appropriate
- Treat concurrent exacerbations with antibiotics and oral steroids
- Stop smoking
- Consider pulmonary rehabilitation
- Opioids (e.g. 2.5–5mg morphine sulfate solution prn/4-hourly) relieve the sensation of dyspnoea without affecting respiratory function. Consider pre-emptive use for known triggers of breathlessness
- O_2 cylinders for intermittent short-burst use may help symptoms. Consider concentrator if multiple cylinders being used.

Hypoxia

- SaO_2 <92%
- LTOT may be appropriate (see p. 709)
- O_2 cylinders for intermittent or ambulatory use may help symptoms, but little data to support their use
- NIV use appropriate for some causes of ventilatory failure (see pp. 700–1).

Anxiety and depression

- May be due to fear and uncertainty over prognosis
- Lead to dyspnoea, which, in turn, worsens anxiety
- Explain they will not suffocate; symptoms will pass
- Benzodiazepines (such as short-acting lorazepam 0.5–1mg sublingually 8–12-hourly) are effective for respiratory panic
- Acute panic may be helped by midazolam 2.5mg IV, increased in steps of 1mg, given in a controlled environment with O_2
- Depression rates are high in patients with COPD. Consider antidepressant treatment and counselling. Amitriptyline or citalopram may be effective at helping anxiety also
- Relaxation exercises, diaphragmatic breathing training, and complementary therapies may help some patients.

Cough

- Treat the underlying cause
- Refer to physiotherapy to improve cough efficacy, particularly if large-volume secretions
- Consider mucolytics, steroids, antibiotics
- Try simple or codeine linctus
- Nebulized saline may help expectoration
- Oral local anaesthetics, such as benzocaine and lidocaine lozenges, may be useful for laryngeal, pharyngeal, or tracheal irritation, but associated risk of aspiration
- Nebulized local anaesthetic may help, e.g. 5mL 2% lidocaine 6-hourly or bupivacaine 5ml 0.25% 6-hourly (avoid in asthmatics, as it causes bronchospasm). Pharyngeal numbness is likely to occur, so avoid fluids for 1–2h afterwards.

Other problems

- Malnutrition, thirst
- Nausea, vomiting, constipation
- Sleep disturbance
- Chest pain
- Fatigue
- Oral candidiasis
- Impact on carers and family of patient with chronic respiratory disease.

Further information

British National Formulary—useful information on prescribing in palliative care in its first section.

Liverpool Care Pathway—used by many hospitals to enable health care workers to deliver optimum hospice-type care to a dying patient, whatever their location or diagnosis. Further information at: ℜ http://www.sii-mcpcil.org.uk/lcp.aspx.

Pulmonary rehabilitation

Aims and patient selection

Pulmonary rehabilitation (PR) is a well-established evidence-based multidisciplinary programme of care for patients with symptomatic chronic respiratory impairment, targeting the extrapulmonary manifestations of the disease. The programme is individually tailored and should contain high-intensity progressive aerobic training, strength training, and self-management education. PR is probably the most cost-effective intervention for COPD. It interrupts the vicious cycle of dyspnoea leading to inactivity, subsequent deconditioning, and further worsening dyspnoea on more minimal exertion.

Aims of rehabilitation

- To reduce disability in people with chronic lung disease
- To improve QoL and restore independence
- To diminish the health care burden of disease.

Early studies demonstrated there were improvements in functional status with PR despite no change in severity of airflow obstruction.

Meta-analysis of 23 RCTs, where PR included exercise training for at least 4 weeks (although the content was varied), confirmed the benefit of rehabilitation, with statistically and clinically significant improvements in functional or maximal exercise capacity and/or QoL. Symptoms of dyspnoea and fatigue are improved, and patients gain an enhanced sense of control over their condition.

Other benefits of PR

- Patients across the disease severity spectrum of COPD (including those with severe airflow obstruction) can benefit from PR
- Studies show patients who completed a rehabilitation course may have fewer hospital admissions for exacerbations than those who had not had rehabilitation, and hospital stays were shorter (10 days vs 21 days)
- Respiratory muscle training improves dyspnoea, but not exercise capacity or health-related QoL, above aerobic training
- High-intensity lower limb aerobic training is recommended, rather than low-intensity training
- Supplemental strength training improves muscle strength but does not provide additional benefit to exercise capacity or health-related QoL than aerobic training alone
- Early PR is recommended after a COPD exacerbation. It is safe and improves exercise tolerance, health-related QoL and reduces hospital admissions
- Short-term programmes achieve overall similar outcome benefits across the spectrum of patient disability. A minimum programme length of 6 weeks is recommended
- Decline in exercise tolerance and health status tends to occur between 6 and 12 months after completion of a course. Sustained improvement with ongoing rehabilitation sessions has yet to be evaluated.

Candidates

- Anyone with chronic lung disease causing functional impairment despite receiving optimum medical treatment
- Well-motivated patients seem to benefit most
- Patients with poor lower limb mobility may still benefit from upper limb exercise and the education package
- O_2 therapy is not a contraindication to rehabilitation
- Recent exacerbation of COPD is not a contraindication
- Stable ischaemic heart disease and heart failure are not contraindications
- Depression should be addressed prior to participation in PR, if possible, to increase the likelihood of benefit.

Candidates in whom rehabilitation may not be indicated

- Unstable ischaemic heart disease, severe valvular heart disease, severe cognitive impairment, or locomotor difficulties
- Poorly motivated people, with geographical or transport problems making attendance difficult, tend to do less well. It may be, however, that different locations (community or home-based) and different interfaces (manuals or web-based) may help these challenges of hospital-based programmes.

Further information

BTS guideline on pulmonary rehabilitation in adults. *Thorax* 2013;**68**(Suppl 2).

Pulmonary rehabilitation: Joint ACCP/AACVPR Evidence-based clinical practice guidelines. *Chest* 2007;**131**(5 Suppl):4S–42S.

Puhan M et al. Pulmonary rehabilitation following exacerbations of chronic obstructive pulmonary disease. *Cochrane Database Syst Rev* 2009;1:CD005305.

Nici L et al. ATS/ERS statement on pulmonary rehabilitation. *Am J Respir Crit Care Med* 2006;**173**:1390–413.

Troosters T et al. Pulmonary rehabilitation in COPD. *Am J Respir Crit Care Med* 2005;**172**:19–38.

Lacasse Y et al. Pulmonary rehabilitation for COPD (Cochrane review). *Cochrane Database Syst Rev* 2002;3:CD003793.

Salman GF et al. Rehabilitation for patients with COPD: meta-analysis of RCTs. *J Gen Intern Med* 2003;**18**(3):213–21.

BTS statement on pulmonary rehabilitation. *Thorax* 2001;**56**:827–34.

Griffiths TL et al. Results at one year of outpatient multidisciplinary pulmonary rehabilitation: a randomised controlled trial. *Lancet* 2000;**355**:362–68.

Programme

Programmes are usually run on an outpatient basis but can be done in the community, home, or as an inpatient. They are run by a multiprofessional team—physician, physiotherapist, occupational therapist, dietician, nurse, pharmacist, social worker, and psychologist. A minimum programme length of 6 weeks is recommended. Programmes should be regularly audited by the department.

- *Physical training* The main component of the programme is progressive high-intensity aerobic exercise, such as walking and cycling, for a minimum of 2–3 times per week, with two supervised/class sessions. The prescription is individualized, and the benefits are improved with higher-intensity training. Upper or lower limb strength exercise with weights is often included. O_2 supplementation may be required if significant desaturation occurs during exercise to below 80% and if exercise tolerance improves with O_2
- Performance enhancement has been investigated. Improvements shown with: tiotropium, in addition to PR, vs PR alone, NIV, partitioned training (single leg cycling), testosterone (improves muscle strength). No improvement with: creatine, O_2. Neutral or subgroups: helium hyperoxia, nutrition
- *Disease education*
- *Psychological and social intervention* with advice on anxiety and depression, smoking cessation, plus physiotherapy and occupational therapy input
- *Nutritional education* to optimize body weight and muscle mass.

Pre-rehabilitation assessment

- Optimize medical treatment
- O_2 saturation on exercise
- ECG may be warranted, especially if history of cardiac disease.

Outcome assessment measures

- *Exercise performance* Often with SWT or 6MWT to assess ability and progress (see Box 60.1)
- *Health status* Disease-specific questionnaires:
  - Chronic Respiratory Questionnaire (CRQ)
  - St George's Respiratory Questionnaire
  - Generic questionnaires, e.g. the Short Form-36 (SF-36)
  - Hospital Anxiety and Depression scores (HADS) are measured
- *Practical* Pedometers can be used for direct feedback and to improve performance.

Future developments

- Access to PR for all who may benefit
- How to optimally maintain the improvements following a rehabilitation programme
- Using technology to enhance compliance and delivery of PR
- Expanding the potential population who may benefit from PR
- Further understanding the mechanisms of health benefits from improving physical activity
- Targeting exercise training earlier in the disease process.

Box 60.1 Shuttle walk test (SWT)

A 10m course between two points (cones). Walking speed is determined by external audio tape signals ('beeps'), and the patient should pace their walk to reach the cone by the next beep. The patient is required to incrementally increase their speed as the beeps occur more frequently each minute. Test finishes when the patient is too breathless or tired to maintain the required pace, and the distance achieved is calculated. The minimum clinically important difference following rehabilitation is 48m (~5 shuttles).

6min walk test (6MWT)

A 30m course between two points on a hard flat surface. Patients do as many 60m laps as they can around the two points in 6min. They determine their pace and intensity of exercise. They are allowed to rest in the time if they need to. Total distance walked in 6min is counted. Results may vary, according to mood and encouragement. An increase from baseline to post-rehabilitation of 35m or more is considered significant.

Cardiopulmonary exercise testing (CPET)

(See ➲ p. 880.)

CPET are rarely used to assess pragmatic PR programmes and have been largely replaced by field testing in the UK. CPET is the gold standard for the assessment of peak O_2 uptake, but they also provide more detailed results on exercise progression and limitations to exercise. Occasionally, they may be performed for safety prior to undertaking PR. CPET are still widely used in a research setting for PR.

Chapter 61

Smoking cessation

Aims and nicotine replacement therapy

Smoking is the main cause of COPD and lung cancer. In 2005, tobacco smoking accounted for ~19% of all UK deaths and cost the NHS at least £5 billion. The UK government has set targets to reduce the number of smokers, with substantial funding for smoking cessation services (£66.4 million in 2011).

- ~22% of men and 20% of women over 16 in England smoked in 2009; 82% of smokers start as teenagers
- The incidence of smoking is increasing, particularly amongst women and in developing countries
- Smoking is associated with cardiovascular and cerebrovascular disease and bladder, oesophageal, cervical, and renal cancers. It is also associated with increased post-operative complications
- Nicotine exerts its effects on the CNS and is very addictive
- Reducing number of cigarettes smoked may not give health benefits, as cigarettes smoked 'harder'—more puffs, greater inhalation
- Peak nicotine withdrawal time is 2–3 days
- 0.4% of smokers manage to stop each year
- Stopping smoking is associated with an average weight gain of 2–5kg, and this deters many, especially women, from quitting
- UK government legislation in 2007 banned smoking in workplaces and public places and increased the age for sale of tobacco from 16 to 18.

Aims of smoking cessation interventions Smoking cessation is a cost-effective treatment (£2,000 per QALY for patients with COPD). To achieve sustained abstinence, the aims are to reduce short-term nicotine cravings (nicotine and non-nicotine replacement therapy) and to modify behaviour in the long term (counselling, telephone or group support-buddy systems). It is vital that the smoker is motivated to quit, or attempts will fail. Health professionals should address smoking cessation at all opportunities, as they can trigger quit attempts by giving brief advice to smokers (advice from doctors often has the strongest impact.). This can lead to 1–3 out of 100 people stopping smoking for 6 months. People may be more receptive to smoking cessation advice during times of concern for their own or their families' health. A guide to approaching the topic is:

- Ask how much a person smokes, and document pack years (number of cigarettes smoked per day ÷ 20 × no of years smoked)
- Ask about non-conventional tobacco smoking, e.g. with cannabis, with a waterpipe (Shisha)
- Advise on risks of continued smoking. Assess commitment to quitting
- Assist by offering behavioural therapy ± pharmacotherapy
- Provide self-help material, and refer to stop smoking services
- Arrange follow-up.

Some hospitals and general practices have smoking cessation counsellors. The best results in terms of quit rates are achieved by combining counselling and nicotine replacement therapy (NRT), bupropion, or varenicline, with regular support and follow-up. These can improve quit rates to around 25%. NICE has issued guidance on the use of NRT, bupropion, and varenicline for smoking cessation. It advises that pharmacotherapy should only be for smokers committed to a target stop date. Choice of therapy is based on a patient's likely compliance, availability of counselling, previous experience of therapies, contraindications, and personal preference. Prescribe 2 weeks of NRT or 3–4 weeks of bupropion/varenicline, and only give further prescription if individual shows a continuing attempt to quit. If they fail to quit, a second attempt within 6 months is not usually funded.

NRT minimizes short- and medium-term nicotine withdrawal symptoms. Should not be used whilst still smoking, as potential for nicotine overdose (symptoms: agitation, confusion, restlessness, palpitations, hypertension, dilated pupils, SOB, abdominal cramps, vomiting). Can be bought over the counter or be prescribed by GP. Cheaper than cigarettes. In 2005, Medicines and Healthcare Regulatory Authority licensed NRT products in pregnancy, breastfeeding mothers, people aged 12–17, and those with cardiovascular disease.

- *Patches* Give small amounts of nicotine via transdermal patch to decrease cravings before they occur. Dose (15, 10, 5mg) depends on amount smoked. Use a higher dose if >10 cigarettes/day smoked. Convenient. Worn continuously throughout day, but removed at night due to vivid dreams. Can get localized irritation at patch site. Patches should be used for 6–8 weeks at the higher dose, then weaned to a lower dose for 2–4 weeks. Available over the counter.
- *Chewing gum* Different strengths of gum that release nicotine as they are chewed (Smoke <20/day—chew one 2mg piece slowly for 30min when urge to smoke occurs. Smoke >20/day or needing >15 pieces of 2mg gum daily—use 4mg strength gum. Max 15 4mg pieces/day). Relieves cravings as they occur. When mouth tingles and has peppery taste, should stop chewing and 'park' the gum inside the cheek. Nicotine is then absorbed through the lining of the mouth. Should not chew continuously or may develop nausea. Nicotine needs to be absorbed through mouth and not swallowed in saliva. Therefore, do not drink with gum. Physical act of chewing can relieve craving. Can taste unpleasant and may need to use several packs of gum a day. Use for 3 months, then reduce the strength and amount of gum used. Available over the counter in a variety of flavours
- *Sublingual tablets* used on demand to help with cravings. Discrete form of treatment. 1–2 tablets should be placed under the tongue every hour when needed. Dissolve over 30min. Licensed for use in pregnancy (one tablet only). Use for 3 months, and then gradually reduce the number of tablets used a day. Available on prescription
- *Lozenges* Suck every 1–2h if urge to smoke (smoke >30/day = 2mg lozenge, <30/day = 1mg lozenge). Available over the counter
- *Inhalator* Cigarette-style appliance giving small amounts of nicotine when used. Useful for people who are habitual or ritualistic in that they have 'restless hands' or want the 'hand to mouth' routine. Nicotine is absorbed through the lining of the mouth, not via the lungs. Use for 2 months, then gradually reduce. Available on prescription
- *Nasal spray* provides rapid relief of craving. Faster absorption than other forms of NRT. May cause local irritation. Use for 2 months, then reduce. Available on prescription.

Non-nicotine replacement therapy

Drugs

Pharmacotherapy should not be used without behavioural support.

Bupropion is promoted as an aid to smoking cessation, in combination with motivational support. It is an antidepressant that was found to reduce the desire to smoke, even in the absence of depression. It weakly inhibits dopamine, serotonin, and noradrenaline reuptake in the CNS. It counteracts nicotine withdrawal symptoms by increasing these levels in the brain. It is suitable for individuals who smoke ≥10 cigarettes a day. Liver metabolism and 20h half-life. Smokers start taking bupropion 1–2 weeks before their intended 'quit day'. Continue for 7–9 weeks after. Leads to improved abstinence rates, compared with placebo or nicotine patch, if associated with counselling (30% 12-month abstinence rate with bupropion, 16% with nicotine patch, 15% with placebo, 35% with patch and bupropion) (*N Engl J Med* 1999;**340**:685–91). Also thought to lessen weight gain associated with stopping smoking. Contraindicated in patients with epilepsy or at risk of fits, those with a CNS tumour, those acutely withdrawing from alcohol or benzodiazepines, pregnancy, those with eating disorders, bipolar disorder, and those on monoamine oxidase inhibitors. Preferentially used in some patient groups, e.g. those with schizophrenia or depression. Reduce dose if elderly or has hepatic or renal impairment. Well tolerated. Recognized adverse effects include dry mouth, hypersensitivity, insomnia, seizures (1:1,000), and death. Prescription only.

Varenicline is a drug also promoted as an aid to smoking cessation, in combination with motivational support. It binds to the A4B2 nicotinic acetylcholine receptor and acts as a partial agonist. Its binding alleviates symptoms of craving and withdrawal. It reduces the rewarding and reinforcing effects of smoking by preventing nicotine binding to the A4B2 receptors. Smokers start taking varenicline 1–2 weeks before their intended 'quit day' and continue for 12–24 weeks. Starting dose is 500 micrograms od for 3 days, 500 micrograms bd for 4 days, then 1mg bd for 11 weeks, if tolerated. If smokers are abstinent after 12 weeks, they should continue for another 12 weeks to avoid relapse. Avoid abrupt withdrawal. Side effects include nausea, vomiting, appetite change, change in taste, headache, difficulty sleeping, abnormal dreams, dry mouth, and tiredness. Use with caution if breastfeeding, in renal impairment, and in those with a history of psychiatric disease. It has been associated with neuropsychiatric disorders (depression, agitation, behavioural changes). RCTs have shown significantly higher quit rates with varenicline than with bupropion or placebo. Quit rates are higher with higher doses (e.g. continuous quit rate for any 4 weeks: 48% with 1mg bd ($p = 0.01$ vs placebo), 37% with 1mg od ($p = 0.01$), 33% with bupropion ($p = 0.02$, 17% with placebo). Adverse drug effects leading to stopping treatment were lower than with bupropion (*Arch Int Med* 2006;**166**:1561–8). Prescription only. Recommended by NICE in 2007.

Hypnosis aims to improve willpower in the subconscious state with therapeutic suggestion. Anecdotal success, but Cochrane review of trials showed no greater abstinence rate with hypnosis than with any other treatment or placebo treatment.

Acupuncture/acupressure No evidence in favour of it over placebo acupuncture. Less effective than NRT.

Electronic cigarettes or e-cigarettes are battery-powered and vaporize nicotine and other chemicals in a liquid solution to an aerosol mist. The nicotine contained is approximately the same amount as in a cigarette. They simulate the act of smoking and are therefore controversial. To be regulated by MHRA from 2014, with all nicotine-containing products requiring a licence from 2016. Not approved by the USA's FDA. Although some studies suggest that they help smokers decrease cigarette consumption, even when they do not intend to quit, the effectiveness of e-cigarettes is unknown, their contents variable, and the short- and long-term effects on pulmonary health unknown. Therefore, should not be recommended as an aid to smoking cessation until a stronger evidence base emerges.

Future developments

- Plain packaging campaign to discourage younger smokers
- Campaign to ban smoking in cars when children present
- Increasing and improving hospital-based smoking cessation services with links to community-based services
- Effectiveness of long-term smoking cessation interventions and relapse rates
- New medications: *clonidine*—approximate doubling of abstinence rates, compared to placebo. However, a high incidence of adverse effects, including significant sedation, postural hypotension, and bradycardia
- *Dopamine D3 antagonists*—the dopamine D3 receptor is involved in mechanisms of nicotine dependence. Trials undergoing
- Nicotine vaccines—induces antibodies directed against nicotine from tobacco smoking, leading to a decrease in the rate and amount of nicotine entering the brain (thus reducing the pleasurable effects of smoking). Phase II trials ongoing.

Further information

Brief interventions and referral for smoking cessation in primary care and other settings. March 2006, NICE PH10 & Smoking cessation services 2008. ℘ http://www.nice.org.uk.

ABC of smoking cessation series. *BMJ* Feb–April 2004.

Riemsma RP *et al.* Systematic review of the effectiveness of stage based interventions to promote smoking cessation. *BMJ* 2003;**326**:1175.

West R *et al.* Smoking cessation guidelines for health professionals. *Thorax* 2000;**55**:987–99. ℘ http://www.nosmokingday.org.uk.

Roy Castle Fag Ends. ℘ http://www.stopsmoking.org.uk.

Quitline ☎ 0800 002200.

BTS Recommendations for Hospital Smoking Cessation Services for Commissioners and Health Care Professionals (with link to BTS website).

Chapter 62

Airway management

Simple airway adjuncts

Simple airway adjuncts are used to overcome backward tongue displacement in an unconscious patient.

▶▶ **Call for anaesthetic help early**

Patients may require support of their airway and ventilation/oxygenation in situations when they are unable to adequately maintain these. Such situations may be related to a GCS of <8, which can cause difficulties with airway maintenance, or related to respiratory compromise or arrest in the critically ill patient.

Oropharyngeal airway (Guedel) A curved plastic tube with a flanged end that is inserted into the mouth. Size is estimated by holding it at the side of the patient's face and estimating required length from incisors to angle of the jaw. Ensure the mouth is clear, then insert the airway 'upside down', with the curved side towards the tongue. When it is in as far as the soft palate, turn it around by 180°, and push it in further so the flange is at the patient's mouth. If the patient has a gag reflex, remove the airway. Suction can be performed through the airway and O_2 administered via a mask.

Nasopharyngeal airway A soft plastic tube, with a bevelled end and a flange at the other end. Better tolerated in the semi-conscious. Avoid use in those with base of skull fractures. Sizes 6–7mm are suitable for adults. Some tubes allow insertion of a safety pin through the flange (prior to use) to prevent insertion beyond nares. Lubricate airway with water-soluble jelly, and insert the bevelled end into right nostril, and gently push back with a twisting action along the floor of the nose. Do not force if obstruction is encountered, but remove and try in the other nostril. Nasal bleeding can be caused if the mucosa is damaged. O_2 can be administered through a mask.

Intubation

Endotracheal tube The optimal method of managing a patient's airway and providing airway protection from aspiration of gastric contents. Requires training in tube insertion. The tube is bevelled at one end with an inflatable cuff and has a connector at the other end. The connector can be removed if the tube needs to be cut but can be replaced.

- Predictors of difficult intubation should be considered, including Mallampati score (see ➲ p. 595), ability to protrude mandible, assessment of neck movements, interincisor distance (<3cm predicts difficulties), thyromental distance (Patil's test; <7cm predicts difficulties), and obesity
- Ensure all equipment is to hand—laryngoscope (usually a size 3/4 curved Macintosh blade; check light source), cuffed endotracheal tube (variety of sizes should be to hand; usually use size 7—♀, size 8—♂; check cuff for leak), syringe for cuff inflation, water-soluble lubricating jelly, Magill's forceps, gum elastic bougie, suitable bandage to secure tube in place, capnography and stethoscope (for confirming tube placement), O_2 and suitable breathing circuit (e.g. self-inflating bag or Water's circuit), suction (Yankauer and flexible catheters), and rescue equipment for failed intubation
- Patient lies flat, with neck flexed and head extended (the 'sniffing the morning air' position). A pillow is placed under the head, not the neck, to aid this
- Pre-oxygenate with bag-and-mask ventilation
- Cricoid pressure (30N over the cricoid cartilage) may reduce gastric inflation and aspiration of gastric contents
- Using the laryngoscope in left hand and standing behind the head, the mouth is opened and the laryngoscope placed over the right side of the tongue and advanced
- It may be necessary to apply suction to clear the mouth of secretions
- When the epiglottis is seen, the laryngoscope is advanced into the vallecula, between the root of the epiglottis and the base of the tongue. Upward pressure in the direction of the laryngoscope handle is applied to lift the jaw slightly, and the cords should come into view, taking care not to damage the teeth. Laryngoscopic views are graded (Cormack and Lehane grading): grade 1, entire laryngeal inlet visible; grade 2, arytenoids and posterior vocal cords visible; grade 3, only epiglottis visible; grade 4, epiglottis not seen
- Slide the tube through the glottis so that the cuff is a few cm past the cords, and then withdraw the laryngoscope
- Inflate the cuff
- Confirm adequate tube position by auscultating for breath sounds over the chest bilaterally (also absence of noise over epigastrium) and using end-tidal CO_2 detection (either waveform capnography or using colorimetric litmus-based detectors); five breaths showing CO_2 confirm an adequate tube position

- If the tube is not in position, usually because it has been passed into the oesophagus, deflate the cuff and remove the tube, then re-oxygenate with the bag and mask before trying again. Pull the tube back slightly if the breath sounds are only on the right, as this suggests the tube is in the right main bronchus
- Secure the tube
- Administer O_2 with a self-inflating bag with O_2 and reservoir bag
- CXR to confirm correct tube position, 2–3cm above the carina
- Suction can be performed through the tube
- Various techniques can be used to assist with difficult tracheal intubation. A gum elastic bougie may be easier to pass through the glottis (allowing endotracheal tube insertion by railroading over the bougie). The BURP technique (external Backward, Upward, and Rightward Pressure on the thyroid cartilage) may improve laryngoscopic view. Other laryngoscope blades (e.g. McCoy levering laryngoscope) and videolaryngoscopes may be useful.

Laryngeal mask airway

A supraglottic airway device used as an alternative to formal intubation. A wide-bore tube with an inflated cuff at one end, which is positioned over the larynx and inflated, hence forming a seal; thus, aspiration of gastric contents and gastric inflation are minimized. It is easy to insert (see Fig. 62.1) and is used in anaesthetic practice and also in emergencies. Requires minimal head tilt so is ideal for use in patients with possible cervical spine injuries. Not suitable for patients with high airway resistance such as pulmonary oedema, bronchospasm, or COPD. Select a size 4 or 5 tube, and, after ensuring the cuff works, deflate it. Put water-soluble lubricating jelly over the cuff. The patient should be lying flat, with head extension, if possible. Hold the tube like a pen, and insert from behind the patient's head, with the point of the cuff positioned to the back of the mouth. Advance along the roof of the mouth, and then press it downwards and backwards until resistance is felt. Inflate the cuff, which will cause the tube to lift out of the mouth a little. Confirm adequate airway position by auscultating for breath sounds over the chest bilaterally. Secure the tube.

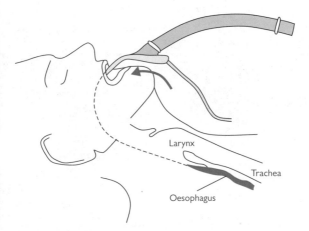

Larynx

Trachea

Oesophagus

Fig. 62.1 Diagram of laryngeal mask airway insertion. Reproduced from Wyatt *et al.* *Oxford Handbook of Emergency Medicine* 3e, 2006, with permission from Oxford University Press.

Chapter 63

Bronchoscopy

Indications and risks

Bronchoscopy is the procedure of passing a telescope or camera into the trachea to inspect the large and medium-sized airways. It may be performed with a flexible scope, using local anaesthetic ± sedation, favoured by physicians, or under a general anaesthetic with a rigid scope, used mostly by surgeons. Airways can be visually inspected, samples taken, and therapeutic procedures can be performed. This chapter focuses on flexible bronchoscopy.

Indications for bronchoscopy

- *Suspected lung cancer* Patients who have a central mass <4cm from the origin of the nearest lobar bronchus, which is likely to be accessible for biopsy at bronchoscopy
- *Suspected pulmonary infection*, such as TB, in a patient who is unable to produce sputum, or in immunocompromised patients, with fever, cough, hypoxia, or CXR changes (induced sputum with hypertonic saline may be an alternative; see ➜ p. 776)
- *Suspected ILD* if a TBB will provide an adequate sample for diagnostic purposes such as in sarcoid. Only indicated in a limited number of ILD, as more adequate biopsies are often obtained through open lung biopsy, which may be preferable
- *Investigation of haemoptysis*
- *Investigation of stridor*
- *Foreign body removal* if this is located proximally
- *Therapeutic indications* include central airway obstruction, sputum plugging, and possibly emphysema (endobronchial lung volume reduction; see ➜ pp. 184–5) and asthma (bronchial thermoplasty; see ➜ p. 143).

Relative contraindications/take care

- If a patient has saturations below 90% on air at rest or <8kPa, the risk of significant hypoxia during bronchoscopy is increased
- FEV_1 <40% predicted
- Blood clotting abnormalities, particularly platelet level <50,000/mm^3
- Uraemia, PHT, SVCO, liver disease, and immunosuppression predispose to haemorrhage
- Recent MI may be associated with cardiac ischaemia during bronchoscopy. Wait until 4 weeks after, if possible (otherwise, liaise with cardiology).

Risks associated with bronchoscopy

Flexible bronchoscopy is a safe procedure, with reported mortality rates in large series being 0.01–0.04% and major complications of 0.08–1.1%. Complications include respiratory depression, pneumonia, pneumothorax, airway obstruction, laryngospasm, cardiorespiratory arrest, arrhythmias, pulmonary oedema, vasovagal episodes, fever (especially following BAL), septicaemia, haemorrhage, nausea, and vomiting.

Bleeding and bronchoscopy

- Significant bleeding occurs in ~0.7% of patients, due to mechanical trauma from the scope, suctioning, brushing, or biopsy, but is more common with TBB (1.6–4.4%). Patients with malignancy, immunocompromise, or uraemia have an increased bleeding tendency
- If bleeding does not stop spontaneously, retract the bronchoscope proximally to maintain vision, and preserve the airway using suction to remove free blood (but do not disturb clot). 1mL aliquots of 1:10,000 adrenaline solution are administered via the bronchoscope as near to the bleeding point as possible, until it stops. 5–10mL iced saline may also be useful. If bleeding does not stop, the bronchoscope should be wedged in the segmental bronchus to tamponade the bleeding for 10–15min
- If massive haemorrhage occurs, the patient should be turned on to the side of the bleeding to protect the other lung. Balloon-tipped vascular catheter may be used to tamponade the bleeding point. If bleeding continues, emergency interventional radiology or thoracic surgery may be indicated.

Further information

Du Rand IA et al. British Thoracic Society guideline for diagnostic flexible bronchoscopy in adults. *Thorax* 2013;**68**:i1–i44.

Lee P et al. Therapeutic bronchoscopy in lung cancer. *Clin Chest Med* 2002;**23**:241–56.

Bungay HK et al. An evaluation of CT as an aid to diagnosing patients undergoing bronchoscopy for suspected bronchial carcinoma. *Clin Radiol* 2000;**55**(7):554–60.

Laroche C et al. Role of CT scanning of the thorax prior to bronchoscopy in the investigation of suspected lung cancer. *Thorax* 2000;**55**(5):359–63.

Patient preparation and procedure

Patient preparation

- *Information* Patients should be given written information about the procedure, ideally >24h prior to the procedure. Provide an information sheet for the patient to take home following the bronchoscopy, with advice about the effects of any sedation and possible complications, as well as telephone numbers in case help is needed
- *Consent* The physician performing the bronchoscopy should obtain written consent, with a description of the procedure and its associated risks
- *Consider stopping anticoagulation* Safe to perform if patient is taking aspirin or prophylactic LMWH, but omit clopidogrel for 7 days prior (may require cardiology discussion), and, if on warfarin, wait until INR <1.5 (may require full-dose LMWH on days prior to bronchoscopy for high-risk conditions, e.g. mitral prosthetic metal valve, prosthetic valve and AF, AF and mitral stenosis, <3 months post-VTE, or thrombophilia syndromes)
- *Risks of sedation* Consider factors which may make sedation more hazardous (see ⊃ p. 796)
- *Nil by mouth* Patients should have no food for 4h beforehand and clear fluids only until 2h beforehand
- *Blood tests* Patients do not need routine pre-procedure blood tests, unless there are specific concerns (active bleeding, uraemia, deranged LFTs, low platelets)
- *Bedside tests* Perform an ECG in patients with a history of cardiac disease. Check blood sugar in patients with diabetes
- *Prophylactic antibiotics* are no longer recommended for the prevention of endocarditis, fever, or pneumonia
- *In those with asthma*, a nebulized bronchodilator should be given before the bronchoscopy
- *Those at high risk of infection (TB)* should be last on the list.

Procedure

- Practices vary between centres. Some perform bronchoscopy with the patient sitting up, facing the operator; some from behind, with the patient lying flat
- *IV access* should be present in all patients
- *Pulse oximetry* ± ECG is monitored throughout. Nasal O2 should be administered if SaO_2 falls by 4%
- *Sedatives* should be offered to provide conscious sedation (verbal contact possible at all times), anxiolysis, and anterograde amnesia, provided no contraindications (see ⊃ p. 796). A benzodiazepine, such as midazolam 1–2mg, with 1mg increments as necessary, may be used with fentanyl/alfentanil. Assess and document sedation depth (see ⊃ p. 793). Some patients and operators prefer not to use sedation, due to concerns particularly in elderly patients, those with COPD, or those with cardiac disease. Midazolam can make some patients more agitated. Premedication with anticholinergics is not beneficial during bronchoscopy

- *Lidocaine* Local anaesthetic 2% gel (6mL = 120mg) is applied to the nostrils, and the vocal cords are anaesthetized by three actuations of local anaesthetic spray (10% lidocaine, 10mg/spray) to the back of the throat during inspiration and time allowed to work (~3–5min)
  - Transcricoid injection may be used to administer 1% lidocaine into the trachea, or this may be anaesthetized under direct vision ('spray-as-you-go') through the bronchoscope
  - Aliquots of 1% lidocaine may be administered to right and left main bronchi via the bronchoscope when it is passed through the vocal cords into the trachea
  - Maximum dose of lidocaine is unclear, but symptoms of toxicity seen at ≥9.6mg/kg delivered to the airways. Use the minimal dose required for cough suppression. Toxic effects include CNS effects (confusion, blurred vision, euphoria, dizziness, myoclonus, seizures) and cardiovascular effects (arrhythmias, cardiac arrest). Risks increased with renal, hepatic, and cardiac dysfunction (see ➔ p. 862)
  - The half-life of lidocaine is 1.5–2h
- Most access the trachea via the nasal route, as this gives increased stability when taking biopsies and allows the patient to cough and spit out secretions more easily. If this is not possible, a mouth guard is used and access obtained through the mouth
- All sections of the bronchial tree should be visually inspected, including the cords and trachea. CXR or CT may help localize the area of concern, so specimen site can then be targeted. This increases the diagnostic yield of bronchoscopy in cases of suspected lung cancer
- Avoid unnecessary suction, as this can increase hypoxia.

Sampling techniques

Bronchial washings are taken by instilling ~10mL of saline and then collecting it in a pot/trap to obtain superficial airway cells.

Bronchial brushings are taken by inserting a covered brush into a bronchial segment, uncovering it, rubbing the bronchial wall, covering it, removing it, and wiping it on a slide. The slide is then sprayed with a cell fixing solution.

Bronchial biopsies are taken with biopsy forceps; 5–7 should be taken to optimize yield. These may be taken blindly or from a visibly abnormal area, which gives a higher diagnostic yield than blind biopsies. They can be placed in formalin or saline solution, depending on whether they are for histology or microbiology.

BAL is performed by instilling 60–180mL of saline through the broncho-scope when it is wedged well in a small airway. Ideally, instill fluid during inspiration, and, after allowing the fluid to dwell for 10–30s, aspirate back into the syringe during expiration or collect in a trap. Best performed in the area of abnormality on CXR or CT or non-dependent lobes such as the right middle lobe or lingula. Poor return if the patient is coughing excessively or if they have emphysema. Can cause hypoxia proportional to amount of lavage fluid used.

TBB Technique of passing TBB forceps down a terminal bronchus until resistance is first felt and taking a sample of parenchymal tissue. Some perform with radiological screening. One technique is to locate the bron-choscope at segmental bronchus of interest and advance forceps (through working channel) as far as possible. Retract forceps by 1cm; open forceps while patients inhaling slowly, then advance and close forceps while exhal-ing. Take biopsy (but stop if pain felt, suggesting that forceps have gathered visceral pleura). Repeat 5–6 times.

Associated with a significant risk of bleeding in 9% and pneumothorax in 1–6%, but up to 14% if patient is mechanically ventilated. Half of all pneu-mothoraces require chest drains. Therefore, perform on one side only, and minimize risk by performing TBB in the lower lobes in dependent segments. Perform CXR after the bronchoscopy if patient symptomatic or clinical suspicion of pneumothorax. Pneumothorax should be managed, according to standard guidelines (see ➔ pp. 374–5). Small pneumothoraces often resolve spontaneously, but the patient may need admission if concerns.

TBNA (see ➔ p. 756) is used to sample mediastinal and hilar lymph nodes in suspected malignancy, TB, or sarcoidosis (see Fig. 63.1). It is also useful in sampling extrabronchial masses or necrotic endobronchial tumour. When added to other sampling techniques in lung cancer, it increases the diagnostic yield by 18%.

When performing bronchoscopy
- Wear gloves, face mask, and eye shields
- Use particulate (duck) masks if there are concerns about TB or HIV.

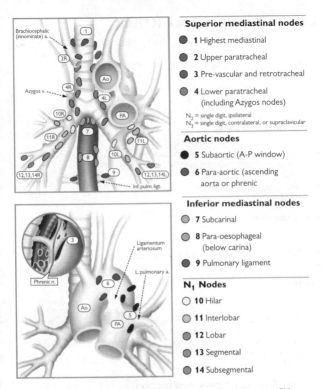

Superior mediastinal nodes

● **1** Highest mediastinal

● **2** Upper paratracheal

● **3** Pre-vascular and retrotracheal

● **4** Lower paratracheal
(including Azygos nodes)

N_2 = single digit, ipsilateral
N_3 = single digit, contralateral, or supraclavicular

Aortic nodes

● **5** Subaortic (A-P window)

● **6** Para-aortic (ascending
aorta or phrenic

Inferior mediastinal nodes

● **7** Subcarinal

● **8** Para-oesophageal
(below carina)

● **9** Pulmonary ligament

N₁ Nodes

○ **10** Hilar

○ **11** Interlobar

● **12** Lobar

● **13** Segmental

● **14** Subsegmental

Fig. 63.1 Mediastinal lymph node stations. Reproduced from Mountain, Clifton, Regional Lymph Node Classification for Lung Cancer Staging, Chest (1997) 111:6 1718-1723, with the kind permission of the American College of Chest Physicians

Central airway obstruction

(See also section on acute upper airway obstruction, Chapter 50, ➔ p. 642.)

Central airway = trachea and main stem bronchi.
Obstruction can be:

- Extrinsic such as tumour pressing on airway causing obstruction
- Intrinsic such as tumour occluding airway lumen
- Mixed, a combination of extrinsic and intrinsic.

Symptoms and signs

- May be asymptomatic if obstruction is mild
- Productive cough, due to mucosal swelling and mucus production
- Wheeze, unilateral wheeze, positional wheeze
- Stridor
- 2° atelectasis and pneumonia
- Dyspnoea.

Investigations

- Flow–volume loops, FEV_1
- CXR—may be normal
- CT chest + 3D airway reconstruction, if possible
- Bronchoscopy to make tissue diagnosis of underlying disease.

Treatment

- Secure airway
- Consider bronchoscopy—senior physician ± anaesthetist should perform. Bronchoscopy itself can cause obstruction in a compromised airway. Adrenaline administered via bronchoscope may be helpful
- Consider endobronchial treatment—core out tumour; dilate a stenosis, or place a stent (see ➔ p. 758)
- Consider heliox (see ➔ p. 643).

Causes of central airway obstruction

- Malignant
    - 1° endoluminal cancer, especially lung cancer or carcinoid
    - Metastatic cancer
    - Laryngeal cancer
    - Oesophageal cancer
    - Mediastinal tumour
    - Lymphadenopathy, lymphoma
- Non-malignant
    - Lymphadenopathy
    - Relapsing polychondritis
    - Tracheomalacia
    - Papilloma
    - Hamartoma
    - Amyloid

- Web
- Goitre
- Foreign body
- Granulation tissue.

Further information

Ernst A et al. Central airway obstruction. Am J Respir Crit Care Med 2004;169:1278–97.

Janssen JP et al. Series: Interventional pulmonology. Eur Respir J 2006;27:1258–71; 28:200–18.

Wood DE et al. Airway stenting for malignant and benign tracheobronchial stenosis. Ann Thorac Surg 2003;76:167–74.

Du Rand IA et al. British Thoracic Society guideline for advanced diagnostic and therapeutic flexible bronchoscopy in adults. Thorax 2011;66:iii1–iii21.

Interventional bronchoscopy 1

Used particularly in the diagnosis and palliative treatment of patients with lung cancer and central airway obstruction due to local tumour growth where the relief of the obstruction will have symptomatic benefits.

Diagnostic procedures

TBNA and EBUS allow mediastinal node sampling without the surgical procedure of mediastinoscopy. Some lymph nodes are accessible for sampling in this way, which cannot be accessed via mediastinoscopy.

TBNA Technique of inserting a biopsy needle (19–22G) blindly through the bronchial wall into an enlarged lymph node or extrabronchial mass and aspirating cells. Used to give additional staging information in lung cancer. Appropriate lymph nodes should be identified on CT first; stations 2R/L, 3P, 4R/L, 7, 10R/L, and 11R/L are accessible. Should be performed initially, so the bronchoscope is not contaminated with malignant cells from the airway, and start with the highest-stage lymph nodes first. Push sheath out through end of bronchoscope until the hub is just visible. Flex the bronchoscope so that the sheath tip lies between cartilaginous rings, directed towards the node/mass. Extend the needle so that it passes through the bronchial wall, and then apply suction. A 'to-and-fro' motion of the needle should allow lymph node 'goo' to be aspirated. Subsequently, the suction is stopped; the needle is withdrawn, and the sheath is removed to allow sample preparation. Subcarinal (7) and right lower paratracheal (4R) nodes are the easiest to sample. Aim for 5–7 needle passes. Malignancy sensitivity 39–78%. Complications rare (0.3%): pneumomediastinum, pneumothorax, minor bleeding, puncture of adjacent structures.

EBUS Technique of visualizing the bronchial wall and the immediate surrounding structures via a convex array ultrasound probe incorporated into the tip of the bronchoscope. A balloon surrounding the probe is inflated with water, in order to achieve close circular contact and view surrounding structures. Useful to assess lymph node involvement in malignancy and for real-time guided TBNA. Possible to sample nodes ≥4mm in short axis. Mediastinal structures or masses next to the airways can be identified, the depth of bronchial wall tumour invasion assessed, or masses within the lung localized for biopsy. Malignancy sensitivity 88–100%. Oesophageal endoscopic ultrasound (EUS) is an alternative strategy, which allows examination of the posterior and inferior mediastinum (particularly useful for stations 8 and 9), the liver, the coeliac axis, and the left adrenal gland. It is more accurate at diagnosing mediastinal metastases than CT and PET.

Autofluorescent bronchoscopy (AFB) Technique to differentiate central malignant areas from normal tissue, including dysplasia and pre-invasive tumours *in situ*. However, the progression of these abnormalities is not known, so the role of AFB is unclear. Used in conjunction with usual white light bronchoscopy. Uses blue light to induce tissue autofluorescence, which means normal and abnormal tissues appear different colours when viewed through a specialized bronchoscope. Airway trauma, however, can also cause a different mucosal appearance, and the test has low specificity. It is being used in some centres as a surveillance tool following surgical resection of lung cancer, or in patients with head and neck cancer suspected of having a lung 1°, or following positive sputum cytology. Its role is not, however, clear, and advances in standard white light bronchoscopes (such as using narrow band imaging) may be found to be as good at identifying abnormal mucosa.

Rigid bronchoscopy Visualizes bronchial tree to level of segmental bronchi. Can remove or core out endobronchial tumours, insert a stent, dilate tracheal or bronchial stenosis, and manage massive haemoptysis. Useful to provide information regarding resectability in lung cancer by measuring airway length. Incidence of serious complications <5%: hypoxia, laryngospasm, pneumothorax, bleeding.

Interventional bronchoscopy 2

Therapeutic procedures

Bronchial laser resection, electrocautery, argon–plasma coagulation (APC), photodynamic therapy (PDT), and cryotherapy/cryoextraction These are all procedures that can be used to debulk obstructing endobronchial lesions or coagulate a bleeding point. The use of an LMA or uncuffed endotracheal tube is recommended to achieve airway control. Electrocautery is the use of a high-frequency electrical current via a probe/snare/needle knife to heat tissue, causing coagulational vaporization, which enables cutting. Nd-YAG Laser achieves the same effect. APC is a non-contact method of electrocautery, using argon gas which causes desiccation and coagulation. These are all effective immediately. These are used predominantly for obstructing malignant lesions but may be used to remove benign lesions, e.g. papilloma, or to treat benign stenoses, e.g. due to intubation, sarcoidosis, granulomatosis with polyangiitis, trauma, etc. Avoid using FiO_2 >0.4 with laser, electrocautery, and APC to minimize the fire risk. Shave skin on thigh, if necessary, before placing electrode for electrocautery, and avoid placing it over metal prosthetic joints. Cryotherapy/cryoextraction is the technique of repeatedly freezing and then thawing an area with a probe in order to destroy tissue such as an endobronchial obstructing lesion. Standard cryotherapy takes hours to days to have its effects, while cryoextraction allows the bronchoscope and cryoprobe to be removed, complete with attached tumour tissue. It can also be used to remove a foreign body, as freezing attaches foreign body to the end of the probe.

PDT IV administration of a photosensitizer drug to the patient (selectively concentrated in tumour tissue), followed 48h later by bronchoscopic exposure of the presensitized tumour to a laser light of specific matching wavelength in order to cause tumour necrosis. Airways cleared of debris immediately after and again a few days later. Skin remains light-sensitive for 8 weeks.

Tracheobronchial stent insertion via the bronchoscope to re-establish airway patency following endobronchial debulking or if there is extrinsic compression. Self-expanding metal airway stents (SEMAS) used in cases of external compression, such as lung cancer, for palliation of breathlessness. Length, diameter, and type of stent need careful selection prior to procedure using CT. Both uncovered stents (for extrabronchial lesions) and covered stents (for tumours with an endobronchial component) are available. These are inserted over a guidewire with flexible bronchoscopic visualization. Repositioning can be tricky after placement. Complications include stent migration or fracture, haemorrhage, mucus impaction, development of granulation tissue, bronchospasm, and even death. Silicone stents are used in mainly benign disease and are inserted via rigid bronchoscopy. They are easily removed and manoeuvred but can migrate and lead to problems with retained secretions.

Brachytherapy Procedure of endobronchial irradiation using iridium-192 via bronchoscope for endobronchial and intramural tumours. A blind-ending catheter (the applicator) is placed within or alongside a tumour, and the bronchoscope is then removed over a long guidewire, which is then replaced by a radio-opaque graduated metal insert. CXR of the insert is used to plan placement of the radioactive source within the applicator. Treatment occurs over a few minutes. Delayed effect, requires several sessions. Complementary to other bronchoscopic therapies. Can cause radiation bronchitis, stenosis, and haemorrhage.

Chapter 64

Chest drains

Indications, drain types, complications

Chest drain insertion is associated with significant morbidity and mortality, and careful consideration should be given to the precise indication for drainage. Out-of-hours drain insertion should be avoided, unless an emergency. Ultrasound guidance should be used for all drains inserted for fluid but is not required for pneumothorax.

Indications

- Tension pneumothorax (following needle decompression)
- Symptomatic pneumothorax with failed aspiration or underlying lung disease or in ventilated patients
- Complicated parapneumonic effusion and empyema
- Malignant pleural effusion for symptomatic relief and/or pleurodesis
- Haemothorax
- Traumatic haemopneumothorax
- Following thoracic surgery
- Rarely, for symptomatic effusions of other aetiology.

Contraindications

- Inexperienced operator
- Lung adherent to chest wall
- Bleeding tendency (a relative contraindication; routine measurement of platelet count and clotting in the absence of risk factors is not required). For anticoagulated patients, do not drain until INR <1.5, unless life-threatening emergency
- Post-pneumonectomy (not a contraindication, but first discuss with cardiothoracic surgical team).

Types of chest drain *Seldinger-style* drains are inserted by sliding the drain into the pleural cavity over a guidewire. Whilst being the most frequently used, they still require experience and care to be inserted safely and comfortably. Sizes up to 36F are available. *Blunt dissection* drains (e.g. *Portex* drains) require gentle dissection of subcutaneous tissue and muscles to gain entry to the pleural space. Drains are then inserted, often over a flexible plastic introducer, into the pleural space. Available in sizes up to 36F. Traditional *trocar* drains should no longer be used, being associated with significant potential complications and even death. These drains consist of a flexible plastic tube surrounding a metal rod with a blunt tip.

Small (10–14F) drains are more comfortable and should be the default choice for the majority of situations. Large-bore chest drains (24–36F) are frequently uncomfortable and only rarely required, e.g. 2° pneumothorax with large air leak and/or surgical emphysema, acute haemothorax, and post-operatively.

Complications

- Pain—insertion should not be painful with good local anaesthetic technique. Subsequent pain common, and opiate analgesia may be required
- Inadequate drain position—may require withdrawal or insertion of new drain

- Surgical emphysema (in pneumothorax)—air leaks into subcutaneous tissues. May occur if tube blocked or positioned with holes subcutaneously, or with very large air leaks. See → p. 381 for management
- Infection—iatrogenic pleural infection rate up to 2%, perhaps higher in trauma patients; wound infection
- Organ damage (e.g. lung, liver, spleen, heart, great vessels, stomach). Intrapulmonary placement results in significant continuous bubbling and bleeding; this may occur in up to 6% of all drain insertions. Drainage of GI contents suggests bowel perforation (or oesophageal rupture as the cause of the effusion)
- Haemorrhage into drain—bloody pleural fluid is a common finding (e.g. in malignant effusions), but unexpected large-volume drainage of frank blood suggests damage to organs or intercostal vessels. Clamp the drain, and leave it in place. Urgent imaging (± interventional radiology) and surgical referral
- Re-expansion pulmonary oedema (see → p. 381)
- Vasovagal reaction
- Sudden death due to vagus nerve irritation reported.

Further information

Havelock T et al. Pleural procedures and thoracic ultrasound: British Thoracic Society pleural disease guideline 2010. Thorax 2010;65(suppl. 2):ii61–76.

New England Journal of Medicine. Videos in clinical medicine. http://www.nejm.org/multimedia/medical-videos.

Insertion technique

An assistant is required. Use a dedicated procedure room when possible.

- Discuss procedure with patient, and obtain written consent (unless emergency situation)
- Insert IV cannula
- Consider giving analgesia. Conscious sedation (e.g. using midazolam) is rarely required and should include O_2 saturation monitoring; be cautious in patients with severe underlying lung disease or respiratory failure; see ➔ p. 794
- Position patient either in lateral decubitus position or lying head elevated at 30°, with insertion side of trunk rotated about 45° upwards and arm on insertion side behind their head. Alternative position is with patient sitting forward, leaning over a table
- Double-check correct side from chest examination and CXR
- Choose insertion site: ideally within 'safe triangle' (see Fig. 64.1), which avoids major vessels and muscles (boundaries: anteriorly, anterior axillary line, and border of pectoralis major; posteriorly, posterior axillary line and border of latissimus dorsi; inferiorly, horizontal to level of nipple in man or fifth intercostal space in woman). Avoid posterior approaches close to spine, as intercostal artery drops medially to lie in mid-intercostal space. Ultrasound guidance should always be used for fluid—either site marking *immediately* prior to drain insertion or real-time needle visualization using sterile ultrasound sheath and gel.
- Sterile skin preparation. Wear sterile gloves and gown
- Infiltrate skin, intercostal muscle, and parietal pleura with 10–20mL of 1% lidocaine (maximum 3mg/kg). Aim just above the upper border of the appropriate rib, avoiding the neurovascular bundle that runs below each rib. The subcutaneous fat lacks pain receptors and does not require anaesthetic. The parietal pleura, however, is extremely sensitive; use the full volume of lidocaine

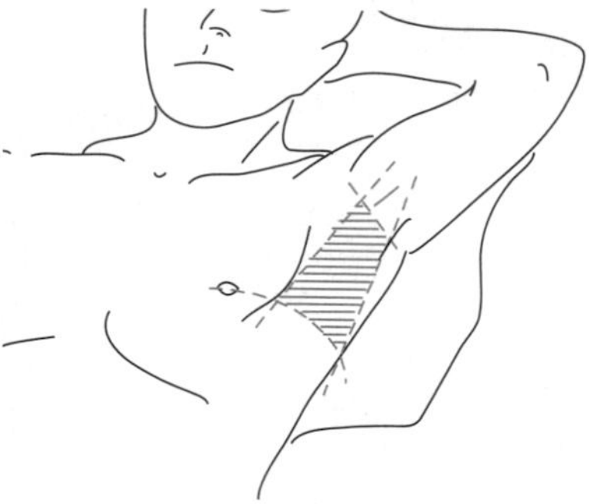

Fig. 64.1 'Safe triangle' for chest drain insertion, bounded anteriorly by pectoralis major, posteriorly by latissimus dorsi, inferiorly by the fifth intercostal space, and superiorly by the axilla. Reproduced from Pleural procedures and thoracic ultrasound: British Thoracic Society pleural disease guidelines 2010, Havelock *et al*, *Thorax* 2010 **65**: i61–i76, Figure 2, with permission from BMJ.

- Verify that the site is correct by aspirating pleural fluid or air. Occasionally, a green (21G) needle may be too short in obese patients, and a longer needle is required. If unable to aspirate fluid or air, do not proceed with drain insertion; consider CT-guided drainage
- Whilst waiting for anaesthetic to work, prepare drain and connections. Assistant should prepare underwater seal
- Insert drain:
  - *Seldinger drains* Gently insert the introducer needle, and check that air or fluid can be easily aspirated with a syringe. Remove syringe. Smoothly insert the guidewire through the introducer needle. Remove introducer needle, taking care not to let go of the guidewire at any time. Make a small skin incision ~5mm. Slide plastic dilator around guidewire to enlarge the entry track. Avoid excessive force; dilator should not be inserted >1cm into the pleural space. Remove the dilator, and slide the drain into the pleural cavity over the guidewire. Remove the wire when the drain is within the chest
  - *Blunt dissection drains* Small (1cm) skin incision parallel to rib. Insert horizontal mattress suture across incision to facilitate later closure. Dissect intercostal muscles with blunt forceps (e.g. Spencer–Wells)—the fibres can be teased apart by opening and then removing the forceps; do not close forceps within the chest; this may damage underlying structures. This blunt dissection may take some time. Insert drain (facilitated by introducer) just into the pleural space smoothly and gently—there should not be any significant resistance. *Never apply force when inserting a chest drain.* Once the pleural space has been entered, insert the drain further while removing the introducer. An alternative approach is to remove any introducer and grip the end of the chest tube with blunt forceps, and use these to guide the tube into the chest. Aim towards the apex for a pneumothorax, and the lung base for a pleural effusion. (Note—in emergencies or in patients with extreme obesity or subcutaneous emphysema, it may be appropriate to make a larger initial incision and insert an index finger to assist the drain track)
- Connect the drain to underwater seal bottle via a three-way tap and tubing. If the drain is correctly positioned in the pleural space, it should swing with respiration and drain air or fluid
- Suture and tape the drain in place on the chest wall
- Ensure adequate analgesia
- Warn the patient not to disconnect the tubing or lift the underwater bottle above the level of the insertion site on the chest; supply a 'chest drain information leaflet'
- Obtain CXR to check position. The 'ideal' tube position (apex for pneumothorax, base for effusion) is not necessary for effective drainage, so do not reposition functioning drains on this basis. CT may be useful in confirming drain position in certain circumstances. Drains are often positioned in fissures, but, in most cases, this does not affect their functioning
- Small drains may need regular flush to ensure patency; prescribe 10mL normal saline flush to drain tds.

Drain management

General points

- Patients should ideally be managed on a specialist ward by experienced nursing staff. 'Chest drain observations' should be charted regularly, including swinging, bubbling, and volume of fluid output
- If drain water level does not swing with respiration, the drain is kinked (check underneath dressing as tube enters skin), blocked, clamped, or incorrectly positioned (drainage holes not in pleural space; check CXR). Occluded drains may sometimes be unblocked by a 30mL saline flush. Non-functioning drains should be removed (risk of introducing infection)
- Suction is sometimes used to encourage drainage, although there is a lack of evidence regarding its use. Consider in cases of pneumothorax with persistent air leak or following chemical pleurodesis. Suction should be high volume/low pressure, typically starting at a level of $5cmH_2O$ and increasing to $10–20cmH_2O$. It may be painful and not tolerated by the patient.

To clamp or not to clamp?

Never clamp a bubbling chest drain (risk of tension pneumothorax). Clamping may be considered in two situations:

- To control the rate of drainage of a large pleural effusion. Rapid drainage of large volumes may result in re-expansion pulmonary oedema; clamping, e.g. for 1h after draining 1.5L, may prevent this
- To avoid inappropriate drain removal in cases of pneumothorax with a slow air leak, when bubbling appears to have ceased. Clamping a drain for several hours, followed by repeat CXR, in such situations may detect very slow or intermittent air leaks. This is controversial, however, and should only ever be considered on a specialist ward with experienced nursing staff. If the patient becomes breathless, the drain should be immediately unclamped.

Drain removal Quickly and smoothly remove the drain, whilst patient is slowly exhaling (although opinions on this differ—some recommend removal in maximal inspiration). Tie previously placed mattress suture, if applicable. Apply dressing. CXR to document lung position.

Indwelling pleural catheters

Predominantly used for domiciliary drainage of recurring malignant effusions, with drainage by patients, family members, or district nurses.

Indications

- Current BTS guidance for malignant pleural effusions advocates IPC use for completely trapped lung (pleurodesis unlikely to be successful) and for recurrent effusions post-pleurodesis
- Use as 1° therapy more controversial, although recent randomized trial (vs talc pleurodesis) demonstrates reduced hospital inpatient time (by 3.5 days) and decreased need for further pleural procedures, with similar improvements in dyspnoea and QoL. However, increased risk of pleural and soft tissue infection, symptomatic loculation, and catheter blockage.

General points

- IPCs are 15.5/16F fenestrated silicone drains with a tunnelled subcutaneous portion and polyester cuff to prevent accidental removal and bacterial ingress
- Inserted as a day case. Essential to consider optimum site for insertion, particularly for women (discomfort with bra straps). Using ultrasound, the Seldinger technique is used to insert pleural portion of drain, and blunt dissection is used to insert subcutaneous portion
- Adapter enables connection of IPC valve to conventional drainage bottles when in hospital. If adapter not available and urgent pleural fluid sampling required (e.g. for possible pleural infection), a large-bore IV cannula *without needle* can be used to aspirate fluid aseptically through the valve mechanism
- To drain at home, a pre-vacuumed 500 or 1,000mL drainage bottle is aseptically connected to the IPC valve, usually 1–3 times/week (dependent on rate of fluid accumulation)
- Spontaneous pleurodesis occurs in 30–70% (dependent on malignancy type and whether lung is trapped). Catheters can be removed if minimal drainage for 3–4 weeks, provided not blocked and minimal fluid remaining on imaging
- Essential for patients to have adequate education and access to support in case of complications
- Not considered a contraindication to chemotherapy.

Further information

Davies HE *et al.* Effect of an indwelling pleural catheter vs chest tube and talc pleurodesis for relieving dyspnea in patients with malignant pleural effusion. *JAMA* 2012;**307**(22):2383–9.

Fysh ETH *et al.* Indwelling pleural catheters reduce inpatient days over pleurodesis for malignant pleural effusion. *Chest* 2012;**142**(2):394–400.

Putnam JB *et al.* A randomized comparison of indwelling pleural catheter and doxycycline pleurodesis in the management of malignant pleural effusions. *Cancer* 1999;**86**(10):1992–9.

Chapter 65

Cricothyroidotomy

General points

In some situations of upper airway obstruction or facial trauma, ventilation and tracheal intubation of a patient is impossible. It may therefore be necessary to create an immediate surgical airway below the level of obstruction.

Cricothyroidotomy technique

See Box 65.1 and Fig. 65.1.

Box 65.1 Cricothyroidotomy

▶▶ *Call for anaesthetic and ENT help.*

- Extend the head, with the patient lying flat. Place a pillow under the patient's shoulders, not their head
- Identify cricothyroid membrane (see Fig. 65.1): soft triangular area above cricoid ring and below the thyroid cartilage. (Put your fingers on the larynx, and move them down to the soft area below where you are aiming for.) Clean with antiseptic swab
- Puncture the membrane in the midline with a large-bore cannula (18G or larger). Remove the needle; attach a syringe, and aspirate air to confirm correct position. Specific cricothyroidotomy kits are available
- Angle the cannula downwards at 45°, and advance. Ensure air can still be aspirated, and then connect to high-pressure O_2 supply, with a Y connector, if possible
- Occlude one limb of Y connector with a finger until chest rises, and then release to allow exhalation, ideally via larynx. Inflate for 1s, and deflate for 4s. Must allow air to be exhaled. If there is no Y connector, a hole is cut in the O_2 tubing, which can be intermittently occluded
- Secure the cannula
- Perform a formal surgical cricothyroidotomy with ENT help, as needle method does not allow adequate ventilation as the tube is too small and the larynx is blocked. Vertical skin incision; press lateral edges outwards to minimize bleeding. Transverse cricothyroid membrane incision (avoids superiorly positioned cricothyroid artery); take care not to damage cricoid cartilage. Dilate tract with tracheal spreader or scalpel handle, and insert a small cuffed endotracheal tube (not too far—carina is near).

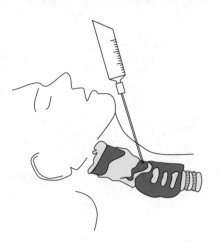

Fig. 65.1 Diagram of needle cricothyroidotomy. Reproduced from Wyatt *et al.* *Oxford Handbook of Emergency Medicine* 3e, 2006, with permission from Oxford University Press.

Further information

Resuscitation Council UK. *Advanced life support provider manual*, 6th edn 2011.

Miscellaneous diagnostic tests

Skin prick tests

These may be useful in identifying specific allergens causing immediate hypersensitivity (IgE-mediated) reactions. They may influence management and guide allergen avoidance. They are also used to help define the presence of atopy. Triggers for contact urticaria, atopic eczema, and suspected food allergy may also be identified. The results are available almost immediately (compared with a RAST test for specific IgE) and correlate well with RAST test results. They should be carried out by staff trained to read the tests and manage adverse reactions.

The allergens tested should be identified from the history and may include common aeroallergens, e.g. pollens (grass, tree, weeds), moulds (*Alternaria alternata, Aspergillus fumigatus, Cladosporium, Penicillium chrysogenum*), house dust mite (*Dermatophagoides pteronyssinus*), and animal dander (dog epithelium, cat pelt).

Practical points

- Testing should be performed off antihistamines (7 days) and omalizumab (≥6 months). Tricyclic antidepressants and phenothiazines may also block response. Oral steroids appear not to suppress test results
- Very small risk of anaphylaxis; adrenaline and resuscitation equipment should be available. Particular care is needed with food and latex testing
- Clean the skin with 70% alcohol solution. Put a drop of allergen on the skin (usually the inside forearm). A range of allergens are available commercially. Fresh produce should be used for suspected fruit and vegetable hypersensitivity
- Prick the skin through the allergen drop, using a needle (do not draw blood). This should be with a calibrated lancet (1mm), held vertically, or a hypodermic needle held at 45° to the skin
- The positive control is usually histamine and the negative control the diluent (usually glycerinated saline)
- Read the histamine control after 10min and the allergen extracts after 15–20min. A positive result is an itchy weal, which should be compared with the controls, as some subjects react to the skin prick alone (dermatographism)
- Different test solutions are standardized to give a mean weal diameter of 6mm across sensitive subjects
- A weal of 3mm or more is considered positive (indicating sensitization)
- A positive result does not prove that the clinical symptoms are due to bronchial hyperresponsiveness to the tested allergen but do raise clinical suspicion. Positive results can occur in those without symptoms, and false negatives do occur.

RAST or radioallergosorbent blood tests are more specific, but less sensitive and more expensive than skin prick tests, but give similar information. There is no risk of anaphylaxis, and the patient does not need to stop antihistamines for the test to be performed.

Unconventional tests Electrodermal allergy testing (using a Vegatest machine) was developed as an aid to homeopathic prescribing and is widely used in complementary medicine to assess allergic status to food and environmental allergens. It is based on small changes in skin electrical impedance at acupuncture points, in response to allergens placed in an electrical circuit. There are no RCT data to show that this method can identify atopic from non-atopic individuals, as identified from skin prick tests.

Technique of induced sputum

- Used to investigate for infection (e.g. TB, PCP) or airway inflammation
- Patients rinse their mouth and clean their teeth to minimize oral contamination. Give inhaled salbutamol to minimize bronchoconstriction
- Nebulized hypertonic (2.7–5%) saline is administered via a face mask. Afterwards the patient expectorates sputum into a sterile pot
- If transmission of infection (e.g. TB) is likely, perform the test in a negative pressure room, with appropriate protection of staff and other patients. Do not perform on the open ward or outpatient department
- Send sputum promptly to microbiology for staining and culture and direct immunofluorescent testing for *Pneumocystis jirovecii* (if indicated). Sputum for differential cell counts is mixed with 0.1% dithiothreitol, diluted with saline, and then filtered and centrifuged.

Bronchoprovocation testing

Several techniques can be used to assess bronchial hyperreactivity, including pharmacological challenges (non-specific bronchoprovocation testing), exercise challenge (for exercise-induced asthma), food additive challenge, and antigen challenge.

Non-specific bronchoprovocation testing

- Helpful if there is diagnostic doubt regarding the diagnosis of asthma
- Typically use inhaled methacholine or mannitol. Methacholine directly stimulates smooth muscle contraction. Mannitol works indirectly via release of endogenous mediators and is more specific but less sensitive
- Should be performed by experienced personnel, with facilities to deal with acute bronchospasm
- Patients need to omit regular asthma therapy (inhaled/oral steroids: 2–3 weeks; antihistamines: 3 days; tiotropium: 1 week; LABA: 2 days)
- Increasing doses of provocation agent are given sequentially, with the FEV_1 measured after each dose
- *Methacholine* Given in a nebulizer using solutions ranging from 0.03mg/mL to 16mg/mL. If there is a 20% fall in FEV_1 or if the highest dose of methacholine has been given, the test is stopped. The concentration of drug causing a 20% fall is known as the PC_{20} and may lie between the concentrations of the last two doses. Asthma is indicated by a PC_{20} ≤8mg/mL. Normal subjects have a PC_{20} >16mg/mL. Intermediate responses may be seen in patients with family history of asthma or in those with COPD or CF or when recovering from viral infections
- *Mannitol* Proprietary dry powder inhaler (Aridol®) used. Provocation dose causing 15% fall in FEV_1 (PD_{15}) is noted. Asthma indicated by PD_{15} at cumulative dose of ≤635mg.

Pleural biopsy

General points

Several techniques can be used to obtain a pleural biopsy.

- Using *image guidance* (either CT or USS), a cutting needle (e.g. 18G Temno® or Cook Quickcore®) takes several 1–2cm cores along the long axis of any parietal pleural pathology. FDG-PET CT may have a role guiding pleural biopsy in patients with diffuse pleural abnormality to increase sensitivity. Malignancy sensitivity >85%
- Using *thoracoscopic biopsy* (medical thoracoscopy/VATS) (see ➲ p. 347). Multiple biopsies are taken of visually abnormal parietal pleura. Malignancy sensitivity >92%
- Using a pleural biopsy needle (e.g. Abrams' or Cope) in a *'blind' percutaneous* fashion to take multiple biopsies. Not advocated for diagnosing malignancy (sensitivity 47%—unsurprising, given patchy nature of pleural malignancy). May have utility in resource-limited settings for diffuse pleural diseases (e.g. TB pleuritis), but thoracoscopy still preferred (TB sensitivity ~100% vs ~80%).

Abrams' pleural needle biopsy

Indications

- Diagnosis of tuberculous pleural effusion when access to other biopsy techniques limited.

Technique

An assistant is required.
- Discuss procedure with patient, and obtain written consent
- Insert IV cannula
- Consider sedation (e.g. midazolam 2–5mg IV, with O_2 saturation monitoring)
- Position patient sitting forward, leaning on a pillow over a table, with their arms folded in front of them
- Double-check correct side from chest examination and CXR
- Choose biopsy site using pleural USS to ensure an adequate volume of pleural fluid under proposed site. Use lateral approach to avoid neurovascular bundle, which lies mid-intercostal space posteriorly
- Sterile skin preparation. Wear sterile gloves and gown
- Infiltrate skin, intercostal muscle, and parietal pleura with 10–20mL (up to 3mg/kg) of 1% lidocaine. Aim just above the upper border of the appropriate rib, avoiding the neurovascular bundle that runs below each rib. Anaesthetize area behind rib below the insertion point. Verify that pleural fluid can be aspirated. If unable to aspirate, do not proceed
- Whilst waiting for anaesthetic to work, assemble Abrams' reverse bevel biopsy needle. The needle consists of an outer sheath with a triangular opening (biopsy port) that can be opened or closed by rotating an inner sheath
- Make small (5mm) skin incision; dissect intercostal muscles with blunt forceps (e.g. Spencer–Wells)
- Insert biopsy needle gently, with biopsy port closed. Do not apply force; the needle should slip into the pleural space without resistance. When in the pleural cavity, fluid can be withdrawn by attaching a syringe to the needle and opening the biopsy port
- To take a biopsy, attach a syringe to the needle. Open the biopsy port and angle it downwards, and then pull the biopsy port firmly against the parietal pleura on the rib beneath the entry point (6 o'clock position relative to entry point). Close the biopsy port, thereby pulling a sample of parietal pleura into the needle
- Remove the biopsy needle; open the biopsy port, and remove biopsy sample
- Repeat procedure 4–6 times in positions 4–8 o'clock; always sampling below the insertion point (to avoid the neurovascular bundle beneath the rib above)
- Send biopsy samples in saline for analysis for TB and in formalin for histological processing
- Apply dressing to biopsy site. May require a single stitch
- CXR to exclude pneumothorax.

Complications include pain (up to 15%), pneumothorax (up to 15%), haemothorax (<2%), and empyema. Haemorrhage from trauma to an intercostal artery may necessitate emergency thoracotomy. Fatalities are well documented but rare.

Further information

Maskell NA et al. Standard pleural biopsy versus CT-guided cutting-needle biopsy for diagnosis of malignant disease in pleural effusions: a randomised controlled trial. Lancet 2003;**361**:1326–31.

Hooper C et al. Investigation of a unilateral pleural effusion in adults: British Thoracic Society pleural disease guideline 2010. Thorax 2010;**65**(Suppl. 2):ii4–17.

Pleurodesis

General points

Aim of pleurodesis is to seal visceral to parietal pleura with adhesions to prevent pleural fluid or air accumulating. Pleurodesis dependent upon:

- Lung re-expansion following removal of pleural fluid or air, which allows the apposition of visceral and parietal pleura. This may be encouraged by applying suction to an intercostal drain
- Inflammation of the pleural surfaces and local activation of coagulation, required to produce pleural fibrosis and adhesions. May be induced by chemical sclerosing agent or by mechanical pleural abrasion at VATS.

Indications

- Recurrent symptomatic pleural effusion (usually malignant, although pleurodesis also rarely used in benign recurrent effusions)
- Recurrent pneumothorax (due to concerns regarding the long-term safety of intrapleural talc, surgical abrasion pleurodesis usually procedure of choice in younger patients; chemical pleurodesis may be used as a last resort in older patients who are unfit for surgery).

Chemical pleurodesis

Types of sclerosant Choice of sclerosing agents varies. The most commonly used agents are sterile talc and bleomycin.

- Talc most effective (success rate ~90%) and usually well tolerated, although risk of ARDS (see later). Administered either as slurry via chest drain or as poudrage at thoracoscopy, with comparable efficacy
- Bleomycin has success rates of only 60%
- Tetracycline successful in 65% cases, but lack of drug manufacture.

Other rarely used agents include doxycycline, minocycline, interferon, interleukins, cisplatin, or patient's own blood.

Corticosteroids may increase failure rate of pleurodesis, by inhibiting inflammatory response and development of adhesions, and should be discontinued. Effect of NSAIDs on pleurodesis efficacy unclear.

Technique Most centres will have written pleurodesis protocol, usually involving premedication and intrapleural local anaesthesia. A typical protocol is set out as follows:

- Discuss procedure with patient, and obtain written consent
- Insert chest drain (see ➲ pp. 764–5): small bore (10–14F) chest tubes sufficient for fluid drainage and pleurodesis and are more comfortable than larger drains. Flush drain with 20mL normal saline 6-hourly
- Commence LMWH thromboembolism prophylaxis (increased risk following pleurodesis, especially in patients with malignancy)
- Drain fluid in a controlled manner. Small risk of re-expansion pulmonary oedema if large effusions drained too quickly; control output by clamping drain; drain a maximum of 1.5L per 2h
- CXR when drain output slows (<150mL/day):
  - Consider pleurodesis if fluid removed and lung fully or partially expanded on CXR (although success rates much lower in the setting of an incompletely expanded lung)
  - Consider trial of suction if lung only partially re-expanded, if pain allows. Aim to increase pressure to −20cmH$_2$O over 2h.

For pleurodesis

- Insert IV cannula, and attach pulse oximeter
- Pleurodesis may be extremely painful. Consider premedication with opioid (morphine sulfate solution 2.5–5mg or IV opioid) and anti-emetic (e.g. metoclopramide 10mg). For significant anxiety, consider a benzodiazepine (e.g. midazolam 1–2mg IV, titrate to conscious level; care in elderly and in patients with respiratory failure). The patient should be comfortable but cooperative
- Administer intrapleural local anaesthetic (e.g. lidocaine 3mg/kg, max 250mg) via chest drain, as intrapleural administration of sclerosants frequently painful. Clamp drain, and wait several minutes
- Prepare talc slurry. Using sterile technique, aspirate 50mL normal saline into a syringe, and carefully remove plunger while keeping gloved finger over end of syringe. Tip 4–5g sterile talc into syringe, and replace plunger gently. Shake syringe for 2–3min to ensure homogeneous slurry. Administer slurry via chest drain over 1–2min

- Flush drain with 20mL saline, and restart 6-hourly flushes
- Further analgesia, if required
- Clamp drain for 1h after administration of sclerosant. Then unclamp, and consider applying suction, increasing to $-20cmH_2O$ over 2h
- Monitor pulse, BP, temperature, RR, and O_2 saturations half-hourly for 2h and then 6-hourly
- Analgesia and antipyretics, as required
- Optimal duration of drainage following pleurodesis unknown; consider drain removal within 24–72h if adequate drainage of fluid and lung expansion on CXR. Can usually remove tube at 48h
- For mesothelioma, arrange drain site prophylactic radiotherapy if large-bore chest drain was used (give total of 21Gy in three fractions over 1 week). Malignant seeding in non-mesothelioma malignant effusions uncommon and prophylactic radiotherapy not required.

Complications All sclerosants may cause chest pain and fever. Sterile talc may rarely (<1%) result in respiratory failure due to ARDS, manifest as hypoxia and diffuse pulmonary infiltrates within 48h of pleurodesis. 'Mixed' talc (containing small particles) appears to be associated with greater systemic inflammation and greater deterioration in gas exchange than 'graded' talc (which has small particles removed), so routine use of graded talc is recommended.

Further information

Maskell NA *et al*. Randomized trials describing lung inflammation after pleurodesis with talc of varying particle size. *Am J Respir Crit Care Med* 2004;**170**:377–82.

Roberts ME *et al*. Management of a malignant pleural effusion: British Thoracic Society pleural disease guideline 2010. *Thorax* 2010;**65**(Suppl 2):ii32–ii40.

Pneumothorax aspiration

Indications

- *1° pneumothorax* Consider aspiration if patient breathless, hypoxic, and pneumothorax large
- *2° pneumothorax* Consider aspiration if evidence of underlying lung disease (or patient with significant smoking history, aged >50y), with small pneumothorax and breathlessness.

Technique

See Chapter 37 for discussion of pneumothorax management. Carefully re-examine the CXR to ensure that the lung is not tethered at any point (may increase procedural risk and require CT-guided intervention). Use a dedicated procedure room when possible.

- Discuss procedure with patient, and obtain written consent (unless emergency situation)
- Consider inserting an IV cannula
- Position patient sitting upright in bed, supported on pillows
- Double-check correct side from chest examination and CXR
- Choose aspiration site: second intercostal space in mid-clavicular line on side of pneumothorax
- Sterile skin preparation. Wear sterile gloves and gown
- Infiltrate skin, intercostal muscles, and parietal pleura with 10mL of 1% lidocaine. Aim just above the upper border of the appropriate rib, avoiding the neurovascular bundle that runs below each rib. Parietal pleura is extremely sensitive; use the full 10mL of lidocaine
- Whilst waiting for anaesthetic to work, connect 50mL syringe to three-way tap, with tap turned 'off' to patient
- Confirm presence of pneumothorax by aspirating air with green (21G) needle
- Insert large-bore (e.g. 16G) cannula over upper border of rib. Remove inner needle; quickly connect cannula to three-way tap and 50mL syringe
- Aspirate 50mL air with syringe; turn tap, and expel air into atmosphere. Repeat until resistance felt or 1.5L of air aspirated (aspiration of >1.5L suggests a large air leak, and aspiration is likely to fail). Halt procedure if painful or patient coughing excessively
- Remove cannula; cover insertion site with dressing
- Repeat CXR
- Aspiration is successful if pneumothorax size has reduced on CXR and patient is symptomatically improved
- If initial aspiration of a 1° pneumothorax fails, a chest drain is likely required. The risks of this procedure need to be outweighed by the clinical necessity (i.e. significant symptoms or adverse physiology).

Further information

Havelock T et al. Pleural procedures and thoracic ultrasound: British Thoracic Society pleural disease guideline 2010. *Thorax* 2010;65(suppl. 2):ii61–76.

Safe sedation—general principles

Administration of sedation

- IV sedation commonly used for bronchoscopy and thoracoscopy and, less frequently, for other procedures, e.g. chest drain insertion. Studies show that both patients and physicians usually prefer the use of sedation for bronchoscopy, although some tolerate unsedated bronchoscopy well; consider patient preference and comorbidities
- Follow *Summary of Safe Sedation Practice* (UK Academy of Medical Royal Colleges) (see Table 70.1)
- Sedation is usually the responsibility of the physician performing a procedure, although some units have anaesthetist-delivered sedation
- Desired depth of sedation is usually *conscious sedation*—patient maintains airway patency and cardiorespiratory function, and verbal contact with the patient is possible at all times. Some procedures (e.g. interventional bronchoscopy) may require deeper sedation provided by anaesthetists, with same level of care and monitoring as for a general anaesthetic
- Significant interpatient variability to IV sedation; therefore, essential to titrate sedatives, using small incremental doses, to avoid oversedation
- Assess (and document) sedation depth. Tools, such as the *Ramsay Scale* (see Table 70.2) and the *Modified Observer's Assessment of Alertness/Sedation (MOAAS)* (see Table 70.3) score, may help documentation.

Table 70.1 Summary of Safe Sedation Practice

Domain	Safe practice
Patient assessment	'Checklist' identification of sedation risk factors prior to procedure
	Provide instructions on activities subsequent to procedure
Level of sedation	Sedation provided only to the level of 'conscious' sedation (verbal contact possible)
IV sedation	Secure venous access mandatory
	Antagonist drugs at hand
	When combination sedation used, give opioids first, and caution to avoid oversedation
Monitoring	Defined professionals have responsibility for monitoring patient safety and making a written record. Pulse oximeter monitoring continued until discharge from unit. Consider monitoring BP and ECG in higher-risk patients
O_2 therapy	Nasal cannula and facial mask O_2 delivery available

Table 70.2 Ramsay scale

Level	Response
1	Anxious and agitated or restless
2	Cooperative, orientated, and tranquil
3	Responds only to commands
4	Brisk response to light glabellar touch or loud noise
5	Sluggish response to light glabellar touch or loud noise

Ramsay MA et al Controlled sedation with alphaxalone-alphadolone. Br Med J 1974;2(5920):656–9.

Table 70.3 Modified Observer's Assessment of Alertness/Sedation (MOAAS) scale

Level	Response
5	Responds readily to name spoken in normal tone
4	Lethargic response to name spoken in normal tone
3	Responds only after name is called loudly or repeatedly
2	Responds only after mild prodding or shaking
1	Does not respond to mild prodding or shaking

Chernik DA et al. Validity and reliability of the Observer's Assessment of Alertness/Sedation Scale: study with intravenous midazolam. J Clin Psychopharmacol 1990;10(4):244–51.

Drugs used for sedation

See Appendix 5 for further details about drug doses, pharmacology, and side effects.

Benzodiazepines

- Benzodiazepines cause sedation, anxiolysis, and anterograde amnesia by binding to, and increasing the activity of, γ-aminobutyric acid (GABA), a brain neuroinhibitory transmitter
- *Midazolam* (used by 78% of bronchoscopists) improves experience of bronchoscopy, reduces procedural discomfort, causes anterograde amnesia, and increases willingness of patients to have further procedures without worsening adverse event profile
- Other benzodiazepines (e.g. diazepam and lorazepam) have also been used, but midazolam has particular suitability with rapid peak effect and relatively short half-life
- Natural variability in action of cytochrome P450 (CYP) 3A4 and 3A5, responsible for benzodiazepine metabolism, may prolong elimination half-life by up to sixfold
- *Flumazenil* (benzodiazepine antagonist) reverses benzodiazepine oversedation and must be immediately available, although administration should not be routine. Flumazenil has a shorter half-life than midazolam, so potential risk of re-sedation
- A 2008 NPSA report documented harm and death from excessive midazolam. To prevent inadvertent injection of high-strength midazolam solution (2 or 5mg/mL), NPSA mandates that only low-strength midazolam solution (1mg/mL) should normally be available in clinical areas
- Following a 2004 NCEPOD report (see Sedation in specific circumstances, ➲ p. 796), no more than 5mg midazolam should be initially drawn up into any syringe prior to a procedure for patients aged <70 (2mg midazolam for patients >70), to reduce likelihood of oversedation.

Opioids

- Mechanism of action of *opioids* are not completely understood, but they are known to be mu-opioid receptor agonists, causing analgesia, sedation, and cough suppression
- *Fentanyl* and *alfentanil* both have favourable pharmacological profiles, having a rapid peak effect and a relatively short half-life
- *Naloxone* (competitive antagonist) reverses opioid-induced respiratory depression and oversedation. For oversedated patients who have received both benzodiazepine and opioid, initial reversal with flumazenil (rather than naloxone) recommended, unless the patient has received particularly high dose of opioid

- Addition of an opioid to midazolam for bronchoscopy improves procedural cough, reduces lidocaine usage, and increases patient procedural tolerance. Most frequent combination agents used for bronchoscopy are midazolam and fentanyl/alfentanil. Opioids should be administered (and allowed to reach maximal effect) prior to administration of midazolam. Risk of oversedation may increase when using combination agents, although several studies fail to show an increase in clinically significant adverse events.

Other drugs
- Propofol (and its pro-drug fospropofol) are sedative-hypnotics that exert their actions partly by increasing GABA activity. Together with ketamine, these drugs have a relatively narrow therapeutic window between 'conscious' sedation and general anaesthesia and are *currently recommended for use solely by anaesthetists in the UK*.

Sedation in specific circumstances

- Risks may be increased when using combined sedation for patients in *respiratory failure*, and caution is recommended
- *Elderly patients* are likely to require lower doses of sedatives and may suffer with prolonged after-effects (e.g. amnesia and coordination impairment). A 2004 NCEPOD report for elderly patients undergoing therapeutic GI endoscopy recommended that no more than 2mg should be initially drawn up for patients aged >70
- *Other comorbidities* likely to require dose modification include hepatic impairment, heart failure, and renal impairment
- *Concomitant medications* (e.g. antifungals, antiretrovirals, CCBs, and macrolide antibiotics) inhibit cytochrome P450 3A4 (which also metabolizes benzodiazepines and opioids) and may prolong sedation.

Further information

Du Rand IA *et al*. British Thoracic Society guideline for diagnostic flexible bronchoscopy in adults. *Thorax* 2013;**68**:i1–i44.

Thoracentesis

General points

Thoracentesis ('pleural tap' or pleural fluid aspiration) may be diagnostic or therapeutic. Site selection using US guidance (see Chapter 72) gives a higher success rate and a better adverse event profile and should be used routinely. Use a dedicated procedure room when possible. Avoid out-of-hours procedures unless an emergency.

Diagnostic thoracentesis

Indication   Undiagnosed pleural effusion.

There are no absolute *contraindications* to pleural aspiration, although, for non-urgent thoracentesis, anticoagulated patients should have their clotting corrected to INR <1.5.

Technique

- Discuss procedure with patient, and obtain written consent.
- Position patient sitting forward, leaning on a pillow over a table, with their arms folded in front of them
- Double-check correct side from chest examination and CXR
- Choose aspiration site using ultrasound, preferably in 'safe triangle' (see ➜ p. 764), unless loculated fluid makes this impossible. Avoid posterior approaches where possible (as the intercostal artery lies in the mid-intercostal space posteriorly)
- Sterile skin preparation and aseptic technique
- Infiltrate skin, intercostal muscle, and parietal pleura with 10mL of 1% lidocaine. Aim just above the upper border of the appropriate rib, avoiding the neurovascular bundle that runs below each rib. The parietal pleura is extremely sensitive; use the full 10mL of lidocaine
- Aspirate pleural fluid with a green (21G) needle and 50mL syringe
- Following diagnostic tap:
  - Record pleural fluid appearance
  - Send sample to biochemistry for measurement of glucose, protein, and LDH
  - Send a fresh 20mL sample in sterile pot to cytology for examination for malignant cells and differential cell count
  - Send samples in sterile pot and blood culture bottles to microbiology for Gram stain and microscopy, culture, and AFB stain and culture
  - Process non-purulent heparinized samples in ABG analyser for pH (consult biochemistry laboratory for local policy of pH analysis beforehand; never put purulent samples in the arterial blood analyser)
  - Consider measurement of cholesterol, triglycerides, chylomicrons, haematocrit, and amylase, depending on the clinical circumstances
- There is no need for a routine CXR following aspiration, unless difficulties were encountered during the procedure
- If unable to obtain fluid, re-ultrasound to confirm depth and conformation of fluid, and consider CT-guided aspiration.

Complications of thoracentesis include pain, failure to obtain fluid, pneumothorax (2–4% with US), cough, bleeding, empyema, spleen or liver puncture, and malignant seeding down aspiration site.

Therapeutic thoracentesis

Indication Symptomatic relief of breathlessness due to a pleural effusion, most commonly due to malignancy.

Technique

- In most cases, can be performed as a day-case procedure. Commercial thoracentesis kits are available, but the following works just as well
- The initial procedure of local anaesthetic infiltration is identical to that of diagnostic thoracentesis. It is important to verify that the insertion site is optimal using US; also always ensure that fluid is first obtained with a green (21G) needle
- Carefully advance an IV cannula (with a syringe on the end) along the anaesthetized track
- When fluid is aspirated, remove the inner needle while fully inserting the plastic cannula. Attach the cannula to a three-way tap
- Aspirate fluid from the chest with a 50mL syringe via the three-way tap, and flush the fluid into a sterile jug through extension tubing (e.g. a blood giving set, cut using sterile scissors). Often, having 'primed' the tubing with pleural fluid, further syringe aspiration is not required, as the fluid siphons down out of the chest itself into the jug. Drain a maximum of 1.5L of fluid on one occasion (risk of re-expansion pulmonary oedema following sudden removal of large volumes). Stop the procedure if resistance is felt or the patient experiences discomfort or severe coughing
- Apply dressing to aspiration site
- CXR is not routinely required post-procedure, unless difficulties were encountered or air was aspirated. Post-procedural US is useful in assessing volume of remaining fluid.

Further information

Havelock T et al. Pleural procedures and thoracic ultrasound: British Thoracic Society pleural disease guideline 2010. Thorax 2010;65(suppl. 2):ii61–76.

Thoracic ultrasound

Diagnostic and therapeutic utility

Thoracic ultrasound (TUS) is increasingly used for bedside evaluation of the pleural space and thorax. Given improved safety, NPSA and BTS guidance 'strongly recommend' TUS for pleural fluid procedure site selection. TUS also gives useful diagnostic information (see Table 72.1) which may alter management (e.g. a patient with a transudative effusion who has pleural nodularity, suggestive of malignancy).

Table 72.1 Diagnostic and therapeutic utility of TUS

Structure	Utility
Pleural fluid	Fluid quantification and characterization. Guided intervention. Obesity and rib crowding cause difficulties
Pleural thickening and nodularity	Detection and guided core biopsy. 'Colour fluid sign' may help differentiate between fluid and thickening
Diaphragm	Assessment of function. Detection of thickening or nodularity (assessment limited by aerated lung)
Pneumothorax	Ruling out post-procedural pneumothorax. Unhelpful for assessing pneumothorax size. COPD, CF, and prior pleurodesis may mimic pneumothorax
Lung	Detection of atelectasis, consolidation, and peripheral lung lesions (abscess/tumour). Guided biopsy. Unable to assess structures deep to aerated lung
Heart	Detection of pericardial fluid, cardiomegaly
Ribs	Rib fracture detection and FNA of metastases
Liver	Metastases/abscess detection
Lymph nodes	Assessment and guided FNA

Training

- Follow the Royal College of Radiology 'level 1' TUS syllabus
  - ℘ http://www.rcr.ac.uk/docs/radiology/pdf/BFCR(12)17_ultrasound_training.pdf
  - ℘ http://www.rcr.ac.uk/docs/radiology/pdf/BFCR(12)18_focused_training.pdf
- Find a suitable mentor (with TUS level 2 or level 1 for ≥2y)
- Keep a log book, and maintain a record of video clips and still images
- Attend a practical and theoretical TUS course
- Level 1 practical training currently requires ≥1 session/week over ≥3 months (~5 scans/session)
- Maintain level 1 competency by: (1) doing ≥20 scans/y (≤3 months between scans), (2) maintaining contact with a named radiologist 'mentor', (3) auditing practice, (4) remaining current with literature and CPD.

Physics of US

Characteristics of the US wave

- US is a longitudinal wave in which particles move in the same direction as the wave (creating successive compressions and rarefactions)
- Frequencies used typically 2.5–12MHz (audible sound 20Hz–20kHz)
- Key formula:
  Frequency (f) = constant (c)/wavelength (λ)

Where c = speed of US in soft tissue (~1,540m/s)

- With a typical frequency of 5MHz, TUS wavelength (which determines resolution) is ~0.3mm.

Changes to the US wave

- US wave can be transmitted, attenuated, or reflected
- *Transmission* occurs when particles in a tissue move together and have coherent vibration
- *Attenuation* (loss of US energy) occurs due to wave absorption, scatter, and refraction. Absorption occurs when particles do not move together and have chaotic vibration, generating heat. Higher frequencies (i.e. shorter wavelengths) are more likely to be absorbed than transmitted, giving poorer depth penetration but better resolution. Deeper structures lead to greater wave attenuation (travels further through tissue), and US machines compensate for this using *time gain compensation* (TGC), which can be fine-tuned using sliders on machine
- *Reflection* occurs at the interface between tissues with different impedance. High impedance at soft tissue-air interface and soft tissue-bone interface causes near-complete reflection (and explains inability to image aerated lung and the acoustic shadow cast behind ribs). Also, reason why coupling US gel required. Partial reflection is required to generate a return of signal to the US probe (and create an image).

Generation of the US wave

- US probes have piezoelectric crystals responsible for wave generation and detection. Timing and power of the returning wave generates the B/2D-mode image
- *Pulse repetition frequency* (PRF) determines interval between successive US pulses (must avoid collision of successive pulses). Slow PRF (e.g. simultaneous 2D/Doppler imaging) causes jerky images. Reducing size of scan field improves PRF.

US artefacts

- Numerous artefacts occur with TUS, including:
  - *Mirror artefact* Smooth curved surfaces (e.g. diaphragm) reflect liver/spleen so that they seem within the thoracic cavity (appearing as consolidated lung)

- *Horizontal reverberation artefact* Tissue interfaces that have significant impedance mismatch (e.g. soft tissue-aerated lung interface) create successive reflections between the interface and the ultrasound probe itself, giving a series of echogenic parallel lines below the pleural stripe
- *Comet tail artefact* Another reverberation artefact seen at the pleural-aerated lung interface, which creates vertical 'comet tails', particularly at the lung bases
- *Posterior acoustic shadowing* Poor visualization of structures deep to interfaces with a high reflection coefficient (e.g. ribs, calcified gallstones) due to complete reflection/absorption
- *Posterior acoustic enhancement* Transmission through a medium which causes minimal attenuation (e.g. fluid-filled cyst) causes apparent enhancement of posterior structures.

Probe choice

- *Curvilinear transducers* (2–6MHz) have a fan-shaped pulse field and give excellent depth penetration and reasonable resolution.
- *Linear transducers* (7–14MHz) have a rectangular pulse field and give excellent near-field resolution but have poor depth penetration.

Performing a TUS examination

Prior to the examination

- Examine any available radiology, particularly CT. Think—are there lesions on the CT which should be visible at TUS (including rib metastases, parenchymal pathology, or liver metastases)?
- Position the patient appropriately. For diagnostic TUS, sat up leaning forward, with arms resting on a table, gives excellent views laterally and posteriorly (where most pleural pathology lies). For pleural procedures, the lateral decubitus position prevents the patient from moving (recommended for real-time US-guided pleural intervention)
- Move the US machine to the patient, taking care not to run over the expensive (~£5,000) probe cables. Think about machine position, particularly if undertaking real-time intervention—the probe and the machine screen should be in a straight line. Clean the US machine and probe with an appropriate wipe.

Operating the US machine

- Confirm and enter patient details on the US machine
- Select 2D/B mode, using 'abdominal' preset if 'thoracic' not available (initial depth ~15cm; ensure that TCG sliders are arranged vertically)
- Use a 5MHz curvilinear probe for routine TUS (good compromise between depth of penetration and resolution). 10MHz linear probe better for vascular access and lymph node/rib metastasis FNA (high resolution but poor depth penetration)
- Hold the probe gently, like a pen. Three movements are important to get the most information from narrow intercostal spaces: rotation, angulation, and translation. TUS is a dynamic process; move the probe over both hemithoraces, while continuously optimizing the image, and make sure to first identify the costophrenic angle and liver/spleen to avoid mimics of a pleural effusion (e.g. ascites and loculated intra-abdominal collections).

Optimize machine controls while imaging

- *Depth* should be changed, depending on structure being imaged. Always ensure that you can initially see the full extent of any effusion and structures deep to the fluid
- *Gain* Avoid the temptation to set the gain too high
- *Focal points* Start with one focal point, positioned at the depth of maximal interest. Multiple focal points, whilst seemingly attractive, reduce the PRF and make the image jerky
- *Frequency* May need to reduce, particularly for larger patients, to increase depth penetration
- *Colour Doppler* Useful for assessing possible vascular structures and differentiating between pleural thickening and fluid ('colour fluid sign')
- *TGC* May need to increase gain at depth, particularly for larger patients. Conversely, a massive effusion (and accompanying posterior acoustic enhancement) may make deeper structures very bright, necessitating reducing gain at depth

- *Sector width* and *zoom*
- *Freeze and store* Always store at least one still image/video clip per patient. If performing an intervention, store a representative image from your intervention site
- *Measure/calipers* Useful for measuring depth of pleural effusion at site of intervention and the distance from skin to pleural effusion (Consider—will a standard 35mm 21G needle reach the fluid?)
- Poor image? Restart using the default settings, and ensure that the TGC sliders are vertical and that depth is appropriate. For larger patients, increase the US power to maximum, and consider reducing US frequency (to ~3MHz). Tissue harmonic imaging may improve tissue boundary differentiation. Some machines have an image 'optimize' button.

TUS appearances 1

Aerated lung

See Fig. 72.1.
- Bright echogenic pleural stripe caused by reflection at the soft tissue-air interface
- Pleural sliding/gliding—a shimmering at the pleural stripe as the visceral pleura slides over the parietal pleura
- Comet tail artefacts—fanning out vertically from the pleural stripe, particularly at the lung bases
- Horizontal reverberation artefacts—repeating periodic horizontal lines below pleural stripe
- Absent deep detail—high reflection coefficient at pleural stripe means that it is impossible to image aerated lung or structures deep to lung. The only apparent structures are artefacts.

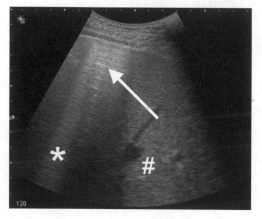

Fig. 72.1 Normal costophrenic angle with aerated lung (left) abutting liver (right, #). Comet tails (*) and horizontal reverberation artefacts (arrow) are seen. Note lack of pleural fluid prevents diaphragm visualization.

Pneumothorax

- TUS may be a useful rule-out test for pneumothorax, but always get a CXR to confirm when pneumothorax suspected
- Absent pleural sliding/gliding
- Absent comet tail artefacts
- Horizontal reverberation artefacts—may be accentuated in pneumothorax
- Absent deep detail.

Pleural effusion

- See Fig. 72.2
- TUS has a higher sensitivity for pleural fluid detection than CXR
- Fluid is seen deep to parietal pleura as a relatively dark (hypoechoic) structure
- *Anechoic effusions* are black and featureless and may be transudative or exudative
- *Echogenic effusions* are exudative and appear speckled, due to protein/ pus/blood/intrapleural air
- *Septated effusions* are also exudative, and septations can be caused by any pleural inflammation (e.g. pleural infection, malignancy)
- Size—measure maximal effusion depth. A variety of formulae have been proposed to estimate pleural fluid volume, particularly in an ITU setting. Practically, the following is suggested—small (only visible at one intercostal space), moderate (less than half the hemithorax), large (greater than half the hemithorax)
- Possible to image structures deep to fluid.

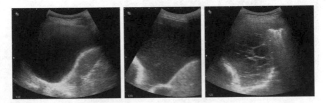
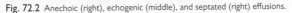

Fig. 72.2 Anechoic (right), echogenic (middle), and septated (right) effusions.

Pleural thickening

- Often relatively hypoechoic and may be difficult to distinguish from pleural fluid. Colour Doppler may help—for fluid, there is a wave-like motion of pleural fluid caused by respiratory/cardiac motion (not seen with thickening).

TUS appearances 2

Diaphragm

- Should be smooth, and it may be possible to discern five alternating hypo- and hyperechoic stripes (see Fig. 72.3; disrupted in pathology)
- Diaphragm poorly visualized without fluid but may be possible by imaging over the liver/spleen and angling probe upwards
- Diaphragm inversion occurs with large effusions and usually associated with significant dyspnoea
- Function may be assessed by watching movement with respiration and sniffing (and comparing both sides).

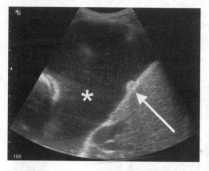

Fig. 72.3 Diaphragmatic nodule (arrow) and echogenic effusion (*).

Abnormal lung

- 'Compressive' atelectasis is commonly seen with pleural fluid. Lung has a concave 'hockey stick' appearance with significant volume loss. Internal structure is visible due to lack of aeration
- Consolidated lung may look similar to liver (or spleen), and parenchymal structure is visible due to lack of aeration (see Fig. 72.4). Minimal volume loss and ill-defined boundaries. Hyperechoic (bright) branching structures and speckles represent air bronchograms. Branching hypoechoic structures are either pulmonary vessels (with demonstrable colour Doppler signal) or fluid bronchograms (without Doppler signal).

TUS features in malignancy

Sonographic features with high specificity (95–100%) for malignancy and overall sensitivity 79%:

- Parietal pleural thickening >1cm
- Nodular pleural thickening
- Visceral pleural thickening
- Diaphragmatic thickening >7mm
- Disruption of five diaphragmatic layers
- Diaphragmatic nodules.

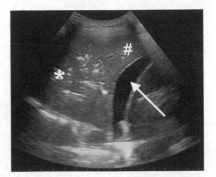

Fig. 72.4 Consolidated lung with visible air bronchograms (*) and pulmonary vessels (#) overlying a subpulmonic effusion (arrow).

TUS features in pleural infection

No sonographic characteristics can rule out pleural infection, and fluid sampling is essential. Septated effusions may drain less well than non-septated effusions (although this should not discourage drain insertion, as many will still drain well). Densely echogenic fluid is likely to be pus or blood.

US-guided intervention

Pleural procedures (aspiration and drainage) can be guided sonographically, either by site marking or using real-time guided intervention. *Site marking* is easier and can be used for most effusions >2–4cm depth but must be performed immediately prior to intervention without patient repositioning. *Real-time visualization* of the needle in the pleural space requires sterile US gel and sheath and is technically more challenging but is required for smaller or loculated effusions. An in-plane oblique course is taken from the side of the probe, and the entire path of the needle is visible. A similar technique is used for *pleural biopsy* (using a Temno® cutting needle) and *lymph node/rib metastasis FNA* (using a linear probe and a 23 or 21G needle).

Cautions

- Avoid risky sampling of small <1cm effusions (which may not even be apparent on CXR), unless there is a genuine diagnostic need
- Always identify the hemidiaphragm to ensure that the pleural space, rather than the upper abdomen, is being imaged
- Avoid posterior approaches for interventions whenever possible (even though this might be the site of maximal fluid depth), due to the relative exposure of the neurovascular bundle. Provided adequate fluid is present, always use the safe triangle.

Further information

Koh DM *et al*. Transthoracic US of the chest: clinical uses and applications. *Radiographics* 2002;**22**(1):e1.

Chapter 73

Thoracoscopy (medical)

General points

Thoracoscopy is the procedure of examining the parietal pleura, visceral pleura, and diaphragm with a thoracoscope and taking biopsies. Chemical pleurodesis can also be performed. Performed by chest physicians using conscious sedation and local anaesthetic. Either a rigid or a 'semi-rigid' flexible thoracoscope (similar to a bronchoscope) is used, dependent on local availability.

There needs to be an adequate space into which the thoracoscope is inserted without damaging the underlying lung. Patients suitable for thoracoscopy are therefore usually those who have an underlying pleural effusion or a pneumothorax where the lung is away from the instrument insertion site (although experts may induce a pneumothorax using a Boutin pleural needle, designed to avoid injuring the visceral pleura).

Indications and risks

Indications

- Undiagnosed pleural effusion—usually an exudate (sensitivity for malignancy >92% and TB ~100%; similar to VATS)
- Suspected mesothelioma
- Staging of pleural effusion in lung cancer
- Treatment of recurrent pleural effusions with pleurodesis
- Pneumothorax requiring chemical pleurodesis, as an alternative to surgery, e.g. patient unfit for surgical thoracoscopy.

Contraindications/proceed with caution

- Obliterated pleural space
- Mature pleural adhesions
- Bleeding disorder
- Hypoxia <92% on air or hypercapnia
- Unstable cardiovascular disease
- Persistent uncontrollable cough
- Severe obesity (thoracoscopy ports not long enough to reach pleura)
- Obstructing central airway tumour.

Risks associated with thoracoscopy

Mortality rates low (0% for diagnostic thoracoscopies; 0.69% when talc also used—but studies included ungraded talc). Major complications <2%.

- Haemorrhage—may need diathermy in the pleural space. Rare
- Pulmonary perforations. Rare
- Air or gas embolism during pneumothorax induction. Rare <0.1%
- Local wound infection
- Empyema
- Fever, ARDS with talc poudrage (see ➔ p. 787)
- Port site tumour seeding.

Thoracoscopy technique

Preparation of patient and consent

- Patient should have written information >24h before the procedure. Written consent taken by doctor performing procedure
- Check recent CXR and any CT scans available
- Check FBC, U&E, and APTT
- Nil by mouth for solids 6h and liquids 2h pre-procedure
- IV cannula in arm on the same side as the thoracoscopy to make repeated sedation/analgesia administration during the procedure easy
- Premedication with analgesia, such as single doses of oral paracetamol and ibuprofen, 1h before. Some centres give a single dose of IV antibiotic as infection prophylaxis (e.g. co-amoxiclav or, if allergic, vancomycin)
- Baseline O_2 saturations, pulse, BP, temperature. Measure oximetry throughout.

Procedure

- The patient is placed in the lateral decubitus position, with the side of the pleural effusion uppermost
- Sedation (IV midazolam) is administered and allowed time to work. O_2 (2–4L/min) is administered via nasal cannulae
- Pleural US is used to define pleural anatomy and optimize location for thoracoscope port insertion
- The skin is cleaned and local anaesthetic inserted, in the same way as for a chest drain. Aspiration of fluid or air from the pleural space confirms it is safe to proceed to thoracoscopy
- An incision is made, and a horizontal mattress suture is inserted (for wound closure post-drain removal). Blunt dissection is performed through the parietal pleura, and the port is inserted
- The pleural effusion is drained via a suction tube through the thoracoscope port. Air is simultaneously allowed to enter the pleural space through this port, and effectively a pneumothorax is created
- The thoracoscope, with its light source, can then be inserted through the port and the pleural cavity inspected. A separate second smaller incision allows forceps or other instruments to be inserted and biopsies taken
- An opioid (e.g. IV fentanyl) is given immediately prior to taking biopsies, as these can be intensely painful
- At the end of the procedure, one port is replaced with a 24F drain, and any further ports are removed and sutures tied
- Thoracoscopic biopsies are usually large and yield good diagnostic results
- If the pleural surfaces have appearances consistent with malignancy, pleurodesis can be performed prior to removing the port, using 4–5g talc administered via an insufflator (poudrage). Talc poudrage efficacy is at least as good as talc slurry via a chest drain, and insufflation during thoracoscopy reduces the number of procedures required.

Post-thoracoscopy care

- Monitor O_2 saturations, pulse, BP, and temperature
- Chest drain on free drainage initially, but suction is started when bubbling stops, incrementing to $-20cmH_2O$ over 2h, as tolerated
- Analgesia, as required, such as IV diamorphine 2.5mg, codeine 30–60mg PO, paracetamol 1g
- DVT prophylaxis with LMWH (increased coagulopathy with talc pleurodesis)
- Mobile CXR the morning after thoracoscopy
- Remove chest drain when the lung is re-inflated on CXR with minimal fluid or air drainage. Trapped lung occurs if the visceral pleura is too thick to allow lung re-inflation (see ➔ pp. 348–9)
- If mesothelioma is diagnosed, refer for radiotherapy to thoracoscopy and chest drain tract sites.

Further information

Rahman NM et al. Local anaesthetic thoracoscopy: British Thoracic Society pleural disease guideline 2010. Thorax 2010;65(Suppl 2):ii54–ii60.

Chapter 74

Tracheostomy

Indications and techniques

Temporary tracheostomy is usually performed as an adjunct to assisted ventilation. Such patients are now often returned to respiratory wards for 'decannulation', with the potential for complications to occur there.

Indications for tracheostomy on the ICU (no uniform agreement).
- After a period of time following intubation with an endotracheal tube
- Improved patient communication (with cuff deflation/tube fenestration)
- Reduced sedation
- Possible reduction in laryngeal damage (the evidence for this is limited)
- Nursing care potentially easier
- Facilitation of weaning.

(*There is no evidence for a reduced incidence of aspiration or pneumonia with tracheostomy vs endotracheal tube.*)
Usual practice is to convert from endotracheal tube to tracheostomy at 7 days if ventilation is likely to be needed beyond 14 days. Earlier conversion for those predicted to require >7 days ventilation is not beneficial, except in reducing sedation. Conversion beyond 14 days is considered best practice and certainly by 21 days.

Percutaneous vs surgical tracheostomy Percutaneous tracheostomy (PT) can be performed on the ICU immediately once the decision is made and is quicker than conventional tracheostomy. There are a variety of PT techniques: Griggs' guidewire with dilating forceps, and the Ciaglia multiple or single (Blue Rhino) dilator approach, preferably with endoscopic verification of placement. In the Blue Rhino system, a curved, cone-shaped dilator is slid over a guidewire and introduced into the tracheal lumen between the second and third tracheal rings until the hole is large enough to accept the required tracheostomy tube. This technique requires controlled force, and there is *significant potential for traumatic damage*. The fit of the tracheostomy tube is tighter, with less stomal infection, less post-operative haemorrhage, but the long-term complications of the two techniques are similar. However, units with prompt access to surgical tracheostomy tend to use this whenever possible, due to the potential traumatic damage from the percutaneous approach. Humidification of the inspired gas is always required to prevent the build-up of thick viscid mucus. Humidification can only be withdrawn in long-term tracheostomy patients after several weeks or months.

Decannulation Tracheostomy may still be required to administer intermittent ventilation, reduce ventilatory dead space, aid respiratory secretion clearance, limit aspiration (when cuffed), and bypass any upper airway obstruction. This is weighed against the consequences of a tracheostomy: increased tendency to aspirate (because of a reduced ability to swallow), reduced ability to talk, and the increased infection brought about from a foreign body in the trachea as well as bypassing the upper airway. Thus, decannulation should be carried out as soon as:
- Adequate clearance of secretions, i.e. good cough and thin secretions
- Low probability that thick mucous plugs will block off large airways and need urgent suctioning

- No upper airway obstruction
- No significant aspiration (can be checked by drinking methylene blue and then suctioning), although a small amount is not an absolute contraindication
- No need to continue ventilation or simply reduce dead space for maintenance of gas exchange
- Conversion to NIV, if necessary, is possible and has been demonstrated to work adequately while tracheostomy capped.

Respiratory physiotherapists can often help with these assessments. The ability to cope adequately without the tracheostomy can be repeatedly determined (and for increasing periods) by capping the tube, with the cuff fully deflated and preferably with a fenestrated tube (to maximally reduce airflow resistance). The addition of a speaking valve does not replicate the physiological challenge of decannulation, as there is still relief from a significant amount of dead space ventilation.

Once a tube has been removed, the stoma can close over very quickly, making reinsertion difficult. Introducing a 'guidewire' (over which the old tube is removed and the new can be inserted) is useful, if there is concern that reinsertion is a possibility (a thin suction tube, with the connector cut off, will suffice as a guide'wire'); alternatively, a mini-tracheostomy can be inserted as an interim measure. The final decision to decannulate is often delayed unnecessarily. Sooner, rather than later, is usually better, as the improved swallowing, reduced aspiration, better coughing, reduced irritation, reduced chance of infection can together outweigh the apparent advantage of easy access to the airway for suction.

Available tube options Tracheostomy tubes can be cuffed or uncuffed. If ventilation is not necessary and aspiration is not a problem, cuffs are not required. Some patients can be adequately ventilated, even with the cuff down (or no cuff at all); this is usually in patients with normal lungs where the compliance is good, inflation pressures therefore low, and only small amounts of air leak upwards through the nose and mouth.

Tracheostomy tubes can be either single or double (i.e. with an inner and outer tube). Double tubes allow better cleaning and therefore reduce the chance of the lumen obstructing, but the diameter of the lumen is of course less for a similar-sized external diameter.

Tracheostomy tubes can be fenestrated to allow exhalation via the larynx to aid talking. The fenestration can be closed off with a non-fenestrated inner tube, should intermittent ventilation still be required.

Speaking valves are available that fit on the tracheostomy, allowing inspiration via the tracheostomy but closing and allowing expiration via the larynx (if cuff down and/or fenestration open!). They effectively still reduce dead space, maintain access for suctioning, but allow talking.

In the very obese, tracheostomy tubes are often too short and too curved to cope with the increased distance between skin and trachea; tubes with adjustable flanges that allow customized intra-tracheal lengths are useful here (but do not usually come with inner tubes, making more difficult the task of keeping the tracheostomy tube free of secretion build-up).

Complications

- *Displacement or obstruction* Evidenced by failing gas exchange, unexpected ventilator pressures; patient may be able to talk despite cuff inflated. If available, use capnography to detect oscillating $FiCO_2$ and determine if obstructed or not. Remove inner tube, and check for secretion build-up. Try passing suction catheter. Fibre-optic inspection. Removal and reinsertion, using fibrescope as guide, to ensure correct placement
- *Infection* Early or late. Good stoma care should prevent this
- *Bleeding* Local erosion at entry site, damage from vigorous suctioning; more seriously, erosion by tracheostomy tip or high-pressure balloon cuff, rarely into the innominate artery which lies anteriorly.

Further information

Commercial video of Cook/Ciaglia Blue Rhino insertion. 🕭
https://www.cookmedical.com/product/-/catalog/display?ds=cc_ptis_webds#tab=resources

McGrath BA et al. Multidisciplinary guidelines for the management of tracheostomy and laryngectomy airway emergencies. *Anaesthesia* 2012;**67**:1025–41.

Royal College of Anaesthetists recommendations on tracheostomy displacement. 🕭 http://www.rcoa.ac.uk/document-store/nap4-section-3-appendices (Appendix 2, p.205).

Young D et al. Effect of early versus late tracheostomy placement on survival in patients receiving mechanical ventilation: the TracMan randomized trial. *JAMA* 2013;**309**:2121–9.

Grant CA et al. Tracheo-innominate artery fistula after percutaneous tracheostomy: three case reports and a clinical review. *Br J Anaesth* 2006;**96**:127–31.

Appendices

Blood gases and acid–base balance

Interpretation of ABGs 1

Normal ranges

Breathing air: PaO_2 >12kPa (>10 in normal elderly), $PaCO_2$ 4.6–5.9.

How to take

- *ABGs* Best taken from radial, rather than brachial, artery due to dual radial/ulnar supply to hand. Use a heparinized syringe; analyse immediately or within 30min if kept on ice.

Always record date, time, and the % inspired O_2.

- *Arterialized capillary sample* An underused technique. Uses small glass pre-heparinized tube to draw up blood from a lancet puncture on the *bottom end* of the ear lobe. Blood gas machine must take microsamples (most do). $PaCO_2$ levels are accurate enough for clinical practice, but good arterialization, with rubefacients (Algipan/Deep Heat) or heat and vigorous rubbing, are required for an accurate PaO_2; the latter is less important, as oxygenation can be assessed by oximetry. Can easily be performed by nursing staff to monitor response to NIV and O_2 therapy.

The three main things blood gases tell you about gas exchange

- How much is the patient ventilating their alveoli? This is derived from the $PaCO_2$. $PaCO_2$ ≥6kPa ≈ underventilating, $PaCO_2$ ≤4.5kPa ≈ overventilating
- Is the PaO_2 high enough to adequately oxygenate tissues and prevent anaerobic metabolism? PaO_2 >6kPa (SaO_2≈ 80%) is probably adequate; PaO_2 >7kPa (SaO_2 >87%) is definitely adequate
- Is there evidence of V/Q mismatch? Evidence of low V/Q units is derived from the calculated A–a O_2 gradient.

The two main things blood gases tell you about acid–base balance

(see later section on acid–base balance)

- What is the respiratory component to an abnormal pH? This is derived from the $PaCO_2$
- What is the metabolic component to an abnormal pH? This is derived from the standard base excess/deficit.

The A–a gradient calculator graph sets out the graphical representation of gas exchange

(see Fig. A1.1)

- Point ① = pO_2 and pCO_2 (virtually zero) of *inspired air* (atmospheric pressure ≈ 100kPa; air is 21% O_2, and air is slightly 'diluted' by water vapour pressure (7kPa) following humidification by upper airways). 21% of 100–7 = 20kPa. (Point ② = pO_2 and pCO_2 when breathing 24% O_2 via a Ventimask, and point ③ = pO_2 and pCO_2 when breathing 28% O_2 via a Ventimask.)
- Point ④ = theoretical pO_2/pCO_2 of *alveolar gas* when breathing air, if all the O_2 removed and replaced by CO_2 (equivalent to extreme hypoventilation and impossible!), when the respiratory quotient (RQ = CO_2 produced/O_2 consumed) is 0.8 (usual value)

- The line between ① and ④ with a gradient of 0.8, describes all possible combinations of alveolar gas, towards ① if ventilating more and towards ④ if ventilating less, called the *alveolar air line*
- Point ⑤ = area in which PaO_2 and $PaCO_2$ of *arterial blood* sit normally. If lungs are perfect gas exchangers, then blood leaving the lungs and entering systemic arterial circulation (④) should be perfectly equilibrated with the alveolar gas (A).

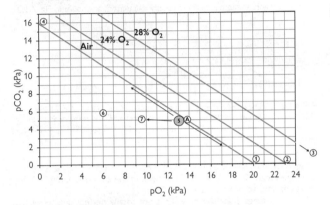

Fig. A1.1 pCO_2 vs pO_2: alveolar air lines and A–a gradient calculator.

- However, the *mixed venous point* = ⑥ (or the *pulmonary arterial* blood) is well to the left of the alveolar air line. This is because capillary PO_2 falls more kPa than the PCO_2 rises during gas exchange in the tissues (CO_2 solubility curve is steeper than PaO_2–SaO_2 solubility, or dissociation curve)
- Thus, if the lungs fail to oxygenate returning mixed venous/pulmonary arterial blood properly (e.g. area of consolidation, or low V/Q due to asthma/COPD), then it is as if mixed venous blood has bypassed the lung and 'leaked' into the arterial blood, which therefore drags the eventual arterial PaO_2/$PaCO_2$ point to the left of the alveolar air line, e.g. point ⑦

Interpretation of ABGs 2

- The horizontal distance between the actual arterial point and the 'ideal' alveolar air line (e.g. ⑤ minus ⑦, 3.5kPa) is called the *alveolar to arterial (A–a) gradient* and is a measure of how efficiently mixed venous blood is equilibrated with alveolar gas, i.e. it is a measure of V/Q mismatch, right-to-left shunts, and very severe lung fibrosis (through reduced diffusion across the alveolar capillary membrane). As well as being read off the graph, it can be mathematically calculated, as shown in Fig. A1.2.

$$A - a \text{ gradient} = PIO_2 - (PaO_2 + \frac{PaCO_2}{0.8})$$

Arterial PO_2 Arterial PCO_2

Inspired PO_2 Respiratory quotient

Fig. A1.2 Calculation of inspired PO_2 breathing air, 24 or 28% O_2. Air, 21% of $(100 − 7) ≈ 20$kPa (where 100kPa is atmospheric pressure, and 7kPa is water vapour pressure due to the inspired air being humidified); **24%**, 24% of $(100 − 7) ≈ 23$kPa; **28%**, 28% of $(100 − 7) ≈ 26$kPa.

In Fig. A1.1, the alveolar air line depends on the % inspired O_2, and the two extra lines for 24% and 28% O_2 are shown. In the calculation, the PIO_2 has to be adjusted accordingly (see Fig. A1.2).

In normal lungs, matching of V/Q is not totally perfect due to relative underperfusion of the apices and overperfusion of the bases (gravity effects on pulmonary arterial blood flow, not fully compensated for by hypoxic vasoconstriction of pulmonary arterioles). These imperfections in V/Q and direct drainage of some of the cardiac muscle venous blood into the LV cavity, and hence systemic arterial circulation, lead to a small A–a gradient, 1–2kPa in the young and middle-aged and 2–3kPa in the elderly. Figures in excess of these values are abnormal and indicate areas of low V/Q or increased shunt.

Use of A–a gradient diagram: examples

Case 1 Consider point W in the pO_2–pCO_2 graph (see Fig. A1.3), the blood gases on air of a young non-smoker complaining of chest pain 7 days post-operatively. The PaO_2 of 13 is normal. Does this reassure you or does it provide supporting evidence for a PE? Ask the following questions:

- How much is the patient ventilating? $PaCO_2 \approx 2$; therefore ≤4.5kPa and indicates hyperventilation
- Is the patient adequately oxygenated? PaO_2 >7kPa; therefore OK
- Is there an abnormal A–a gradient? Read off graph, horizontal line between W and alveolar line, or calculate:

$$20 - [13 + (2/0.8)] \approx 4.5\text{kPa}$$

>2kPa, hence yes; therefore, the V/Q matching is not normal.

This provides supporting evidence for a PE but could just as well be due to consolidation from pneumonia, for example.

- Remember, PaO_2 cannot be used to assess V/Q matching in the lung without an associated $PaCO_2$ to tell you 'what the PaO_2 ought to be'.

Case 2 Consider point X on the pO_2–pCO_2 graph (see Fig. A1.3). These are the gases on air from a young man following an overdose of methadone tablets.

- How much is the patient ventilating? $PaCO_2 \approx 11$; therefore ≥6kPa and indicates hypoventilation
- Is the patient adequately oxygenated? PaO_2 only 6kPa; therefore not enough and needs extra O_2
- Has the patient got an A–a gradient?

$$20 - [6 + (11/0.8)] \approx 0.8\text{kPa}$$

<2kPa, hence no; therefore, there is nothing wrong with the lungs, despite the abnormal gases; this represents pure hypoventilation.

After a messy stomach washout, he is sent to the ward and 24h later is febrile. Gases on 24% O_2 are point Y on the graph; thus, both $PaCO_2$ and PaO_2 are better.

- How much is the patient ventilating? $PaCO_2$ just ≥6kPa; therefore is still hypoventilating a bit
- Is the patient adequately oxygenated? PaO_2 >7kPa; therefore adequately oxygenated
- Has the patient got an A–a gradient?

$$23 - [11 + (6.5/0.8)] \approx 4.2\text{kPa}$$

(remember, the PIO_2 is 23kPa, because he is on 24% O_2.)

>2kPa, hence yes; therefore may have developed an aspiration pneumonia.

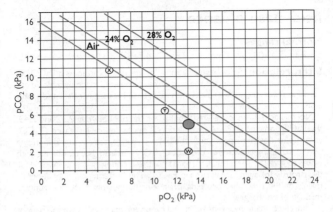

Fig. A1.3 Examples of using A–a gradient.

Three things blood gases tell you about gas exchange
- How much is the patient ventilating their alveoli?—$PaCO_2$
- Is the PaO_2 high enough to adequately oxygenate tissues and thus prevent anaerobic metabolism?
- Is there any evidence of a V/Q mismatch, assessed from the A–a gradient for O_2?

Acid–base balance

Normal ranges

pH 7.37–7.43 (H^+ 37–43nmol/L), $PaCO_2$ 4.7–5.9, base excess ± 3mmol/L.

Interpretation Acid–base relationships are best plotted as a $PaCO_2$ vs pH graph, because these are the two 1°measurements made by a blood gas machine (everything else to do with acid–base balance is calculated). This is shown in Fig. A1.4.

Normal acid–base is the area labelled N, the pH between 7.37 and 7.43, the $PaCO_2$ around 5kPa. As ventilation is decreased or increased ($PaCO_2$ going up or down, respectively), the pH will change, the amount depending on the buffering capacity of the blood (CO_2 is an acid gas, combining with water to give $[H^+]$ and $[HCO_3^-]$ ions). Without buffering, the pH would fall disastrously following small rises in $PaCO_2$. This buffering capacity depends mainly on Hb and other proteins, producing the normal buffer line running through N on the graph.

Therefore, *acute hypoventilation and hyperventilation* will move the patient up and down this line, in the direction *b* or *c*, respectively. If the *hypoventilation* at point *b* becomes *chronic* (e.g. as it may in COPD), then the kidney retains bicarbonate (by excreting $[H^+]$) to try and correct the pH towards normal, and the patient moves onto a new iso $[HCO_3^-]$ buffer line displaced to the right, e.g. the one labelled +10meq/L (35meq/L). The degree of displacement represents the *metabolic component to the acid–base status* and, in this case, because the $[HCO_3^-]$ has risen, will be higher than the normal figure of about 25meq/L. When the raised figure is quoted relative to the normal 25meq/L (by subtracting 25), this is called the *base excess*. Thus, buffer lines to the right of the normal buffer line represent a metabolic alkalosis or base excess.

These figures are calculated, assuming a normal or 'standard' $PaCO_2$, called the 'standard bicarbonate' (SBC on the blood gas machine printout) or 'standard base excess' (usually BE). The other similar figures on some printouts (usually HCO_3^- and TCO_2) are calculated at the patient's actual $PaCO_2$ and are not much use.

Chronic hyperventilation (e.g. at altitude due to the hypoxia) produces the opposite, a resorption of $[H^+]$ by the kidney, and the buffer line shifts to the left, giving a negative value for the 'base excess', a *base deficit*. Thus, a metabolic acidosis compensates for a respiratory alkalosis. Note that these corrections rarely bring the pH back to normal, as there needs to be an error signal to keep the correction process going.

A *metabolic acidosis* (such as in ketoacidosis) will also move the line to the left (*a*), producing a base deficit (or negative base excess), followed by hyperventilation to try and correct it (i.e. a respiratory alkalosis to correct a metabolic acidosis). This pure ventilatory stimulation in the absence of abnormal lungs often produces deep breathing, with little increase in rate, and is called *Kussmaul's breathing*. Thus, lines to the left of the normal buffer line represent a metabolic acidosis or base deficit.

Important point—a metabolic acidosis, e.g. due to anaerobic metabolism (and hence lactic acid production), can reverse the compensatory metabolic alkalosis 2° to chronic hypercapnia, e.g. during a COPD exacerbation with severe hypoxia, thus removing the 'evidence' for previous chronic CO_2 retention.

Finally, a *metabolic alkalosis*, e.g. during hypokalaemia (when the kidney is forced to use $[H^+]$, instead of $[K^+]$, to swap for the sodium that needs resorbing from the tubular fluid), moves the buffer line to the right (*d*) but with only limited hypoventilation available to compensate, due to the inevitable ventilatory stimulation the attendant hypoxaemia produces.

Thus, the mixture of respiratory and metabolic contributions to a patient's acid–base disturbance can be established by plotting the $PaCO_2$ and pH on the graph.

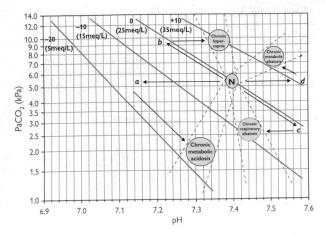

Fig. A1.4 Acid–base balance: $PaCO_2$–pH. Lines running top left to bottom right are the iso-bicarbonate lines labelled as absolute $[HCO_3^-]$ (in brackets) or as a base excess/deficit (relative to a $[HCO_3^-]$ of 25meq/L), hence can be – (metabolic acidosis) or + (metabolic alkalosis).

Anion gap

The anion gap $[(Na^+ + K^+) - (Cl^- + HCO_3^-)]$ shows the amount of other anions, apart from $[Cl^-]$ and $[HCO_3^-]$, that exists and helps differentiate the cause of any metabolic acidosis. Depending on methods of measurement, the normal value is between 8 and 16mmol/L (or meq/L) and mainly due to albumin. High anion gap indicates loss of $[HCO_3^-]$ without a subsequent increase in $[Cl^-]$. Electroneutrality is maintained by increase in anions such as ketones, lactate, $[PO_4^-]$, and $[SO_4^-]$. Because these anions are not part of the anion gap calculation, a high anion gap results.

An acidosis with a normal anion gap will be a simple HCO_3^-/Cl^- exchange such as might occur, e.g. in:
- Renal tubular acidosis
- Acetazolamide therapy
- [HCO_3^-] loss from profuse diarrhoea.

An anion gap is likely to be present, e.g. when the metabolic acidosis is due to:
- Diabetes, starvation, or alcohol-induced ketoacidosis (ketones are acids)
- Renal failure (although can be in the normal range too)
- Lactic acidosis
- Salicylate poisoning
- Methanol poisoning
- Ethylene glycol (antifreeze) poisoning.

Three things arterial samples tell you about acid–base balance

- Is there a ventilatory/respiratory component from an abnormally high or low $PaCO_2$?
- Is there a metabolic component evidenced by a shift of the buffer line to the left or right, numerically the base excess (or deficit)?
- If there is a metabolic acidosis, is there an increased anion gap?

Further information

Williams AJ. ABC of O_2. ℅ http://www.bmj.com/cgi/content/full/317/7167/1213.

Conversion between arterial O₂ saturation and O₂ tension (Hb dissociation curve)

See Fig. A1.5 and Table A1.1.

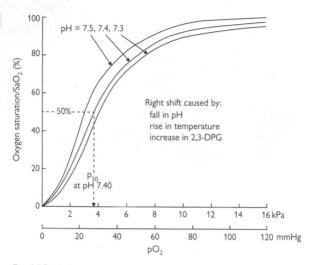

Fig. A1.5 Hb dissociation curve.

A *fall in pH* (more acidic) or a rise in *body temperature* will move the dissociation curve to the *right*. This has the effect of making the *PaO2 higher for any given SaO2*, e.g. at pH 7.20, a measured saturation (e.g. by oximetry) of 90% is equivalent to a higher PaO₂ of 9.7kPa (73mmHg) than the usual 7.7kPa (58mmHg); a rise in body temperature to 41°C will do the same, and the effects of pH and temperature are additive.

Conversely, for a given PaO₂, pyrexia and acidosis will *lower the SaO2* and thus O₂ carriage to the tissues. A PaO₂ of 7.7kPa (58mmHg) will normally give an SaO₂ of 90%, but, if the temperature rises to 41°C and pH falls to 7.20, then the SaO₂ falls to 70%.

Increasing 2,3-DPG levels shift the curve to the right, but levels fluctuate unpredictably and any changes are small.

Changes in body temperature are often the reason why measured pulse oximetry saturations apparently 'do not agree' with the measured blood gases (pH is taken into account in the *theoretical* calculation of SaO₂ by blood gas analysers, but the patient's correct body temperature is rarely entered and thus is not taken into account). This is particularly important in hypothermia when the curve is left-shifted, leading to impaired O_2 unloading. Furthermore, an apparently adequate oximetry reading can mask a low PaO_2, which will further lessen O_2 availability to the tissues (although somewhat mitigated by the reduced metabolic rate of hypothermic tissues).

Table A1.1 Conversion chart*

% saturation	kPa	mmHg
98	15.0	112
97	12.2	92
96	10.8	81
95	9.9	74
94	9.3	70
93	8.8	66
92	8.4	63
91	8.1	60
90	7.7	58
88	7.3	55
86	6.8	51
84	6.5	49
82	6.2	47
80	5.9	45
75	5.4	40
70	4.9	37
65	4.5	34
60	4.2	31
55	3.8	29
50	3.5	27

* Assumes a normal position of the Hb dissociation curve; kPa and mmHg conversion factor: 7.5 × kPa ≈ mmHg.

BMI calculator; height and weight converter

For BMI calculator, see Fig. A2.1.

BMI ≈ weight in kilograms, divided by height in metres squared.
For example, 70kg man, 1.8m tall:

BMI ≈ 70 / (1.8 × 1.8) ≈ 21.6

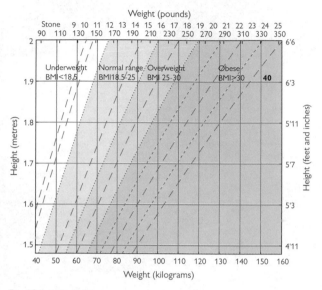

Fig. A2.1 BMI calculator.

CT anatomy of the thorax

These are *not* standard images set for mediastinal or lung viewing but have been adjusted to aid anatomical labelling (see Fig. A3.1 to Fig. A3.6). Contrast was used to highlight the vessels.

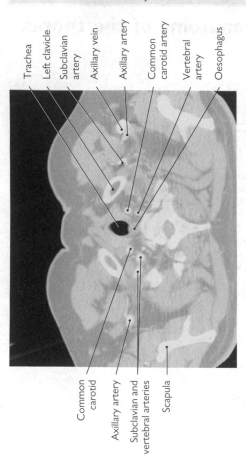

Fig. A3.1 CT anatomy of the thorax: level of C7.

Trachea
Left clavicle
Subclavian artery
Axillary vein
Axillary artery
Common carotid artery
Vertebral artery
Oesophagus

Common carotid
Axillary artery
Subclavian and vertebral arteries
Scapula

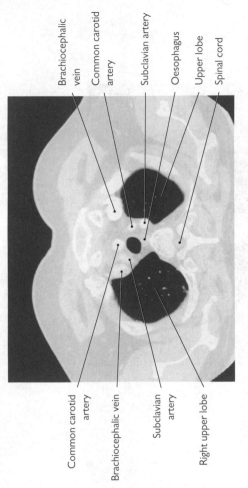

Brachiocephalic vein

Common carotid artery

Subclavian artery

Oesophagus

Upper lobe

Spinal cord

Common carotid artery

Brachiocephalic vein

Subclavian artery

Right upper lobe

Fig. A3.2 CT anatomy of the thorax: level of T2.

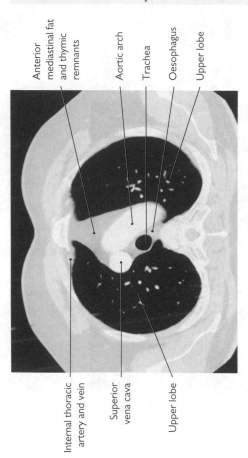

Fig. A3.3 CT anatomy of the thorax: level of T4.

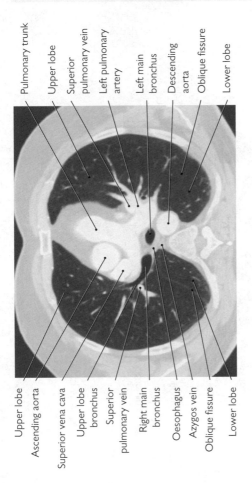

Pulmonary trunk
Upper lobe
Superior pulmonary vein
Left pulmonary artery
Left main bronchus
Descending aorta
Oblique fissure
Lower lobe

Upper lobe
Ascending aorta
Superior vena cava
Upper lobe bronchus
Superior pulmonary vein
Right main bronchus
Oesophagus
Azygos vein
Oblique fissure
Lower lobe

Fig. A3.4 CT anatomy of the thorax: level of T6.

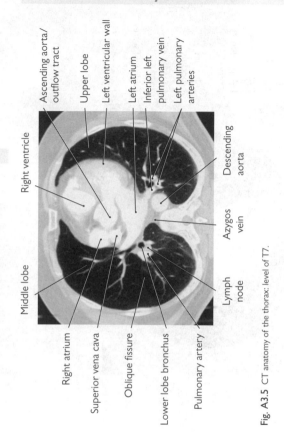

Right ventricle

Ascending aorta/ outflow tract

Upper lobe

Left ventricular wall

Left atrium

Inferior left pulmonary vein

Left pulmonary arteries

Descending aorta

Azygos vein

Lymph node

Middle lobe

Right atrium

Superior vena cava

Oblique fissure

Lower lobe bronchus

Pulmonary artery

Fig. A3.5 CT anatomy of the thorax: level of T7.

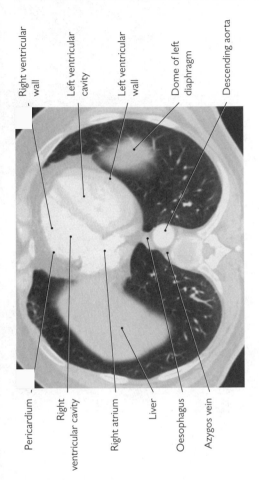

Right ventricular wall

Left ventricular cavity

Left ventricular wall

Dome of left diaphragm

Descending aorta

Pericardium

Right ventricular cavity

Right atrium

Liver

Oesophagus

Azygos vein

Fig. A3.6 CT anatomy of the thorax: level of T9.

CT patterns of lung disease

Airspace consolidation

Process	Causes
Fluid/secretion accumulation in alveoli	Pneumonia, pulmonary oedema or haemorrhage, ARDS, COP, lymphoma, drugs, bronchoalveolar cell carcinoma, eosinophilic pneumonia

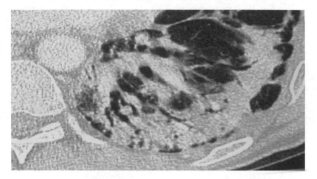

Fig. A4.1 Chronic organizing pneumonia (COP). Air bronchograms clearly present.

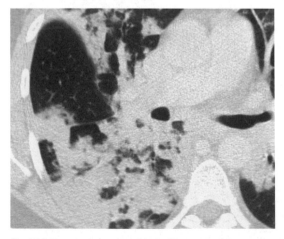

Fig. A4.2 Extensive airspace consolidation due to eosinophilic pneumonia.

Air trapping

Process	Causes
Partial small airway obstruction	Asthma, obliterative bronchiolitis, COPD

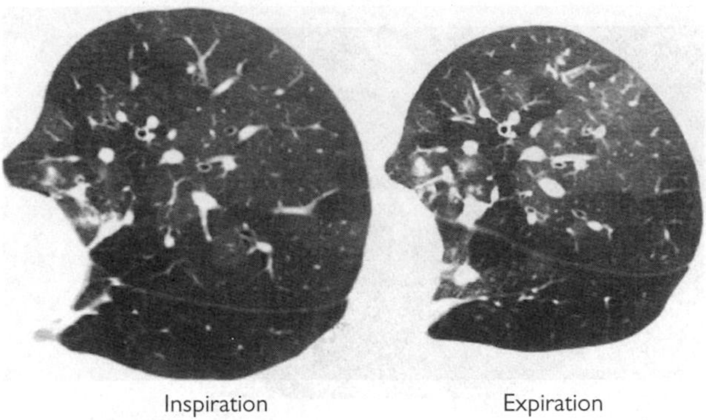

Inspiration   Expiration

Fig. A4.3 Subject prone. On expiration, the denser area becomes more dense, indicating the lung has deflated; other parts of the lung remain lucent, indicating that air is trapped behind narrowed airways.

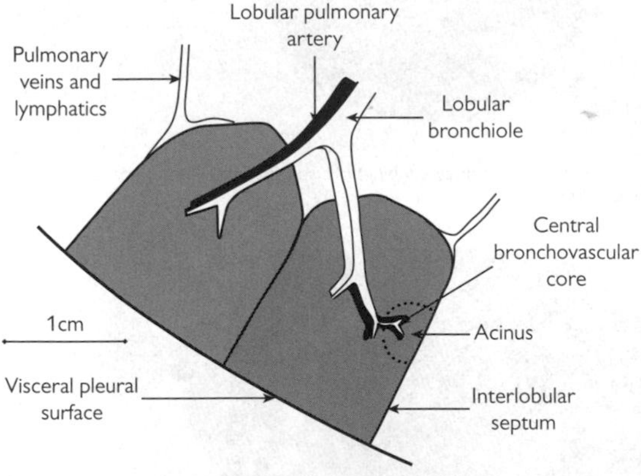

Fig. A4.4 Structure of two 2° pulmonary lobules abutting the pleural surface. The 2° pulmonary lobule is the smallest anatomical area visible on CT. Tree-in-bud appearance will be in the acinus around the central bronchovascular core. Reticular patterns will be centred on the interlobular septae and/or draining lymphatics. Mosaic patterns and air trapping will tend to follow outlines of the lobule or sets of lobules.

Cystic airspaces

Process	Causes
Clearly defined air-containing space with definable wall	LAM, LCH, end-stage UIP, PCP, LIP, septic emboli

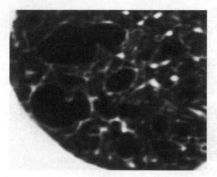

Fig. A4.5 Langerhans cell histiocytosis (LCH). Walls are thin, but more pronounced, irregular, and widely spread than emphysematous holes.

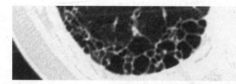

Fig. A4.6 Peripheral cysts (honeycombing) of usual interstitial pneumonitis (UIP). Characteristic subpleural distribution.

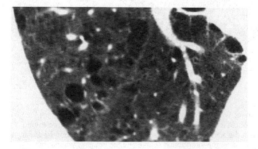

Fig. A4.7 Holes in the lungs due to emphysema. No real 'walls'.

Fissural, bronchovascular, and subpleural nodularity

Process	Causes
Nodules seen along the pulmonary fissures, along the bronchovascular bundles, and subpleurally	Sarcoidosis. Also described in Kaposi's sarcoma

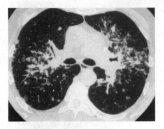

Fig. A4.8 Sarcoidosis, perihilar, and bronchovascular distribution of nodularity.

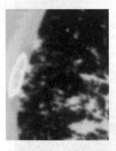

Fig. A4.9 Sarcoidosis, subpleural nodules.

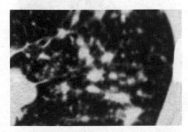

Fig. A4.10 Irregular/nodular thickening of fissures and bronchovascular bundles.

Ground-glass shadowing

Process	Causes
Grey appearance to lung interstitium; air in bronchus looks blacker	Parenchymal inflammatory conditions such as sarcoidosis, alveolitis, early UIP and other IIPs, HP, pulmonary oedema or haemorrhage, PCP, alveolar proteinosis, drug/radiation injury

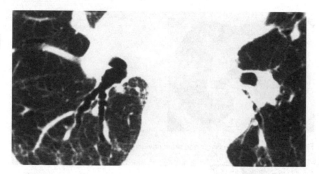

Fig. A4.11 Subtle ground-glass shadowing in early UIP. Airways appear blacker, but lung is diffusely more dense. Early reticular pattern at right base also.

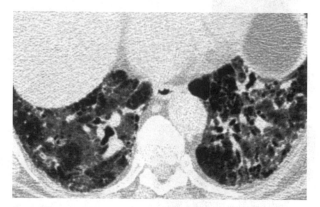

Fig. A4.12 More marked ground-glass shadowing in UIP. Very early honeycombing and traction bronchial dilatation (bronchiectasis) as well.

Honeycomb lung

Process	Causes
End-stage fibrotic lung	UIP, asbestosis

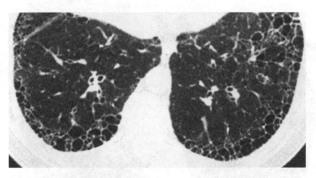

Fig. A4.13 Honeycombing in UIP. Usually mainly peripheral.

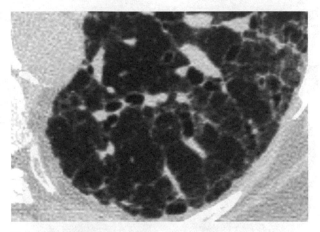

Fig. A4.14 More subtle honeycombing at the lung periphery with other features of UIP. Traction bronchial dilatation due to surrounding lung fibrosis and a reticular pattern beginning to outline the 2° pulmonary lobule.

Mosaic attenuation pattern

Process	Causes
Well-defined areas of normal lung abutting abnormal lung, giving a mosaic pattern. Seen particularly in expiration	Indicates small airways disease, such as asthma, vascular disease, such as PE, or infiltrative disease such as obliterative bronchiolitis, HP

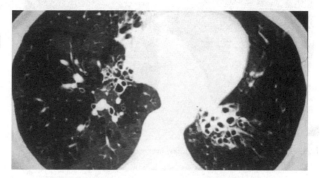

Fig. A4.15 Bronchiectasis with small airways disease that is causing the mosaic pattern. In addition, there are markedly bronchiectatic airways in the left lower lobe, with considerable airway crowding due to distal lung collapse.

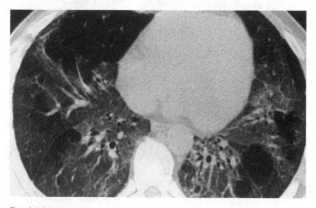

Fig. A4.16 Non-specific interstitial pneumonitis (NSIP), showing patchy and mosaic-like pattern of increased attenuation.

Nodularity

Process	Causes
Small discrete dots 1–10mm, may be in airspaces or interstitium	Metastases, sarcoidosis, pneumoconiosis, HP, miliary TB, fungal infection, idiopathic pulmonary haemorrhage, alveolar microlithiasis, varicella pneumonitis

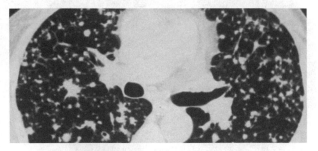

Fig. A4.17 Multiple dense nodules of varying size due to metastases.

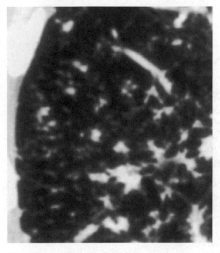

Fig. A4.18 Sarcoid. Multiple small nodules throughout lung but usually associated with other features of sarcoid such as fissural nodularity and bilateral hilar node enlargement.

Poorly defined centrilobular nodules

Process	Causes
Peribronchiolar inflammation in the absence of intraluminal secretion	HP, RB-ILD

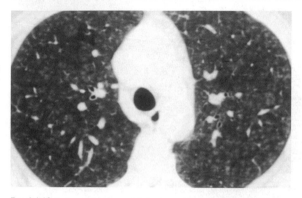

Fig. A4.19 Soft centrilobular nodularity due to HP (also called extrinsic allergic alveolitis, EAA).

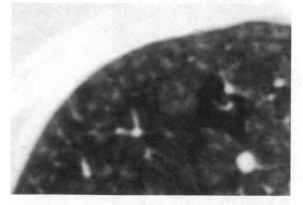

Fig. A4.20 Another example of HP, enlarged to show position of soft nodules in the centre of the 2° pulmonary lobules.

Reticular (or linear) pattern

Process	Causes
Linear fine lines, indicating thickened interlobular septa. Subpleural reticulation	ILD (e.g. UIP, asbestosis), pulmonary oedema, drug-induced fibrosis, pulmonary haemorrhage, lymphangitis

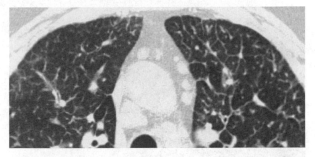

Fig. A4.21 Lymphangitis carcinomatosis. Infiltrated lymphatics widen and thicken the interlobular septa.

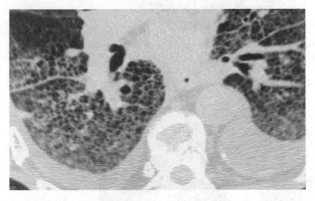

Fig. A4.22 Pulmonary oedema due to left heart failure. Fluid-distended lymphatics outlining the 2° pulmonary lobules. Worse in dependent areas. Fluid in the fissures, bilateral pleural effusions, and some airspace filling with pulmonary oedema.

Tree in bud

Process	Causes
Mucus/pus/secretions filling bronchioles and causing dilatation	Small airways disease, particularly infection, including mycobacteria, *Haemophilus influenzae*, diffuse pan-bronchiolitis, CF, yellow nail syndrome, 1° pulmonary lymphoma

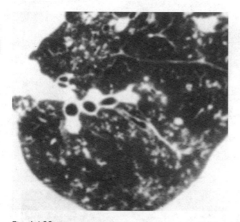

Fig. A4.23 Extensive tree-in-bud appearance in the left lower lobe from opportunistic mycobacterial disease.

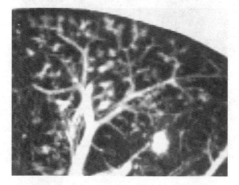

Fig. A4.24 Tree-in-bud appearance, enhanced by a post-processing technique called 'maximum intensity projection'. Effectively, this squashes denser structures from several thin cuts into one, allowing branching structures to be viewed in their entirety.

Drugs used for bronchoscopy and sedation

Table A5.1 Commonly used drugs for sedation and bronchoscopy (continued on ↪ p. 863). Adapted from *BTS guideline for diagnostic flexible bronchoscopy in adults, Thorax* (2013);68:i1–i44, with permission from BMJ.

Drug	Dose	Pharmacology	Side effects
Midazolam	Slow IV injection—maximum rate 2mg/min Initial dose: 2–2.5mg (0.5–1mg in the frail or elderly), given 5–10min before procedure Supplemental doses, if required: 1mg (0.5–1mg in frail or elderly), at 2–10min intervals Usual maximum total dose: 3.5–7mg (3.5mg in frail or elderly) for standard bronchoscopic procedures. May be higher in longer procedures	Onset within 2min, with maximum effect at 5–10min (may be longer in frail or elderly or those with chronic illnesses) Duration of action variable, but typical range is 30–120min Approximate half-life 1.5–2.5h	Respiratory depression, apnoea, bronchospasm, laryngospasm, hypotension, heart rate alterations, cardiac arrest Life-threatening side effects and prolonged sedation are more likely in the elderly and those with impaired respiratory or cardiovascular status, hepatic impairment, renal impairment, myasthenia gravis, and with rapid IV injection
Fentanyl	Slow IV injection—usually over 1–3min Initial dose: 25 micrograms Supplemental doses, if required: 25 micrograms Usual maximum total dose: 50 micrograms	Onset almost immediate, with maximum effect at 5min Duration of action variable, but typical range is 30–60min Approximate half-life 2–7h	Nausea, vomiting, and other GI upset, myoclonic movements, respiratory depression, apnoea, bronchospasm, laryngospasm, hypo/hypertension, arrhythmia, cardiac arrest Caution in elderly patients and those with impaired respiratory or cardiovascular status, hepatic impairment, and myasthenia gravis

Alfentanil	Slow IV injection—usually over 30s Initial dose: 250 micrograms Supplemental doses, if required: 250 micrograms Usual maximum total dose: 500 micrograms	Onset almost immediate onset and maximum effect Duration of action variable, but usually shorter than fentanyl Approximate half-life 1–2h	See Fentanyl
Lidocaine (during bronchoscopy)	*Intranasal* Lidocaine 2% gel: 6mL (120mg) *Oropharynx* Lidocaine 10% spray: three actuations (30mg) *Vocal cords, tracheobronchial tree* Lidocaine 1% solution: 2mL boluses applied topically, as required Use minimum dose to achieve effective cough suppression and patient comfort. Subjective symptoms of lidocaine toxicity are common when ≥9.6mg/kg is used; much lower doses are usually sufficient	Onset 3–5min. Common mistake not to wait long enough for maximal effect, leading to unnecessary extra doses Duration of action variable, but typical range is 60–90min Approximate half-life 1.5–2h	CNS effects (confusion, blurred vision, dizziness, drowsiness, light-headedness, myoclonus, nausea, nystagmus, paraesthesiae, restlessness, tremulousness, coma, convulsions, respiratory failure) CVS effects (hypotension, bradycardia, arrhythmia, cardiac arrest) Methaemoglobinaemia (rare) Caution in those with hepatic and cardiac dysfunction, and with significant renal impairment
Adrenaline (during bronchoscopy)	Topical Adrenaline 1:10,000: 2–10mL		Hypertension, tachycardia, arrhythmia, tremor

Table A5.2 Antagonists available for sedative drugs (adapted from BTS guideline for diagnostic flexible bronchoscopy in adults with permission)

Drug	Dose	Pharmacology	Side effects
Flumazenil	To reverse midazolam Initial dose: 200 micrograms IV over 15s Supplemental doses: 100 micrograms every 60s if inadequate response Typical cumulative dose range: 300–600 micrograms Maximum total dose: 1mg Note—when combined midazolam-opioid sedation used and reversal required, use flumazenil first (unless large dose of opioid given)	Onset 1min Duration of action 1–4h Approximate half-life 40–80min Duration of action may be shorter than midazolam → care to ensure sedation does not recur	Nausea, vomiting, anxiety, agitation, dizziness, hypertension, tachycardia May lower seizure threshold May cause withdrawal in chronic benzodiazepine users
Naloxone	To reverse opioids Initial dose: 100–200 micrograms IV Supplemental dose: 100 micrograms every 2min, if inadequate response	Onset 2–3min Duration of action 45min to 4h Approximate half-life 1–1.5h Duration of action may be shorter than opioid → care to ensure sedation does not recur	Nausea, vomiting, dizziness, headache, tachycardia, hypo/hypertension May cause withdrawal in chronic opioid users

Table A5.3 Doses and concentrations of lidocaine used for bronchoscopy (adapted from BTS guideline for diagnostic flexible bronchoscopy in adults with permission)

Drug	Dose per unit volume	Site of application	Comments
Lidocaine 2% gel	20mg/mL	Nasal	Gel preparation syringe typically contains 6mL (120mg)
Lidocaine 10% aerosol spray	10mg/actuation	Oropharynx	Three actuations (30mg) often sufficient
Lidocaine 10% aerosol spray	10mg/mL	Vocal cords, trachea, and bronchial tree	

Further information

Du Rand IA *et al*. British Thoracic Society guideline for diagnostic flexible bronchoscopy in adults. *Thorax* 2013;**68**:i1–i44.

Lung function and cardiopulmonary exercise testing

Flow–volume loop 1

A good start to understanding lung function tests is the flow–volume loop (see Fig. A6.1). This plots inspiratory and expiratory flow against lung volume during a maximal expiratory and maximal inspiratory manoeuvre.

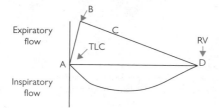

Expiratory
flow

Inspiratory
flow

Fig. A6.1 Flow–volume loop.

At the beginning of *expiration* from a full breath in, the expiratory muscles are at their strongest, the lungs at their largest, and hence the airways are at their most open (*A*). Because the lungs are at their largest, the radial attachments to the airways, effectively the alveolar/capillary membranes and their connective tissue, are pulling the hardest and supporting the airways against *dynamic compression* during the exhalation manoeuvre.

This means that the highest flow rates are possible at the beginning of the blow, hence the sudden rise to a *PEFR* in the first 100ms or so of the forced breath out (*B*). This is the *peak flow* and is essentially what a peak flow meter measures (see Fig A6.5).

As the lung empties and the lung volume drops, the dilatory pull on the airways from the radial attachments of the surrounding lung tissue reduces (*C*). Hence, the airways narrow and become less supported and are less able to resist dynamic compression. This means that the maximal airflow obtainable, regardless of effort, falls too.

Eventually, the expiratory muscles come to the end of their 'travel' and cannot squeeze the chest anymore. Also, increasingly with age, the small airways may actually close off, preventing any more emptying (*D*). The volume at which this begins to happen is called the *closing volume*.

As maximal *inspiration* starts, although the inspiratory muscles are at their strongest, the airways are at their smallest. Thus, flow rates start low and increase as the airways open up. However, as the lung expands, the inspiratory muscles are approaching the end of their 'travel' and are weakening; this means the flow rates fall again, hence the different rounded appearance of the inspiratory limb of the flow–volume curve.

Thus, normally, the inspiratory and expiratory flow rates depend on lung volume and are termed 'volume-dependent'. If there is a *fixed upper airway narrowing*, such as from a solid hard tumour partially blocking the trachea, then the size of the airway at this point may become so narrow that it now limits maximal flows. However, its diameter will *vary very little* with lung volumes, and hence flow will become 'volume-independent'. Fig. A6.2 shows this.

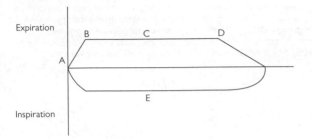

Fig. A6.2 Volume-independent flow.

At (A), the rise in flow will initially be normal, but, at some point, the maximum flow imposed by the upper airway narrowing will cut in (B). From that point onwards, the flow rate will be fixed at this maximum (C) until, at much lower lung volumes, the lower recoil and narrowing of the small airways again determine the maximum flow (D). The flow–volume curve has been severely 'clipped', with a square-ish appearance. The same clipped appearance will be present on the inspiratory limb (E), giving rise to the so-called 'square box' appearance.

Sometimes, such upper airways restriction may be *variable*, rather than *fixed*, and only obstruct during inspiration (e.g. paralysed and collapsing vocal cords), due to the obstructing elements being sucked in and then blown open again on expiration.

- Thus, a square inspiratory limb, but normal expiratory limb, provides evidence of a mobile **extrathoracic** *upper airways obstruction.*

Conversely, a mobile intrathoracic upper airway obstruction (e.g. soft fleshy tumour at the carina or retrosternal thyroid) may obstruct more during expiration (when the expiratory effort is compressing the lung), compared with inspiration when the chest is being expanded.

- Thus, a square expiratory limb, but normal inspiratory limb, is evidence of a *variable* **intrathoracic** *upper airways obstruction.*

Sometimes, ratios of maximal inspiratory to maximal expiratory flows are used to characterize the intra- or extrathoracic airway obstruction.

Flow–volume loop 2

The other, more common, causes of airway obstruction are due to narrowing of the lower airways (asthma, COPD). In these conditions, the airway calibre (and thus flow rates) still remains dependent on lung volume. Hence, the flow rates decrease, as the lung volume decreases, but particularly decrease at low lung volumes. This is because resistance to flow is proportional to the airway radius raised to the power of 4 (r^4) and therefore most significant when airways are already small. Hence, increasing airflow obstruction produces expiratory flow–volume curves like those in Fig. A6.3. This greater effect of small airways narrowing at low lung volumes has led some to report flow rates at, for example, 25% expired lung volume or averaged between 25% and 75% of the total expired lung volume.

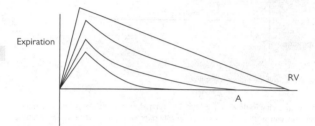

Fig. A6.3 Expiratory flow–volume curves—lower airways obstruction.

Airways can be so small that, during expiration, they begin closing off earlier than normal (the *closing volume*); hence, a full breath out is not possible, producing air trapping and a raised RV (A). Sensitive tests of small airways narrowing have to concentrate on flows at low lung volumes, and peak flow measurements are relatively insensitive.

- Note, however, that peak flow measurements are the most sensitive to *upper airway narrowing* and a good way to follow changes in upper airway narrowing during, for example, radiotherapy for a central airway obstructing lung cancer.

Spirometry, peak flow measurements, and CO transfer

- The ordinary spirometer (mechanical or electronic) records *volume against time*, rather than *flow against volume*
- The two essential measures are *FEV1* and *VC*.

The VC is the maximum amount of air that can be blown out completely. This will be *reduced* if the lungs are *stiff* (preventing a full breath in), the *inspiratory muscles are weak* (preventing a full breath in), or the *airways are narrowed* such that the small airways collapse during expiration (preventing a full breath out).

The FEV_1 is the amount (forced expiratory volume) that can be blown out in 1s. Because the value is taken over a second, a much longer period of flow is being captured during the breath out than the PEFR, but, despite this, the measurement is still being made when the airways are larger. It is less dependent on effort and generally more robust. The ratio of the two figures (FEV_1/VC) tells us about the degree of airflow obstruction.

- A ratio of FEV_1/VC of less than about 70–75% indicates airflow *obstruction*.

This ratio is very useful because it is hardly affected by age, sex, height, ethnic origin, etc.—it is self-normalizing. The individual measures of FEV_1 and VC *do* need corrections for the above factors and are usually quoted as % predicted. The range of normality is considerable, and it may not be clear if results are simply at the bottom end of normal or considerably reduced from the patient's normally much higher figures. Serial measurements indicating continuing deterioration may be the first clue. Only if the FEV_1/VC ratio is *normal*, can the VC be confidently used to infer whether there is a reduced total lung volume such as from ILD. A low VC with normal FEV_1/VC ratio is called a *restrictive* pattern. A *low* FEV_1/VC ratio is called an *obstructive* pattern, and a reduced VC *cannot* then be confidently used to infer that the total lung volume is also reduced and indeed may even be increased because of air trapping. A small print fact is that the FEV_1/VC ratio may actually be raised in ILD, as the airways are better supported by the fibrosed radial attachments, which reduces dynamic compression, thus increasing expiratory flow, compared to that expected for the lung volume.

The *slope* of the volume–time plot from a spirometer is effectively the *flow* at any particular point; because flow is dropping during expiration, the slope progressively flattens off. However, if there is any fixed upper airways obstruction (as previously discussed), the expiratory flow rate will be constant for a while, and hence the spirometer line will be straighter than usual. An interesting index to detect possible upper airway obstruction the *Empey index* has been described:

Empey Index $\approx$ [FEV_1 (mL) / PEFR (L/min)]

Because PEFR is clipped first by the presence of upper airflow obstruction, relative to the FEV_1, the above index gets larger with such a problem. A figure over 10 is suggestive of upper airflow obstruction, but it is only a pointer, and there will be false positives and negatives.

Although one-off measures of lung function can be made, more interesting information comes from serial measurements, e.g. in asthma, PEFR will fluctuate with characteristic morning 'dips'.

Spirometry—how to do it

Everyone has their own way to do spirometry (see Table A6.1), but this is a way that works for the authors. Say to the patient, 'This is a test of how big your lungs are and how fast you can empty them. What I would like you to do is take an enormous breath in, the biggest you can manage, then seal your lips around the tube, and blow as hard and as fast and as long as you possibly can'. Then demonstrate the manoeuvre yourself with a spare tube (not necessarily connected to the spirometer) so that they can then mimic it. Whilst they are blowing, say 'excellent, well done, keep blowing, come on, come on, come on, keep blowing'. There are various recommendations as to numbers of blow, etc. these are the arguments.

Table A6.1 Spirometer tips

Standing or sitting?	High intrathoracic pressure generated may cause the patient to pass out. Therefore, sitting down is safer, but better and more consistent figures are obtained standing. Have a chair behind patient to sit on, if dizzy.
Nose clip?	Prevents escape through the nose which would give falsely low figures but is uncomfortable. Vast majority of patients do not need it, but, if the line appears to fall off towards the end of the blow or inconsistent volumes, try a nose clip.
Best of three blows?	Needed to demonstrate that maximal blow has been consistently achieved, usually by seeing two identical tracings. A device showing the actual spirometer tracing is extremely helpful. If two tracings are identical, this is probably enough but may need more if blowing is erratic, until satisfied it is maximal.
Keep going to end of page (6s) or not?	Needed to establish correct VC. Therefore, if line still rising, then VC not reached, but have to stop somewhere. In restrictive disease or normals, usually maximal by 3s; in obstructive disease, may need to do a slow VC to establish 'real' value, which can be much larger than the forced VC (FVC) due to dynamic compression.
Repeat with a submaximal effort?	Similar to above, it is sometimes useful to ask patient to repeat the expiratory manoeuvre with slightly less effort, when emphysema suspected. This will often give better expiratory volume in 1s and the VC, which would suggest major dynamic airways compression.

CO transfer

Usually done in the lung function laboratory, and it essentially measures the amount of *gas-exchanging surface area* available. A gas mixture containing CO is inhaled, the breath held for 10s, and then exhaled. The amount of CO that has disappeared (by crossing the alveolar capillary membrane and being taken up by red cells) is calculated. A correction for the Hb concentration is required, as the amount of CO transferred will fall as the available Hb is reduced. The *total amount of CO transferred is the TLCO* (total lung, TL). When divided by the total lung volume during the breath-hold, it is called the *kCO, gas transfer per unit lung volume*. The total lung volume 'reached' by the CO is the amount breathed in *plus* the amount of air already in the lung at the start of the breath in. This is measured by including helium in the inhaled gas mixture that is diluted by the air already in the lung; by comparing inspired helium concentration with expired, this total lung volume can be calculated.

- The TLCO and kCO are *reduced* most in emphysema when alveoli have been destroyed
- The TLCO and kCO are *reduced* in ILD where the alveolar capillary membrane may be thick enough to reduce CO passage
- The kCO may also be *raised* (and TLCO normal) when lungs are poorly expanded by, say, weak respiratory muscles, because the lung is 'more concentrated' and transfers CO *better* when quoted per unit volume
- The kCO may also be *raised* for a few days when there has been profuse lung haemorrhage, as can occur in, e.g. SLE, Wegener's, and Goodpasture's. This is because the free red cells lining the alveoli take up CO directly and 'falsely' elevate the figure. As the Hb is broken down, the kCO returns to normal, unless there is another bleed. This helps to distinguish re-bleeding from other causes of lung infiltrates such as infection.

This test requires more cooperation than simple spirometry, as well as a minimum inspired volume, and therefore cannot always be obtained.

Respiratory muscle function, body plethysmography, and lung volumes

Respiratory muscle function

Respiratory failure and small VCs may be due to weak respiratory muscles. It is therefore useful to be able to assess inspiratory and expiratory muscle power. There may be global weakness or specific inspiratory weakness, usually due to diaphragm paralysis. In the clinic, the simplest test is a *lying and standing VC*. If the diaphragm is paralysed, then, on lying down, the abdominal contents will push up the diaphragm and limit inspiration. On standing, the abdominal contents drop and aid inspiration.

- A fall in VC of <10% on lying down is probably normal
- A fall of 10–20% is suspicious of diaphragm paralysis
- A fall of >20% is abnormal and suggests significant, usually bilateral, diaphragm paralysis.

In the laboratory, there are various ways to test respiratory muscle function. The patient can blow against a *pressure meter* after a maximum inspiration and inspire against the meter after a full expiration. This is, of course, highly effort-dependent. A manoeuvre, such as a *sniff*, is very stereotypic, and patients can reproduce this. Measuring the inspiratory pressure produced at the nose during this manoeuvre is a rough and ready way of screening for inspiratory muscle weakness. More accurate assessments of inspiratory muscle function, particularly the diaphragm, can be obtained using two semi-inflated balloons, introduced via the mouth and oesophagus, placed above and below the diaphragm, and connected to pressure transducers. The *transdiaphragmatic pressures* during maximal inspiratory efforts, sniffing, and breathing to TLC all provide reproducible measures of diaphragm function but depend on good cooperation and effort by the patient. Activating the phrenic nerve directly with a superficial electrical stimulator, or by using high-intensity magnetic stimulation over the nerve roots of C3–C5, whilst measuring transdiaphragmatic pressures, provides a non-effort-dependent way to test diaphragm function.

Body plethysmography requires the patient to climb into an airtight cabinet and breathe through a shuttered mouthpiece connected to the outside world. It has two particular advantages over simpler lung function tests. It is able to measure the total lung volume or capacity (TLC) in the thorax, and it provides a measure of airways obstruction, involving little or no effort by the patient.

The other main method of measuring TLC involves helium dilution, as described during the TLCO measurement above. However, in the presence of lower airways obstruction, the helium may not 'reach' all parts of the lung during the 10s breath-hold, and the volume calculated from this dilution will therefore be lower than the real TLC. The body plethysmograph relies on the pressure changes that occur when all the air in the chest is alternately compressed and expanded by the patient making breathing efforts against an airway closed by a shutter at the mouth. The pressure changes produced in the oral cavity vs those in the box are then proportional to the volume of air being compressed and rarefied, thus allowing calculation of the volume in the chest at the time. Note that this volume will include any bullae or pneumothorax, and the difference between the plethysmographic lung volume and the helium dilution volume will reflect the bullae/pneumothorax volumes, as well as areas not reached by the helium due to increased airways resistance.

Measurement of *airways resistance* with the body box relies on a similar principle. If there were no airways resistance, then breathing in and out would not compress or rarefy the air in the chest. With increasing resistance, the air in the chest will be compressed during expiration and rarefied on inspiration. It is this phenomenon that allows calculation of the airways resistance during quiet breathing or panting (the latter ensures the vocal cords are fully open and not contributing to the measured resistance). See Fig. A6.4 and Table A6.2.

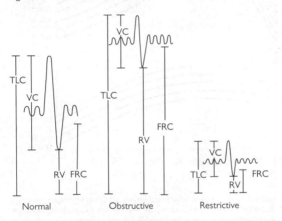

Fig. A6.4 Lung volumes in normal, obstructive, and restrictive lung conditions. TLC, total lung capacity (not always increased when obstructive pattern); VC, vital capacity; RV, residual volume; FRC, functional residual capacity; FEV$_1$, forced expiratory volume in 1s.

Table A6.2 Lung volume patterns

Derivative	Obstructive	Restrictive
FEV$_1$ (% predicted)	↓↓	↓
VC (% predicted)	↓ or →	↓
FEV$_1$/VC ratio	↓	→ or ↑ (increased recoil)
TLC (% predicted)	↑ or →	↓
RV (% predicted)	↑	↓
FRC (% predicted)	↑	↓
RV/TLC ratio	↑ (gas trapping)	→ or ↓

Further information

Gibson GJ. *Clinical tests of respiratory function*, 3rd edn. Hodder Arnold, 2008.

Peak flow reference ranges

See Fig. A6.5.

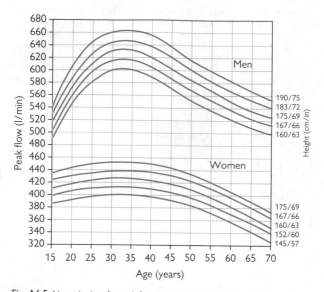

Fig. A6.5 Normal values for peak flow, based on original Gregg and Nunn values (*BMJ* 1973) but corrected for new EU scale peak flow meters. Normal range extends about ± 15% or roughly 100L/min in men and 50L/min in women.

Note: old Wright peak flow meters over-read in the middle of the scale (e.g. reading about 400 when actual value was 350L/min) and were replaced from October 2004 by a corrected scale.

Cardiopulmonary exercise testing (CPET)

General points

- An exercise test, with additional measurement of ventilatory gases
- Useful for assessing:
  - Cardiorespiratory fitness
  - Relative contribution of cardiovascular (CV) and respiratory (RS) disease to exercise limitation
  - Disease severity assessment and prognostication
  - Risk stratification pre-lung resection, lung and cardiac transplantation, cardiac medical device therapy, other surgical evaluations
  - Response to an intervention.

Undertaking CPET

- Baseline spirometry and maximum voluntary ventilation (MVV)
- Measurements include serial ECGs, SaO_2, BP, HR, expired concentrations of O_2 and CO_2, tidal volume, and breathing frequency (via face mask or mouthpiece with nose clips)
- Calculation of V_E (minute ventilation), VO_2 (O_2 consumption), VCO_2 (CO_2 production) at rest and throughout exercise
- Ventilatory threshold represents a point where several ventilatory parameters show a threshold-like behaviour, related to the onset of anaerobic respiration and lactic acidosis. Many ways of estimating; look for the inflection point on plots of VCO_2 vs VO_2 or V_E vs VCO_2
- ABGs (via an arterial line) are occasionally taken
- Usually performed on a cycle ergometer (alternatively, a treadmill)
- Cycle is initially unloaded, and then work is ramped (based on usual activity level; pre-test FEV_1 and MVV results can also be helpful)
- Doctor and physiologist monitor patient during test and ensure mask/ mouthpiece closely fitting. Patient encouragement during testing enhances performance and can make results more meaningful
- Test usually stopped due to exhaustion (e.g. tired legs or too dyspnoeic). Stop immediately with significant arrhythmias, ST depression ≥2mm, heart block, significantly falling BP, ischaemic-sounding chest pain, severe symptomatic hypoxaemia, or near syncope
- Unloaded pedalling at end of test.

Interpreting variables

- See Table A6.3.

Patterns in unexplained exertional dyspnoea

- Decreased VO_2 peak/max—defines degree of impairment, independent of mechanism
- V_E/VCO_2 slope increase and $P_{ET}CO_2$ decrease—consider causes of exercise-related PHT
- SaO_2 fall—suggests V/Q mismatching
- FEV_1 or PEF decreases, V_E/MVV increases—suggests respiratory cause
- Lack of ventilatory threshold—suggests cause related to ventilation.

Further information

Guazzi M et al. Clinical recommendations for cardiopulmonary exercise testing data assessment in specific patient populations. *Eur Heart J* 2012;**33**:2917–27.

Table A6.3 Interpreting CPET variables

Variable	Interpretation	Normal values
Peak VO_2 (mL/kg/min) (or VO_2 max)	Maximum O_2 utilization Global prognostic marker/severity assessment. Influenced by CV, RS, and muscular function	Influenced by age and sex (15–80mL/kg/min) Reported as % predicted
VO_2 at ventilatory threshold (VT) (mL/kg/min)	Associated with anaerobic threshold. Limit of workload sustainable for prolonged periods	± 50–65% peak VO_2 Influenced by training and genetic predisposition
Peak respiratory exchange ratio (RER)	RER = VCO_2/VO_2 ratio ↑work → ↑VO_2 but ↑↑VCO_2 → ↑RER Marker of effort during exercise	Good effort suggested by RER ≥1.1
V_E/VCO_2 slope (V_E on y-axis; VCO_2 on x-axis)	Determined by V/Q matching Marker of disease severity	<30 normal. Particularly high in PHT
V_E/VO_2 at peak exercise	Ventilatory cost of O_2 uptake at peak exercise	≤40 normal
End-tidal CO_2 partial pressure $P_{ET}CO_2$	Determined by V/Q matching and cardiac function Marker of disease severity	Rest: 4.8–5.6kPa At VT: ↑ 0.4–1.1kPa Above VT: ↓ due to increased ventilatory response to metabolic acidosis
V_E/MVV V_E measured at peak exercise, MVV at rest	Helps determine if dyspnoea is related to a pulmonary cause	≤0.8 normal >0.8 suggests pulmonary limitation
O_2 pulse (mL O_2/beat)	O_2 pulse = VO_2/HR Surrogate for stroke volume response to exercise Helpful for assessing possible myocardial ischaemia	Normally rises during exercise, reduced rise in chronic heart failure
Change in VO_2/change in workload ($\Delta VO_2/\Delta W$)	Helpful for assessing possible myocardial ischaemia	Normally linear rise of VO_2 with work Average 10mL/min/W
FEV_1 and PEF (L/min)	Compare pre- and post-exercise Changes suggest respiratory cause of dyspnoea (not asthma-specific)	<15% reduction with exercise
Heart rate recovery (HRR)	Compares max HR with HR after 1min recovery. Related to parasympathetic activation	Normally HRR >12 beats lower at 1min. If <12, suggests cardiac cause
Exercise BP	CV response to exercise	Usual to have modest increase in SBP with exercise. DBP usually static or decreases due to vasodilatation
SaO_2	Useful for assessing for respiratory causes of exertional dyspnoea	Should not fall >5%. Greater fall in RS disease and PHT

Plain radiograph and lobar collapses

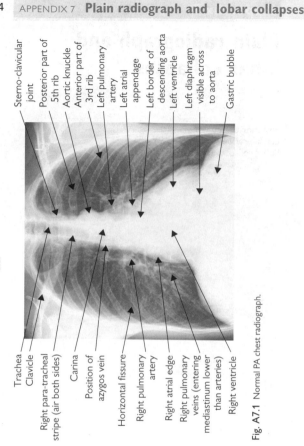

Sterno-clavicular joint
Posterior part of 5th rib
Aortic knuckle
Anterior part of 3rd rib
Left pulmonary artery
Left atrial appendage
Left border of descending aorta
Left ventricle
Left diaphragm visible across to aorta
Gastric bubble

Trachea
Clavicle
Right para-tracheal stripe (air both sides)
Carina
Position of azygos vein
Horizontal fissure
Right pulmonary artery
Right atrial edge
Right pulmonary veins (entering mediastinum lower than arteries)
Right ventricle

Fig. A7.1 Normal PA chest radiograph.

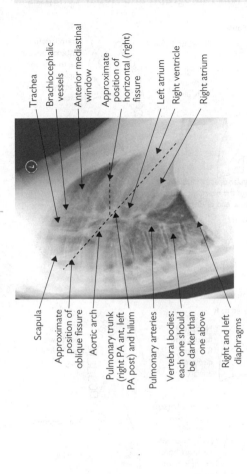

Trachea

Brachiocephalic vessels

Anterior mediastinal window

Approximate position of horizontal (right) fissure

Left atrium

Right ventricle

Right atrium

Scapula

Approximate position of oblique fissure

Aortic arch

Pulmonary trunk (right PA ant, left PA post) and hilum

Pulmonary arteries

Vertebral bodies: each one should be darker than one above

Right and left diaphragms

Fig. A7.2 Normal left lateral chest radiograph.

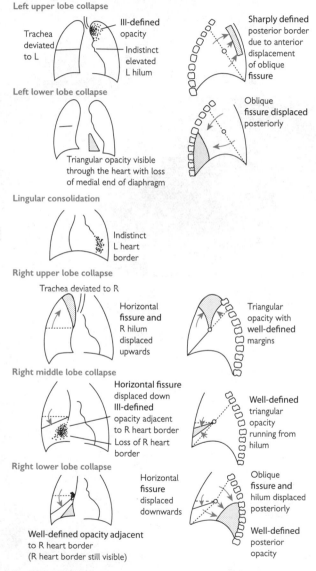

Left upper lobe collapse

Trachea deviated to L — Ill-defined opacity — Indistinct elevated L hilum

Sharply defined posterior border due to anterior displacement of oblique fissure

Left lower lobe collapse

Triangular opacity visible through the heart with loss of medial end of diaphragm

Oblique fissure displaced posteriorly

Lingular consolidation

Indistinct L heart border

Right upper lobe collapse

Trachea deviated to R — Horizontal fissure and R hilum displaced upwards

Triangular opacity with well-defined margins

Right middle lobe collapse

Horizontal fissure displaced down Ill-defined opacity adjacent to R heart border Loss of R heart border

Well-defined triangular opacity running from hilum

Right lower lobe collapse

Horizontal fissure displaced downwards

Well-defined opacity adjacent to R heart border (R heart border still visible)

Oblique fissure and hilum displaced posteriorly

Well-defined posterior opacity

Fig. A7.3 Lobar collapse.

Radiological investigations and radiation exposure

Table A8.1 Common radiological investigations used in respiratory practice (continued on ➡ p. 889)

Investigation	Plain CXR (AMBER), one view	Staging chest and abdo CT	HRCT	CTPA	Low-dose CT	V/Q scan 99mTcMAA and 133Xe	PET scan	MRI	Head CT
Indication	Best technique for plain chest radiography	For example, for staging lung cancer, usually with IV contrast to identify vascularity of structures	For diffuse lung disease, giving good resolution at level of s pulmonary lobule	For PE and visualization of pulmonary vasculature	Used in lung cancer screening	For identifying perfusion defects without accompanying ventilation defects, as in PE	For detection of malignant deposits and increasingly for areas of inflammation	Better detection of malignant tissue invasion	For example, for brain metastases
Technique	Multiple beam equalization improves contrast by varying beam intensity, depending on tissue density	Commonly, 5mm slices at 5mm intervals, with thinner slices reconstructed from same data. Whole lung scanned. 200–400mA beam intensity	1.25mm at 10mm intervals, i.e. only about 10% of the lung scanned	72mm slices at 2mm intervals	0.6mm slices at 0.6mm intervals, i.e. whole lung scanned at approx ¼ standard beam intensity (50mA)	IV radiolabelled albumin macro-aggregates that lodge in the pulmonary arterioles to image vasculature, and inhaled xenon gas to image ventilated areas	Radiolabelled glucose (18 F-FDG) – uptake proportional to metabolic activity		5 or 10mm slices at 5 or 10mm intervals, i.e. whole brain scanned

Radiation dose mSv or mGy (x100 for mrad)	0.04	Variable, 74-8 (higher in USA where 400mA more common). Larger doses of contrast medium scatter more radiation into nearby tissues	4 / Probable higher effective dose due to contrast medium scattering of radiation	Variable, 71	1.5-2	7		0	2
Radiation dose (time equivalent to background radiation in the UK)	5 days	2y	4 months	1.3y	4 months	7 months	2.3y	0	8 months
Radiation dose (equivalent to numbers of CXRs)	1	150	25	100	23	44	175	0	50
Limitations	Poorer resolution, so s pulmonary lobule cancers may be not visualized	8.5mm gaps, so s early cancers may be missed	Same as ordinary CT	Lower beam intensity produces lower resolution	No structural information or the ability to make alternative diagnoses	Usually combined with resolution CT, so add on up to another 6mSv			Lower resolution

Different departments/countries will use different protocols, e.g. some will always do a standard CT as well as an HRCT in case a malignant nodule is missed.

Radiation dose estimates are fraught with many assumptions, and there is significant uncertainty in some areas.

1mSy is the dose of absorbed radiation produced by exposure to 1mGy of radiation.

1mSy = 100mrad absorbed dose (mSy includes quality factor (type of radiation and nature of tissue), but, for X-rays and most tissues, mSy and mGy are numerically identical (for alpha emitters, 1mGy causes 20mSy)).

Background radiation ~3mSy/y (mainly from radiation in the home and varies across the country); transatlantic flight = extra 0.03mSy.

Useful websites

Thoracic societies

American College of Chest Physicians ℘ http://www.chestnet.org
American Thoracic Society ℘ http://www.thoracic.org
British Society for Allergy and Clinical Immunology ℘ http://www.bsaci.org
British Thoracic Society ℘ http://www.brit-thoracic.org.uk
Canadian Thoracic Society ℘ http://www.lung.ca
European Respiratory Society ℘ http://www.ersnet.org
Society of Thoracic Surgeons ℘ http://www.sts.org
Thoracic Society of Australia and New Zealand ℘ http://www.thoracic.org.au

Thoracic journals

American Journal of Respiratory and Critical Care Medicine ('Blue journal') ℘ http://www.atsjournals.org
Chest ℘ http://www.chestjournal.org
European Respiratory Journal access via ℘ http://www.ersnet.org
Thorax ℘ http://thorax.bmj.com

General journals

British Medical Journal ℘ http://www.bmj.com
Free medical journals site ℘ http://www.freemedicaljournals.com
Journal of the American Medical Association ℘ http://jama.ama-assn.org
The Lancet ℘ http://www.thelancet.com
National Library of Medicine (Pub Med) ℘ http://www.ncbi.nlm.nih.gov/pubmed
New England Journal of Medicine ℘ http://www.nejm.org/

Teaching resources

Drugs that cause respiratory disease ℘ http://www.pneumotox.com
Evidence-based medicine site ℘ http://www.bestbets.org
Supercourse lectures on public health ℘ http://www.pitt.edu/~super1

Fitness to drive

Driver and Vehicle Licensing Agency ℘ https://www.gov.uk/government/organisations/driver-and-vehicle-licensing-agency

Charities

British Lung Foundation ℘ http://www.lunguk.org
Charity Commission directory of charities ℘ http://www.charitycommission.gov.uk/find-charities/

Index

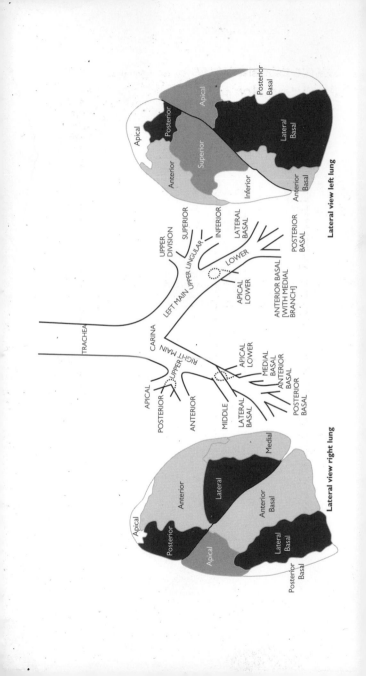

Lateral view left lung

Lateral view right lung

Apical
Posterior
Anterior
Superior
Inferior
Posterior Basal
Lateral Basal
Anterior Basal

TRACHEA
CARINA
APICAL
POSTERIOR
ANTERIOR
MIDDLE
LATERAL BASAL
POSTERIOR BASAL
ANTERIOR
MEDIAL BASAL
APICAL LOWER
UPPER
RIGHT MAIN
LEFT MAIN
UPPER DIVISION
UPPER LINGULAR
SUPERIOR
INFERIOR
LATERAL BASAL
LOWER
APICAL LOWER
ANTERIOR BASAL [WITH MEDIAL BRANCH]
POSTERIOR BASAL

Apical
Posterior
Anterior
Lateral
Medial
Apical
Anterior Basal
Lateral Basal
Posterior Basal